Inner Ear Diseases: A Clinical Guide

Inner Ear Diseases: A Clinical Guide

Editor: Sacha Forte

AMERICAN
MEDICAL PUBLISHERS
www.americanmedicalpublishers.com

AMERICAN
MEDICAL PUBLISHERS
www.americanmedicalpublishers.com

Cataloging-in-Publication Data

Inner ear diseases : a clinical guide / edited by Sacha Forte.
p. cm.
Includes bibliographical references and index.
ISBN 979-8-88740-215-4
1. Labyrinth (Ear)--Diseases. 2. Labyrinth (Ear)--Diseases--Treatment. 3. Labyrinth (Ear)--Diseases--Diagnosis.
4. Ear--Diseases. I. Forte, Sacha.
RF260 .I56 2023
617.8--dc23

American Medical Publishers,
41 Flatbush Avenue,
1st Floor, New York,
NY 11217, USA

ISBN 979-8-88740-215-4 (Hardback)

Contents

Preface

This book aims to highlight the current researches and provides a platform to further the scope of innovations in this area. This book is a product of the combined efforts of many researchers and scientists, after going through thorough studies and analysis from different parts of the world. The objective of this book is to provide the readers with the latest information of the field.

The inner ear is located in the petrous area of the temporal bone. It is divided into two major sections, namely, semicircular canals and cochlea. Various inner ear diseases include Ménière's disease, drug-induced ototoxicity, vestibular neuronitis, benign paroxysmal positional vertigo, vestibular schwannoma, herpes zoster oticus and purulent labyrinthitis. There are several symptoms of these diseases, such as vertigo, hearing loss, imbalance and tinnitus. A focused physical examination can be used to diagnose inner ear diseases. Electronystagmography (ENG) can be used to diagnose vertigo, and audiometry is used to diagnose hearing loss. Intratympanic steroid therapy and intratympanic gentamicin are the two forms of drugs that are commonly used to treat inner ear diseases. This book aims to shed light on some of the clinical aspects of inner ear diseases. From theories to research to practical applications, case studies related to all contemporary topics of relevance to these diseases have been included herein. Those in search of information to further their knowledge will be greatly assisted by this book.

I would like to express my sincere thanks to the authors for their dedicated efforts in the completion of this book. I acknowledge the efforts of the publisher for providing constant support. Lastly, I would like to thank my family for their support in all academic endeavors.

Editor

1

Middle Ear Administration of a Particulate Chitosan Gel in an *in vivo* Model of Cisplatin Ototoxicity

Pernilla Videhult Pierre[1]*, Anette Fransson[2], Marta Alina Kisiel[2†], Peter Damberg[3], Sahar Nikkhou Aski[3], Mats Andersson[4], Lotta Hällgren[4] and Göran Laurell[2]

[1] Division of Audiology, Department of Clinical Science, Intervention and Technology, Karolinska Institutet, Stockholm, Sweden, [2] Department of Surgical Sciences, Uppsala University, Uppsala, Sweden, [3] Karolinska Experimental Research and Imaging Center, Karolinska University Hospital, Stockholm, Sweden, [4] Division of Bioscience and Materials, RISE Research Institutes of Sweden, Södertälje, Sweden

****Correspondence:***
Pernilla Videhult Pierre
pernilla.videhult-pierre@ki.se

†Present address:
Marta Alina Kisiel,
Department of Medical Sciences,
Occupational and Environmental
Medicine, Uppsala University
Hospital, Uppsala, Sweden

Background: Middle ear (intratympanic, IT) administration is a promising therapeutic method as it offers the possibility of achieving high inner ear drug concentrations with low systemic levels, thus minimizing the risk of systemic side effects and drug drug interactions. Premature elimination through the Eustachian tube may be reduced by stabilizing drug solutions with a hydrogel, but this raises the secondary issue of conductive hearing loss.

Aim: This study aimed to investigate the properties of a chitosan-based particulate hydrogel formulation when used as a drug carrier for IT administration in an *in vivo* model of ototoxicity.

Materials and Methods: Two particulate chitosan-based IT delivery systems, Thio-25 and Thio-40, were investigated in albino guinea pigs ($n = 94$). Both contained the hearing protecting drug candidate sodium thiosulfate with different concentrations of chitosan gel particles (25% vs. 40%). The safety of the two systems was explored *in vivo*. The most promising system was then tested in guinea pigs subjected to a single intravenous injection with the anticancer drug cisplatin (8 mg/kg b.w.), which has ototoxic side effects. Hearing status was evaluated with acoustically evoked frequency-specific auditory brainstem response (ABR) and hair cell counting. Finally, *in vivo* magnetic resonance imaging was used to study the distribution and elimination of the chitosan-based system from the middle ear cavity in comparison to a hyaluronan-based system.

Results: Both chitosan-based IT delivery systems caused ABR threshold elevations ($p < 0.05$) that remained after 10 days ($p < 0.05$) without evidence of hair cell loss, although the elevation induced by Thio-25 was significantly lower than for Thio-40 ($p < 0.05$). Thio-25 significantly reduced cisplatin-induced ABR threshold elevations ($p < 0.05$) and outer hair cell loss ($p < 0.05$). IT injection of the chitosan- and hyaluronan-based systems filled up most of the middle ear space. There were no significant differences between the systems in terms of distribution and elimination.

Conclusion: Particulate chitosan is a promising drug carrier for IT administration. Future studies should assess whether the physical properties of this technique allow for a smaller injection volume that would reduce conductive hearing loss.

Keywords: auditory brainstem response, particulate chitosan, cisplatin, hair cell, hearing loss, intratympanic administration, magnetic resonance imaging, sodium thiosulfate

INTRODUCTION

Cisplatin is a first-generation, platinum-based chemotherapeutic agent widely used in solid tumor treatment. However, cisplatin may cause permanent hearing loss and tinnitus, limiting its therapeutic use. There is no established pharmacological method to prevent or treat cisplatin-induced ototoxicity.

At the cellular level, cisplatin-induced ototoxic effects are often manifested as loss of the cochlear outer hair cells (OHCs), as shown in experimental animals (Rybak et al., 2007). Excessive levels of reactive oxygen species play a key role in cisplatin-induced ototoxicity (Sheth et al., 2017), while systemic co-administration of cisplatin with antioxidants can reduce ototoxicity in experimental animals (Campbell et al., 1996; Dickey et al., 2004; Fransson et al., 2017). However, developing a safe antioxidant treatment to protect the hearing of cancer patients subjected to cisplatin therapy is more complicated. Antioxidant treatment can reduce cisplatin's antineoplastic efficacy since antioxidants may chemically interact with cisplatin (Videhult et al., 2006) and/or promote tumor growth (Sayin et al., 2014) and/or tumor metastasis (Le Gal et al., 2015). Another issue is that at least two barrier systems, the blood-perilymph barrier and intrastrial fluid-blood barrier, limit transportation of otoprotectors from systemic circulation to the cochlear compartments (Cohen-Salmon et al., 2007; Shi, 2016). Both of these problems may be circumvented by middle ear (intratympanic, IT) drug administration.

The round and oval windows are the main routes of drug transport from the tympanic cavity to the inner ear (Salt et al., 2016). Some drugs are likely also absorbed by the middle ear mucosa, which may provide an alternative transportation route to the inner ear. One problem with IT drug delivery is that a large portion of the solution may flow through the Eustachian tube and be swallowed. There are several potential methods to increase the amount of drug reaching the cochlea. However, repeated IT application may be limited by round window edema (Saber et al., 2009) and is associated with increased risks of middle ear infection and chronic perforation of the tympanic membrane. Direct administration of a drug onto the round window membrane involves unnecessary surgical trauma and may have deleterious effects on the inner ear. In the present study, the risk of premature elimination from the tympanic cavity was reduced by using a hydrogel as a drug carrier.

IT administration induces temporary conductive hearing loss, a factor which must be accepted by patients. Furthermore, ideally, a drug carrier should degrade in a controlled manner without inducing any side effects in the middle and inner ears. Here, we assessed the protective effects of a chitosan-based delivery system for sodium thiosulfate to inhibit cisplatin-induced ototoxicity over a 10-day period. The carrier was a homogenously deacetylated chitosan with physical and immunological properties different to those of traditional, heterogeneously deacetylated chitosans. The specific aim of the present study was to investigate a chitosan formulation, based on a dispersed particulate hydrogel in an aqueous suspension, as a drug carrier for IT administration in an *in vivo* model of ototoxicity.

MATERIALS AND METHODS

Study Design

The study consisted of three parts. The first part investigated the safety of a chitosan-based delivery system for IT administration by exploring its effects on auditory brainstem responses (ABRs) to air-conducted pure tones and on hair cells. Two different candidate gel formulations were used, herein referred to as Thio-25 and Thio-40. These formulations differed in terms of the concentration of chitosan particles: 25% in Thio-25 and 40% in Thio-40. Guinea pigs were randomly assigned to one of two treatment groups: Thio-25 (n = 15) or Thio-40 (n = 15). Both groups received a single unilateral IT injection of sodium thiosulfate (100 mM) in a chitosan-based hydrogel formulation. The contralateral ear served as a control (no IT injection). ABR was measured prior to and 7 and 10 days after IT injection. Neither formulation caused hair cell loss, and ABR threshold shifts in the Thio-25 group were milder than in the Thio-40 group. Thio-25 was therefore used in the second part of the study.

The second part investigated the protective effects of Thio-25 IT administration on cisplatin-induced ototoxicity. Guinea pigs were randomly assigned to three treatment groups: Thio-25-cispt (n = 15), Placebo-25-cispt (n = 15), or NaCl-cispt (n = 15). All three groups received a single intravenous (i.v.) injection of cisplatin [8 mg/kg body weight (b.w.)]. One hour earlier, the Thio-25-cispt group was given a single unilateral IT injection of Thio-25, while the Placebo-25-cispt group received the vehicle only (Placebo-25), i.e., the same gel formulation (25% chitosan gel particles) but without sodium thiosulfate. The NaCl-cispt group was given an IT injection of sodium chloride (9 mg/mL; NaCl). The contralateral ears were not injected in any group. Auditory function was evaluated by measuring ABR prior to injection and then 10 days later.

Animals were euthanized after the final ABR measurement in both study parts. The cochleae of animals in the Thio-25, Thio-40, and Thio-25-cispt groups were collected for histological analyses.

The third part investigated the behavior of a chitosan-based formulation in the tympanic cavity compared with a hyaluronan-based formulation. Guinea pigs (n = 19) received single IT injections of a paramagnetic gel based on chitosan (Chito-Dota) and hyaluronan (Hya-Dota). All animals received Chito-Dota in one ear and Hya-Dota in the contralateral ear. The gels were then visualized *in vivo* using magnetic resonance imaging (MRI), which was carried out on three occasions per animal over a 2-week period after gel injection. The animals were euthanized immediately after the final MRI session.

Animals

Our experiments involved 94 guinea pigs (Duncan-Hartley, Lidköpings Kaninfarm, Lidköping, Sweden). Both sexes were utilized, and b.w. ranged from 263 to 413 g. Animals were maintained in an enriched environment in small groups on a 12-h light/12-h dark cycle at a temperature of 21°C and 60% humidity. They were given access to water and standard chow *ad libitum* and were allowed to acclimatize for a minimum of 10 days prior to the first experimental procedure. At baseline, all guinea pigs had normal tympanic membranes and hearing as determined by otoscopic examination and ABR assessment. During the experimental procedures, the animals were placed on a homeothermic pad. Animals subjected to cisplatin administration were weighed and hydrated with NaCl (37°C) subcutaneously (s.c., 5 mL) each day after cisplatin exposure. All animal procedures were performed under anesthesia and aseptic conditions and were in accordance with the Swedish national regulations for animal care and use. The experimental protocol was approved by the Regional Ethical Review Board in Uppsala (No. C5/15) and the Regional Ethical Review Board in Stockholm (No. 138/15).

Anesthesia

In parts one and two of the study, general anesthesia was produced with ketamine [intramuscular (i.m.), 40 mg/kg b.w.; Ketalar, 50 mg/mL; Pfizer AB, Sollentuna, Sweden] and xylazine (i.m.; 10 mg/kg b.w.; Rompun, 20 mg/mL; Bayer Health Care AG, Copenhagen, Denmark). Anesthesia depth was assessed by measuring the pedal reflex, and additional doses of ketamine (25 mg/kg b.w.) were given if needed. Bupivacaine (s.c.; Marcain, 2.5 mg/mL; AstraZeneca, Södertälje, Sweden) was used for local anesthesia. Buprenorphine (s.c.; 0.06 mg; Temgesic, 0.3 mg/mL; Schering-Plow, Kenilworth, NJ, United States) was used as a post-treatment analgesia in animals subjected to cisplatin administration.

In part three of the study, general anesthesia was induced in an induction box using 4–5% isoflurane in a 3:7 oxygen:air gas mixture after pretreatment with atropine (s.c.; 0.02–0.05 mg/kg b.w.; Atropine Mylan, 0.5 mg/mL; Mylan, Stockholm, Sweden) and 100% oxygen for 30 min to reduce respiratory tract secretions. The animal was then quickly transferred to an MRI-compatible rig where anesthesia was maintained using 2–3% isoflurane. Lidocaine (s.c.; Lidocaine Accord, 10 mg/mL; Accord Healthcare AB, Solna, Sweden) was used for local anesthesia. Anesthesia depth was monitored by measuring the pedal reflex and visual inspection of the respiratory rate. Under MRI, anesthesia depth was monitored by automatic assessment of heart and breathing rates.

Gel Preparation

Thio-25, Thio-40, and Placebo-25

To prepare Thio-25, chitosan (4.4 g, degree of N-deacetylation 49%, viscosity 365 mPas; Viscosan^{TM}, Flexichem AB, Uttran, Sweden) was suspended in 185 mL of distilled water (Baxter Medical AB, Kista, Sweden) and dissolved in 2 M aqueous HCl, which was added dropwise. The pH of the solution was adjusted to neutral with 1 M aqueous NaOH. The total volume was then adjusted to 200 mL with distilled water. The solution was filtered through a 5-μm syringe filter and heat-sterilized at 121°C for 20 min. Then, 12 g of this solution was mixed with a solution of sodium thiosulfate (4.8 g, 100 mM; Acros Organics, Thermo Fisher Scientific, Göteborg, Sweden) and another 7.2 g of distilled water. The resultant solution was then filtered through a 5 μm syringe filter. 3,4-Diethoxy-3-cyclobutene-1,2-dione [Aldrich Merck KGaA, Darmstadt, Germany; 41 μL of a 10% (v/v) solution in ethanol] was then added to 22.8 mL of the chitosan solution, and the mixture was stirred for 15 min at room temperature. The solution was then placed in a heating cabinet at 40°C for 14 days, after which the solidified gel was mechanically processed into 10-μm particles. Then, 1.29 g of gel particles were added to 3.87 g of a 30 mM phosphate buffer containing 100 mM of sodium thiosulfate to yield a 25% (w/w) ViscoGel^{TM} suspension. Thio-40 was prepared using the same method but by mixing 2.08 g particles with 3.12 g of the phosphate/thiosulfate buffer. A placebo gel to Thio-25, referred to as Placebo-25, was prepared in a similar way as Thio-25 but without the addition of sodium thiosulfate.

Chito-Dota

Chitosan (609.95 mg, degree of N-deacetylation 49%, viscosity 49 mPas; Viscosan^{TM}, Flexichem AB, Uttran, Sweden) was suspended in 90 mL of distilled water. Then, 530 μL of 2 M aqueous HCl was added, and the chitosan concentration adjusted to 0.5% with water. DOTA-NHS-ester (117.16 mg; Macrocyclics, Plano, TX, United States) was dissolved in 20.0 mL of distilled water. Then, 14.0 mL of this solution was added to 23.51 mL of the chitosan solution. The pH was adjusted to 7.02 with 1 M NaOH, and the mixture stirred for 2 days. Gadolinium (III) acetate hydrate (216.5 mg; Aldrich, Merck KGaA) was dissolved in distilled water (20.0 mL); 14.6 mL of this solution was then added to the chitosan-DOTA solution, and the mixture was stirred overnight. Then, 270 mg of EDTA (Scharlau, Scharlab, Barcelona, Spain) was added, and the mixture stirred for 30 min. The solution was dialyzed against 3 × 3 L distilled water (Spectra/Por Membrane molecular weight cut-off [MWCO]: 6–8,000). Subsequently, the dialysate was lyophilized; 86.8 mg of the lyophilized powder was dissolved in distilled water, the pH adjusted to 6.7, and the volume adjusted to 6.5 mL. To 3.75 g of this solution, diethoxy-3-cyclobutene-1,2-dione

[Acros, Organics, Thermo Fisher Scientific; 14 μL of a 6.5% (v/v) solution in ethanol] was added while stirring. After 15 min of stirring at room temperature, the solution was placed in a heating cabinet at 40°C for 14 days. Finally, the solidified gel was mechanically processed into 10-μm particles, and 2.068 g of gel particles were mixed with 6.2 mL of 30 mM phosphate buffer.

Hya-Dota

Ethylene diamine (62.2 mg; Sigma-Aldrich; Merck KGaA) was dissolved in 20 mL of distilled water, pH was adjusted to 6.0 with 2 M HCl, and the volume was adjusted to 25.0 mL. *N*-hydroxy succinimide (23.3 mg; Aldrich, Merck KGaA) was then added under vigorous stirring to 209 mg of sodium hyaluronate (Fluka, Merck KGaA). Then, *N*-dimethylaminopropyl-*N* ethyl carbodiimide hydrochloride (10.7 mg; Sigma, Merck KGaA) was added under continuous stirring. This solution was slowly added to the ethylene diamine solution under vigorous stirring, and the reaction mixture was left at room temperature for 4 h. The solution was then dialyzed against 4 × 5 L distilled water (Spectra/Por Membrane MWCO: 2,000), after which the dialysate was lyophilized. Then, 138 mg of the lyophilized powder was dissolved in distilled water; 34.1 mg of DOTA-NHS-ester was added, the pH was adjusted to 6.9, and the mixture was stirred overnight. Then, 41 mg of gadolinium (III) acetate hydrate in 4 mL distilled water was added, and the mixture was stirred overnight. Finally, 270 mg of EDTA was added, and the mixture was stirred for 30 min followed by dialysis against 3 × 4 L of distilled water (Spectra/Por Membrane MWCO: 2,000). The dialysate was subsequently lyophilized, and 54.4 mg of the lyophilized powder was dissolved in 5.44 mL of 30 mM phosphate buffer.

IT Administration

All animals were subjected to a single gel injection (approximate volume: 0.15 mL) into the auditory bulla following a small paracentesis of the tympanic membrane.

Cisplatin Administration

Cisplatin (8 mg/kg b.w.; Platinol 1 mg/mL; Bristol-Myers Squibb AB, Solna, Sweden) was injected at a rate of 0.2 mL/min through a catheter (PE50, inner diameter 0.58 mm, outer diameter = 0.965 mm; Intramedic, Becton Dickinson, Franklin Lakes, NJ, United States) inserted into the right jugular vein toward the heart. To rinse the catheter, 1 mL of sterile saline was administered immediately after cisplatin injection. The catheter was subsequently removed, the jugular vein was ligated, and the skin was sutured.

Hearing Thresholds

Auditory function was quantified by determining the hearing thresholds at 12.5, 20.0, and 30.0 kHz with air-conducted acoustically evoked ABR. Each animal was placed in a soundproof box. The frequency-specific stimulus signal was generated through a signal analyzer (Tucker-Davis Technologies, Alachua, FL, United States) controlled by a computer and presented through an electrostatic speaker (EC1, Tucker-Davis Technologies). The speaker was connected to a 10-cm tube positioned in the ear canal of each guinea pig. Neural responses were then collected using three subdermal electrodes: one placed at the vertex (active), one on the mastoid (reference), and a ground electrode on the lower back. The ABR threshold was defined as the lowest stimulus intensity that produced a reproducible response for ABR wave II, which was visualized at the same latency after an average of 1,000 recordings.

Morphology

After the final ABR assessment, animals were deeply anesthetized with sodium pentobarbital [25 mg/kg, intraperitoneal (i.p.); Allfatal vet., 100 mg/mL; Omnidea AB, Stockholm, Sweden] and subsequently decapitated. In the Thio-25, Thio-40, and Thio-25-cispt groups, the temporal bones were removed and the bulla opened to expose the cochleae. Small fenestrations were made in the apex and round window, and 4% phosphate-buffered formaldehyde was gently flushed through the cochlea. Surface preparation was performed as previously described (Fransson et al., 2017). After analyzing all inner hair cells (IHCs), OHCs, and scar formations, the proportion (%) of hair cell loss per millimeter distance from the round window was calculated and plotted in cytocochleograms.

MRI

As described in section "Study Design", guinea pigs (n = 19) received a single IT injection of Chito-Dota in one ear and Hya-Dota in the contralateral ear. Each animal underwent MRI immediately after injection and on two more occasions over 2 weeks. Anesthetized animals were placed in the supine position with the middle ear cavity situated within the sensitive region of a four-channel phased array coil originally designed for rat heart imaging (Rapid Biomedical, Würzburg, Germany) within an MR-compatible animal holder. The bed was positioned in the isocenter of a horizontal 9.4 T Agilent magnet equipped with a 12-cm inner diameter gradient system with a maximum gradient strength of 6000 mT/m and an actively tuned birdcage coil (RAPID Biomedical, Würzburg, Germany). Respiration rate was monitored throughout the experiment, and core body temperature was maintained at 37°C using feedback-controlled warm air (SA Instruments, Stony Brook, NY, United States). T1-weighted 3D images were acquired with a gradient echo 3D (GE3D) sequence: repetition time, 5.16 ms; echo time, 2.60 ms; number of averages, 4; flip angle, 20°; data matrix, 256 × 256 × 348; field of view (FOV), 38.4 × 38.4 × 57.6 mm^3; resolution scan duration, 33 min and 51 s including two dummy scans.

The bias field was characterized from the ratio of blurred (1.6% of FOV) 3D images acquired separately with the surface and volume coils using identical parameters as for the high-resolution images, apart from a reduced matrix size of 256 × 192 × 192.

After imaging, the animals were sacrificed by an i.p. injection of sodium pentobarbital, followed immediately by decapitation.

All MRI images were bias-field corrected using low-resolution and blurred volume and surface coil images. Intensities and volumes were estimated by segmenting areas in the image where there was a contrast difference using ImageJ (version 1.43;

National Institutes of Health, Bethesda, MD, United States) and ITK-snap [version 3.4[1] (Yushkevich et al., 2006)].

Statistics

To investigate effects on hearing thresholds, mixed linear modeling was used to account for heteroscedasticity and autocorrelation in terms of time point, frequency, and IT administration (when both ears of an animal were included in the analysis). Frequency was included as a continuous variable. The model with the lowest maximum likelihood and fewest estimated parameters was considered to have the best fit; this was determined with a likelihood ratio chi-square test.

Repeated measures analysis of variance (ANOVA) was used to analyze the percentage loss of OHCs in each row (three levels: rows 1, 2, and 3) as the within-subjects effect and the two types of IT administration (two levels: Thio-25 and none) as the within-subjects effect.

An alpha level of 0.05 was used throughout, and all tests were two-sided. All calculations were performed in IBM SPSS Statistics (v. 23, release 23.0.0.0, 64-bit edition for Mac; Armonk, NY, United States).

RESULTS

Study Part One

Hearing Thresholds

The first part of the study investigated conductive hearing loss induced by unilateral IT injection of two sodium thiosulfate-containing particulate chitosan gels, Thio-25 and Thio-40. The hearing thresholds of each animal measured before and after injection are presented in **Figure 1**. Mixed linear modeling was performed using hearing threshold as the outcome variable and IT administration (two levels: Thio-25 and Thio-40) as the effect, and frequency and time point (three levels: pretreatment, day 7, and day 10) as repeated effects. In the final model, time point was also used to model a random slope. There was a significant main effect of frequency ($F = 146.18$, $p < 0.0001$) and significant interactions between frequency and IT administration ($F = 14.87$, $p < 0.001$), frequency and time point ($F = 69.00$, $p < 0.0001$), and IT administration and time point ($F = 24.85$, $p < 0.0001$). The estimates of fixed effects are given in **Table 1A**, and pairwise comparisons are shown in **Tables 1B,C**. Both Thio-25 and Thio-40 increased the electrophysiological hearing thresholds, although Thio-25 did this to a significantly lesser extent than Thio-40. The hearing thresholds of both groups were significantly higher on days 7 and 10 compared to pretreatment.

Morphology

No significant IHC or OHC loss was found in the first five animals of the Thio-25 (**Supplementary Table S1**) and Thio-40 (**Supplementary Table S2**) groups. As the morphological procedure is very laborious, we decided not to count the remaining cochleae. These results indicate that the elevated hearing thresholds presented in section "Hearing Thresholds" were caused by conductive hearing loss.

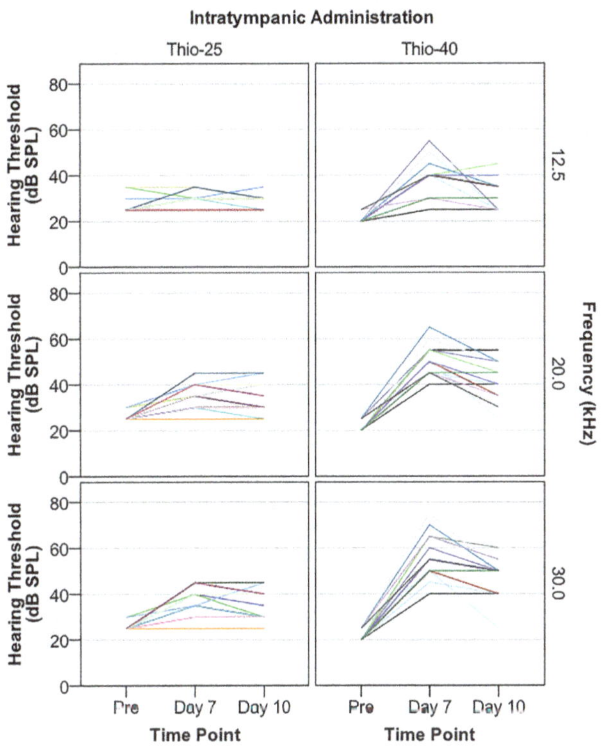

FIGURE 1 | Guinea pigs were subjected to a single, unilateral intratympanic (IT) injection of sodium thiosulfate (100 mM) in a particulate chitosan gel with a gel particle concentration of 25% (Thio-25 group, $n = 15$) or 40% (Thio-40 group, $n = 15$). Electrophysiological hearing thresholds assessed with air-conducted acoustically evoked auditory brainstem response (ABR) were measured at 12.5, 20.0, and 30.0 kHz before (pre) and 7 and 10 days after IT administration. Hearing threshold (decibel sound pressure level, dB SPL) vs. time point stratified by IT administration and frequency is shown. Each color represents one animal. Fewer colors than 15 per graph are due to overlapping lines.

Study Part Two

Hearing Thresholds

As the IT administration of Thio-25 induced less conductive hearing loss than Thio-40 and because neither treatment caused hair cell loss, the protective effects of Thio-25 on cisplatin-induced ototoxicity were explored. Electrophysiological hearing thresholds before and 10 days after IT administration of Thio-25 followed by i.v. cisplatin injection are shown in **Figure 2**. Mixed linear modeling was then carried out using hearing threshold as the outcome variable and IT administration (two levels: Thio-25 and none), frequency, and time point (two levels: pretreatment and day 10) as repeated effects. In the final model, time point was also used to model a random slope. A significant main effect of IT administration ($F = 56.68$, $p < 0.0001$) and frequency ($F = 126.06$, $p < 0.0001$), and significant interactions between time point and IT administration ($F = 33.76$, $p < 0.0001$) and between time point and frequency ($F = 126.38$, $p < 0.0001$) were found. The fixed

[1] www.itksnap.org

TABLE 1A | Mixed linear modeling of associations of the hearing thresholds presented in **Figure 1** with IT administration, frequency, and time point.

Estimates of fixed effects on hearing threshold (dB SPL)						
Parameter		**β**	**SE of β**	**t**	***p*-value**	**95% CI**
Intercept		23	1.9	12.51	< 0.0001	20 to 27
Frequency#		0.72	0.08	8.59	< 0.0001	0.55 to 0.89
Interactions						
Time Point and IT	*Pre and Thio-25*	4.6	2.1	2.17	0.03	0.38 to 8.9
	Pre and Thio-40	−3.4	1.9	−1.75	NS	−7.23 to 0.48
	Day 7 and Thio-25	−2.9	2.8	−1.03	NS	−8.54 to 2.69
	Day 7 and Thio-40	8.2	2.5	3.37	0.001	3.4 to 13
	Day 10 and Thio-25	−2.0	2.0	−1.01	NS	−6.1 to 2.0
	Day 10 and Thio-40	Ref				
Time Point and Frequency#	*Pre and Frequency*	−0.65	0.08	−7.73	< 0.0001	−0.82 to −0.48
	Day 7 and Frequency	0.11	0.11	1.04	NS	−0.11 to 0.33
	Day 10 and Frequency	Ref				
IT and Frequency#	*Thio-25 and Frequency*	−0.14	0.04	−3.86	< 0.001	−0.21 to −0.07
	Thio-40 and Frequency	Ref				

Estimates of fixed effects on the outcome variable, hearing threshold (dB SPL) are shown. Results obtained with mixed linear modeling using electrophysiological hearing threshold based on acoustically evoked ABR as the outcome variable, IT administration as an effect, frequency as a repeated effect, time point as a repeated effect, and time point as an effect for random slope. Covariate type: compound symmetry heterogeneous (fixed effects) and variance components (random effect). #In kHz. ABR, auditory brainstem response; β, coefficient of regression; CI, confidence interval; dB SPL, decibel sound pressure; IT, intratympanic; NS, non-significant; Pre, before IT administration; Ref, reference category.

TABLE 1B | Pairwise comparisons of the analysis results presented in **Table 1A**.

Pairwise comparisons of effects for hearing threshold (dB SPL)						
Time point	**(I) IT**	**(J) IT**	**Mean difference (I-J)**	**SE**	***p*-value**	**95% CI**
Pre	Thio-25	Thio-40	5.1*	1.0	<0.0001	3.1 to 7.1
Day 7	Thio-25	Thio-40	−14*	1.9	<0.0001	−18 to −10
Day 10	Thio-25	Thio-40	−4.9*	2.0	0.02	−8.9 to −1.0

*CI, confidence interval; dB SPL, decibel sound pressure level; NS, non-significant; pre, before IT administration; SE, standard error of mean difference. * signifies $p < 0.05$ (Bonferroni adjusted).*

TABLE 1C | Pairwise comparisons of the analysis results presented in **Table 1A**.

Pairwise comparisons of effects for hearing threshold (dB SPL)						
IT	**(I) Time point**	**(J) Time point**	**Mean difference (I-J)**	**SE**	***p*-value**	**95% CI**
Thio-25	Pre	Day 7	−8.4*	1.3	<0.0001	−12 to −5.1
	Pre	Day 10	−6.9*	1.4	<0.0001	−10 to −3.3
	Day 7	Day 10	1.5	1.4	NS	−1.9 to 4.9
Thio-40	Pre	Day 7	−28*	1.3	<0.0001	−31 to −24
	Pre	Day 10	−17*	1.4	<0.0001	−21 to −13
	Day 7	Day 10	11*	1.4	<0.0001	7.3 to 14

*CI, confidence interval; dB SPL, decibel sound pressure level; NS, non-significant; pre, before IT administration; SE, standard error of mean difference. * signifies $p < 0.05$ (Bonferroni adjusted).*

effects estimates are given in **Table 2A**, and pairwise comparisons are given in **Tables 2B,C**. In summary, cisplatin injection induced a significant increase in electrophysiological hearing threshold; however, this effect was significantly lower in ears treated with Thio-25 compared to no IT administration.

This experiment was repeated using Placebo-25 (the chitosan-based vehicle without sodium thiosulfate) instead of Thio-25. Ten days after cisplatin administration, animals in the Placebo-25 group had symmetrical, bilateral electrophysiological hearing threshold elevations (**Supplementary Figure S1**), suggesting that the vehicle itself did not offer any otoprotection.

The experiment was then repeated a third time, using NaCl instead of Thio-25. Ten days after cisplatin administration, the animals had symmetrical, bilateral electrophysiological hearing

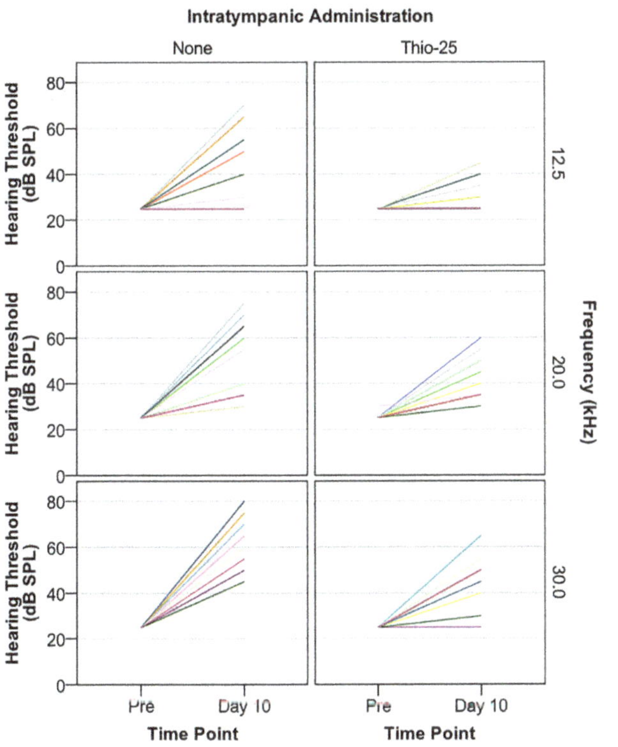

FIGURE 2 | Guinea pigs were subjected to a single, unilateral IT injection of a sodium thiosulfate-containing chitosan-based gel (Thio-25, $n = 15$), while the other ear was left untreated, serving as a control (None). The animals received a single high dose of cisplatin (8 mg/kg b.w., i.v.) 1 h later. Electrophysiological hearing thresholds (in decibel sound pressure level, dB SPL) assessed with air-conducted acoustically evoked auditory brainstem response (ABR) at 12.5, 20, and 30 kHz before and 10 days after IT administration are shown. Each color represents one animal. Fewer colors than 15 per graph are due to overlapping lines.

threshold elevations (**Supplementary Figure S2**). Thus, IT administration had no effect on hearing thresholds.

Morphology

A representative example of the hair cell loss observed in cisplatin-injected animals that were unilaterally pretreated with IT Thio-25 (group Thio-25-cispt) is shown in **Figures 3A,B**. One animal showed marked bilateral hair cell loss (**Figures 3C,D**). The mean percentage losses of OHCs and IHCs in all animals are presented in **Table 3**. Repeated measures ANOVA revealed a statistically significant difference in terms of OHC loss across rows 1 [$F(1,14) = 35.868$, $p < 0.001$], 2 [$F(1,14) = 19.368$, $p < 0.001$], and 3 [$F(1,14) = 18.145$, $p < 0.001$], as well as statistically significant differences in terms of IT administration [$F(2,13) = 27.310$, $p < 0.001$]. The *post hoc* analysis results are shown in **Figure 4**. In summary, cisplatin-induced loss of OHCs was significantly less severe in ears subjected to IT Thio-25 compared to no IT administration, which agreed with our electrophysiological hearing threshold results.

Study Part Three

Gel Distribution and Clearance

In the last part of the study, serial MRI was performed to monitor the middle ear distributions of chitosan and hyaluronan, including clearance from the middle ear cavity over a period of 14 days. The polymers were conjugated with a paramagnetic contrast agent to further improve detection and enable estimation of gel clearance over time. Minutes after injection, the contrast-enhanced gel appeared hyperintense and its location in the middle ear cavity was clearly seen, as seen in **Figures 5A–C**, which show different orthogonal viewing planes of 3D data from an animal with IT administration of Chito-Dota and Hya-Dota in the right and left middle ears, respectively. At subsequent time points, the intensities were similar to nearby brain tissue,

TABLE 2A | Mixed linear modeling of associations of the hearing thresholds in the Thio-25-cispt group ($n = 15$) presented in **Figure 2** with IT administration, frequency, and time point.

		Estimates of fixed effects on hearing thresholds (dB SPL)				
Parameter		β	**SE OF** β	**t**	***p*-value**	**95% CI**
Intercept		21	2.0	10.80	<0.0001	17 to 25
IT	*None*	16	1.9	8.26	<0.0001	12 to 19
	Thio-25	Ref				
Frequency[#]		0.96	0.06	14.79	<0.0001	0.83 to 1.1
Interactions						
Time point and IT	*Pre and None*	−12	3.6	−3.26	<0.005	−19 to −4.40
	Pre and Thio-25	4.0	2.6	1.51	NS	−1.3 to 9.2
	Day 10 and None	Ref				
	Day 10 and Thio-25	Ref				
Time point and frequency	*Pre and Frequency*	−0.96	0.09	−11.24	<0.0001	−1.1 to −0.79
	Day 10 and Frequency	Ref				

Estimates of fixed effects on the outcome variable, hearing threshold (decibel sound pressure level; db SPL), are shown. Results obtained with mixed linear modeling using electrophysiological hearing threshold based on acoustically evoked ABR as the outcome variable, IT administration as a repeated effect, frequency as a repeated effect, time point as a repeated effect, and time point as an effect for random slope. Covariate type: first-order factor analytic (repeated effects) and variance components (random effect). [#]*In kHz; ABR, auditory brainstem response; β, coefficient of regression; CI, confidence interval; dB SPL, decibel sound pressure; IT, intratympanic; NS, non-significant; Pre, before IT administration; Ref, reference category; SE, standard error of β.*

TABLE 2B | Pairwise comparisons of the analysis results presented in **Table 2A**.

Pairwise comparisons of effects for hearing threshold (dB SPL)						
Time point	**(I) IT**	**(J) IT**	**Mean difference (I-J)**	**SE**	***p*-value**	**95% CI**
Pre	None	Thio-25	−0.1	0.8	NS	−1.7 to 1.5
Day 10	None	Thio-25	16*	1.9	<0.0001	12 to 19

*CI, confidence interval; dB SPL, decibel sound pressure level; NS, non-significant; Pre, before IT administration; SE, standard error of mean difference. * signifies p < 0.05 (Bonferroni adjusted).*

TABLE 2C | Pairwise comparisons of the analysis results presented in **Table 2A**.

IT	(I) Time point	(J) Time point	Mean difference (I-J)	SE	*p*-value	95% CI
None	Pre	Day 10	−31.6*	2.7	<0.0001	−37 to −26
Thio-25	Pre	Day 10	−16.0*	1.9	<0.0001	−20 to −12

*CI, confidence interval; NS, non-significant; Pre; before IT administration; SE, standard error of mean difference. * signifies p < 0.05 (Bonferroni adjusted).*

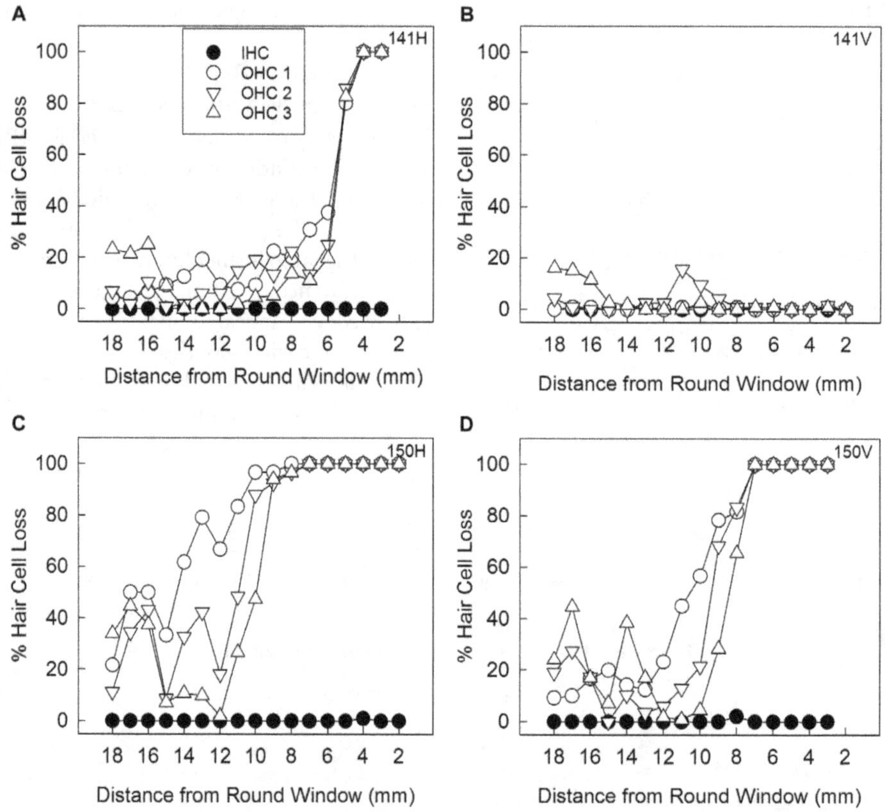

FIGURE 3 | Animals in the Thio-25-cispt group (shown in **Figure 2**) were euthanized after hearing threshold assessment on day 10. Their cochleae were collected to quantify loss of inner hair cells (IHCs) and outer hair cells (OHCs) in the first (OHC1), second (OHC2), and third (OHC3) rows. Cytocochleogram results from an animal with a loss pattern that was representative of most of the cisplatin-treated guinea pigs subjected to no IT administration **(A)** and to IT administration of Thio-25 **(B)**. Cytocochleogram results from the only cisplatin-treated animal with a large loss in the untreated ear **(C)** and the Thio-25-treated ear **(D)**.

as seen in **Figures 5D–F**, which were taken 4 days after gel administration and show an empty right middle ear and a mostly fluid-filled left middle ear. **Figure 6** shows gel volume vs. time (A and B) and intensity vs. time (C and D) curves of all middle ears. The volume occupied by the gel was larger at the earliest second scanning, i.e., two days after gel administration, compared to the scanning performed immediately after administration of Chito-Dota (**Figure 6A**) and Hya-Dota (**Figure 6B**). At later time points, there was a trend for a successive decrease in gel volume. However, there was considerable interindividual variability (represented by the spread shown in **Figures 6A,B**) at each time point. For example, in 3 of 9 middle ears monitored

TABLE 3 | Quantification of hair cell loss in Thio-25-cispt group described in **Figure 2**.

	Hair cell loss (%)							
	OHC1		OHC2		OHC3		IHC	
IT	Mean	SD	Mean	SD	Mean	SD	Mean	SD
None	36	24	26	21	23	18	0.0	0.1
Thio-25	11	15	7.6	12	6.8	12	0.8	1.8

IHC, inner hair cells; IT, intratympanic; OHC1, -2, and -3, outer hair cells by row; SD, standard deviation.

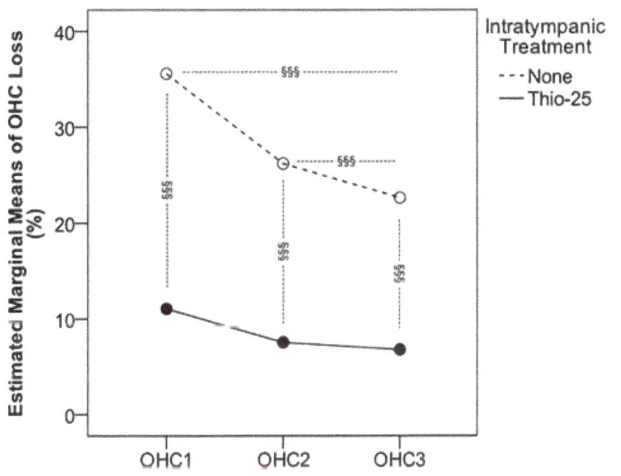

FIGURE 4 | Animals in the Thio-25-cispt group (presented in **Figure 2**) were euthanized after hearing threshold assessment on day 10. Their cochleae were collected to quantify hair cell loss. Repeated measures ANOVA of the percentage loss of outer hair cells (OHCs) in the first (OHC1), second (OHC2), and third (OHC3) rows are shown for ears injected with a thiosulfate-containing gel (Thio-25) and for the contralateral, non-injected ear (None). §§§ signifies $p < 0.001$.

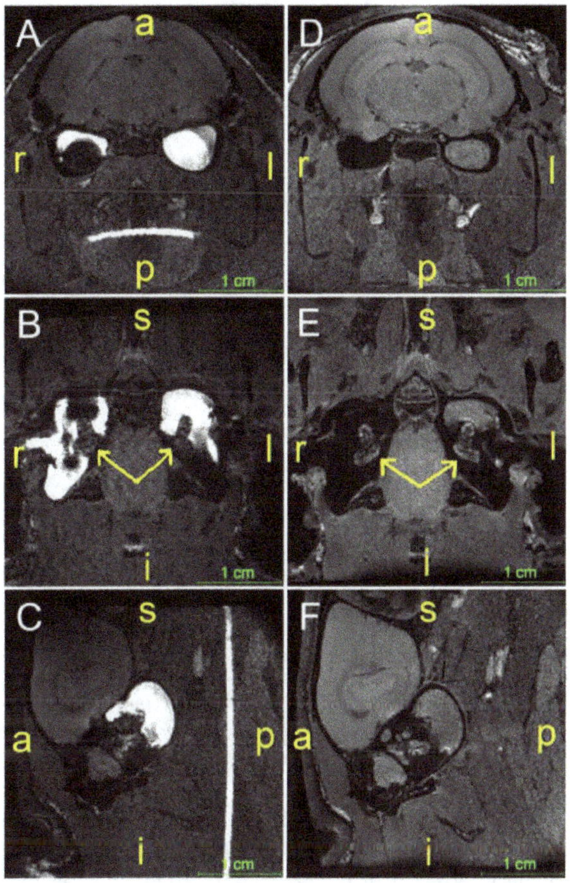

FIGURE 5 | Guinea pigs ($n = 19$) were subjected to IT administration of a paramagnetic chitosan based gel (Chito-Dota) in one ear and a hyaluronan-based gel (Hya-Dota) in the contralateral ear. The gels were then visualized by magnetic resonance imaging. Different orthogonal viewing planes of 3D data from one animal taken immediately after **(A–C)** and 4 days after **(D–F)** injection of Chito-Dota into the right ear and Hya-Dota into the left ear. The position of each cochlea is indicated with a yellow arrow in **B** and **E**. The sagittal plane in **C** and **F** shows the left ear. Keys (in yellow): a, anterior; i, inferior; l, left; p, posterior; r, right; s, superior.

6 days after gel injection in each of the Chito-Dota and Hya-Dota groups, the gel volume was larger than immediately after gel injection and thereafter decreased. T1-weighted MR image intensity was dramatically decreased when comparing images acquired at the time of gel administration with those acquired 2 days later (**Figures 6C,D**). Presumably, the increase in volume and reduction in intensity reflect an initial accumulation of water from the surrounding tissues, thus diluting the contrast agent. Both the distribution and elimination of the chitosan- and hyaluronan-based gels appear to follow similar patterns, and a clear difference between the two forms could not be identified.

DISCUSSION

IT administration is commonly used in preclinical research. The present large-scale *in vivo* study in guinea pigs provides key data relating to the safety, efficacy, and elimination of an IT drug delivery system composed of an antioxidant incorporated in a particulate hydrogel drug carrier. A sodium thiosulfate-containing, chitosan-based system reduced ototoxic injury induced by a single high dose of cisplatin. Cisplatin is a common anticancer agent that predominantly exerts its effects through DNA-dependent mechanisms (Ghosh, 2019). Evidence from preclinical studies demonstrates that the cisplatin ototoxicity is primarily caused by OHC damage in the cochlea (Laurell and Bagger-Sjöbäck, 1991), and the underlying mechanisms include oxidative stress and mitochondrial dysfunction (Giari et al., 2012; Sheth et al., 2017). Drugs that up-regulate the antioxidant system are therefore considered promising candidates for otoprotection. Two measures were used to explore the ototoxic effects of cisplatin and the efficacy of middle ear administration: assessment of ABR and counting of cochlear hair cells. The primary outcome measure to verify toxicity and assess protective effects was hair cell counting, while the functional capacity of the ear following IT administration was better reflected by ABR

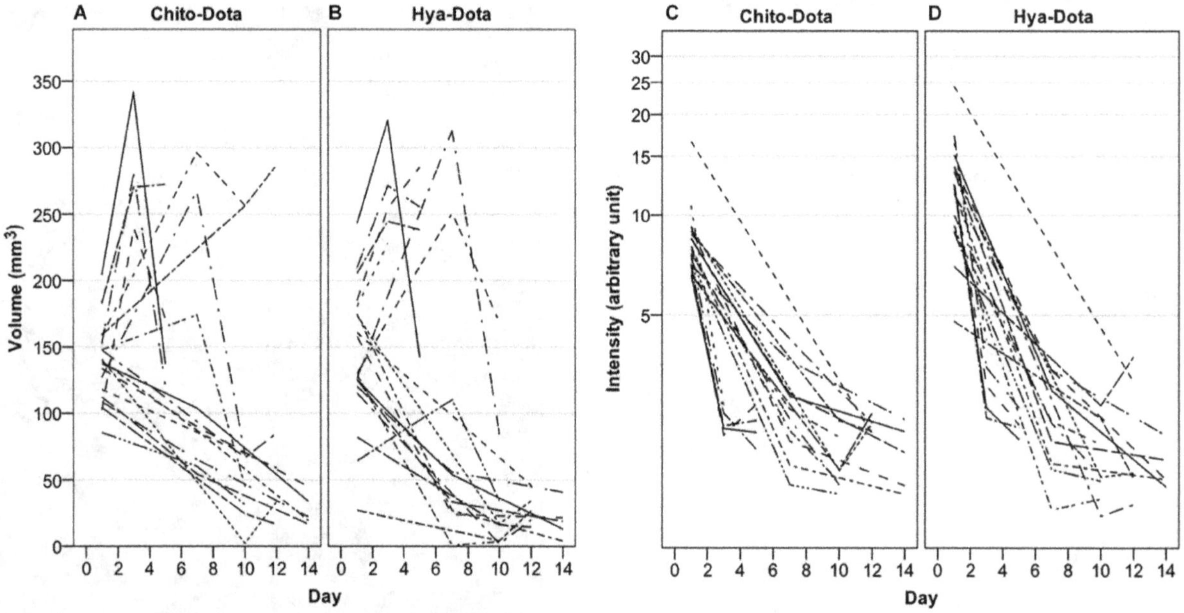

FIGURE 6 | Guinea pigs were subjected to intratympanic IT administration of two different paramagnetic gels, one based on chitosan (Chito-Dota) in one ear and one based on hyaluronan (Hya-Dota) in the contralateral ear. Volume and intensity in the middle ear were explored with magnetic resonance imaging performed on three different occasions in each guinea pig. The volume **(A,B)** and intensity **(C,D)** in the middle ear vs. time curves for each guinea pig are shown. $n = 19$ on day 1, $n = 5$ on day 3, $n = 4$ on day 5, $n = 9$ on day 7, $n = 8$ on day 10, $n = 5$ on day 12, and $n = 5$ on day 14 for both Chito-Dota and Hya-Dota.

assessment. Under normal physiological conditions, the middle ear cavity is filled with gas to optimize sound conduction to the cochlea. When a drug carrier is inserted into the middle ear cavity, air-conducted sound might temporarily be obstructed (conductive hearing loss). Therefore, it is generally desirable to use a technique to estimate bone conduction frequency-specific ABRs as this could provide useful information about middle ear function. However, assessing bone thresholds is difficult in the guinea pig. The first part of the study investigated hair cell loss induced by the drug delivery system. Although ABR assessment showed significantly increased thresholds on days 7 and 10, hair cell counting did not reveal any OHC or IHC loss. This finding corroborates previous results (Saber et al., 2010; Lajud et al., 2015). Taken together, the observed effects of the drug delivery system on hearing thresholds are largely due to conductive hearing loss and agree with a number of earlier *in vivo* studies (Engmér Berglin et al., 2015; Cole et al., 2018). In the second part of the study, the utility of particulate chitosan as a drug carrier for an antioxidant to protect inner ear structures was examined. The choice of sodium thiosulfate was based on positive results from earlier studies (Videhult et al., 2006; Videhult Pierre et al., 2009; Berglin et al., 2011). Sodium thiosulfate (100 mM), in a formulation containing 25% of thiosulfate-containing chitosan gel particles in suspension was used to protect the hearing end organ via a simple injection to the middle ear cavity 1 h before cisplatin administration. As conductive hearing loss did not completely recover within 10 days in the first part of the study, it was evident that hair cell counting represented a more reliable measure of ototoxicity. A partial protective effect on all three OHC rows was observed. Although some OHC loss occurred, it is important to consider that this is the first evidence of otoprotection observed 10 days after a single i.v. administration of cisplatin. On the other hand, short-term *in vivo* studies reported partial protection against cisplatin ototoxicity [see e.g., (Ghosh et al., 2018; Wang et al., 2018)]. Unfortunately, findings from many preclinical studies cannot be translated into clinical trials because of drug toxicity, drug-drug interaction, or the impermeability of the blood-labyrinth barriers. For example, Roldán-Fidalgo et al. (2016) reported that lutein exerted significant otoprotective effects *in vitro* but not *in vivo*. Earlier studies on drug delivery involved short follow-up periods, multiple dosing strategies, and more unreliable methods for administering cisplatin (i.p.). In the second part of the study, the effects of the drug carried itself on cisplatin-induced ototoxicity was also investigated. ABR assessment showed no significant difference between vehicle-treated and untreated ears. Therefore, hair cell loss in vehicle-treated ears was not assessed, largely because the technique is very laborious. As chitosan exhibits antioxidant properties (Ngo and Kim, 2014), it cannot be excluded that chitosan reduced hair cell loss in vehicle-treated ears but the effect was masked by the conductive hearing loss induced by IT administration. In the last part of the study, MRI was used to examine the distribution and elimination of particulate chitosan in comparison to hyaluronan, which is a frequently used vehicle for IT drug delivery [see e.g., (Arriaga and Goldman, 1998; Berglin et al., 2011; Rolland et al., 2019)]. To the best of our knowledge, no previous study has investigated these properties in two gels in the same animal for up to 14 days. Both polymers were conjugated with a gadolinium-containing contrast agent to improve detection. Gel volume changes in the middle ear varied between animals. A typical pattern was increase in gel volume the first days after IT injection, followed by a decrease. At 2 weeks (4 days longer than the protective study in part two), the middle ear was typically clear of fluid, and the MR signal in the inner ear had returned to baseline.

Two major treatment approaches have been employed to circumvent ototoxicity in patients receiving cisplatin-based chemotherapy: systemic and local administration of otoprotector drug candidates. Drugs can be systemically administered during a time window that achieves otoprotection hopefully without compromising antineoplastic efficacy (Brock et al., 2018), or IT injection can deliver otoprotector drugs directly to the inner ear (Marshak et al., 2014; Sarafraz et al., 2018; Rolland et al., 2019). There has been much interest in improving formulations for IT drug delivery. The most appropriate formulation would facilitate drug transport of an otoprotector into the inner ear compartments while minimizing negative effects in the middle ear, including conductive hearing loss. In the present study, the entire middle ear was filled with chitosan. Injecting a smaller volume could be one way to improve chitosan-based delivery systems. Future research should address the effects of injection volume on conduction following IT delivery of a gel. Furthermore, little is known about drug absorption in the middle ear mucosa and how it affects drug transport to the inner ear; future research should address this shortfall. Longitudinal studies for longer than 10 days after cisplatin administration should also be performed to determine whether IT administration can sustain otoprotective effects.

Chitosan is a water-soluble polymer formed by deacetylation of the linear, naturally occurring polymer chitin, which is built up by 1-4-b-linked *N*-acetyl-glucosamine (Ways et al., 2018). Chitosan is biodegradable with low toxicity, and its cationic nature makes it mucoadhesive (Ways et al., 2018). It has been investigated in many types of pharmaceutical formulations (Ways et al., 2018), including drug delivery to the inner ear (Paulson et al., 2008; Lajud et al., 2013). Technically speaking, there are two types chitosans: those with heterogeneous or homogenous acetylation patterns (Sannan et al., 1976). For decades, only heterogeneously deacetylated chitosans were available on the market. They are typically 70–95% deacetylated, which limits their solubility, and precipitate from solution at pH > 6. Heterogeneously deacetylated chitosans are therefore less suitable for IT administration. Although the pH in the middle ear cavity was not measured in the present study, a pH > 6 is expected in the steady-state conditions established in the guinea pig model. Moreover, IT administration of an acidic formulation can exacerbate cisplatin ototoxicity (Tanaka et al., 2003, 2004). The present study use a formulation with homogenously deacetylated chitosan and a pH of 7.4. These chitosans have recently become available and have lower degrees of deacetylation at 35–80%. In addition to the advantageous properties of heterogeneously deacetylated chitosans, new products have additional features including more rapid biodegradation (Shigemasa et al., 1994) and solubility at physiological pH (Vårum et al., 1994). In contrast to the heterogeneously deacetylated chitosans, the homogenously deacetylated chitosans enable the formation of a viscoelastic hydrogel, so called "crushed gels" or "ringing gels." These gels are slightly cross-linked and form rigid constructs, which can be loaded with drugs, and after solidification they can be mechanically processed into well-separated particles of defined size. ViscoGel^{TM} is an example of such a particulate hydrogel (Franzen et al., 2015) and was clinically evaluated in a vaccine study where it showed a good safety profile Neimert-Andersson et al., 2014). The present investigation used a chitosan-based, cross-linked sodium thiosulfate-loaded viscoelastic gel suspended in an aqueous thiosulfate-containing buffer. The formulation was designed to combine the most attractive properties of chitosan hydrogels and drug release functionality. We hypothesized that the aqueous phase would enable rapid transport of thiosulfate to the inner ear, while the gel particles would achieve more sustained thiosulfate delivery by increasing its time in the middle ear cavity. The formulations were easily injected into the middle ear cavity and also offer the possibility of fine-tuning drug-release properties by altering gel particle size and/or concentration.

Minimizing cisplatin-induced ototoxicity is of great clinical importance. Many physicians would like to avoid systemic protective treatment as it may interfere with the antineoplastic efficacy of cisplatin (Freyer et al., 2017). A prerequisite for developing otoprotection strategies is knowledge of the inner ear pharmacokinetics of cisplatin. It is well recognized that cisplatin-induced hearing loss is primarily seen in the high-frequency area corresponding to the basal turn of the cochlea. The drug is not uniformly distributed throughout the cochlea; instead, the highest concentration is found in the basal turn (Hellberg et al., 2013), in the vicinity of the round and oval windows. The findings above support the development of local protective treatment via IT administration of one or more otoprotectors. Previous studies suggest that cisplatin is not just transported by passive diffusion; enhanced uptake to inner ear targets involves active transport mechanisms, such as the organic cation 2 and the copper transporter 1 (Ciarimboli et al., 2010; More et al., 2010). IT administration of a drug that could block these transporters in the inner ear might represent an alternative method to reduce cisplatin-induced ototoxicity.

CONCLUSION

The results of this preclinical *in vivo* study show that cisplatin ototoxicity can be reduced by the localized administration of the antioxidant sodium thiosulfate in a suspension of a particulate, homogenously deacetylated chitosan. The IT drug delivery system induced conductive hearing loss that was not completely resolved within the 10-days study period, probably due to gel residue remaining in the middle ear. Future research will determine whether the properties of particulate chitosan for drug delivery to the inner ear can be further improved.

AUTHOR CONTRIBUTIONS

All authors listed have made a substantial, direct and intellectual contribution to the work, and approved it for publication.

ACKNOWLEDGMENTS

Mrs. Louise Zettergren and Birgitta Linder, Ph.D. are acknowledged for excellent laboratory work.

REFERENCES

Arriaga, M. A., and Goldman, S. (1998). Hearing results of intratympanic steroid treatment of endolymphatic hydrops. *Laryngoscope* 108 (11 Pt 1), 1682–1685.

Berglin, C. E., Pierre, P. V., Bramer, T., Edsman, K., Ehrsson, H., Eksborg, S., et al. (2011). Prevention of cisplatin-induced hearing loss by administration of a thiosulfate-containing gel to the middle ear in a guinea pig model. *Cancer Chemother. Pharmacol.* 68, 1547–1556. doi: 10.1007/s00280-011-1656-2

Brock, P. R., Maibach, R., Childs, M., Rajput, K., Roebuck, D., Sullivan, M. J., et al. (2018). Sodium thiosulfate for protection from cisplatin-induced hearing loss. *N. Engl. J. Med.* 378, 2376–2385. doi: 10.1056/NEJMoa1801109

Campbell, K. C. M., Rybak, L. P., Meech, R. P., and Hughes, L. (1996). D-methionine provides excellent protection from cisplatin ototoxicity in the rat. *Hear. Res.* 102, 90–98.

Ciarimboli, G., Deuster, D., Knief, A., Sperling, M., Holtkamp, M., Edemir, B., et al. (2010). Organic cation transporter 2 mediates cisplatin-induced oto- and nephrotoxicity and is a target for protective interventions. *Am. J. Pathol.* 176, 1169–1180. doi: 10.2353/ajpath.2010.090610

Cohen-Salmon, M., Regnault, B., Cayet, N., Caille, D., Demuth, K., Hardelin, J. P., et al. (2007). Connexin30 deficiency causes instrastrial fluid-blood barrier disruption within the cochlear stria vascularis. *Proc. Natl. Acad. U.S.A.* 104, 6229–6234. doi: 10.1073/pnas.0605108104

Cole, L. K., Rajala-Schultz, P. J., and Lorch, G. (2018). Conductive hearing loss in four dogs associated with the use of ointment-based otic medications. *Vet. Dermatol.* 29:341. doi: 10.1111/vde.12542

Dickey, D. T., Muldoon, L. L., Kraemer, D. F., and Neuwelt, E. A. (2004). Protection against cisplatin-induced ototoxicity by N-acetylcysteine in a rat model. *Hear. Res.* 193, 25–30.

Engmér Berglin, C., Videhult Pierre, P., Ekborn, A., Bramer, T., Edsman, K., Hultcrantz, M., et al. (2015). Local treatment of the inner ear: a study of three different polymers aimed for middle ear administration. *Acta Otolaryngol.* 135, 985–994. doi: 10.3109/00016489.2015.1058534

Fransson, A. E., Kisiel, M., Pirttilä, K., Pettersson, C., Videhult Pierre, P., and Laurell, G. F. E. (2017). Hydrogen inhalation protects against ototoxicity induced by intravenous cisplatin in the guinea pig. *Front. Cell. Neurosci.* 11:280. doi: 10.3389/fncel.2017.00280

Franzen, H. M., Draget, K. I., Langebäck, J., and Nilsen-Nygaard, J. (2015). Characterization and properties of hydrogels made from neutral soluble chitosans. *Polymers* 7, 373–389.

Freyer, D. R., Chen, L., Krailo, M. D., Knight, K., Villaluna, D., Bliss, B., et al. (2017). Effects of sodium thiosulfate versus observation on development of cisplatin-induced hearing loss in children with cancer (ACCL0431): a multicentre, randomised, controlled, open-label, phase 3 trial. *Lancet Oncol.* 18, 63–74. doi: 10.1016/S1470-2045(16)30625-8

Ghosh, S. (2019). Cisplatin: the first metal based anticancer drug. *Bioorg. Chem.* 88:102925. doi: 10.1016/j.bioorg.2019.102925

Ghosh, S., Sheth, S., Sheehan, K., Mukherjea, D., Dhukhwa, A., Borse, V., et al. (2018). The endocannabinoid/cannabinoid receptor 2 system protects against cisplatin-induced hearing loss. *Front. Cell. Neurosci.* 12:271. doi: 10.3389/fncel.2018.00271

Giari, L., Dezfuli, B. S., Astolfi, L., and Martini, A. (2012). Ultrastructural effects of cisplatin on the inner ear and lateral line system of zebrafish (*Danio rerio*) larvae. *J. Appl. Toxicol.* 32, 293–299. doi: 10.1002/jat.1691

Hellberg, V., Wallin, I., Ehrsson, H., and Laurell, G. (2013). Cochlear pharmacokinetics of cisplatin: an in vivo study in the guinea pig. *Laryngoscope* 123, 3172–3177. doi: 10.1002/lary.24235

Lajud, S. A., Han, Z., Chi, F. L., Gu, R., Nagda, D. A., Bezpalko, O., et al. (2013). A regulated delivery system for inner ear drug application. *J. Control. Release* 166, 268–276. doi: 10.1016/j.jconrel.2012.12.031

Lajud, S. A., Nagda, D. A., Qiao, P., Tanaka, N., Civantos, A., Gu, R., et al. (2015). A novel chitosan-hydrogel-based nanoparticle delivery system for local inner ear application. *Otol. Neurotol.* 36, 341–347. doi: 10.1097/MAO.0000000000000445

Laurell, G., and Bagger-Sjöbäck, D. (1991). Dose-dependent inner ear changes after i.v. administration of cisplatin. *J. Otolaryngol.* 20, 158–167.

Le Gal, K., Ibrahim, M. X., Wiel, C., Sayin, V. I., Akula, M. K., Karlsson, C., et al. (2015). Antioxidants can increase melanoma metastasis in mice. *Sci. Transl. Med.* 7:308re8. doi: 10.1126/scitranslmed.aad3740

Marshak, T., Steiner, M., Kaminer, M., Levy, L., and Shupak, A. (2014). Prevention of cisplatin-induced hearing loss by intratympanic dexamethasone: a randomized controlled study. *Otolaryngol. Head Neck Surg.* 150, 983–990. doi: 10.1177/0194599814524894

More, S. S., Akil, O., Ianculescu, A. G., Geier, E. G., Lustig, L. R., and Giacomini, K. M. (2010). Role of the copper transporter. *J. Neurosci.* 30, 9500–9509. doi: 10.1523/JNEUROSCI.1544-10.2010

Neimert-Andersson, T., Binnmyr, J., Enoksson, M., Langeback, J., Zettergren, L., Hallgren, A. C., et al. (2014). Evaluation of safety and efficacy as an adjuvant for the chitosan-based vaccine delivery vehicle ViscoGel in a single-blind randomised Phase I/IIa clinical trial. *Vaccine* 32, 5967–5974. doi: 10.1016/j.vaccine.2014.08.057

Ngo, D. H., and Kim, S. K. (2014). Antioxidant effects of chitin, chitosan, and their derivatives. *Adv. Food Nutr. Res.* 73, 15–31. doi: 10.1016/B978-0-12-800268-1.00002-0

Paulson, D. P., Abuzeid, W., Jiang, H., Oe, T., O'Malley, B. W., and Li, D. (2008). A novel controlled local drug delivery system for inner ear disease. *Laryngoscope* 118, 706–711. doi: 10.1097/MLG.0b013e31815f8e41

Roldán-Fidalgo, A., Martin Saldaña, S., Trinidad, A., Olmedilla-Alonso, B., Rodríguez-Valiente, A., García-Berrocal, J. R., et al. (2016). In vitro and in vivo effects of lutein against cisplatin-induced ototoxicity. *Exp. Toxicol. Pathol.* 68, 197–204. doi: 10.1016/j.etp.2016.01.003

Rolland, V., Meyer, F., Guitton, M. J., Bussieres, R., Philippon, D., Bairati, I., et al. (2019). A randomized controlled trial to test the efficacy of trans-tympanic injections of a sodium thiosulfate gel to prevent cisplatin-induced ototoxicity in patients with head and neck cancer. *J. Otolaryngol. Head Neck Surg.* 48:4. doi: 10.1186/s40463-019-0327-x

Rybak, L. P., Whitworth, C. A., Mukherjea, D., and Ramkumar, V. (2007). Mechanisms of cisplatin-induced ototoxicity and prevention. *Hear. Res.* 226, 157–167. doi: 10.1016/j.heares.2006.09.015

Saber, A., Laurell, G., Bramer, T., Edsman, K., Engmér, C., and Ulfendahl, M. (2009). Middle ear application of a sodium hyaluronate gel loaded with neomycin in a Guinea pig model. *Ear Hear.* 30, 81–89. doi: 10.1097/AUD.0b013e31818ff98e

Saber, A., Strand, S. P., and Ulfendahl, M. (2010). Use of the biodegradable polymer chitosan as a vehicle for applying drugs to the inner ear. *Eur. J. Pharm. Sci.* 39, 110–115. doi: 10.1016/j.ejps.2009.11.003

Salt, A. N., Hartsock, J. J., Gill, R. M., King, E., Kraus, F. B., and Plontke, S. K. (2016). Perilymph pharmacokinetics of locally-applied gentamicin in the guinea pig. *Hear. Res.* 342, 101–111. doi: 10.1016/j.heares.2016.10.003

Sannan, T., Kurita, K., and Iwakura, Y. (1976). Studies on chitin, 2. Effect of deacetylation on solubility. *Macromol. Chem. Phys.* 177, 3589–3600.

Sarafraz, Z., Ahmadi, A., and Daneshi, A. (2018). Transtympanic Injections of N-acetylcysteine and dexamethasone for prevention of cisplatin-induced ototoxicity: double blind randomized clinical trial. *Int. Tinnitus J.* 22, 40–45. doi: 10.5935/0946-5448.20180007

Sayin, V. I., Ibrahim, M. X., Larsson, E., Nilsson, J. A., Lindahl, P., and Bergo, M. O. (2014). Antioxidants accelerate lung cancer progression in mice. *Sci. Transl. Med.* 6:221ra15. doi: 10.1126/scitranslmed.3007653

Sheth, S., Mukherjea, D., Rybak, L. P., and Ramkumar, V. (2017). Mechanisms of cisplatin-induced ototoxicity and otoprotection. *Front. Cell. Neurosci.* 11:338. doi: 10.3389/fncel.2017.00338

Shi, X. (2016). Pathophysiology of the cochlear intrastrial fluid-blood barrier (review). *Hear. Res.* 338, 52–63. doi: 10.1016/j.heares.2016.01.010

Shigemasa, Y., Saito, K., Sashiwa, H., and Saimoto, H. (1994). Enzymatic degradation of chitins and partially deacetylated chitins. *Int. J. Biol. Macromol.* 16, 43–49.

Tanaka, F., Whitworth, C. A., and Rybak, L. P. (2003). Influence of pH on the ototoxicity of cisplatin: a round window application study. *Hear. Res.* 177, 21–31.

Tanaka, F., Whitworth, C. A., and Rybak, L. P. (2004). Round window pH manipulation alters the ototoxicity of systemic cisplatin. *Hear. Res.* 187, 44–50.

Vårum, K. M., Ottoy, M. H., and Smidsrod, O. (1994). Water-solubility of partially N-acetylated chitosans as a function of pH: effect of chemical composition and depolymerisation. *Carbohyd. Polym.* 25, 65–70.

Videhult, P., Laurell, G., Wallin, I., and Ehrsson, H. (2006). Kinetics of cisplatin and its monohydrated complex with sulfur-containing compounds designed for local otoprotective administration. *Exp. Biol. Med.* 231, 1638–1645.

Videhult Pierre, P., Engmér, C., Wallin, I., Laurell, G., and Ehrsson, H. (2009). High concentrations of thiosulfate in scala tympani perilymph after systemic administration in the guinea pig. *Acta Otolaryngol.* 129, 132–137. doi: 10.1080/00016480802116232

Wang, X., Chen, Y., Tao, Y., Gao, Y., Yu, D., and Wu, H. (2018). A666-conjugated nanoparticles target prestin of outer hair cells preventing cisplatin-induced hearing loss. *Int. J. Nanomed.* 13, 7517–7531. doi: 10.2147/IJN.S170130

Ways, T. M. M., Lau, W. M., and Khutoryanskiy, V. V. (2018). Chitosan and its derivatives for application in mucoadhesive drug delivery systems. *Polymers* 10:267. doi: 10.3390/polym10030267

Yushkevich, P. A., Piven, J., Hazlett, H. C., Smith, R. G., Ho, S., Gee, J. C., et al. (2006). User-guided 3D active contour segmentation of anatomical structures: significantly improved efficiency and reliability. *Neuroimage* 31, 1116–1128. doi: 10.1016/j.neuroimage.2006.01.015

2

Investigations of the Microvasculature of the Human Macula Utricle in Meniere's Disease

Gail Ishiyama[1], Ivan A. Lopez[2]*, Dora Acuna[2] and Akira Ishiyama[2]

[1] *Department of Neurology, David Geffen School of Medicine at UCLA, Los Angeles, CA, United States,*

[2] *Department of Head and Neck Surgery, David Geffen School of Medicine at UCLA, Los Angeles, CA, United States*

Correspondence:
Ivan A. Lopez
ilopez@ucla.edu

The integrity and permeability of the blood labyrinthine barrier (BLB) in the inner ear is important to maintain adequate blood supply, and to control the passage of fluids, molecules and ions. Identifying the cellular and structural components of the BLB, the vascular endothelial cells (VECs), pericytes, and the perivascular basement membrane, is critical to understand the pathophysiology of the inner ear microvasculature and to design efficient delivery of therapeutics across the BLB. A recent study of the normal and pathological ultrastructural changes in the human macula utricle microvasculature demonstrated that the VECs are damaged in Meniere's disease (MD), and further studies identified oxidative stress markers (iNOS and nitrotyrosine) in the VECs. Using fluorescence microscopy, the microvasculature was studied in the macula utricle of patients diagnosed with MD that required transmastoid labyrinthectomy for intractable vertigo ($n = 5$), and patients who required a translabyrinthine approach for vestibular schwannoma (VS) resection ($n = 3$). Normal utricles (controls) were also included ($n = 3$). VECs were identified using rabbit polyclonal antibodies against the glucose transporter-1 (GLUT-1) and pericytes were identified using mouse monoclonal antibodies against alpha-smooth muscle actin (α-SMA). Immunofluorescence (IF) staining was made in half of the utricle and flat mounted. The other half was used to study the integrity of the BLB using transmission electron microscopy (TEM). GLUT-1-IF, allowed delineation of the macula utricle microvasculature (located in the stroma underneath the sensory epithelia) in both MD and VS specimens. Three sizes of vessels were present in the utricle vasculature: Small size (<15 μm), medium size (15–25 μm) and large size >25 μm. α-SMA-IF was present in pericytes that surround the VECS in medium and thick size vessels. Thin size vessels showed almost no α-SMA-IF. AngioTool software was used for quantitative analysis. A significant decreased number of junctions, total vessel length, and average vessel length was detected in the microvasculature in MD specimens compared with VS and control specimens. The deeper understanding of the anatomy of the BLB in the human vestibular periphery and its pathological changes in disease will enable the development of non-invasive delivery strategy for the treatment of hearing and balance disorders.

Keywords: microvasculature, macula utricle, pericytes, Meniere's disease, blood labyrinthine barrier, vascular endothelial cells, glucose transporter-1

INTRODUCTION

The inner ear cochlear and vestibular function is dependent on the integrity of the vasculature for the maintenance of an adequate blood supply, control of metabolism, and fluid homeostasis (Shi, 2016). The blood labyrinthine barrier (BLB) plays a critical role in the ionic transport needed to maintain the highly differing ionic composition of the endolymph and the perilymph, creating the electrophysiological gradient necessary for hearing and balance function. Recent studies in the blood brain barrier (BBB) demonstrate that several environmental factors, mental stress, noise exposure, air pollution affects vascular endothelial function (Daiber et al., 2017), and a similar pathophysiology may occur in the inner ear vasculature in response to environmental insults.

The anatomy of the human inner ear vasculature has been recently described (Mei et al., 2018) and a detailed anatomical review was given by Mudry and Tange (2009). In their review, they confirmed the spatial organization of the inner ear vasculature illustrated by Nabeya in 1923 (Nabeya, 1923). Mazzoni describes in detail the vascular anatomy of the normal vestibular labyrinth in humans using 1 mm thick sections of decalcified temporal bones stained with osmium tetroxide and cleared with methylsalycylate Mazzoni (1990).

In the last 20 years considerable advances have been made to understand the physiology and cellular, molecular structural organization of the BLB in animal models (Shi, 2016). The BLB in the rodent model is a complex structure formed by VECs, pericytes, and the underlying perivascular basement membrane (Shi et al., 2008; Neng et al., 2013a,b; Zhang et al., 2013). The first detailed anatomical and ultrastructural study of the human vestibular BLB demonstrated similarities of the human BBB and the animal BLB (Ishiyama et al., 2017).

Our recent studies have demonstrated pathology of the BLB in MD (Ishiyama et al., 2017, 2018), a disabling inner ear disorder characterized by incapacitating attacks of vertigo, hearing loss, and tinnitus (Baloh, 2001; Ishiyama et al., 2001). Histopathological studies have demonstrated a nearly universally associated hydrops of the endolymphatic system of the inner ear, a ballooning of the endolymph structures (Hallpike and Cairns, 1938; Yamakawa, 1938; Schuknecht, 1993). However, the role of hydrops in MD remains unknown (Merchant et al., 2005; Semaan et al., 2005; Semaan and Megerian, 2010; Foster and Breeze, 2013; Ishiyama et al., 2015). While it has been proposed that hydrops is an epiphenomenon (Merchant et al., 2005), we believe that given the near universality of hydrops in cases of MD, that hydrops is a necessary but not sufficient factor for MD. The lack of an animal model for MD that fully exhibits the clinical features hampers the identification of the cellular and molecular pathophysiological mechanisms.

Several studies using MRI with gadolinium in patients diagnosed with MD have demonstrated endolymphatic hydrops of the affected inner ear of MD subjects (Ishiyama et al., 2015; Sepahdari et al., 2015, 2016; Pakdaman et al., 2016). In these studies which utilize gadolinium enhanced MRI protocols to image endolymphatic hydrops, patients with MD exhibit significantly greater contrast enhancement in the affected ear perilymph (Tagaya et al., 2011; Yamazaki et al., 2012; Barath et al., 2014; Pakdaman et al., 2016). Intravenous gadolinium is taken up into the perilymph, presumably via perfusion through the BLB, specifically the blood-perilymph barrier. In animal studies, substances that break down the BLB when introduced intratympanically, such as lipopolysaccharide, cause ipsilateral increased perilymph (LeFloc'h et al., 2014) or increased entry of serum fluorescein into the perilymph (Hirose et al., 2014), demonstrating that an increase in BLB permeability can cause ipsilateral increased perilymph gadolinium signal on MRI.

Histopathological studies of the morphological alterations of the inner ear vasculature from MD patients have revealed basement membrane pathology in the BLB (McCall et al., 2009). Further evaluations demonstrated epithelial and perivascular basement membrane constituent protein alterations (Calzada et al., 2012), suggesting that the pericytes of the BLB may be affected in MD. The pericytes surround the abluminal face of the VECs tube and extend long cellular processes along the abluminal face of the VECs. In the rodent BLB, pericytes contain contractile proteins and have the ability to contract to control the diameter of the capillary (Shi et al., 2008). To the date there are not specific markers for pericytes, however, several antibodies have been used to identify them: α-smooth muscle actin (α-SMA), platelet-derived growth factor receptor-β (PDGFRβ), NG2, desmin and other markers (Shi et al., 2008). The ultrastructure of blood vessels located in the stroma of the MD human macula utricle has demonstrated increased vesicle formation and degeneration of the VECs of the BLB (Ishiyama et al., 2017). The expression of two oxidative stress markers: inducible nitric oxide synthase (iNOS) and nitrotyrosine in VECs of the BLB of the human vestibular utricle from Meniere's patients implicates oxidative stress as mediating the disruption of the BLB (Ishiyama et al., 2018).

In the present study we hypothesize that the vasculature of the BLB of the macula utricle will exhibit structural alterations and constrictions in MD, and that the cellular components of the BLB will exhibit degenerative changes. There is evidence that leakage of the microvasculature of the inner ear may result in edema triggering MD symptoms (Ishiyama et al., 2015). Recent progress on BLB pathophysiology in animal models highlights the importance of the BLB integrity for ion homeostasis, prompting us to question whether dysfunction of the BLB is key to understand the pathophysiology of MD (Shi, 2011, 2016; Hirose et al., 2014). We detected increased transcellular vesicular transport across VECs, detachment of pericyte processes, and disruption of perivascular basement membrane in the stroma beneath the macula and cristae vestibular sensory epithelia in MD patients (Ishiyama et al., 2017, 2018).

We have examined and described in detail the histopathology of vestibular endorgans (macula and cristae) obtained from MD patients (McCall et al., 2009; Ishiyama et al., 2017, 2018). In the prior histopathological studies of the BLB microvasculature in MD, we noted a narrowing of the lumen which may affect the perfusion of the auditory and vestibular neuroepithelium and nerve (Ishiyama et al., 2017, 2018). However, these observations were made in thin cross sections, making it difficult to identify the extent of alterations in the vasculature in the whole endorgan. Whole mount immunofluorescence staining and quantification of changes in the vascular network using AngioTool software (Zudaire et al., 2011) was made in the macula utricle obtained by ablative surgery from MD and vestibular schwannoma (VS) patients and normal (control) utricles obtained from microdissected temporal bones obtained at autopsy. The specimens were immunostained with antibodies against glucose transporter-1 (GLUT-1) to visualize VECs and α-SMA to identify pericytes in the utricle microvasculature.

MATERIALS AND METHODS

Sources of Specimens

Appropriate informed consent for inclusion in the study was obtained from each donor. Approval was obtained from the University of California at Los Angeles Institutional Review Board (IRB protocol # 10-001449). Vestibular endorgans were acquired at surgery from patients diagnosed with MD that required transmastoid labyrinthectomy for intractable vertigo (n = 5, 2 male: 43 and 58 years old (specimen #1 and #2; female: 52, 61 and 69 years old: specimens #3, #4 and #5), patients who required a translabyrinthine approach for VS resection (n = 3, male: 60 years old, specimen # 6; female: 53 and 58 years old: specimens #7 and #8). Normal utricles microdissected from temporal bones obtained at autopsy (2 females age 68, 70 years old, specimen #9 and #10 respectively, and 1 male 75 years old, specimen #11) were also included in this study (**Table 1**).

Inclusion Criteria

The following criteria were required for surgical specimens diagnosed with MD: (1) Documentation that the patient meets the 1995 AAO-HNS criteria for definite MD. (2) Ipsilateral non-serviceable hearing. (3) Intractable to medical therapy including low salt diet and diuretics.

Tissue Processing

Utricles obtained from ablative surgery or microdissected from temporal bones were fixed in 10% formalin overnight, washed with phosphate buffered saline solution (PBS, 0.1M, pH 7.4) and cut in two halves under the dissecting microscope (**Figure 1A**). The cut was made from the medial (nerve stump) to the lateral portion. One half was used for immunofluorescence staining and one half was processed for transmission electron microscopy (TEM). Tissue used for immunofluorescence staining was immersed in 30% sucrose in PBS for 1 day for cryoprotection. The following day the tissue was snap frozen in liquid nitrogen, thawed (Lopez et al., 2005) and processed for immunofluorescence staining (Lopez et al., 2016).

Immunofluorescence (Whole Mount Preparation)

Tissue was placed in a rotary shaker and incubated for 3 h in a blocking solution containing 2% bovine serum albumin fraction V (Sigma, SLM), 0.1% Triton X-100 (Sigma, SLM) diluted in PBS at 4–6°C. Subsequently, the blocking solution was removed and the half utricles are incubated for 72 h with the primary antibodies, placing the vials in the rotatory shaker in a cold room. At the end of the incubation, the blocking solution was removed and the primary antibodies against GLUT-1 (1:1000 in PBS) and α-SMA (1:1000 in PBS) were incubated 48 h at 4°C in a humidity chamber. GLUT-1 (Abcam, is a rabbit polyclonal antibody with specific reactivity for human and rat, raised against a synthetic peptide), α-SMA is a mouse monoclonal antibody (SIGMA-ALDRICH, specific reactivity for human, mouse and rat, generated with an N-terminal synthetic decapeptide of α-SMA). The secondary antibodies against rabbit or mouse labeled with Alexa 488 or 594 (1:1000, Molecular Probes, Carlsbad, CA, United States) were applied and incubated for 2 h at room temperature in the dark. At the end of the incubation, the whole endorgans or sections were washed with PBS (20 min × 5) and mounted flat on glass slides with Vectashield solution containing DAPI (Vector Labs, Burlingame, CA, United States) to visualize all cell nuclei. Specimens #3, #4, #5, and #8 were cut in two halves. One half was used for IF and the second half was used for TEM.

Positive Controls

Cryostat sections were obtained from the macula utricle microdissected from temporal bones (contralateral side, specimens #9, #10, and #11 (IRB protocol # 10-001449). Sections were immunostained as described above. GLUT-1-IF delineate VECs and α-SMA-IF pericytes in the blood vessels located in the stroma utricle (same immunolocalization as shown in Ishiyama et al., 2018).

Negative Controls

As negative controls, the primary antibody was omitted or preabsorbed with the antigen as described previously (Lopez et al., 2016; Ishiyama et al., 2018) and the immunoreaction was performed as described above. No immunoreaction was detected in both types of negative controls.

Confocal Imaging

Fluorescent images were acquired using a high-resolution laser confocal microscope light-sheet (Leica, model SP8). For the region of interest (illustrated in new **Figure 1A**), series of approximately 50 digital GLUT-1-IF images (0.5 micron thick) were collected by the confocal microscope, and individual stacks were obtained. The first image was collected from the top of the stack where GLUT-1-IF blood vessels begin to appear (flat mount preparation) (generally below the sensory epithelia) until the bottom of the stack where the GLUT-1-IF blood vessels are no longer visible. Then a maximum projection image was created from each stack and this maximum projection image was used for quantification. All images were prepared using the Adobe Photoshop software program run in a Dell OptiPlex 3020 computer.

Quantitative Analysis of the Vascular Network Using AngioTool Software

This software allows the quantification of vascular networks in microscopic immunofluorescence stained images and computes

TABLE 1 | Parameters computed by AngioTool.

Specimen	Type	Vessels area (mm^2)	Vessels % area	Number of junctions	Total vessels length (mm)	Average vessels length (mm)	Total number of end points
1	MD	0.064	20.13	46	5.32	0.10	139
2	MD	0.098	30.08	63	8.05	0.14	158
3	MD	0.043	15.35	18	3.84	0.10	87
4	MD	0.086	27.90	57	6.96	0.11	159
5	MD	0.11	35.92	92	9.70	0.08	106
6	VS	0.13	39.88	201	11.71	0.18	262
7	VS	0.11	34.78	119	11.16	0.13	313
8	VS	0.10	25.55	239	12.64	0.19	252
9	C	0.113	23.33	133	13.37	0.17	274
10	C	0.105	32.14	205	13.15	0.13	251
11	C	0.121	20.30	234	12.85	0.16	343

MD, Meniere's disease; VS, vestibular schwannoma; C, control. Total area analyzed 0.578 × 0.578 mm = 0.334 mm^2.

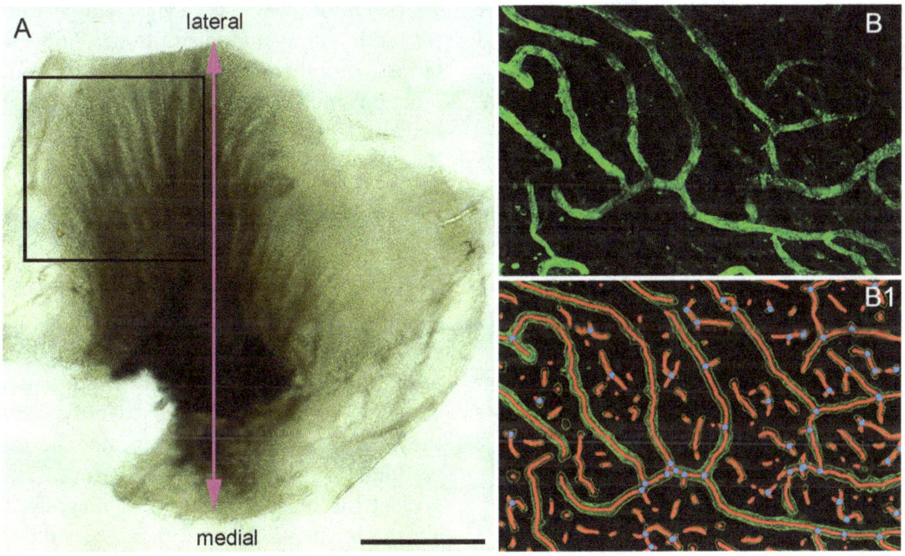

FIGURE 1 | (A) The macula utricle was cut into two halves. The black color rectangular frame shows the area analyzed for quantitative immunoflurescence. **(B)** A small immunostained area of the macula utricle (Specimen on **Figure 4C**) and **(B1)** shows the resulting segmented and skeletonized image from **(B)**. Blue dots showed the branching index. Bar in **(A)** is 1 mm.

several morphological and spatial parameters: area covered by the vasculature vascular network, the number of vessels, vessels length, vascular density and lacunarity, and branching index. Confocal images of immunostained utricles with GLUT-1 were analyzed using this program (Open source)[1] and processed as described (Zudaire et al., 2011). Images for quantitative analysis were acquired with the confocal microscope using a 20× objective (oil) at 1 zoom (200×). The image is immediately segmented, skeletonized and the analysis of the vasculature is performed automatically, the resulting image shows the overlay of the area of all vessels and shows also the computed branching points inside the area imaged. **Figure 1A** indicates the region of interest (ROI) analyzed (black color frame to the left side of the utricle). **Figure 1B**, illustrates the blood vessels immunostained with antibodies against GLUT-1. **Figure 1B1** shows the segmented and skeletonized (delineated) blood vessels from which quantitative analysis was made. Branching points are seen in blue color. The image generated by the software was saved as TIFF file and an Excel file containing the computed results was generated.

Quantification was made double blinded, i.e., the researcher performing the immunostaining and the quantification was only given the specimen number (**Table 1**). At the end of the analysis each specimen was identified as MD, VS or control. The area examined per specimen (image field) used was 0.578 × 0.578 mm = 0.335 mm^2. The GLUT-1-IF green color (channel) was selected because of the consistent delineation of the blood vessels (VECs). The following parameters were quantified: vessels area (the area of the segmented vessels), vessel percentage area (the percentage of area occupied by vessels inside

[1] http://angiotool.nci.nih.gov

the area examined), total number of junctions (the total number by vessels inside the explant area), total vessel length (the sum of Euclidean distances between pixels of all the vessels in the image), average vessel length (the mean length of all the vessels in the image and the total number of endpoints (the number of open ended segments).

Statistics

Comparisons of the parameters described above were made as follow: Meniere's vs. VS, MD vs. controls and VS vs. controls (**Tables 2A–C**). A student *t*-test for two independent means was obtained using the IBM SPSS statistics software program version 25 (IBM Corporation, Armonk, NY, United States). A value of $p < 0.05$ was denoted as a statistically significant difference.

TEM Processing

Macula utricles halves (specimens #3, #4, and #5 are from Meniere's utricles and specimen #8 is from an VS utricle) were immersed in 4% paraformaldehyde, 2.5% glutaraldehyde for 1 day and then immersed in the following solutions: 2% OsO4 and 2% potassium ferricyanide (EMS, Fort Washington, PA, United States), 0.1% thio-carbohydrazide for 1 h, 2% OsO4 for 30 min, uranyl acetate 1% overnight, and 0.1% lead aspartate for 30 min (Ishiyama et al., 2017). Tissue was dehydrated in ascending ethyl alcohols and embedded in resin (Epon®, EMS). One-micron thick sections were made to identify the blood vessels at light microscopy, when the area of interest was visible, ultrathin 100 nm sections were obtained, and mounted on formvar coated single slot copper grids.

TEM Qualitative Study

Systematic analysis was made in tissue sections containing the microvasculature in the stroma of the macula utricle. TEM observations and digital image capture were made using a FEI Tecnai transmission electron microscope T20 TEM -200 KV (Hillsboro, OR, United States). All sections are systematically analyzed at low (×3,500–5,000), and higher magnification view (×19,000–25,000). All sections were studied for the presence of vesicles in the VECs, pericytes, and perivascular BM alterations (i.e., thickening and disruption). TEM was used to identify ultrastructural changes, the distribution and alterations of tight junction morphology, abnormalities of cellular interactions between VEC and pericytes.

TABLE 2A | Statistical comparisons MD vs. VS (*t*-test for 2 independent means).

Parameter	*t*-value	*p*-value	Statistical significance at $p < 0.05$
Vessels area	−1.91966	0.051658	No
Vessels% area	−1.30905	0.119207	No
Number of junctions	−4.31097	0.002516	Yes
Total vessels length	−3.61488	0.005583	Yes
Average vessels length	−3.22271	0.009038	Yes
Total number of end points	−6.178	0.000413	Yes

TABLE 2B | Statistical comparisons MD vs. Control (*t*-test for 2 independent means).

Parameter	*t*-value	*p*-value	Statistical significance at $p < 0.05$
Vessels area	−2.00431	0.045939	Yes
Vessels% area	0.11231	0.457121	No
Number of junctions	−4.98871	0.00124	Yes
Total vessels length	−4.63808	0.001774	Yes
Average vessels length	−3.00747	0.011889	Yes
Total number of end points	−5.73169	0.000612	Yes

TABLE 2C | Statistical comparisons VS vs. Control (*t*-test for 2 independent means).

Parameter	*t*-value	*p*-value	Statistical significance at $p < 0.05$
Vessels area	0.03348	0.487447	No
Vessels% area	1.48253	0.10617	No
Number of junctions	−0.09334	0.46506	No
Total vessels length	−2.81273	0.024092	Yes
Average vessels length	0.60302	0.289508	No
Total number of end points	−0.40821	0.352014	No

RESULTS

Whole Mount Immunofluorescence

Using immunofluorescence labeling and high-resolution laser confocal microscopy on whole mount preparations of the macula utricle obtained at surgery from patients diagnosed with MD and VS it was possible to identify VECs and pericytes of the microvascular network located in the stroma below the vestibular sensory epithelia. **Figure 2A** shows a representative area of the macula utricle (low magnification view) from one VS specimen. VECs were identified with antibodies against the glucose transporter-1 (GLUT-1). Uniform GLUT-1 labeling was observed in blood vessels (thick arrowheads). Three sizes of blood vessels were identified: Small size (<15 μm), medium (>15 to <25 μm) and large size (>25 μm).

αSMA-IF was seen in pericytes that surround in medium and large size vessels (>15 μm). The αSMA-IF pericytes in the large size vessels showed a protuberant soma and encircling circumferential processes (arrows in **Figure 2A**). The lack of αSMA-IF around GLUT-1 blood vessels of small size suggest that pericytes in these vessels express a different immunomarker as it has been seen in animal models (Shi et al., 2008). **Figure 2B**, shows the normal appearance of the blood vessels (high magnification view from **Figure 2A**).

Pericytes and VECs Showed Marked Alterations in the Blood Vessels of Meniere's Specimens

Using double immunolabeling and high-resolution laser confocal microscopy we identified pericytes in a thick sized blood vessel from a VS patient in **Figure 3A**. The pericytes showed protuberant soma and encircling circumferential processes that

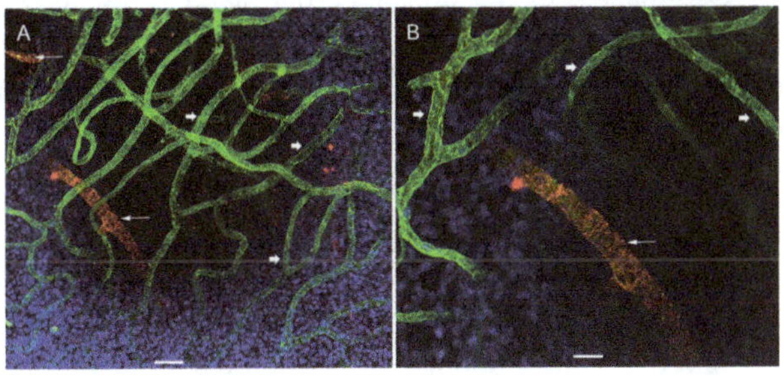

FIGURE 2 | Whole mount preparation of the human macula utricle (VS) immunoreacted with antibodies against GLUT-1 and αSMA. **(A)** Shows a representative area of the macula utricle (low magnification view, 200×) from an VS patient (Specimen 6). Glucose transporter-1-IF (GLUT-1, green color, arrowheads), allowed to identify VECs in thin blood vessels (approximately 10–15 μm), αSMA-IF (red color) was seen in thick vessels (approximately 25 μm) were visualized (white thin arrows). DAPI stain cell nuclei (blue). **(B)** Is a high magnification view from **(A)**. Bar in **(A)** is 50 μm, in **(B)** is 25 μm.

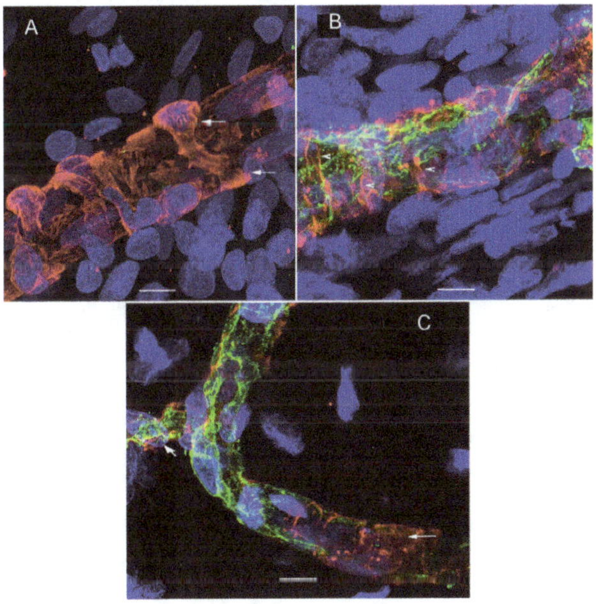

FIGURE 3 | Double immunolabeling and high-resolution laser confocal microscopy we detected alterations in the macula utricle BLB. **(A)** Shows αSMA-IF (red) in thick vessels from an VS utricle (Specimen 6), small arrows point to a wrapping pericyte, IF is uniform through the blood vessel. **(B)** Shows a thick vessel from a Meniere's patient (Specimen 1), there is disorganization of the pericyte processes (arrowheads) and there is evidence of degeneration of the VECs with an uneven lumen and the vessel wall exhibits areas of severe thinning (green color). **(C)** Shows constriction in the blood vessels (diagonal arrowhead). Small white arrow point to the blood vessel pericyte. DAPI stain cell nuclei (blue). Bar in **(A,B)** is 10 μm, in **(C)** is 15 μm.

nearly cover the vessel uniformly. In contrast, there were signs of damage in the pericytes and VECs of the macula utricle from two MD patients (**Figures 3B,C**). The pericytes in the Meniere's specimen do not uniformly encircle the vessel and the pericyte processes are thinner and there are areas of the vessel unprotected by the pericyte processes. The pericyte processes appear to be disorganized and there were fewer pericyte soma present. **Figure 3C** shows an area of constriction within the blood vessel, and at this region there were few encircling pericytes, and the VECs were disorganized forming an uneven lumen of the vessel.

Whole Mount Preparation Allows a Quantitative Analysis of Vascular Network

Using GLUT-1-IF to delineate the vasculature it was possible to identify and quantify changes in the different specimens. **Figure 4**, shows one VS and two MD specimens. Qualitative analysis showed a differential pattern of organization of the vasculature. The vasculature in Specimen 1 (VS) was well-organized, forming uniform patterns of branching and of size

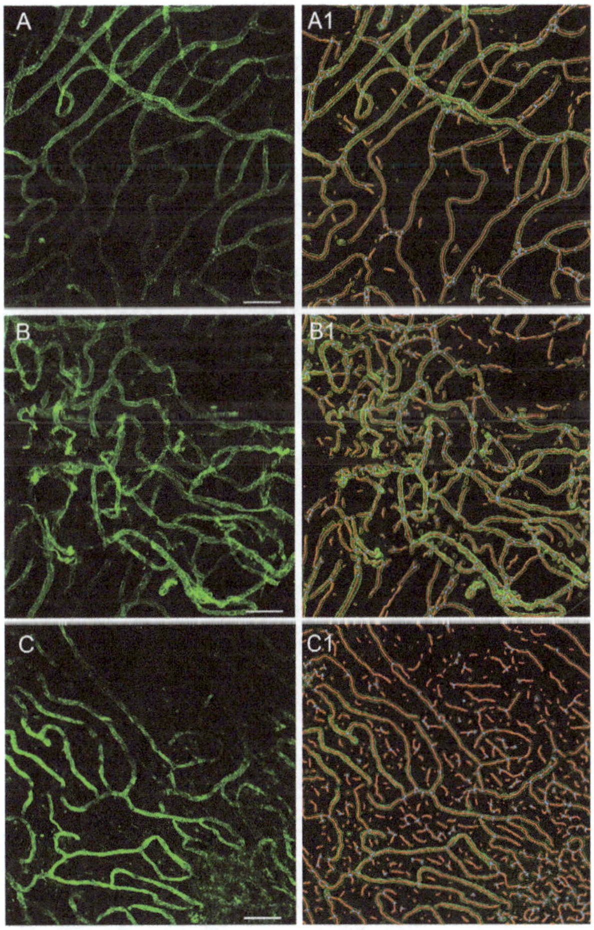

FIGURE 4 | Whole mount preparation of the macula utricle allows a quantitative analysis of vascular network. Using GLUT-1-IF (green color) to delineate the vasculature it was possible to identify changes in the different specimens using AngioTool software. **(A–C)** Shows GLUT-1-IF in one VS utricle (Specimen 1), and two Meniere's utricles (Specimen 2 and 3 respectively). **(A1–C1)** Shows the corresponding segmented images (From the left) created by the software. The segment images are then subjected to quantitative analysis (**Table 1**). Bar is 100 μm.

(**Figure 4A**). In contrast, in one of the Meniere's utricle (Specimen 2), there were distorted vessels with an overall appearance of non-uniform bent and misshapen vessels, some shortened and twisted (**Figure 4B**). In contrast, there was a relatively normal appearance of blood vessels in specimen 3 (**Figure 4C**). Quantitative results are seen in **Table 1**. **Figures 4A1–C1** shows the corresponding segmented images obtained with the software. Analysis of each image was achieved in less than 3 min, and the following the parameters were obtained: the vessels area, vessels percentage area, number of junctions, total vessels length, average vessel length and total number of endpoints (**Table 1**). Comparisons of the quantitative results were made as follow: MD vs. VS, MD vs. controls, and VS vs. controls. **Tables 2A–C**, shows that the number of junctions, total vessels length and average, and the number of endpoints were significantly smaller in MD specimens compared with VS specimens and controls. There were not statistical differences when we compared VS vs. controls, the only difference was in vessel length (**Table 2C**).

Transmission Electron Microscopy

TEM analysis allowed the identification of changes in pericytes and VECs (**Figures 5, 6**). The blood vessels from the VS specimen showed an almost normal organization (**Figure 5A**, from Specimen #8). The lumen of the blood vessel is open and uniform, the VECs showed no cytoplasmic vacuolization and the pericytes are also normal. In the VS specimens, the perivascular basement membrane is well delineated and the stroma shows no signs of edema. In contrast the blood vessels of Meniere's specimens showed consistently a narrow luminal space and the VECs showed vacuolization and swollen cytoplasm (**Figures 5B, 6A,B**), the pericytes processes showed also vacuolization. The perivascular basement membrane is disorganized and the vestibular stroma showed signs of edema. **Figures 5B, 6A,B** were obtained from Specimens #3, #4, and #5 respectively.

DISCUSSION

In the present study, we characterize and quantify the pathological changes in the microvasculature of patients diagnosed with MD. We have previously identified the cellular components of the BLB vasculature using antibodies against GLUT-1 and αSMA in formalin fixed cryostat sections of the utricular macula (Ishiyama et al., 2018). We were able to identify changes in the expression of these two proteins and other cellular markers (Ishiyama et al., 2018). However, it was not possible

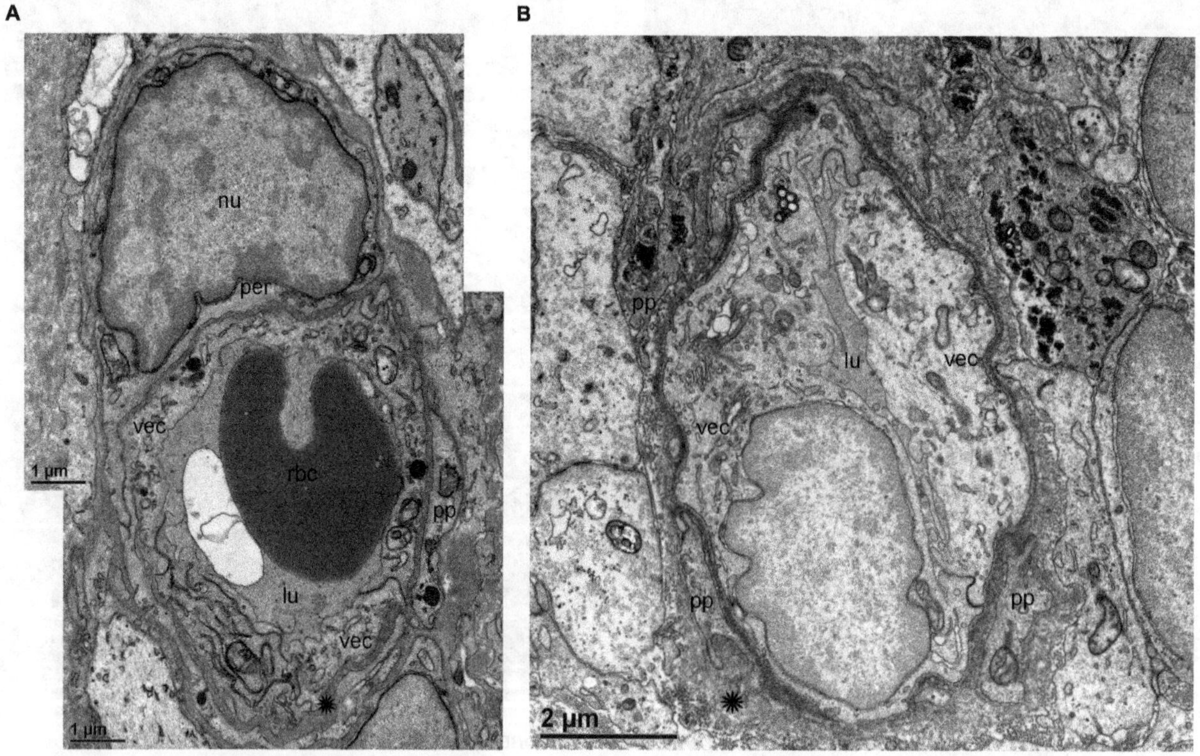

FIGURE 5 | Transmission electron microscopy (TEM) of blood vessels from an VS and MD specimens. **(A)** Shows the normal organization of a blood vessel from an VS specimen. The lumen (lu) of the blood vessel is open and uniform, VECs (vec) showed no cytoplasmic vacuolization, and the pericytes (per) and processes (pp) are also normal, the perivascular basement membrane is compact with no vacuolization and compact (asterisk). **(B)** In contrast, the blood vessels of MD specimens showed consistently a narrow luminal space (lu) and the VECs (vec) showed vacuolization (thin arrow) and swollen cytoplasm, the pericytes processes (pp) showed also vacuolization, and the perivascular basement membrane shows disorganization, nu, cell nucleus; rbc, red blood cell. **(A)** Was obtained from specimen #8, and **(B)** from specimen #3. Thin sections (90 nm) were counterstained with uranyl acetate and lead nitrate.

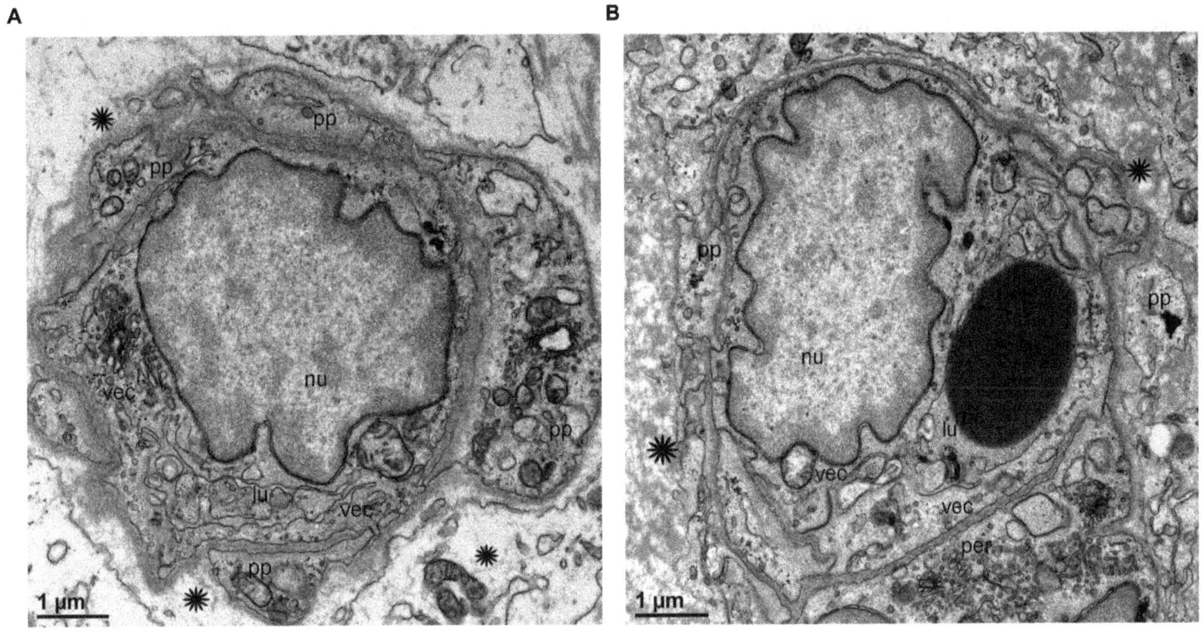

FIGURE 6 | Transmission electron microscopy of blood vessels from MD specimens. **(A,B)** Showed a narrow luminal space (lu) and VECs (vec) showed swollen cytoplasm. The pericytes processes were vacuolated (thick arrowheads) **(A)**. The perivascular basement membrane is disorganized (asterisk). **(A)** Is from specimen #4, and **(B)** is from specimen #5 (respectively). Thin sections (90 nm) were counterstained with uranyl acetate and lead nitrate.

to identify differences in the vascular network as the analysis was limited to a select of sample of thin cross-sections of the utricle. For this reason, in the present study we used whole mount immunostained preparations to investigate changes in the microvasculature of the utricular macula in MD and compared with VS and control specimens.

There were similar changes in the expression of cellular markers and consistent ultrastructural alterations of the VECs, pericytes and perivascular basement membrane.

We also evaluated the degree of alteration in VECs and surrounding pericytes using TEM in these specimens. The ultrastructural changes correspond with the areas that our prior studies had demonstrated an upregulation of iNOS and the presence of nitrotyrosine, markers of oxidative stress (Ishiyama et al., 2017, 2018). In prior studies, we have detected downregulation of two basement membrane proteins in utricles of MD patients: collagen IV and laminin-beta, and upregulation of cochlin, the most abundant protein in the inner ear in the utricular stroma (Calzada et al., 2012). These results support the pathological leakage of the BLB in the vestibular endorgans from patients diagnosed with MD as a likely physiological mechanism causing vestibular and auditory dysfunction.

Quantification of Alterations in the Vasculature

GLUT-1-IF was an excellent marker of VECs, that allow for the performance of automated assessment of the utricular macula vascular network. The use of this software allowed to determine that the number of junctions, total vessels length and average, and the number of endpoints were significantly smaller in Meniere's specimens compared with VS and control specimens. An increase of the number of specimens for both groups would help to determine to what extent the vessels are affected in Meniere's patients. These findings confirm the qualitative analysis of the visualization of the vasculature within the whole mounted specimens. The vasculature in the Meniere's specimens exhibited disorganization, shortened and distorted vessels, quantified as a decrease in total vessel length, average vessel length. A significant decrease in the number of junctions and the total number of end points was found in MD specimens when compared with VS and control specimens. The information obtained with this preparation allowed comparison of the overall organization of the microvasculature, identify regional damages, atrophy and degree of vascularization. Quantitative changes using TEM will help to identify changes in discrete structures like tight junctions and vesicular transport.

Mechanism for BLB Disruption in MD

Based on these results and our previous reports (Ishiyama et al., 2017, 2018) we suggest a possible mechanism for BLB disruption in MD and the subsequent signs of edema, that disrupt the homeostasis of the vestibular and auditory endorgans: (1) VECs exhibit signs of increased cellular permeability with increased transcytosis, possibly due to an ototoxic effect by an infection, noise or genetic predisposition. (2) Abnormally permeable VECs allow the transport of solutes to the abluminal portion of the capillary, sending signaling to the pericyte processes that are in close contact to the VECs (Ishiyama et al., 2017). (3) The morphological alterations and upregulation of oxidative stress marker iNOS and nitrotyrosine may be the pathophysiological change supporting the cellular damage of the VECs and pericytes (Ishiyama et al., 2018). MRI-FLAIR studies confirm the ipsilateral disruption of the BLB in MD to a much greater extent than that seen in sudden sensorineural hearing loss (Pakdaman et al., 2016). (4) The transport of solutes also affects the perivascular membranes which exhibit evidence of structural damage in the present study. (5) The leakage of fluids and ion homeostasis disruption affects the surrounding extracellular matrix which had been documented in our prior immunohistochemical studies of collagen IV in MD (Calzada et al., 2012). (6) These changes in the extracellular matrix, which is essential to protect and maintain the surrounding basement membrane, allows for abnormal thickening of the basement membrane noted in our early histopathological studies (McCall et al., 2009). (7) The alterations in the basement membranes of the vasculature may affect the transport of solutes from the basal to the apical portion of the supporting cells via disruption of the expression of aquaporins 4 and 6 (Ishiyama et al., 2010).

It is important to mention that the mechanisms of BLB dysfunction are likely far more complex, as other components of the BLB in the human remains to be investigated. The expression of tight junction proteins and the expression of proteins involved in transcellular transport have not yet been investigated as potential players in the abnormally high permeability of the vasculature in the BLB of MD, and these may reveal further target areas for treatment. Also, our study is focused on MD, however, the mechanism of damage to the BLB in other conditions such as noise induced hearing loss, exposure to ototoxic agents, and age related otopathologies remain to be investigated.

Implications in Therapeutics

The delivery of local therapeutics to the inner ear is an active field for treating different types of disorders (Nyberg et al., 2019) and clinical trials begin to be implemented for different types of inner ear disorders. The challenge remains as there are several types of barriers in the cochlea and vestibular system (Rybak et al., 2019). Our results and previous studies in animal models on the normal organization of the utricle microvasculature shows that the organization of the BLB is quite similar, suggesting that the microvasculature could be used to deliver therapeutics into the inner ear. For the normal BLB, the delivery of therapeutics to the inner ear should be possible using the VECs transcellular transport mechanisms. As we have identified damage to the VECs it would be possible to use drugs that prevent or delay deterioration of these cells. Recent studies by Glueckert et al. (2015) proposed the use of nanoparticles in inner ear mouse explants. Nanoparticles could be applied systemically and VECs could internalize them via transcytosis. The knowledge of both normal and pathological organization of the microvasculature and the BLB is also relevant for local delivery because the inner ear blood supply is so intricate and varies in the different compartments.

The present study results demonstrate pathological changes in the microvasculature of the macula utricle from Meniere's patients including disorganization of the vasculature, with abnormally shaped vessel lumen, uneven lumen with areas of constriction, abnormal branching and pericyte processes with decreased abluminal coverage and thinning, leaving the VECs exposed and unprotected. Quantitative analysis indicates that there are structural changes in the microvasculature of MD specimens, with a significantly decreased total vessel length and decreased average vessel length, and number of junctions and end points. This indicates that interventions aimed at preventing the damage to the microvasculature may help stop the progression of damage to the vestibular system, restoring balance and preventing vertigo spells. We believe that a similar process occurs in the cochlea of MD patients, and interventions aimed at preventing damage to the microvasculature may also help preserve hearing. The pathological changes found in the microvasculature of Meniere's patients noted in this report and in our prior studies (Ishiyama et al., 2017, 2018) suggest that amelioration of vasoconstriction and BLB leakage may prevent chronic damage to vestibular endorgans. This may explain in part the temporary relief from vestibular symptoms when steroids are administered in MD.

Limitations of This Study and Future Directions

Given the limited availability of human tissue specimens we did not perform quantitative immunohistochemistry to investigate changes with age, disease condition, or gender. There is also the need to identify VECs and pericytes in temporal bones from patients diagnosed with Meniere's using celloidin embedded sections. The quantitative differences between specimens from patients with MD vs. VS must be interpreted with caution, given the small sample of patients analyzed, in addition VS vestibular endorgans are pathological specimens and thus are not true "normal" specimens, however, comparison with controls showed a similar vasculature organization.

Our study suggests that human inner ear tissue could be used to compare and contrast findings in animal models to design better therapies for vestibular and auditory disorders. The development of novel methods to identify and quantify blood vessels will allow the investigation of changes in the inner ear microvasculature in different animal models (Alves et al., 2018; Jiang et al., 2019) or pathological conditions.

CONCLUSION

In the present study, we identified the microvasculature of patient's diagnose with MD using whole mount preparations immunoreacted with antibodies against GLUT-1-IF and αSMA-IF. GLUT-1-IF was an excellent marker of VECs that allow to perform automated assessment of the macula utricle vascular network. αSMA-IF allowed to identify pericytes in large sized vessels, in contrast most of thin sized vessels were almost devoid of IF. The understanding of the complex intercellular communication between the VECs and pericytes would give directions to design potential drug therapies that alleviate and or prevent BLB disruption. The results allowed us to investigate the extent of intercellular disruption in the microvasculature of the macula utricle from Meniere's patients. Our study suggest that human inner ear tissue could be used to compare and contrast findings in animal models to design better therapies for vestibular and auditory disorders.

ETHICS STATEMENT

The studies involving human participants were reviewed and approved by the University of California, Los Angeles Institutional Review Board. The patients/participants provided their written informed consent to participate in this study.

AUTHOR CONTRIBUTIONS

GI designed the project, wrote the first draft of the manuscript, interpreted the histopathology and clinical data, and worked on the final manuscript. AI designed the project, collected the specimens at surgery, selected the patients, and reviewed the final manuscript. DA performed all the immunofluorescent staining and processed the tissue for TEM. IL developed all methodologies, collected all images, performed the quantitative analysis, wrote the results, edited the final manuscript, and coordinated all work related to the manuscript.

ACKNOWLEDGMENTS

Thanks to Dr. Matthew Schibler from the Advanced Microscopy Laboratory and Spectroscopy (AMLS) of California Nanosystems Institute at UCLA (CNSI) for allowing the use of SP8 Leica laser confocal high-resolution microscope, and Mr. Ivo Atasanov for the use of the T12 (FEI) transmission electron microscope located at the Electron Imaging Center for NanoMachines (EICN)-CLMS-UCLA.

REFERENCES

Alves, A. P., Mesquita, O. N., Gomez-Gardenes, J., and Agero, U. (2018). Graph analysis of cell clusters forming vascular networks. *R. Soc. Open Sci.* 5:171592. doi: 10.1098/rsos.171592

Baloh, R. W. (2001). Prosper Meniere's and his disease. *Arch. Neurol.* 58, 1151–1156.

Barath, K., Schuknecht, B., Monge Naldi, A., Schrepfer, T., Bockisch, C. J., and Hegemann, S. C. A. (2014). Detection and grading of endolymphatic hydrops in Meniere's disease using MR imaging. *AJNR* 35, 1–6. doi: 10.3174/ajnr.A3856

Calzada, A., Lopez, I. A., Ishiyama, A., Beltran Parrazal, L., and Ishiyama, G. (2012). The expression of cochlin and extracellular matrix proteins in vestibular endorgans obtained from Meniere's disease patients. *Cell Tissue Res.* 350, 373–384. doi: 10.1007/s00441-01201481-x

Daiber, A., Steven, S., Weber, A., Shuvaev, V. V., Muzykantos, V. R., Laher, I., et al. (2017). Targeting vascular endothelial dysfunction. *Br. J. Pharmacol.* 174, 1591–1619. doi: 10.1111/bph.13517

Foster, C. A., and Breeze, R. E. (2013). The Meniere's attack: an ischemia/reperfusion disorder of inner ear sensory tissues. *Med. Hypotheses* 81, 1108–1115. doi: 10.1016/j.mehy.2013.10.015

Glueckert, R., Pritz, C. O., Roy, S., Dudas, J., and Schrott-Fischer, A. (2015). Nanoparticle mediated drug delivery of rolipram to tyrosine kinase B positive cells in the inner ear with targeting peptides and agonistic antibodies. *Front. Aging Neurosci.* 7:71. doi: 10.3389/fnagi.2015.00071

Hallpike, C. S., and Cairns, H. (1938). Observations on the pathology of Meniere's síndrome: section of otology. *Proc. R. Soc. Med.* 31, 1317–1336. doi: 10.1080/0001640801901774

Hirose, K., Li, S. Z., Hartsock, J. J., Johnson, S., Santi, P., and Salt, A. N. (2014). Systemic lipopolysaccharide compromises the blood-labyrinth barrier and increases entry of serum, fluorescein into the perilymph. *J. Assoc. Res. Otolaryngol.* 15, 707–719. doi: 10.1007/s10162-014-0476-476

Ishiyama, G., Ishiyama, A., Jacobson, K., and Baloh, R. W. (2001). Drop attacks in older patients secondary to an otologic cause. *Neurology* 57, 1103–1106. doi: 10.1212/WNL.57.6.1103

Ishiyama, G., Lopez, I. A., Beltran-Parrazal, L., and Ishiyama, A. (2010). Immunohistochemical localization and mRNA expression of aquaporins in the macula utricle of patients with Meniere's disease and acoustic neuroma. *Cell Tissue Res.* 340, 407–419. doi: 10.1007/s00441-010-0975-977

Ishiyama, G., Lopez, I. A., Ishiyama, P., and Ishiyama, A. (2017). The blood labyrinthine barrier in the human normal and Meniere's macula utricle. *Sci. Rep.* 7:253. doi: 10.1038/s41598-017-00330-335

Ishiyama, G., Lopez, I. A., Sepahdari, A. R., and Ishiyama, A. (2015). Meniere's disease: histopathology, cytochemistry, and imaging. *Ann. N. Y. Acad. Sci.* 1343, 49–57. doi: 10.1111/nyas.12699

Ishiyama, G., Wester, J., Lopez, I. A., Beltran-Parrazal, L., and Ishiyama, A. (2018). Oxidative stress in the blood labyrinthine barrier in the macula utricle of Meniere's disease patients. *Front. Physiol.* 9:1068. doi: 10.3389/fphys.2018.01068

Jiang, H., Wang, X., Zhang, J., Kachelmeier, A., Lopez, I. A., and Shi, X. (2019). Microvascular networks in the area of the auditory peripheral nervous system. *Hear. Res.* 371, 105–116. doi: 10.1016/j.heares.2018.11.02

LeFloc'h, J., Tan, W., Telang, R. S., Vlajkovic, S. M., Nuttall, A., Rooney, W. D., et al. (2014). Markers of cochlear inflammation using MRI. *J. Magn. Reson. Imaging.* 39, 150–161. doi: 10.1002/jmri.24144

Lopez, I., Ishiyama, G., Tang, Y., Frank, M., Baloh, R. W., and Ishiyama, A. (2005). Estimation of the number of nerve fibers in the human vestibular endorgans using unbiased stereology and immunohistochemistry. *J. Neurosci. Methods* 145, 37–46. doi: 10.1016/j.neumeth.2004.11.024

Lopez, I. A., Ishiyama, G., Hosokawa, S., Hosokawa, K., Acuna, D., Linthicum, F. H., et al. (2016). Immunohistochemical techniques for the human inner ear. *Histochem. Cell Biol.* 146, 367–387. doi: 10.1007/s00418-016-1471-1472

Mazzoni, A. (1990). The vascular anatomy of the vestibular labyrinth in man. *Acta Otolaryngol.* 472, 1–83. doi: 10.3109/00016489009121137

McCall, A., Ishiyama, G., López, I. A., Sunita, B., and Ishiyama, A. (2009). Histopathological and ultrastructural analysis of vestibular endorgans obtained from patients with Meniere's disease. *BMC Ear Nose Throat Disord.* 9:4. doi: 10.1186/1472-6815-94

Mei, X., Atturo, F., Wadin, K., Larsson, S., Agrawal, S., Ladak, H. M., et al. (2018). Human inner ear blood supply revisited: the uppsala collection of temporal bone- an international resource of education and collaboration. *Ups. J. Med. Sci.* 123, 131–142. doi: 10.1080/03009734.2018.1492654

Merchant, S. N., Adams, J. C., and Nadol, J. B. (2005). Pathophysiology of Meniere's syndrome: are symptoms caused by endolymphatic hydrops? *Otol. Neurotol.* 26, 74–81. doi: 10.1097/00129492-200501000-00013

Mudry, A., and Tange, R. A. (2009). The vascularization of the human cochlea: its historical background. *Acta Oto. Laryngol.* 129(Suppl. 561), 3–16. doi: 10.1080/00016480902924469

Nabeya, D. (1923). A study in the comparative anatomy of the blood-vascular system on the internal ear in mammalian and in homo (Japanese). *Acta Sch. Med. Univ. Imp. Kyoto* 6, 1–127.

Neng, L., Zhang, F., Kachelmeier, A., and Shi, X. (2013a). Endothelial cell, pericytes, and perivascular macrophage-type melanocyte interactions regulate cochlear intrastrial fluid-blood barrier permeability. *JARO* 14, 175–185. doi: 10.1007/s10162-012-0365-369

Neng, L., Zhang, W., Hassan, A., Zemla, M., Kachelmeier, A., Fridberger, A., et al. (2013b). Isolation and culture of endothelial cells, pericytes and perivascular resident macrophage-like melanocytes from the young mouse ear. *Nat. Protoc.* 8, 709–720. doi: 10.1038/nprot.2013.033

Nyberg, S., Abbott, N. J., Shi, X., Steyger, P. S., and Dabdoub, A. (2019). Delivery of therapeutics to the inner ear: the challenge of the blood-labyrinth barrier. *Sci. Transl. Med.* 11:eaao0935. doi: 10.1126/scitranslmed.aao0935

Pakdaman, M. N., Ishiyama, G., Ishiyama, A., Peng, K. A., Kim, H. J., Pope, W. B., et al. (2016). Blood-labyrinth barrier permeability in Meniere's disease and idiopathic sudden sensorineural hearing loss: findings on delayed contrast 3D-Flair MRI. *AJNR Am. J. Neuroradiol.* 37, 1903–1908. doi: 10.3174/ajnr.A48822

Rybak, L. P., Dhukhwa, A., Mukherjea, D., and Ramkumar, V. (2019). Local drug delivery for prevention of hearing loss. *Front. Cell. Neurosci.* 13:300. doi: 10.3389/fncel.2019.00300

Schuknecht, H. F. (1993). *Pathology of the Ear*, 2nd Edn. Philadelphia, PA: Lea and Febiger.

Semaan, M. T., Alagramam, K. N., and Megerian, C. A. (2005). The basic science of Meniere's disease and endolymphatic hydrops. *Curr. Opin. Otolaryngol. Head Neck Surg.* 13, 301–307. doi: 10.1097/01.moo.0000186335.44206.1c

Semaan, M. T., and Megerian, C. A. (2010). Contemporary perspectives on the pathophysiology of Meniere's disease: implications for treatment. *Curr. Opin. Otolaryngol. Head Neck Surg.* 18, 393–398. doi: 10.1097/MOO.)b)13e32833d3164

Sepahdari, A. R., Ishiyama, G., Vorasubin, N., Peng, K. A., Linetsky, M., and Ishiyama, A. (2015). Delayed intravenous contrast-enhanced 3D FLAIR MRI in Meniere's disease: correlation of quantitative measures of endolymphatic hydrops with hearing. *Clin. Imaging* 39, 26–33.

Sepahdari, A. R., Vorasubin, N., Ishiyama, G., and Ishiyama, A. (2016). Endolymphatic hydrops reversal following acetazolamide therapy: demonstrated with delayed intravenous contrast-enhanced 3D-FLAIR MRI. *Am. J. Neuroradiol.* 37, 151–154. doi: 10.3174/ajnr.A4462

Shi, X. (2011). Physiopathology of the cochlear microcirculation. *Hear. Res.* 282, 10–24. doi: 10.1016/j.heares.2011.08.006

Shi, X. (2016). Pathophysiology of the cochlear intrastrial fluid-blood barrier (review). *Hear. Res.* 338, 52–63. doi: 10.1016/j.hearres.2016.01.010

Shi, X., Han, W., Yamamoto, H., Tang, W., Lin, X., Xiu, R., et al. (2008). The cochlear pericytes. *Microcirculation* 15, 515–529. doi: 10.1080/10739680802047445

Tagaya, M., Yamazakim, M., Teranishi, M., Naganawa, S., Yoshida, T., Otake, H., et al. (2011). Endolymphatic hydrops and blood-labyrinthine barrier in Meniere's disease. *Acta Otolaryngol.* 131, 474–479. doi: 10.3109/00016489.2010.534114

Yamakawa, K. (1938). Uber die pathologisch veranderung bei einem Meniere's-kranken. *J. Otorhinolaryngol. Soc. Japn.* 4, 2310–2312.

Yamazaki, M., Naganawa, M., Tagaya, M., Kawai, H., Ikeda, M., Sone, M., et al. (2012). Comparison of contrast effect on the cochlear perilymph after intratympanic and intravenous gadolinium injection. *AJNR* 33, 773–778. doi: 10.3174/ajnr.A2821

Zhang, F., Zhang, J., Neng, L., and Shi, X. (2013). Characterization and inflammatory response of perivascular macrophage-resident macrophage-like melanocytes in the vestibular system. *JARO* 14, 635–643.

Zudaire, E., Gambardella, L., Kurcz, C., and Vermen, S. (2011). A computational tool for quantitative analysis of vascular networks. *PLoS One* 6:e27385. doi: 10.1371/journal.pone.0027385

3

Forgotten Fibrocytes: A Neglected, Supporting Cell Type of the Cochlea with the Potential to be an Alternative Therapeutic Target in Hearing Loss

*David N. Furness**

School of Life Sciences, Keele University, Keele, United Kingdom

Correspondence:
David N. Furness
d.n.furness@keele.ac.uk

Cochlear fibrocytes are a homeostatic supporting cell type embedded in the vascularized extracellular matrix of the spiral ligament, within the lateral wall. Here, they participate in the connective tissue syncytium that enables potassium recirculation into the *scala media* to take place and ensures development of the endolymphatic potential that helps drive current into hair cells during acoustic stimulation. They have also been implicated in inflammatory responses in the cochlea. Some fibrocytes interact closely with the capillaries of the vasculature in a way which suggests potential involvement, together with the *stria vascularis*, also in the blood-labyrinth barrier. Several lines of evidence suggests that pathology of the fibrocytes, along with other degenerative changes in this region, contribute to metabolic hearing loss (MHL) during aging that is becoming recognized as distinct from, and potentially a precursor for, sensorineural hearing loss (SNHL). This pathology may underlie a significant proportion of cases of presbycusis. Some evidence points also to an association between fibrocyte degeneration and Ménière's disease (MD). Fibrocytes are mesenchymal; this characteristic, and their location, make them amenable to potential cell therapy in the form of cell replacement or genetic modification to arrest the process of degeneration that leads to MHL. This review explores the properties and roles of this neglected cell type and suggests potential therapeutic approaches, such as cell transplantation or genetic engineering of fibrocytes, which could be used to prevent this form of presbycusis or provide a therapeutic avenue for MD.

Keywords: cochlear fibrocyte, cochlear lateral wall, metabolic hearing loss, Ménière's disease, cell replacement therapy

INTRODUCTION

The major tissues of the cochlea are notable for their discrete functional roles and the diversity of cell types that each possesses. At the same time, these tissues display a complex interdependence in which their disruption, either singly or in different combinations, leads to hearing impairment. There are three main tissues: the sensory epithelium (organ of Corti), located on the basilar membrane, that detects and transduces sound energy into an electrical response; the neural component, i.e., auditory nerve fibers and spiral ganglion, that conveys the responses of the organ of Corti along the auditory pathway; and the lateral wall, a homeostatic tissue that maintains electrochemical conditions within the cochlea favorable to the optimal function, and potentially survival of the sensory organ and the neural elements. In addition to these, there are also other tissue components whose functions are probably less directly involved in hearing, such as the endolymphatic sac and various periosteal linings (see for example Standring, 2015).

The diversity of functions and cell types present in these tissues means that there is a range of ways that degeneration affecting different targets contributes to hearing loss. The purpose of this review is to raise the profile of one cell type whose importance has been underestimated and contribution often neglected: the fibrocytes of the spiral ligament. A simple search of PubMed using the search terms "cochlear hair cell" and "cochlear fibrocyte" makes this neglect clear as the former (at the time of writing) obtained 11,557 hits whilst the latter obtained 262, a ratio of 44:1. On the basis of scientific endeavor, then, this might imply that fibrocytes contribute very little to cochlear function. On the basis of human pathological studies (Schuknecht and Gacek, 1993), however, the reality is that in fact, a significant proportion of hearing loss cases are likely to have either directly or indirectly a major contribution from lateral wall, and likely fibrocyte, dysfunction.

THE DIFFERENT TYPES OF HEARING LOSS

Five-hundred million people worldwide have some form of hearing loss. Hearing loss is often subdivided into sensorineural (SNHL) and conductive (CHL; Sheffield and Smith, 2018). Around 90% is generally attributed to inner ear damage of some type, due primarily to aging, ototoxic drugs (chemotherapy/aminoglycoside antibiotics) and loud noises (e.g., soldiers, miners) and using the definition above, this would thus be considered SNHL where the sensory hair cells in the organ of Corti and/or spiral ganglion nerve (SGN) cells that form the auditory nerve are affected. SNHL also includes the recently described "hidden hearing loss" resulting from synaptopathy at the level of auditory nerve input (Viana et al., 2015). The problem with this definition, however, is that hearing loss can also result from cellular degeneration in the cochlea in the other tissues noted above, sometimes separately, sometimes together. Thus, some definitions include metabolic hearing loss (MHL), where lateral wall structures (spiral ligament and *stria vascularis*) are affected as distinct from SNHL (Schuknecht and Gacek, 1993; Dubno et al., 2013). Currently, no cure exists either for MHL or SNHL, though hearing loss, in general, is managed by prosthetics (hearing aids and cochlear implants).

The relative proportion of MHL and SNHL in age-related hearing loss patients, and with what frequency both may be present at some point in the patient's disease progression, is uncertain. Because SNHL is often quoted as the major cause of hearing loss, hair cell repair or regeneration is the commonest target of most research in cochlear therapies. However, the pathological studies of human temporal bones by Schuknecht and Gacek (1993) suggest that the greater proportion of such acquired hearing loss could be MHL on the basis of a pattern of lateral wall atrophy. Whilst this is likely to be contentious, if correct, this would change our general perception of hearing loss. As it stands, however, there is insufficient evidence to be certain, so this needs to be confirmed.

The lack of data on the relative proportion of MHL compared with SNHL is presumably because there are no good diagnostic techniques to distinguish clearly between these disorders. Such techniques are being developed on the basis of animal models (Dubno et al., 2013; Vaden et al., 2017, 2018) and are likely to be in place in the relatively near future. More refined diagnostic techniques would enable the clinician to determine, with greater accuracy than presently possible, the form of the hearing loss and therefore identify patients who would be amenable to appropriately targeted treatment.

THE STRUCTURE AND FLUID COMPOSITION OF THE COCHLEAR DUCT

To understand the concept of lateral wall-based MHL, it is necessary to review briefly the structure of the cochlea and cochlear homeostasis, with an emphasis on the region of the spiral ligament. The spiral cochlea contains the sensory organ of Corti located in the cochlear duct which is the middle chamber of three fluid-filled chambers (**Figure 1**) that run longitudinally along the cochlea. These are the *scala vestibuli* and *scala tympani*, which are in continuity at the cochlear apex and are filled with perilymph, a solution high in sodium ions and containing a number of other ions and substances, and the *scala media* that contains endolymph which is high in potassium ions. The *scala media* is separated from the other two compartments by a lining of epithelial cells of various types, all of which are connected by tight junctions that prevent paracellular translocation of ions and other substances, thus forming a complete electrochemical barrier between the inside of the *scala media* and the surrounding tissues and extracellular spaces.

The tight junction barrier on the inside of the *scala media* lining ensures that the composition of cochlear fluids is under the control of the cells lining the epithelium, in the sense that the only access between the inside of the duct and the outside is through the plasma membranes of the cells facing the inside. Hence the transfer of ions or substances of any kind is limited to apical membrane channels or transporters on these cells. Maintenance of the correct fluid composition in the different compartments is thus dependent on each cell type contributing to the re-distribution of ions in an appropriate manner. This is vital for normal auditory function, specifically in providing support for the function of the sensory hair cells (see review by Wangemann, 2006).

The tight junctions in the organ of Corti occur between the adjoining apical surfaces of hair cells and supporting cells, which form a region called the reticular lamina. Each hair cell is characterized by a sensory hair bundle that projects into the endolymph in the *scala media*, whilst the cell bodies below the reticular lamina are bathed in perilymph. During the sensory functioning of the hair cells, the only route for transfer of ions across this surface is through channels located in the hair bundles; stimulation by sound causes these mechanotransducer channels to open resulting in entry predominantly of K^+, but also Ca^{2+}, which depolarizes the

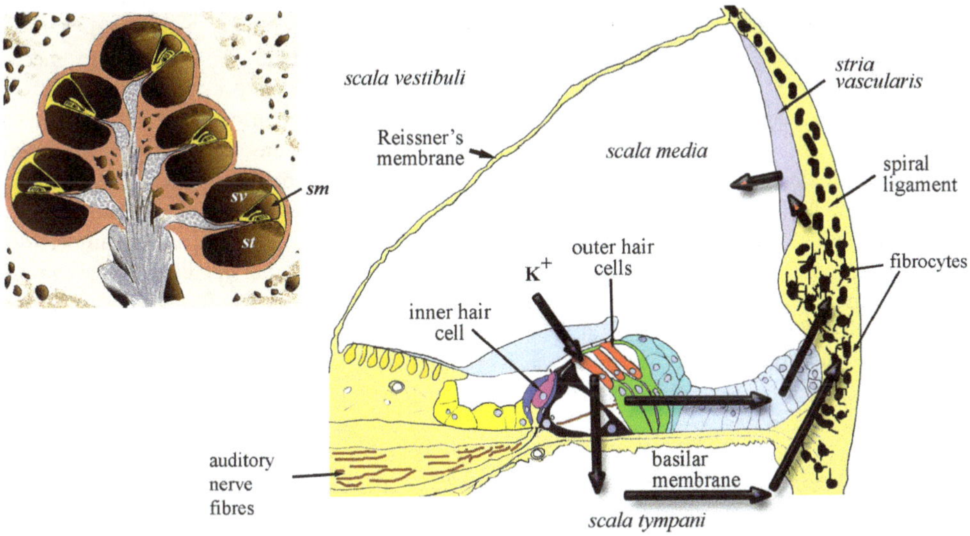

FIGURE 1 | Diagrammatic representation of the cochlea in section (inset) showing the chambers of the spiral and the location of *scala media* (sm) *scala vestibuli* (sv) and *scala tympani* (st). The main panel shows a cross-section of the sm and the arrows indicate the two probable routes of recycling potassium through the organ of Corti, perilymph and lateral wall, including the fibrocytes.

hair cells, resulting in the release of the neurotransmitter glutamate at synapses between auditory nerve fibers and the basal pole of the hair cells. This, in turn, leads to stimulation of spiral ganglion neurons (SGNs) which then signal the hair-cell response to the brain. Potassium ions exit the hair cells into perilymph *via* basolateral potassium channels (see review by Wangemann, 2006). To our knowledge, the supporting cell apical surfaces do not express ion channels or transporters, but the cells are connected sub-apically by gap junctions which help to form an epithelial gap junction network as described below.

In essence, continued active redistribution of the K^+ ions results in a powerful battery, the endocochlear (or endolymphatic) potential (EP) that drives current into the hair cells whilst their transduction channels are open. Exhaustion of K^+ ions would reduce the magnitude of transduction; thus loss of EP results in loss of auditory nerve function (Lang et al., 2010). In addition, excessive K^+ in hair cells appears to result in hair-cell death (Nouvian et al., 2003). This toxicity can be avoided only because potassium is continuously pumped out of the perilymph. Failure to maintain the correct balance of fluids within these compartments might also lead to volumetric changes that result in endolymphatic hydrops, a likely origin of Ménière's disease (MD). The lateral wall tissue is of prime importance in this process by contributing to two major routes for recycling the K^+ ions released into perilymph from the hair cells (**Figure 1**). These routes involve transcellular relocation of the K^+ ions through the ligament. The source of the ions is either directly from perilymph or *via* the gap-junction connected supporting cells of the organ of Corti. The breakdown of these homeostatic mechanisms can result in failure to recycle this crucial ion between the different fluid-filled compartments of the cochlea.

LATERAL WALL STRUCTURE AND FUNCTION

The two major components of the lateral wall: the *stria vascularis* and the spiral ligament, function together to maintain the EP during K^+ recycling. As shown in **Figure 1**, the recycling occurs *via* the two main routes from the perilymph around the hair cell bases. The first of these is a transcellular route (the epithelial gap-junction network) *via* the cells of the outer sulcus which are connected to each other by gap junctions composed of connexins such as Cx26, Cx30 and Cx31 (Xia et al., 1998; Forge et al., 1999; Mei et al., 2017). This is the epithelial gap junction network and the cells involved form an epithelial syncytium where their cytoplasmic compartments are in direct contact. Its importance is exemplified by the fact that genetic mutations in these genes are significant contributors to genetic hearing loss, for example, GJB2 (Cx26), GJB6 (Cx30) and GJB3 (Cx31; see for example Forge et al., 2003). Gap junctional proteins have also been confirmed directly in histological studies to occur in the human spiral ligament (Liu et al., 2017).

The second route for potassium transfer is through perilymph. This also ends up at the lateral wall where potassium ions enter the lateral wall gap-junction system (the connective tissue gap junction network or syncitium).

The *stria vascularis* is a heavily vascularized three-cell layered tissue composed of marginal cells facing the *scala media*, intermediate cells and basal cells. This tissue lines the inner curved surface of the spiral ligament between a spiral ridge of tissue (the spiral prominence) and the junction of the ligament with the upper boundary of the cochlear duct, Reissner's membrane. The ligament itself is longer, extending above and below the *stria vascularis*; at its lower end is the anchor point of the basilar membrane, whilst extending above Reissner's membrane it lines the bony external wall to the upper boundary of the spiral chamber (**Figure 2**). The ligament varies in width in different cochlear turns, becoming wider towards the basal end of the cochlea. Cell types and densities thus vary along the cochlear duct, but quantitative information about these changes is, thus far, limited.

The cell types of the ligament include perivascular endothelial cells around capillaries, root cells (a large, branched cell type projecting from near the basilar membrane anchorage and midway into the ligament) and fibrocytes. There are five main types of fibrocyte in mice, with differential morphology, protein expression and location (**Figure 2**; Furness et al., 2009; Mahendrasingam et al., 2011a,b) although in other studies, for example in gerbil, these have been divided into several further subtypes (Spicer and Schulte, 1996).

From electron microscopic studies, the fibrocytes are distinguished by fine structural characteristics such as the density of cytoplasm, content of cell organelles and the extent to which the plasma membrane is folded (**Figure 2**). Thus, the least complex of the cells structurally is the type I fibrocyte which has an elongated shape, relatively light cytoplasm and few organelles, and a minimal number of plasma membrane folds. Type II and type V are structurally very similar to each other, have relatively dense cytoplasm and multiple membrane folds. Type III tend to have elaborately branched surfaces, and very dense cytoplasm, with narrow cell bodies. Type IV cells are similar to but generally larger than type III with intermediate amounts of surface elaborations between type III and type II or type V.

The role of these various fibrocyte types is uncertain, but they show other differences in characteristics in terms of protein expression (**Table 1**). As with the epithelial syncitium, the gap junction network of the ligament comprises several connexins (Cx26, Cx30, Cx31 and Cx43). It is known that type I fibrocytes are connected by gap junctions to the basal cells of the *stria vascularis* (Forge et al., 2003), and that type II and type V cells possess high levels of the Na, K, ATPase transporter, whilst type I cells have less and type III and type IV cells have little (Mahendrasingam et al., 2011a). To some extent, these distributions have been confirmed in human tissues as well (Liu et al., 2017), although type I cells were not found to express the NaKATPase. This perhaps reflects age or sampling issues of human tissues. Type II cells appear to be connected to type I cells in the gap junction network. Other proteins expressed in fibrocytes include the potassium channel Kir5.1 (Hibino et al., 2004), BK channels (Liang et al., 2003; Shen et al., 2004), L-type $Ca2^{+}$ channel (Liang et al., 2004) and Na-K-Cl co-transporter 1 (NKCC1; Crouch et al., 1997) which are likely to be involved in the recycling of K^{+}. Type III cells (alternatively called tension fibroblasts) contain prominent cables of actin filaments and may modulate tension between the basilar membrane and the bony wall of the cochlea (Henson and Henson, 1988), but they also, uniquely amongst fibrocytes of the cochlea, express aquaporin 1, implicating them in water homeostasis (Mahendrasingam et al., 2011a).

Root cells have extensive broad processes penetrating into the lower part of the ligament. They also have gap junctions communicating with the surrounding cells and are supported by a tubulin/microtubular cytoskeleton, presumably to maintain the extensive branches (Jagger et al., 2010).

The homeostatic K^{+} recycling mechanism involving fibrocytes is generally presumed necessary to ensure maximum sensitivity of the sensory hair cells (Wangemann, 2006) and also to maintain the conditions which ensure the continued survival of other cochlear tissues. The K^{+} then travels to the *stria vascularis* basal cells lying adjacent to the spiral ligament. *Stria vascularis* function is perhaps better understood than that of the ligament. The molecular players involved in the redistribution of ions suggest a kidney like function, with concentration gradients that drive the relocation of potassium. This is thought to be initiated by transport into the basal cells *via* the gap junction connections with type I fibrocytes (**Figure 3**). The *stria vascularis* is also compartmentalized from the ligament by tight junctions composed of claudin 11 in both humans and rodents (Kitajiri et al., 2004; Liu et al., 2017), ensuring that cellular ion transport mechanisms are the route for K^{+}.

PHYSIOLOGICAL PROPERTIES OF FIBROCYTES

Electrophysiological studies of fibrocytes have been fairly limited, but there is evidence that they have unusual properties that may be associated with a potassium recycling role. Typically eukaryotic cells have a negative resting membrane potential, but fibrocytes have been reported to possess positive potentials *in vivo* of up to +12 mV (Yoshida et al., 2016). It has been suggested that this contributes to the establishment of appropriate ionic gradients inside the lateral wall that enable the development of the EP through the *stria vascularis*. Studies of the potentials within the ligament suggest it is slightly positive compared with perilymph. Blockers of Na, K, ATPase decrease K^{+} concentration within the fibrocytic zone and reduce EP (Adachi et al., 2013) providing evidence for the role of fibrocytes in maintaining EP.

Our study of glutamate transport properties of fibrocytes in slices from rat pups (Furness et al., 2009) established that the cells had a glutamate transporter-associated current that corresponded with the amount of GLAST in them—i.e., type II fibrocytes which express GLAST more than other fibrocytes had greater glutamate transport capability than type I fibrocytes which express less GLAST. Since GLAST is a co-transporter of Na^{+} and K^{+}, it may also contribute to the recirculation of K^{+}. However, during glutamate uptake, K^{+} is transported out of the cytoplasm—thus GLAST would in principle be operating in an opposing direction to the Na, K, ATPase with respect to K^{+}.

Other physiological properties that have been directly measured have been noted in *in vitro* studies of fibrocyte cultures. These suggest that fibrocytes also possess chloride channels (Qu et al., 2006).

A ROLE FOR FIBROCYTES IN INFLAMMATORY RESPONSES

Cochlear inflammation is often triggered by middle ear infection or damage caused by environmental insults such as acoustic

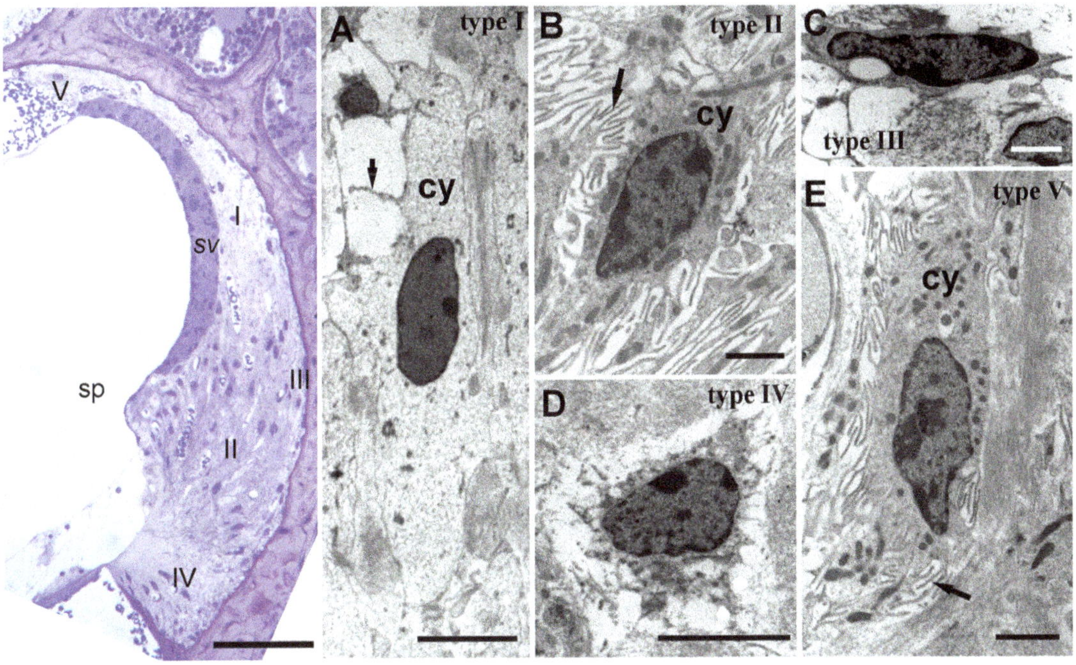

FIGURE 2 | Lateral wall structure in a CD/1 mouse. The left panel shows a light microscopy section of *stria vascularis* (sv) spiral prominence (sp) and the spiral ligament containing five types of fibrocyte (I—V). Scale bar = 50 μm. Panels **(A–E)** show fibrocyte types I to V by transmission electron microscopy. They have varying numbers of small processes (arrows) and differences in the density of cytoplasm (cy) and organelle content. Scale bars: **(A,C)** = 5 μm; **(B,D,E)** = 2 μm (adapted with permission from Mahendrasingam et al., 2011a).

TABLE 1 | Characteristic proteins of fibrocytes.

Protein	Function	Strongly expressing	References
Caldesmon	Calcium modulation	Type III	Mahendrasingam et al. (2011a)
S-100	Calcium modulation	Type I, II and V	Suko et al. (2000) and Mahendrasingam et al. (2011a)
Na, K-ATPase	Sodium/potassium transport	Type II and V	Suko et al. (2000) and Mahendrasingam et al. (2011a)
Ca, ATPase	Calcium transport	Type I	Ichimiya et al. (1994)
Na, K, Cl-cotransporter	Sodium/potassium/chloride transport	Type II, IV and V	Qu et al. (2006)
NCBE	Bicarbonate transporter		Huebner et al. (2019)
GLAST	Glutamate transport		Jin et al. (2003) and Furness et al. (2009)
Kir5.1	Potassium channel	Type II, IV, and V	Hibino et al. (2004)
Ether-a-gogo	Potassium channel		Nie et al. (2005)
Kv3.1	Potassium channel		So et al. (2001)
BK channels	Potassium channel		Liang et al. (2003)
ClC	Chloride channels		Qu et al. (2006)
Connexin 26, 30, 31, 43	Gap junction channel		Forge et al. (2003)
AQP1	Water channel	Type III	Miyabe et al. (2002) and Mahendrasingam et al. (2011a)
Carbonic anhydrase	Carbon dioxide-water converter	Type I, III, IV and V	Spicer and Schulte (1991)
Creatine kinase	ADP-ATP cycling	Type I, III, IV and V.	Spicer and Schulte (1991)
Connective tissue growth factor (CTGF)	Collagen metabolism	Type IV	Adams (2009)

Table illustrating some of the proteins known to be of functional relevance in fibrocytes and often used to characterize the different types.

trauma or ototoxic drugs. Fibrocytes are thought to play a role in inflammatory responses in the cochlea and to offer a potential for protection from inflammation that could lead on to SNHL. In experimental models of inflammatory triggers, immunostaining for Na, K, ATPase and Cx26 have been shown to be decreased in labyrinthitis while in otitis media Cx26 is reduced (Ichimiya et al., 2000). The same authors showed that cultured spiral ligament fibrocytes release chemokines after stimulation by proinflammatory cytokines, TNF-α or IL-1β. IL-10 mediated protection from ototoxic drugs has also been observed (So et al., 2001), suggested to be associated with an anti-inflammatory response in fibrocytes (Woo et al., 2015). Hence it is likely that as part of their homeostatic role, the fibrocytes have anti-inflammatory capabilities that have the potential to protect the cochlea from inflammation leading to deafness.

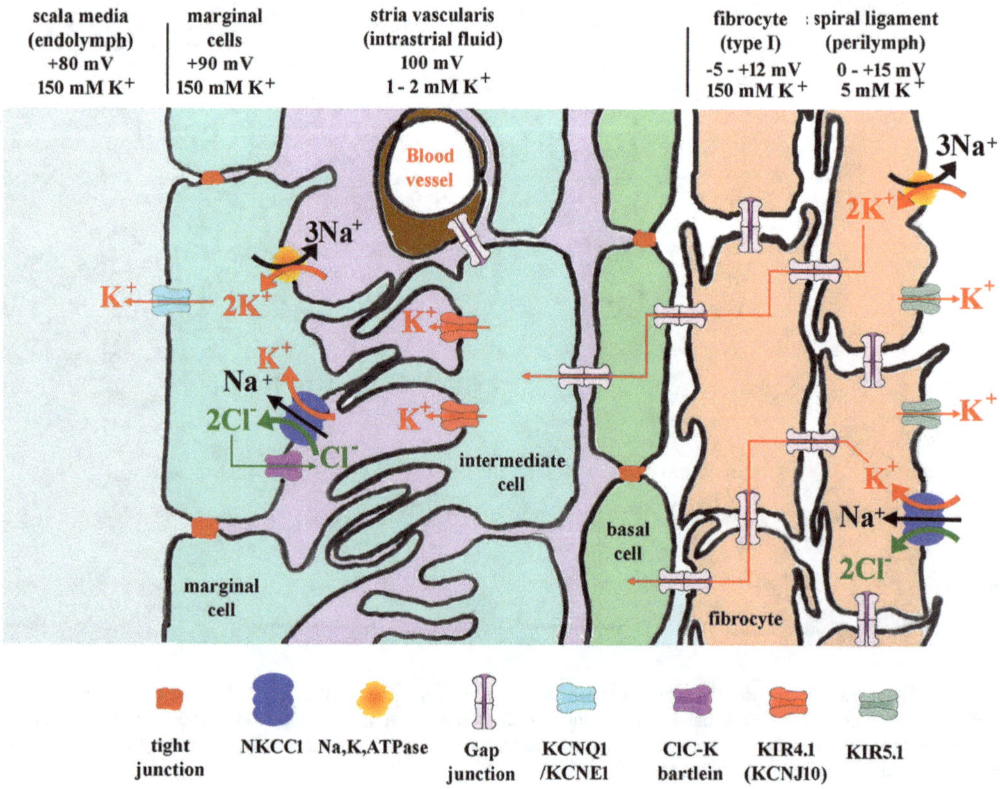

FIGURE 3 | Diagram showing potassium and other ion circulation and the formation of the EP within the lateral wall. In the stria vascularis and the spiral ligament, K^+ concentration gradients ($[K^+]$) and potentials vary at different points in the tissue as shown. Gap junctions connect the spiral ligament fibrocytes together and also connect them to basal cells and then intermediate cells of the stria vascularis. K^+ entering from outer sulcus cells of the organ of Corti or directly from perilymph *via* Na, K, ATPase or NKCC1 then flows through the syncytium of the ligament into the stria vascularis where it is transported to marginal cells and secreted into endolymph. For protein identity, see key below diagram. Modified figure based on Hibino and Kurachi (2006) with additional data from Adachi et al. (2013).

LATERAL WALL AND THE BLOOD-LABYRINTH BARRIER

As well as K^+ recycling, the lateral wall is a major contributor to the blood supply of the cochlea. In this context, the functional relationship of lateral wall fibrocytes to the blood-labyrinth barrier is of potentially great interest, but as yet is unclear. It is likely that the *stria vascularis* is the main site of the blood-labyrinth barrier, as indicated by its heavy vascularization. It is perhaps less well known that the spiral ligament is well vascularized (Carraro et al., 2016). Indeed, ultrastructural studies suggest a close association between some fibrocyte types and the blood vessels of the ligament (Spicer and Schulte, 1996) including endfeet-like processes (Dai and Shi, 2011), where material transport between blood and labyrinth tissue is likely to be tightly controlled. Furthermore, tracer studies showed that spiral ligament vessels have lower permeability than those of *stria vascularis*, with tight junctional barriers between the endothelial cells of the blood vessels (Sakagami et al., 1982). How this influences the homeostatic activities and barrier properties of the lateral wall remains to be established.

More indirectly, a role for fibrocytes in vascular control of the cochlear blood supply has been suggested. The study by Dai and Shi (2011) found elevation of Ca^{2+} in fibrocytes generates a Ca^{2+} signal to nearby vascular cells causing vasodilation of capillaries. This coupling was also found to mediate sound-stimulated cochlear blood flow increases.

LATERAL WALL PATHOLOGY IN HEARING LOSS

Evidence from both animal and human deafness studies suggests that degeneration of the lateral wall fibrocytes is associated with hearing loss and a contributor probably to MHL. Time course studies suggest that fibrocyte degeneration can precede hair cell loss (Hequembourg and Liberman, 2001; Mahendrasingam et al., 2011b), so it is possible to surmise that it could also lead to SNHL by giving rise to a change in the composition of cochlear fluids that negatively affect hair cells and neural elements. One human deafness gene (DFN3) has been identified that has degeneration of fibrocytes as its major pathology, accompanied by severe reduction of the EP in an animal model (Minowa et al., 1999), and fibrocyte degeneration has been reported in mice showing age-related hearing loss (Hequembourg and Liberman, 2001). We found early fibrocyte pathology, including damaged and degenerating cells, in CD/1 mice that show accelerated age-related hearing loss (Mahendrasingam et al., 2011b). The degeneration was primarily, in its initial stages, in the form of mitochondrial damage, as is found in other types of age-related degeneration (see review by Zhu et al., 2019). These findings led us to hypothesize that fibrocyte degeneration is a significant cause of MHL leading to SNHL.

In their study of human temporal bones of a range of ages, Kusunoki et al. (2004) found significant early loss of types II and IV fibrocytes followed by types I and III, respectively. From the ultrastructural studies noted above Spicer and Schulte (1996), loss of type II cells and their association with blood vessels might well compromise the blood-labyrinth barrier in the type II location. This could lead to disturbances of cochlear fluid composition, increased vulnerability to toxins, and deleterious changes leading to further pathological alterations, potentially loss of EP and hearing loss.

It should be noted, however, that it is not always clear that loss of EP produces hearing loss. Although measurements of EP in some cases of threshold elevation show EP losses (Mei et al., 2017) others do not (Lukashkina et al., 2017). This lack of consistency in data from the literature makes it harder to make the case for MHL through *stria* or ligament dysfunction. Nevertheless, the temporal bone studies showing that lateral wall pathology is seen with deafness in older people remains a good indicator that there is a link.

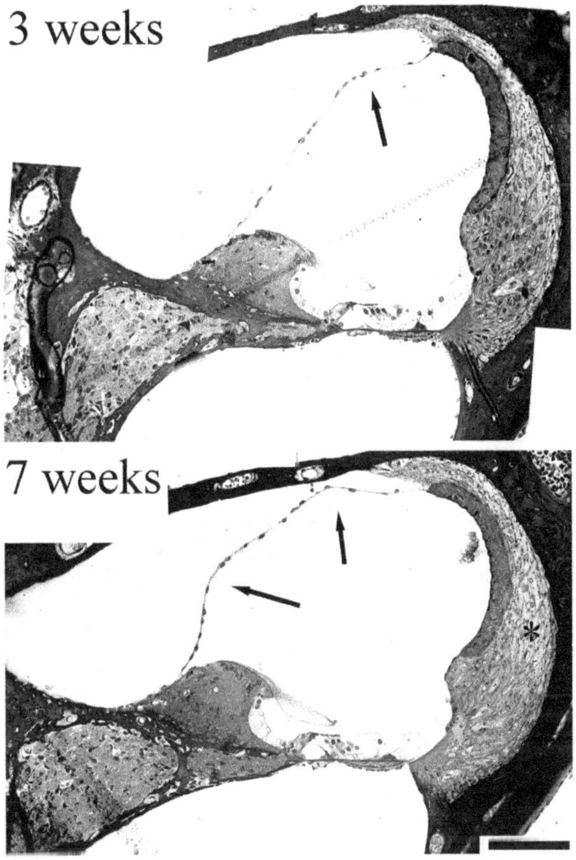

FIGURE 4 | Sections from a 3 week and 7 week CD/1 mouse cochlea showing accelerated age-related hearing loss. Fibrocyte degeneration in these mice has been reported (Mahendrasingam et al., 2011b) and can be seen as loss of cell nuclei/thinning of the tissue (*). The evidence for progressive hydrops is indicated by the arrows, where Reissner's membrane is distorted at 3 weeks, but this distortion becomes more exaggerated at 7 weeks, implying an increase in volume. Scale bar = 50 μm (adapted with permission from Mahendrasingam et al., 2011b).

LATERAL WALL AND MÉNIÈRE's DISEASE

As well as hearing loss, lateral wall pathology has been implicated in MD. Whilst some of the symptoms of MD can be attributed to a loss of the sensory hair cells in the inner ear, other pathological changes have also been noted in endolymphatic hydrops, a feature of MD. In a study of experimental (surgically induced) endolymphatic hydrops in guinea pig, Nadol et al. (1995) evaluated pathological changes throughout the cochlea over a period of time up to 6 months. They found that type I fibrocytes showed early changes with downregulation of expression of a variety of proteins tested (e.g., S-100, Ca, ATPases and other enzymes) and later type I and type II fibrocytes showed reduction in Na, K, ATPases and connexin 26, along with structural degeneration. This led Merchant et al. (2005) to evaluate the relationship between endolymphatic hydrops and MD in a human temporal bone archive. They found hydrops in all MD cases, although not always MD in hydrops cases, and concluded that spiral ligament pathology was clearly involved with both hydrops and MD.

An evaluation of the CD/1 mice in our studies (Mahendrasingam et al., 2011b) also hinted at a link between MD and fibrocyte pathology. Although we did not report the pathology at the time, it is evident that sections of the cochlea show a distended cochlear duct, with Reissner's membrane being deformed (**Figure 4**) to an increasing extent with age, a possible indicator of MD. Although this distortion was not always present in older CD/1 mice, it might suggest that fibrocyte degeneration contributes to fluid changes in the cochlea.

Aquaporin 4 and 6 (proteins involved in water homeostasis) expression also seem to be affected in MD (Ishiyama et al., 2015) although aquaporin 1 (expressed by type III fibrocytes) was not reported to be affected. Nevertheless, degeneration of type III fibrocytes seems likely to occur along with the other fibrocytes, as we have seen in our studies of CD/1 mouse lateral wall degeneration, and this would cause loss of aquaporin 1 and potentially osmotic changes. The role of aquaporin 1, therefore, needs further investigation. The distribution of the glutamate transporter GLAST, presumed to be involved in glutamate recycling, is altered in the lateral wall in Ménière's patients (Ahmed et al., 2013). Build-up of glutamate in perilymph could potentially lead to excitotoxicity in the cochlea, affecting the SGNs nerve terminals with the hair cells; indeed glutamate based excitotoxicty of SGN terminals on hair cells has been demonstrated in a number of studies (see review by Pujol and Puel, 1999). Finally, Ishiyama et al. (2007) found a significant reduction against age-matched controls in both *stria* and spiral ligament volume in five temporal bones from humans suffering from MD.

Thus, although a direct, causal link between any specific pathology and MD has yet to be established, there is good evidence that fibrocyte degeneration is highly likely to be a contributory factor.

FIBROCYTES AS A POTENTIAL TARGET FOR THERAPY IN HEARING LOSS AND MD

The lateral wall of the cochlea is relatively superficial as a structure, compared with hair cells or SGN. Substances could potentially be introduced into this area through the round window or an opening in the cochlear bony wall. Its superficial location also means it is more accessible than deeper structures for surgical intervention. The tough ligament itself is likely to be better able to withstand surgical procedures or physical manipulation than other more delicate tissues in the cochlea, although with the proviso that disruption of the blood-labyrinth barrier in the ligament, or of the tight junction network on the inner surface of the *scala media*, might prove damaging. It has proved possible to make a small opening in the bony wall of the guinea pig cochlea through which electrodes can be introduced into the ligament and *stria vascularis* (Yoshida et al., 2016). The question then is what might be introduced into the ligament that could assist in the repair and restoration of homeostasis, or prevention of hearing loss?

Intervention in spiral ligament degeneration could take several forms: (i) stimulation of the fibrocytes' natural proliferative capacity to increase repair potential; (ii) alteration of the physiology of the cells to enhance their homeostatic activities, e.g., through transfection with genes to overexpress functional proteins, or even to express new proteins that might support other cells in the cochlea (e.g., growth factors); and (iii) direct replacement of fibrocytes through cellular transplantation. These options require a better knowledge of the functions of fibrocytes and ways to manipulate them, as well as a source of fibrocytes *in vitro*. The latter provides not only an experimental platform in which to study them (see for example Qu et al., 2006) but also a possible source of cells for transplantation therapy.

Accordingly, stem cells that have the potential to form fibrocytes, or direct culture of cochlear fibrocytes are possible ways forward in achieving the options suggested above. The developmental germ layer of origin of fibrocytes is mesoderm, and as cochlear fibrocytes form part of a connective tissue, they are thus considered to be mesenchymal cells. Such cells commonly retain a proliferative capacity throughout life and can thus be stimulated to grow; a related cell type, circulating fibrocytes in blood, are involved in wound healing and scar formation, producing myofibroblasts in fibrotic lesions (Quan et al., 2006). However, although a small degree of proliferation has been detected within the lateral wall in adult cochlea (Li et al., 2017), this proliferative capacity seems to be insufficient to maintain fibrocyte populations or reverse the degenerative processes. One positive outcome though of this proliferative capacity is that once removed from the lateral wall it has proved possible to grow fibrocytes *in vitro* (Gratton et al., 1996; Suko et al., 2000; **Figure 5**). Alternatively, they could be derived from mesenchymal stem cells (MSCs) that are repurposed into fibrocytes (Kamiya et al., 2007).

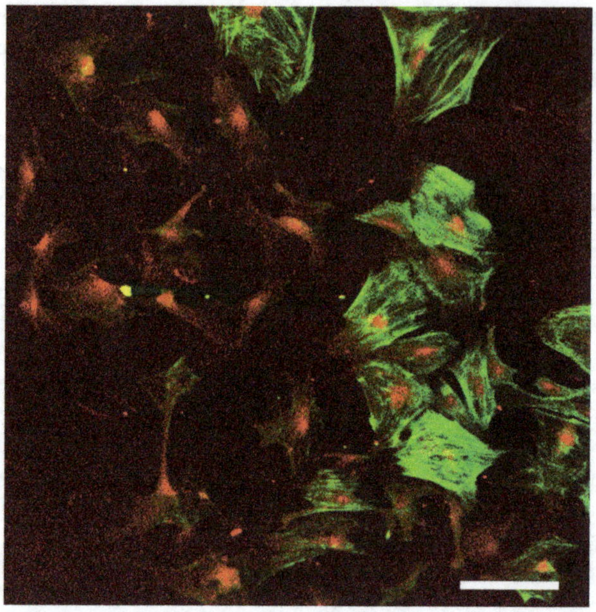

FIGURE 5 | Monolayer fibrocyte culture after immunofluorescence labeling for caldesmon (green) and Na, K, ATPase (red). The cells exhibit a mixed phenotype with some cells labeled strongly for both, and others labeled primarily for the Na, K, ATPase. Scale bar = 100 μm.

Fibrocyte monolayer cultures are obtained by extracting pieces of spiral ligament and placing them in culture wells with a coverslip over the top (**Figure 5**). After a few days, the cells appear in the well around the ligament pieces (Gratton et al., 1996) and these can then be passaged into sub-cultures. Characterization of these cultures at first suggested that they contained type I fibrocytes as they were negative for Na, K, ATPase but positive for other markers suggested being characteristic of type I cells (Gratton et al., 1996; Suko et al., 2000). However, such classification is difficult to verify as it relies on visual confirmation and is not quantitative. For example, semi-quantitative analysis has shown that type I fibrocytes do express moderate levels of Na, K, ATase relative to type III and type IV fibrocytes which express none, whilst type II and type V express the most (Mahendrasingam et al., 2011b). Other substrates are also possible, and 3D culturing of fibrocytes is another way forward. Preliminary work in our lab (Furness, 2014) has shown that fibrocytes can be grown on a variety of substrates and 3D culturing of type III fibrocytes from guinea pig in hydrogels has been successful (Kelly et al., 2012). This paves the way for novel strategies to grow fibrocytes and use of an appropriate matrix that could direct the phenotypes of the cultured cells, even to potentially "bioprinting" a replacement ligament *in vitro*.

The use of MSCs as an alternative to cultured fibrocytes also has some evidence to support it. It has been shown in one mouse model where the cochlear lateral wall was damaged by a mitochondrial toxin, that transplantation of MSCs by injection into the semi-circular canal located near to the cochlea produced some recovery of hearing function after loss (Kamiya et al., 2007). In this study, the MSCs were postulated to become fibrocytes once they had been integrated into the lateral wall and other regions containing fibrocytes (e.g., the spiral limbus running along the organ of Corti—**Figure 1**). Although there was no ultrastructural evidence that these transplanted MSCs had become fibrocytes, nevertheless they were in the correct locations and expressed connexin 26 and 30 as found in native fibrocytes. Whilst the mitochondrial toxin approach used in their study is not a natural degenerative process, nevertheless a hallmark of the degeneration we have observed is mitochondrial damage (Mahendrasingam et al., 2011b), hence giving confidence to the notion that a cell-replacement therapy for fibrocytes is a practical way forward.

Genetic engineering of fibrocytes is a relatively novel concept and there are a lot of unknowns as it is a strategy that has not been explored to any great extent. Cultures of fibrocytes can be used to test transfection strategies and develop either genetically engineered fibrocytes for transplantation or transfection methods that could be applied to native cells *in vivo*. For example, using cultured fibrocytes, we can test whether transfection will enable them to generate survival factors and release them. If genetically engineered cells are successfully incorporated into the lateral wall, they could be used to enhance the survival of other cell types in the cochlea (see below). Fibrocytes have been targeted in a very limited number of studies for transfection (only two to our knowledge: Zhuo et al., 2008; Oh et al., 2012).

Finally, it may also be possible to functionalize the fibrocytes in novel ways, e.g., by optogenetics to enable them to be more effective in potassium transport. A recently developed light-sensitive potassium channel shows that it may be possible to alter their potassium transport ability in response to light (Alberio et al., 2018). This could potentially be used to manipulate EP generation by stimulating fibrocytes through an external route *in vivo*. These approaches are clearly speculative, but there is much to be gained from exploring these potential new avenues.

OTHER ADVANTAGES OF FIBROCYTE MANIPULATION

Arresting the degeneration of the lateral wall is likely to have other consequences for hearing function if the degeneration of hair cells and/or the spiral ganglion in SNHL is, to some extent, triggered by fibrocyte degeneration (Mahendrasingam et al., 2011b). Thus, lateral wall repair could potentially prevent subsequent SNHL. Furthermore, engineering fibrocytes to express certain growth factors could increase the longevity of the replacement fibrocytes and also be used to support long-term survival of both hair cells and supporting cells in the organ of Corti. Insulin-like growth factor 1 (IGF1) is thought to be a survival factor for hair cells and is currently undergoing clinical trials as a therapeutic agent (Yamamoto et al., 2014; Yamahara et al., 2015). Another growth factor that is potentially useful is brain-derived neurotrophic factor (BDNF) which helps to support SGNs (Leake et al., 2011). Survival of the SGNs is a requirement for the successful use of a cochlear implant long term after profound hearing loss caused by hair cell loss. This prosthetic device produces electrical pulses that stimulate SGNs and provides a signal that preserves some of the frequency content of the stimulus, replacing that derived from the missing hair cells, which normally are innervated by the neurons. The implant is amenable to working together with biological regenerative therapies (Roemer et al., 2017).

CONCLUSIONS

The fibrocytes of the lateral wall of the cochlea are known to go missing in certain forms of hearing loss, and temporally, show early signs of loss of degeneration in humans and animal models. This leads to potential breakdown of cochlear homeostatic mechanisms and loss of the endocochlear potential. An under-recognized category of hearing loss—MHL—seems to be the likely consequence of this degeneration, and it may lead to SNHL in later stages. Fibrocytes thus constitute a relatively novel target in strategies to prevent hearing loss. Another positive attribute of these cells is that they are especially amenable to both investigation *in vitro* and enhancement or replacement *in vivo* because of their proliferative capacity which enables them to be grown in culture from adult cochleae. Therapeutic strategies involving fibrocytes thus hold great potential for the future.

AUTHOR CONTRIBUTIONS

DF conceived the topic area and wrote the review in its entirety.

ACKNOWLEDGMENTS

I would like to thank Dr. S Mahendrasingam and Mrs. K Walker who have contributed to this work and to remember my wife and colleague, Professor Carole M Hackney who passed away in February 2015.

REFERENCES

Adachi, N., Yoshida, T., Nin, F., Ogata, G., Yamaguchi, S., Suzuki, T., et al (2013). The mechanism underlying maintenance of the endocochlear potential by the K+ transport system in fibrocytes of the inner ear. *J. Physiol.* 591, 4459–4472. doi: 10.1113/jphysiol.2013.258046

Adams, J. C. (2009). Immunocytochemical traits of type IV fibrocytes and their possible relations to cochlear function and pathology.

J. Assoc. Res. Otolaryngol. 10, 369–382. doi: 10.1007/s10162-009-0165-z

Ahmed, S., Vorasubin, N., Lopez, I. A., Hosokawa, S., Ishiyama, G., and Ishiyama, A. (2013). The expression of glutamate aspartate transporter (GLAST) within the human cochlea and its distribution in various patient populations. *Brain Res.* 1529, 134–142. doi: 10.1016/j.brainres.2013.06.040

Alberio, L., Locarno, A., Saponaro, A., Romano, E., Bercier, V., Albadri, S., et al. (2018). A light-gated potassium channel for sustained neuronal inhibition. *Nat. Methods* 15, 969–976. doi: 10.1038/s41592-018-0186-9

Carraro, M., Park, A. H., and Harrison, R. V. (2016). Partial corrosion casting to assess cochlear vasculature in mouse models of presbycusis and CMV infection. *Hear. Res.* 332, 95–103. doi: 10.1016/j.heares.2015.11.010

Crouch, J. J., Sakaguchi, N., Lytle, C., and Schulte, B. A. (1997). Immunohistochemical localization of the Na-K-Cl co-transporter (NKCC1) in the gerbil inner ear. *J. Histochem. Cytochem.* 45, 773–778. doi: 10.1177/002215549704500601

Dai, M., and Shi, X. (2011). Fibro-vascular coupling in the control of cochlear blood flow. *PLoS One* 6:e20652. doi: 10.1371/journal.pone.0020652

Dubno, J. R., Eckert, M. A., Lee, F. S., Matthews, L. J., and Schmiedt, R. A. (2013). Classifying human audiometric phenotypes of age-related hearing loss from animal models. *J. Assoc. Res. Otolaryngol.* 14, 687–701. doi: 10.1007/s10162-013-0396-x

Forge, A., Becker, D., Casalotti, S., Edwards, J., Evans, W. H., Lench, N., et al. (1999). Gap junctions and connexin expression in the inner ear. *Novartis Found. Symp.* 219, 134–150. doi: 10.1002/9780470515587.ch9

Forge, A., Becker, D., Casalotti, S., Edwards, J., Marziano, N., and Nevill, G. (2003). Gap junctions in the inner ear: comparison of distribution patterns in different vertebrates and assessement of connexin composition in mammals. *J. Comp. Neurol.* 467, 207–231. doi: 10.1002/cne.10916

Furness, D. N. (2014). Abstracts of the fourth joint annual conference, experimental and clinical short papers meetings of the british society of audiology. *Int. J. Audiol.* 53, 641–696. doi: 10.3109/14992027.2014.938194

Furness, D. N., Lawton, D. M., Mahendrasingam, S., Hodierne, L., and Jagger, D. J. (2009). Quantitative analysis of the expression of the glutamate-aspartate transporter and identification of functional glutamate uptake reveal a role for cochlear fibrocytes in glutamate homeostasis. *Neuroscience* 162, 1307–1321. doi: 10.1016/j.neuroscience.2009.05.036

Gratton, M. A., Schulte, B. A., and Hazen-Martin, D. J. (1996). Characterization and development of an inner ear type I fibrocyte cell culture. *Hear. Res.* 99, 71–78. doi: 10.1016/s0378-5955(96)00080-9

Henson, M. M., and Henson, O. W.Jr. (1988). Tension fibroblasts and the connective tissue matrix of the spiral ligament. *Hear. Res.* 35, 237–258. doi: 10.1016/0378-5955(88)90121-9

Hequembourg, S., and Liberman, M. C. (2001). Spiral ligament pathology: a major aspect of age-related cochlear degeneration in C57BL/6 mice. *J. Assoc. Res. Otolaryngol.* 2, 118–129. doi: 10.1007/s101620010075

Hibino, H., and Kurachi, Y. (2006). Molecular and physiological bases of the K^+ circulation in the mammalian inner ear. *Physiology* 21, 336–345. doi: 10.1152/physiol.00023.2006

Hibino, H., Higashi-Shingai, K., Fujita, A., Iwai, K., Ishii, M., and Kurachi, Y. (2004). Expression of an inwardly rectifying K+ channel, Kir5.1, in specific types of fibrocytes in the cochlear lateral wall suggests its functional importance in the establishment of endocochlear potential. *Eur. J. Neurosci.* 19, 76–84. doi: 10.1111/j.1460-9568.2004.03092.x

Huebner, A. K., Maier, H., Maul, A., Nietzsche, S., Herrmann, T., Praetorius, J., et al. (2019). Early hearing loss upon disruption of Slc4a10 in C57BL/6 mice. *J. Assoc. Res. Otolaryngol.* 20, 233–245. doi: 10.1007/s10162-019-00719-1

Ichimiya, I., Adams, J. C., and Kimura, R. S. (1994). Immunolocalization of Na+, K+-ATPase, Ca++-ATPase, calcium-binding proteins and carbonic anhydrase in the guinea pig inner ear. *Acta Otolaryngol.* 114, 167–176. doi: 10.3109/00016489409126037

Ichimiya, I., Yoshida, K., Hirano, T., Suzuki, M., and Mogi, G. (2000). Significance of spiral ligament fibrocytes with cochlear inflammation. *Int. J. Pediatr. Otorhinolaryngol.* 56, 45–51. doi: 10.1016/s0165-5876(00)00408-0

Ishiyama, G., Lopez, I. A., Sepahdari, A. R., and Ishiyama, A. (2015). Meniere's disease: histopathology, cytochemistry and imaging. *Ann. N. Y. Acad. Sci.* 1343, 49–57. doi: 10.1111/nyas.12699

Ishiyama, G., Tokita, J., Lopez, I. A., Tang, Y., and Ishiyama, A. (2007). Unbiased stereological estimation of the spiral ligament and stria vascularis volumes in aging and Meniere's disease using archival human temporal bones. *J. Assoc. Res. Otolaryngol.* 8, 8–17. doi: 10.1007/s10162-006-0057-4

Jagger, D. J., Nevill, G., and Forge, A. (2010). The membrane properties of cochlear root cells are consistent with roles in potassium recirculation and spatial buffering. *J. Assoc. Res. Otolaryngol.* 11, 435–448. doi: 10.1007/s10162-010-0218-3

Jin, Z. H., Kikuchi, T., Tanaka, K., and Kobayashi, T. (2003). Expression of glutamate transporter C24GLAST in the developing mouse cochlea. *Tohoku J. Exp. Med.* 200, 137–144. doi: 10.1620/tjem.200.137

Kamiya, K., Fujinami, Y., Hoya, N., Okamoto, Y., Kouike, H., Komatsuzaki, R., et al. (2007). Mesenchymal stem cell transplantation accelerates hearing recovery through the repair of injured cochlear fibrocytes. *Am. J. Pathol.* 171, 214–226. doi: 10.2353/ajpath.2007.060948

Kelly, J. J., Forge, A., and Jagger, D. J. (2012). Contractility in type III cochlear fibrocytes is dependent on non-muscle myosin II and intercellular gap junctional coupling. *J. Assoc. Res. Otolaryngol.* 13, 473–484. doi: 10.1007/s10162-012-0322-7

Kitajiri, S., Miyamoto, T., Mineharu, A., Sonoda, N., Furuse, K., Hata, M., et al. (2004). Compartmentalization established by claudin-11-based tight junctions in stria vascularis is required for hearing through generation of endocochlear potential. *J. Cell Sci.* 117, 5087–5096. doi: 10.1242/jcs.01393

Kusunoki, T., Cureoglu, S., Schachern, P. A., Baba, K., Kariya, S., and Paparella, M. M. (2004). Age-related histopathologic changes in the human cochlea: a temporal bone study. *Otolaryngol. Head Neck Surg.* 131, 897–903. doi: 10.1016/j.otohns.2004.05.022

Lang, H., Jyothi, V., Smythe, N. M., Dubno, J. R., Schulte, B. A., and Schmiedt, R. A. (2010). Chronic reduction of endocochlear potential reduces auditory nerve activity: further confirmation of an animal model of metabolic presbyacusis. *J. Assoc. Res. Otolaryngol.* 11, 419–434. doi: 10.1007/s10162-010-0214-7

Leake, P. A., Hradek, G. T., Hetherington, A. M., and Stakhovskaya, O. (2011). Brain-derived neurotrophic factor promotes cochlear spiral ganglion cell survival and function in deafened, developing cats. *J. Comp. Neurol.* 519, 1526–1545. doi: 10.1002/cne.22582

Li, Y., Watanabe, K., Fujioka, M., and Ogawa, K. (2017). Characterization of slow-cycling cells in the mouse cochlear lateral wall. *PLoS One* 12:e0179293. doi: 10.1371/journal.pone.0179293

Liang, F., Hu, W., Schulte, B. A., Mao, C., Qu, C., Hazen-Martin, D. J., et al. (2004). Identification and characterization of an L-type Cav1.2 channel in spiral ligament fibrocytes of gerbil inner ear. *Brain Res. Mol. Brain Res.* 125, 40–46. doi: 10.1016/j.molbrainres.2004.03.003

Liang, F., Niedzielski, A., Schulte, B. A., Spicer, S. S., Hazen-Martin, D. J., and Shen, Z. (2003). A voltage- and Ca2+-dependent big conductance K channel in cochlear spiral ligament fibrocytes. *Pflugers Arch.* 445, 683–692. doi: 10.1007/s00424-002-0976-9

Liu, W., Schrott-Fischer, A., Glueckert, R., Benav, H., and Rask-Andersen, H. (2017). The human "Cochlear Battery"-claudin-11 barrier and ion transport proteins in the lateral wall of the Cochlea. *Front. Mol. Neurosci.* 10:239. doi: 10.3389/fnmol.2017.00239

Lukashkina, V. A., Levic, S., Lukashkin, A. N., Strenzke, N., and Russell, I. J. (2017). A connexin30 mutation rescues hearing and reveals roles for gap junctions in cochlear amplification and micromechanics. *Nat. Commun.* 8:14530. doi: 10.1038/ncomms14530

Mahendrasingam, S., Bebb, C., Shepard, E., and Furness, D. N. (2011a). Subcellular distribution and relative expression of fibrocyte markers in the CD/1 mouse cochlea assessed by semiquantitative immunogold electron microscopy. *J. Histochem. Cytochem.* 59, 984–1000. doi: 10.1369/0022155411421801

Mahendrasingam, S., Macdonald, J. A., and Furness, D. N. (2011b). Relative time course of degeneration of different cochlear structures in the CD/1 mouse model of accelerated aging. *J. Assoc. Res. Otolaryngol.* 12, 437–453. doi: 10.1007/s10162-011-0263-6

Mei, L., Chen, J., Zong, L., Zhu, Y., Liang, C., Jones, R. O., et al. (2017). A deafness mechanism of digenic Cx26 (GJB2) and Cx30 (GJB6) mutations: reduction of endocochlear potential by impairment of heterogeneous gap junctional function in the cochlear lateral wall. *Neurobiol. Dis.* 108, 195–203. doi: 10.1016/j.nbd.2017.08.002

Merchant, S. N., Adams, J. C., and Nadol, J. B.Jr. (2005). Pathophysiology of Meniere's syndrome: are symptoms caused by endolymphatic hydrops? *Otol. Neurotol.* 26, 74–81. doi: 10.1097/00129492-200501000-00013

Minowa, O., Ikeda, K., Sugitani, Y., Oshima, T., Nakai, S., Katori, Y., et al. (1999). Altered cochlear fibrocytes in a mouse model of DFN3 nonsyndromic deafness. *Science* 285, 1408–1411. doi: 10.1126/science.285.5432.1408

Miyabe, Y., Kikuchi, T., and Kobayashi, T. (2002). Comparative immunohistochemical localizations of aquaporin-1 and aquaporin-4 in the cochleae of three different species of rodents. *Tohoku J. Exp. Med.* 196, 247–257. doi: 10.1620/tjem.196.247

Nadol, J. B.Jr., Adams, J. C., and Kim, J. R. (1995). Degenerative changes in the organ of Corti and lateral cochlear wall in experimental endolymphatic hydrops and human Menière's disease. *Acta Otolaryngol. Suppl.* 519, 47–59. doi: 10.3109/00016489509121870

Nie, L., Gratton, M. A., Mu, K. J., Dinglasan, J. N., Feng, W., and Yamoah, E. N. (2005). Expression and functional phenotype of mouse ERG K+ channels in the inner ear: potential role in K+ regulation in the inner ear. *J. Neurosci.* 25, 8671–8679. doi: 10.1523/jneurosci.1422-05.2005

Nouvian, R., Ruel, J., Wang, J., Guitton, M. J., Pujol, R., and Puel, J. L. (2003). Degeneration of sensory outer hair cells following pharmacological blockade of cochlear KCNQ channels in the adult guinea pig. *Eur. J. Neurosci.* 17, 2553–2562. doi: 10.1046/j.1460-9568.2003.02715.x

Oh, S., Woo, J. I., Lim, D. J., and Moon, S. K. (2012). ERK2-dependent activation of c-Jun is required for nontypeable Haemophilus influenzae-induced CXCL2 upregulation in inner ear fibrocytes. *J. Immunol.* 188, 3496–3505. doi: 10.4049/jimmunol.1103182

Pujol, R., and Puel, J. L. (1999). Excitotoxicity, synaptic repair and functional recovery in the mammalian cochlea: a review of recent findings. *Ann. N Y Acad. Sci.* 884, 249–254. doi: 10.1111/j.1749-6632.1999.tb08646.x

Qu, C., Liang, F., Hu, W., Shen, Z., Spicer, S. S., and Schulte, B. A. (2006). Expression of CLC-K chloride channels in the rat cochlea. *Hear. Res.* 213, 79–87. doi: 10.1016/j.heares.2005.12.012

Quan, T. E., Cowper, S. E., and Bucala, R. (2006). The role of circulating fibrocytes in fibrosis. *Curr. Rheumatol. Rep.* 8, 145–150. doi: 10.1007/s11926-006-0055-x

Roemer, A., Staecker, H., Sasse, S., Lenarz, T., and Warnecke, A. (2017). Biological therapies in otology. *HNO* 65, 87–97. doi: 10.1007/s00106-016-0306-8

Sakagami, M., Matsunaga, T., and Hashimoto, P. H. (1982). Fine structure and permeability of capillaries in the stria vascularis and spiral ligament of the inner ear of the guinea pig. *Cell Tissue Res.* 226, 511–522. doi: 10.1007/bf00214780

Schuknecht, H. F., and Gacek, M. R. (1993). Cochlear pathology in presbycusis. *Ann. Otol. Rhinol. Laryngol.* 102, 1–16. doi: 10.1177/00034894931020s101

Sheffield, A. M., and Smith, R. J. H. (2018). The epidemiology of deafness. *Cold Spring Harb. Perspect. Med.* 9:a033258. doi: 10.1101/cshperspect.a033258

Shen, Z., Liang, F., Hazen-Martin, D. J., and Schulte, B. A. (2004). BK channels mediate the voltage-dependent outward current in type I spiral ligament fibrocytes. *Hear. Res.* 187, 35–43. doi: 10.1016/s0378-5955(03)00345-9

So, E., Kikuchi, T., Ishimaru, K., Miyabe, Y., and Kobayashi, T. (2001). Immunolocalization of voltage-gated potassium channel Kv3.1b subunit in the cochlea. *Neuroreport* 12, 2761–2765. doi: 10.1097/00001756-200108280-00033

Spicer, S. S., and Schulte, B. A. (1991). Differentiation of inner ear fibrocytes according to their ion transport related activity. *Hear. Res.* 56, 53–64. doi: 10.1016/0378-5955(91)90153-z

Spicer, S. S., and Schulte, B. A. (1996). The fine structure of spiral ligament cells relates to ion return to the stria and varies with place-frequency. *Hear. Res.* 100, 80–100. doi: 10.1016/0378-5955(96)00106-2

Standring, S. (2015). *Gray's Anatomy: The Anatomical Basis of Clinical Practice* 41st edn. New York, NY: Elsevier Limited.

Suko, T., Ichimiya, I., Yoshida, K., Suzuki, M., and Mogi, G. (2000). Classification and culture of spiral ligament fibrocytes from mice. *Hear. Res.* 140, 137–144. doi: 10.1016/s0378-5955(99)00191-4

Vaden, K. I.Jr., Matthews, L. J., and Dubno, J. R. (2018). Transient-evoked otoacoustic emissions reflect audiometric patterns of age-related hearing loss. *Trends Hear.* 22:2331216518797848. doi: 10.1177/2331216518797848

Vaden, K. I.Jr., Matthews, L. J., Eckert, M. A., and Dubno, J. R. (2017). Longitudinal changes in audiometric phenotypes of age-related hearing loss. *J. Assoc. Res. Otolaryngol.* 18, 371–385. doi: 10.1007/s10162-016-0596-2

Viana, L. M., O'Malley, J. T., Burgess, B. J., Jones, D. D., Oliveira, C. A., Santos, F., et al. (2015). Cochlear neuropathy in human presbycusis: confocal analysis of hidden hearing loss in post-mortem tissue. *Hear. Res.* 327, 78–88. doi: 10.1016/j.heares.2015.04.014

Wangemann, P. (2006). Supporting sensory transduction: cochlear fluid homeostasis and the endocochlear potential. *J. Physiol.* 576, 11–21. doi: 10.1113/jphysiol.2006.112888

Woo, J. I., Kil, S. H., Oh, S., Lee, Y. J., Park, R., Lim, D. J., et al. (2015). IL-10/HMOX1 signaling modulates cochlear inflammation *via* negative regulation of MCP-1/CCL2 expression in cochlear fibrocytes. *J. Immunol.* 194, 3953–3961. doi: 10.4049/jimmunol.1402751

Xia, J. H., Liu, C. Y., Tang, B. S., Pan, Q., Huang, L., Dai, H. P., et al. (1998). Mutations in the gene encoding gap junction protein beta-3 associated with autosomal dominant hearing impairment. *Nat. Genet.* 20, 370–373. doi: 10.1038/3845

Yamahara, K., Yamamoto, N., Nakagawa, T., and Ito, J. (2015). Insulin-like growth factor 1: a novel treatment for the protection or regeneration of cochlear hair cells. *Redox Biol.* 330, 2–9. doi: 10.1016/j.heares.2015.04.009

Yamamoto, N., Nakagawa, T., and Ito, J. (2014). Application of insulin-like growth factor-1 in the treatment of inner ear disorders. *Front. Pharmacol.* 5:208. doi: 10.3389/fphar.2014.00208

Yoshida, T., Nin, F., Murakami, S., Ogata, G., Uetsuka, S., Choi, S., et al. (2016). The unique ion permeability profile of cochlear fibrocytes and its contribution to establishing their positive resting membrane potential. *Pflugers Arch.* 468, 1609–1619. doi: 10.1007/s00424-016-1853-2

Zhu, Y., Liu, X., Ding, X., Wang, F., and Geng, X. (2019). Telomere and its role in the aging pathways: telomere shortening, cell senescence and mitochondria dysfunction. *Biogerontology* 20, 1–16. doi: 10.1007/s10522-018-9769-1

Zhuo, X. L., Wang, Y., Zhuo, W. L., Zhang, Y. S., Wei, Y. J., and Zhang, X. Y. (2008). Adenoviral-mediated up-regulation of Otos, a novel specific cochlear gene, decreases cisplatin-induced apoptosis of cultured spiral ligament fibrocytes *via* MAPK/mitochondrial pathway. *Toxicology* 248, 33–38. doi: 10.1016/j.tox.2008.03.004

4

Gene Therapy for Human Sensorineural Hearing Loss

*Yin Ren[1,2], Lukas D. Landegger[1,2,3] and Konstantina M. Stankovic[1,2,4,5]**

[1] Department of Otolaryngology, Harvard Medical School, Boston, MA, United States, [2] Eaton Peabody Laboratories, Department of Otolaryngology, Massachusetts Eye and Ear, Boston, MA, United States, [3] Department of Otolaryngology, Vienna General Hospital, Medical University of Vienna, Vienna, Austria, [4] Program in Speech and Hearing Bioscience and Technology, Harvard Medical School, Boston, MA, United States, [5] Harvard Program in Therapeutic Science, Harvard University, Boston, MA, United States

***Correspondence:**
Konstantina M. Stankovic
konstantina_stankovic@meei.harvard.edu

Hearing loss is the most common sensory impairment in humans and currently disables 466 million people across the world. Congenital deafness affects at least 1 in 500 newborns, and over 50% are hereditary in nature. To date, existing pharmacologic therapies for genetic and acquired etiologies of deafness are severely limited. With the advent of modern sequencing technologies, there is a vast compendium of growing genetic alterations that underlie human hearing loss, which can be targeted by therapeutics such as gene therapy. Recently, there has been tremendous progress in the development of gene therapy vectors to treat sensorineural hearing loss (SNHL) in animal models *in vivo*. Nevertheless, significant hurdles remain before such technologies can be translated toward clinical use. These include addressing the blood-labyrinth barrier, engineering more specific and effective delivery vehicles, improving surgical access, and validating novel targets. In this review, we both highlight recent progress and outline challenges associated with *in vivo* gene therapy for human SNHL.

Keywords: gene therapy, adeno-associated virus (AAV), nanoparticles, blood labyrinth barrier, Anc80L65, tumor penetrating peptide, round window niche

INTRODUCTION

Hearing loss is the most common sensory impairment in humans and currently disables 466 million people across the world; this number is expected to rise to nearly 1 billion by 2050 (WHO Deafness and Hearing Loss, 2018). It is especially prevalent in the aging population as nearly two-thirds of the U.S. population over the age of 70 years are affected by disabling hearing loss (Lin et al., 2011). Furthermore, congenital deafness affects at least 1 in 500 newborns, with over 50% of these being hereditary in nature. Most of this burden is due to sensorineural hearing loss (SNHL) which originates from defects in the cochlea, the spiraling organ of the inner ear.

The human inner ear is a small, three-dimensionally complex, fluid-filled structure encased in the densest bone in the body and located deep in the base of skull. Acoustic energy from sound is transmitted to the fluids of the cochlea via vibrations of the tympanic membrane and ossicular chain in the middle ear, producing a traveling wave along the basilar membrane. The length of the cochlea and stiffness of the basilar membrane enables the differentiation of sound frequencies (Manoussaki et al., 2006). This in turn leads to activation of mechanotransduction by hair cells, specialized sensory cells located in the organ of Corti, which turn mechanical stimulation into electrical depolarization. The electrical signal initiated by the inner hair cells (IHCs) is then processed by spiral ganglion neurons (SGNs) that make up the auditory nerve and ultimately decoded in the auditory cortex of the temporal lobe (Rubel and Fritzsch, 2002).

The genetic basis for human hearing loss has been under intensive investigation for the past two decades. Initially noted by Gorlin et al. (1995) that a significant portion of hearing loss has an underlying genetic etiology, the number of distinct genes associated with inherited hearing loss has since rapidly expanded with the advent of advanced sequencing technologies. A list of human loci linked with hearing loss has been compiled and regularly updated[1]. Broadly speaking, genetic hearing loss is subcategorized into Mendelian inheritance including both syndromic and non-syndromic cases, or complex inheritance which includes both genetic and environmental factors. Today, there are 115 genes responsible for non-syndromic hearing loss, with 45 autosomal dominant genes, 73 autosomal recessive genes, 5 X-linked genes, and additional loci for modifiers, Y-linked, and auditory neuropathy, respectively. On a global scale, the prevalence of hearing loss is highest in Eastern Europe, Central and South Asia, and Asia Pacific approaching 10%. Regions with lower income and literacy levels also tend to have higher rates of hearing loss (Sheffield and Smith, 2018). Further characterizations of the molecular pathways defined by these genes and loci have been reviewed elsewhere (Dror and Avraham, 2010; Stamatiou and Stankovic, 2013).

Despite our growing knowledge of the molecular underpinnings of auditory development, as well as an expanding armamentarium of deafness genes identified to date, there are no pharmacotherapies clinically approved for SNHL. Current treatments focus on amplification of sound through hearing aids, or via electrical stimulation of auditory neurons through cochlear implantation (CI) for severe to profound deafness. Nevertheless, neither approach restores the native inner ear sensory epithelium. Given the genetic basis underlying many forms of hearing loss and progress in our understanding of the mechanisms of hair cell regeneration and neuronal synapse repair, targeted modulation of affected genes in specific cell types of the inner ear could be a powerful therapeutic strategy. There have been numerous recent reports highlighting the complexity of genetic hearing loss and both non-viral and viral delivery approaches for therapeutic delivery (Chang, 2015; Ahmed et al., 2017; Devare et al., 2018; Lustig and Akil, 2018). In this review, we focus on (1) transport barriers to inner ear drug delivery, (2) viral and nanotechnology carriers that target the inner ear with high precision and efficiency, (3) adult animal models for clinically translatable hearing restoration, and (4) practical surgical challenges in navigating the middle and inner ear.

TRANSPORT BARRIERS TO THE INNER EAR

The translation of modern molecular therapy into clinical use is hindered by the so-called "delivery" challenge. To engineer a precise and effective inner ear delivery system, one must first develop a comprehensive understanding of the anatomic and physiologic barriers that isolate labyrinthine organs from the middle ear space and the brain. The perilymphatic space communicates via the round and oval windows to the middle ear, and via the cochlear aqueduct and cochlear modiolus to the cerebral spinal fluid (CSF) space (**Figure 1**). The arterioles and venules are located inside bony channels within the scala vestibuli and scala tympani, respectively, with the major capillary beds located in the stria vascularis, spiral ligament, and spiral ganglion (Axelsson, 1988). A lymphatic system is also thought to provide clearance and drainage of the middle and inner ear (Lim and Hussl, 1975). On a microscopic scale, specialized cell layers consisting of tight junctions and endothelial cells lining cochlear blood vessels form the blood-labyrinth barrier (BLB), an intricate network that tightly regulates the transport of macromolecules and ions between the vascular compartment and the inner ear.

The BLB has been compared to the blood–brain barrier (BBB), a complex system of endothelial cells, basement membrane, pericytes, and astrocytes that isolates and protects the central nervous system (CNS). While the complexity of the BBB renders delivery of macromolecule therapeutics challenging, it also presents unique opportunities for drug delivery across the barrier (Pardridge, 2016). Novel ways to improve therapeutic delivery include modifications of the drug to improve pharmacokinetics and lipophilicity, development of "Trojan horse" carriers or analogs for endogenous ligands, inhibition of drug efflux, and modulation of BBB permeability (Banks, 2016). Recent promising work in nanotechnology has overcome this bottleneck and bypass the BBB in pathologic conditions such as traumatic brain injury (Smith et al., 2016). These promising strategies should be emulated and adapted to enhance drug delivery across the BLB into the inner ear.

Under physiologic conditions, the intact BLB is thought to maintain ionic homeostasis, isolate from pathogens in the blood, and thereby contribute to the semi immune-privileged nature of the inner ear (Salt and Hirose, 2018). By contrast, this barrier can become "leaky" upon exposure to toxic levels of noise or ototoxic medications through activated macrophages (Kopke et al., 1999; Suzuki et al., 2002). Interestingly, evidence suggests that a compromised BLB through systemic exposure to lipopolysaccharide does not correlate with a loss of hearing (Hirose et al., 2014; Hirose and Li, 2019). Therefore, the dynamic nature of the BLB's permeability could be harnessed as a window for intracochlear therapeutic delivery. Indeed, strategies to temporarily enhance the permeability of tissue barriers have seen success in delivering macromolecule drugs to tumors or the brain that would be otherwise difficult to traverse (Ren et al., 2012; Kwon et al., 2016). Future experimental animal models will need to specifically and precisely alter the permeability of the BLB and identify new epitopes that are unveiled in the cochlear sensory epithelium or neurons. Strategies to reduce lymphatic or macrophage-mediated clearance of delivered drugs could effectively improve the biodistribution of the drug within the desired tissue. Future interventions that transiently enhance macromolecule transport across the BLB without causing significant cellular damage may serve as useful adjuncts to improve drug penetration.

[1] http://hereditaryhearingloss.org/

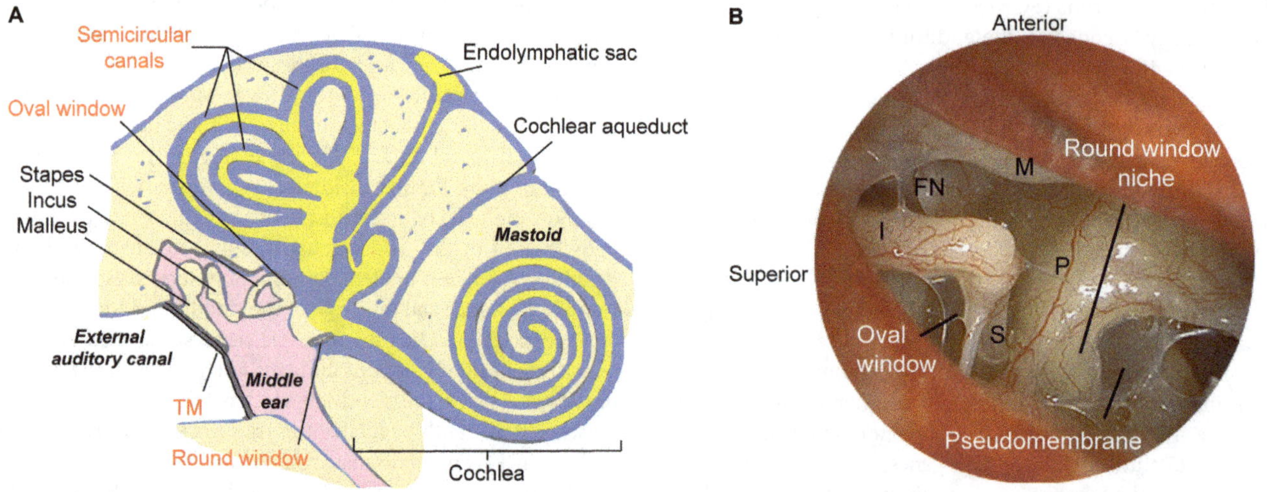

FIGURE 1 | Schematic illustrating methods of delivering therapeutics to the human ear. **(A)** The relevant structures through which drugs such as gene therapy agents, nanoparticles, or biologics are introduced into the inner ear are labeled in red, and include both indirect and direct approaches. The indirect approach is through the tympanic membrane (transtympanic or intratympanic) to deposit the therapeutic in the middle ear and allow it to diffuse into the inner ear via the oval and round windows. Direct approaches include delivery into the cochlea through application over or through the round window membrane, through a surgically drilled cochleostomy adjacent to the round window, a fenestra in the bony oval window, or a semicircular canal. Approaches for drug/gene delivery also include combining existing technologies such as cochlear implant electrodes or stapes prosthesis during stapedotomy. **(B)** Endoscopic view of the anatomy of the human middle ear. The round window niche consists of bony overhang, and the round window is often obscured by a pseudomembrane. M, malleus manubrium; I, incus; P, cochlear promontory; S, stapes; FN, facial nerve; TM, tympanic membrane. Image reproduced with permission from Medscape Drugs & Diseases (https://emedicine.medscape.com/), Surgical Treatment of Meniere Disease, 2018, available at: https://emedicine.medscape.com/article/856658-overview.

MODEL SYSTEMS FOR GENE THERAPY

While optimization and characterization of gene therapy vectors could be done in cell cultures and cochlear explants *in vitro*, animal studies are required to understand the full panoply of the gene's effects in the inner ear microenvironment. Furthermore, the long-term therapeutic effects, interactions with other organ systems and organ toxicities can only be characterized in a living host. Historically, *in vivo* gene delivery experiments have been carried out in zebrafish, birds, and rodents. Both zebrafish and birds have well-characterized genomes and robust regenerative capacity in the inner ear sensory epithelium after injury (Daudet et al., 2009; Cotanche and Kaiser, 2010); nevertheless, these non-mammalian model systems are rarely utilized for gene transfer research due to dissimilarities from mammals and humans.

Rodents are the preferred animal models due to their well-characterized genomes, robustness to manipulations, cost-effectiveness, and close resemblance to the human inner ear and potential for pre-clinical testing. While the human inner ear is larger than that of rodents, the cochlea of rodents such as guinea pigs can be more accessible due to their unique anatomy where the otic capsule protrudes into the middle ear space and contains thin bony walls (Mikulec et al., 2009; Jawadi et al., 2016). Today, transgenic mouse models capturing various genetic alterations that mimic human disease are well characterized, and mutant mice carrying simultaneous mutations in multiple genes crucial for normal hearing function have been established using CRISPR/Cas-9 technology (Zhang et al., 2018). However, experiments involving delivery of gene therapy using novel AAV systems to the cochlea have been performed largely in neonatal mice (Landegger et al., 2017; Pan et al., 2017). In a mouse model of hereditary deafness through a null mutation in the vesicular glutamate transporter-3 (VGLUT3) responsible for IHC-afferent nerve synaptic transmission, early intervention using AAV-mediated gene delivery at postnatal days 1–3 led to more efficient and longer duration of hearing recovery than intervention at postnatal day 10 (Akil et al., 2012). While these results are exciting, they may have limited potential for direct clinical correlation and translation to treatments of newborns and adult patients with hearing loss.

Unlike humans, mice are born deaf and begin to hear at approximately 2 weeks of age. Therefore, delivery of therapeutics to neonates would be equivalent to *in utero* therapy in humans, and thereby pose additional significant technical challenges. In mouse models of progressive hearing loss, gene therapy is typically administered prior to organ of Corti beginning to degenerate in the early postnatal period. By contrast, in many forms of hereditary deafness, there is likely already degeneration of the sensory epithelium and neurons which occurred early *in utero*, thereby rendering postnatal therapy targeting either hair cells or SGNs futile.

To address these concerns, recent reports utilizing common AAVs, Anc80L65, and 7m8 vectors showed efficient transduction of vestibular hair cells in adult mice ranging from P15 to P60, without jeopardizing their cochlear function (Suzuki et al., 2017; Yoshimura et al., 2018; Isgrig et al., 2019). Therefore, future studies should continue to focus on expanding the therapeutic window and developing cochlear gene therapies for adult-stage hearing loss, which would be equivalent to the clinical scenario of treating patients with hearing loss months to even years after the initial insult.

Prior to conducting human clinical trials, it is also critically important to test the efficacy and safety of hearing-restoration therapeutics in non-human primates. Inner ear volumes (including soft tissue and fluid) correlate with body mass across species, with an estimated volume of 2.3–2.5, 59.4–63, and 191.1–237 μL for mouse, rhesus monkey, and human, respectively (Ekdale, 2013; Dai et al., 2017). While it is tempting to apply results from mouse studies to human clinical trials, the large discrepancies in inner ear volumes may make such direct extrapolations challenging. Since the human cochlea and labyrinth measures approximately two orders of magnitude larger than that in rodents and only three- to fourfold larger than monkeys, it may be easier to extrapolate successful technical implementation of gene delivery in rhesus monkeys to humans. To achieve this goal, Dai et al. (2017) assessed rhesus audiovestibular functions after mock saline injections via either the oval or round windows. Encouragingly, nearly all animals tolerated the injections with no evidence of toxicity in histological, audiometric, and behavioral analyses (Dai et al., 2017). Based on these results, György et al. (2019) performed the first transmastoid injection of an AAV9 variant via the round window membrane (RWM) in a cynomolgus monkey, which appeared to mediate efficient transduction of both inner and outer hair cells (György et al., 2019). Nevertheless, results were inconsistent as a second monkey showed significantly limited transduction at a lower dose. Future studies utilizing a larger number of animals are required to understand variables such as pre-existing immunity to the AAV vector (Louis Jeune et al., 2013), the dose-dependency of transduction efficiency, and the technical reproducibility of RWM injections in larger mammals (György et al., 2019).

VEHICLES AND TARGETS

Nearly half of all congenital hearing loss arises from genetic factors, and approximately two-thirds of these are inherited. Most non-syndromic deafness is autosomal recessive (75–90%) with mutations in *GJB2* and *SLC26A4* responsible for the majority of cases; most of the remaining cases are inherited in an autosomal dominant pattern, and a small fraction of up to 1.5% are either X-linked or mitochondrial (Dror and Avraham, 2010; Stamatiou and Stankovic, 2013; Chang, 2015). Compared to gene therapy for acquired hearing loss after mechanical or pharmacological insults, genetic hearing loss poses greater challenges in that successfully regenerated hair cells or neurons would still harbor the causative genetic defect. Therefore, targeted correction of the underlying genetic mutation in all affected cell populations in the cochlea is paramount. Fortunately, with advent in modern sequencing technologies and prenatal testing, it is now becoming possible to detect genetic defects and intervene on them at an earlier stage.

The choice of delivery vector for *in vivo* gene therapy depends on many factors including the cell type being targeted, route of administration, and therapeutic potency. Delivery platforms can be broadly classified into viral vectors including adenoviruses (AdVs), adeno-associated viruses (AAVs), and retroviruses including lentiviruses (Kiernan and Fekete, 1997; Pietola et al., 2008); versus non-viral vectors such as nanoparticles and exosomes. In theory, viral vectors generally enable more stable and durable expression of the transgene. However, the complex immune response to viruses and the safety of long-term transgene expression are unknown and can be challenging to assess. By contrast, non-viral delivery vehicles are less immunogenic and can be engineered to satisfy the exact therapeutic need. A summary of the viral and non-viral vectors reported in the literature over the last 10 years for *in vivo* delivery in mature animals is shown in **Table 1**.

Viral Delivery Agents

Much of the pre-clinical success in gene therapy for hearing loss is owing to the use of viral vectors to carry payloads into the inner ear. Popular viral vectors include variants of AdV and AAV, both of which have excellent tropism toward a number of cell types in the cochlea and relatively high transduction efficiency in animal models (Akil et al., 2012; Askew et al., 2015). AdV-mediated delivery results in transient expression of the transgene, whereas AAV-mediated delivery could lead to long-lasting gene expression. A summary of the advantages and disadvantages of both AdV and AAV vectors for cochlear gene therapy have been the topics of many recent reviews (Husseman and Raphael, 2009; Ahmed et al., 2017; Lustig and Akil, 2018).

Of note, a particular synthetic "ancestral" AAV subtype, Anc80L65, was able to efficiently transduce over 90% of both inner and outer hair cells at a dose that is two to three times lower than conventional AAV counterparts (Landegger et al., 2017). In a mouse model of Type I Usher syndrome due to mutations in *Ush1c* encoding the protein harmonin, wild-type harmonin was successfully delivered into the inner ear after RW membrane injection using the Anc80 vector. In neonatal P0-1 mice, the delivered gene product was found to be localized to the stereocilia near tip-link insertions on hair cells. Ultrastructural studies using scanning electron microscopy showed normal hair cell morphology and decreased hair cell loss. The treatment not only restored mechanotransduction, but also led to dramatic improvements in complex audiovestibular functions to near wild-type levels for at least 6 months (Pan et al., 2017). These results suggest that virally mediated expression of the transgene can rescue hair cell function if they are present before hair cells degenerate as the animal matures, and such effects could be long-lasting for the duration of development.

Another unresolved question in viral-mediated cochlear gene therapy is whether stable levels of transgene expression can be sustained, and if so, for how long. Since many genes implicated in human deafness are only transiently expressed during normal development, how severe are the negative effects from over-expression? As cells in the sensory epithelium do not typically divide, expression of exogenously transduced genes is not diluted from cell division and could theoretically remain stable over time (Bainbridge et al., 2015). Previous studies in mice have shown stable treatment efficacy with follow-ups of 3–6 months (Akil et al., 2012; Chang et al., 2015; Isgrig et al., 2017;

TABLE 1 | A summary of the viral vectors recently reported in the literature in the last 10 years for *in vivo* gene delivery in adult animals.

Model (References)	Age	Follow-up	Sex (*n*)	Vector(s)	Route	Outcome
Guinea pig (pigmented) (Shibata et al., 2009)	N/A	2 weeks	M ($n = 20$)	BAAV-CMV-β-actin-GFP	Cochleostomy	Cochlea: Transduced the supporting cells of both normal and deafened animals
Mouse (CBA/CaJ) (Kilpatrick et al., 2011)	2–12 months	5 months	M&F ($n = 120$)	AAV2/1-CMV-EGFP (also AAV2/2, 5, 6, 8)	Cochleostomy	Cochlea: Efficient AAV inoculation (via the scala media) can be performed in adult mouse ears, with hearing preservation
Guinea pig (pigmented) (Budenz et al., 2015)	1–2 months	3 months	M&F ($n = 46$)	AAV2/2-CBA-EGFP, AAV2/2-CBA-NTF3, AAV2/2-CBA-BDNF	Cochleostomy	Cochlea: Transient elevation in neurotrophin levels can sustain the cochlear neural substrate in the long term
Mouse (CBA/J) (Chien et al., 2015)	1–2 months	4 weeks	M&F ($n = 66$)	AAV2/8-CMV-GFP	Cochleostomy and RWM	Cochlea: Cochleostomy and RWM approach can both be used. The RWM approach results in less hearing loss vs. cochleostomy
Mouse (CBA/CaJ) (Shu et al., 2016)	6 weeks	3 months	M ($n = 4$)	AAV2/1-CAG-EGFP (also AAV2/2, 5, 6, 6.2, 7, 8, 9, rh.8, rh.10, rh.39, rh.43)	Cochleostomy	Cochlea: AAV1, 2, 6.2, 7, 8, 9, rh.39, rh.43 transduced IHCs, but no OHCs – even partial OHC loss.
Guinea pig (pigmented) (Lee et al., 2016)	1–2 months	3 weeks	M&F ($n = 26$)	Ad5-Empty, Ad5-NTF3, AAV2/2-CBA-NTF3	Cochleostomy	Cochlea: Hearing threshold shifts, disorganization of peripheral nerve endings, and synaptic disruption with both vectors. Elevation of NT3 levels in cochlear fluids can disrupt innervation and degrade hearing.
Mouse (CBA/CaJ) (Suzuki et al., 2017)	7 weeks	2 weeks	M ($n = 13$)	AAV2/Anc80L65-CASI-EGFP-RBG	PSCC	Cochlea: Successful transduction of all IHCs, majority of OHCs especially at apex, and 10% of SGNs. Vestibular: Maculae and cristae transduced. Transduction of many hair cells, all supporting cells.
Mouse (C57BL/6) (Gao et al., 2018)	6 weeks	2 weeks	M&F ($n = 3$)	Cas9:GFP sgRNA:lipid complex	PSCC	Cochlea: Target gene disruption at 25 ± 2.1% efficiency, i.e., probably applicable to dominant genetic deafness manifested with late-onset hearing loss
Mouse (C57BL/6J and CD1) (Tao et al., 2018)	8–10 weeks	7 weeks	M ($n = 29$)	AAV2/1-CAG-EGFP (also AAV2/2, 6.2, 8, 9, rh.39, rh.43), AAV2/Anc80L65-CMV-EGFP-WPRE, Ad5-CMV-EGFP	PSCC	Cochlea: Most AAVs transduce IHCs efficiently, but are less efficient at transducing OHCs. Subset of AAVs transduces other cell types. Canalostomy can be a viable delivery route.
Mouse (FVB/N) (Guo et al., 2018)	5–6 weeks	1 week	F ($n = 1$)	AAV2/8-GFP	PSCC	Canalostomy is an effective and safe approach to drug delivery into the inner ears of adult mice.
Mouse (C57BL/6) (György et al., 2019)	4 weeks	2 weeks	M&F ($n = 2$)	AAV2/9-PHP.B-CBA-GFP	PSCC	Cochlea: Almost all IHCs from apex to base transduced, no OHC transduction. Vestibular: Robust transduction.
Mouse (C57BL/6J) (Nist-Lund et al., 2019)	4 weeks	7 weeks	M&F ($n = 12$)	AAV2/Anc80L65-CMV-TMC1-WPRE, AAV2/Anc80L65-CMV-TMC2-WPRE, AAV2/Anc80L65-CMV-TMC1EX1-WPRE, AAV2/Anc80L65-CMV-EGFP-WPRE	RWM	Cochlea: Gene therapy rescue of sensory function in mature hair cells. Vestibular: Gene therapy recovery of balance even possible at mature stages.
Mouse (CBA/J) (Isgrig et al., 2019)	1–6 months	4 weeks	M&F ($n = 6$)	AAV2/7m8-CAG-EGFP	PSCC	Cochlea: Successful transduction of IHCs (84.5%) and OHCs (74.9%). Vestibular: Only data for neonatal animals – less efficient in vestibular organs than cochlea.

In case of neonatal and adult injections in the same study, only the adult ages are mentioned in the table. If the n for a specific experiment wasn't explicitly stated, figures were analyzed to infer the minimal n (listed). When no sex was mentioned, it was assumed that male and female animals were used. When detailed vector information was not available, the listed vector in the table was assumed based on other information in a given paper or information provided by a study author who was individually contacted.

Pan et al., 2017), but few studies have examined the phenotype after this time point.

A related field where rapid progress in gene therapy has occurred in the last decade is the treatment of inherited retinal dystrophies. Importantly, the first successful clinical application of gene therapy involved treatment of inherited blindness (Dalkara et al., 2016). AAV-mediated delivery of *RPE65* gene for treatment of Leber's congenital amaurosis received FDA approval in January 2018. This represented the first directly administered clinical gene therapy in the United States that targets a disease caused by mutations in a single gene. Interestingly, long-term studies in patients who underwent gene therapy showed a decline in vision improvement at the 3-year time point, possibly due to the decline in RPE65 expression below a certain threshold level (Bainbridge et al., 2015). Lessons from these studies, along with new data generated in adult animal models, will help better inform the optimal treatment conditions that will maximize successful hearing outcomes.

While equivalent data do not yet exist in human inner ear gene therapy, preclinical animal studies have indicated secondary benefits associated with long-term hearing restoration. A recent study by Nist-Lund et al. (2019) examined the breeding efficiency and survival in a mouse model of recessive *TMC1* deafness. Animals injected with AAVs carrying *Tmc1* transgene at P1 not only showed improvements in auditory function and balance behavior, but also produced higher number of litters with significantly higher survival rates and near-normal growth rates. Follow-up studies should not only continue to examine the treatment effects of restoring gene expression at longer time points, but also probe the dynamics of gene expression and effects on normal inner ear development.

A potential shortcoming of AAV-mediated gene delivery is the limited cargo size of approximately 4.7–5 kb. As such, delivery of large gene sequences using viral vectors can be challenging. This problem can be partially overcome by dual-AAV systems, where each of the two AAV vector carries a fragment of the large transgene and the two vectors are reassembled to reconstitute the full-length expression cassette in the target cell (Ghosh et al., 2008). Two recent studies used split viral vectors carrying otoferlin cDNA in otoferlin knock-out mice. This led to dual transduction in nearly half of the target IHCs, restoration of protein expression to 30% of wild-type levels, and partial rescue of auditory function (Akil et al., 2019; Al-Moyed et al., 2019). These results provide proof-of-concept evidence that large gene constructs can be transduced to the cochlear sensory epithelium to at least partially restore hearing in animals. The use of different AAV serotypes and variations in injection timing and dosage may further optimize outcomes in the future.

Non-viral Approaches

Non-viral vectors, including liposomes, polymeric nanoparticles, and synthetic peptides, offer a powerful alternative strategy for delivery of therapeutics to the inner ear. Compared to viruses, nanomaterials have several distinct advantages. They can be engineered to precisely target a specific cell subpopulation, exhibit low immunogenicity and toxicity, and multiplex in a high-throughput manner to simultaneously address multiple gene targets and pathways. Nanotechnology tools have been employed extensively in fields such as cancer therapeutics to improve the efficacy and accuracy of delivery of small molecules, biologics, and nucleic acid drugs. Nanomaterial-based cochlear delivery systems using liposomes, peptides, or polymers have been developed in recent years and have shown limited success in applications including genetic hearing loss.

Liposomal agents consisting of cationic lipids, which form a bi-layered structure that protects nucleic acids from degradation and antibody neutralization, have enabled cytosolic delivery of nucleic acids into the cytosol for therapeutic applications. Delivery of cre-recombinase and genome editing agents by lipid complexes resulted in 90% recombination and 20% genomic editing in neonatal mouse OHCs *in vivo* (Zuris et al., 2015). Gao et al. (2018) recently developed cationic lipid nanoparticles that encapsulated CRISPR/Cas-9 complexes targeting the $Tmc1^{Bth}$ allele. In a mouse model of dominant genetic deafness, injection into the cochlea of neonatal mice resulted in moderate reduction of progressive hearing loss and improved hair cell survival *in vivo* (Gao et al., 2018). Of note, Cas9-single guide RNA was coupled to the cationic lipid formulation, Lipofectamine 2000®, an unmodified commercially available lipid transfection reagent that does not have any specificity toward a cell subpopulation. As many commercial lipid-based reagents have been shown to mediate significant non-specific modulation of gene expression and cytotoxicity, further work is needed to optimize the efficacy of delivery and minimize off-target effects (Lv et al., 2006). Furthermore, positively charged lipid nanoparticles could evoke a dramatic pro-inflammatory response marked by upregulation of Th1 cytokines, such as IL-2, IFN-γ, and tumor necrosis factor alpha (TNF-α), when administered systemically into mice (Kedmi et al., 2010). While therapeutics delivered to the cochlea are thought to remain localized to the inner ear and isolated from systemic circulation by the BLB, any immunostimulatory effects through potential systemic exposure could significantly confound the experimental results. Future studies must carefully assess and minimize the effects from off target immune stimulation while maintaining the efficiency and tissue specificity of delivery. Chemical modifications to lipid molecules could be designed in a rational fashion using computational approaches. Furthermore, high-throughput screening technologies of large combinatorial libraries of lipid-like materials should be utilized to identify *in vivo* carriers that specifically target hair cells or supporting cells in the organ of Corti (Whitehead et al., 2014).

A distinct advantage of nanoparticle systems is their "tunability" toward a specific delivery need. By modifying the surface chemistry and altering biophysical properties of nanomaterials, one can optimize inner ear bioavailability, reduce clearance, and improve drug targeting. Polymers such as chitosan-glycerophosphate that slowly degrade over time have been customized to enable the sustained-release of dexamethasone and gentamicin into perilymph over several days in mice (Lajud et al., 2015), and deliver a small molecule to protect mice from noise-induced hearing loss (Kayyali et al., 2018). Elsewhere, targeting ligands such as peptides improved the specificity of nanoparticles toward OHCs (Surovtseva et al., 2012;

Kayyali et al., 2018), spiral ganglion cells (Roy et al., 2010), or cochlear nerve cells (Zhang et al., 2011).

Recently, a new class of peptides carrying short interfering RNAs (siRNA) against TNF-α, known as tumor-penetrating nanocomplexes, was used to actively target primary vestibular schwannoma cultures *in vitro* (Ren et al., 2017). These nanoparticles are based on a new class of tissue-targeting and tumor-penetrating peptides, where the RGD-motif bind to integrins overexpressed on the surface of cancer cells and endothelial cells and subsequently undergo proteolytic processing to unveil a cryptic RXXR domain, which ultimately increases tissue permeability and enables translocation of delivered cargo (Ruoslahti et al., 2010; Liu et al., 2017). By engineering a peptide consisting of a tandem tumor-penetrating and membrane-translocating/siRNA-binding domain, the resulting nanoparticles can penetrate tumor tissue when administered systemically. This platform holds great promise to gain access across the BLB, by increasing the permeability through barriers such as the RWM or oval window. Future work should be directed toward utilizing these novel tumor-penetrating nanomaterials to optimize the *in vivo* delivery of gene editing or gene silencing agents through the RWM.

SURGERIES FOR GENE THERAPY DELIVERY

To obtain surgical access to the inner ear in patients, two principal approaches employed clinically include intra- or trans-tympanic delivery, where the therapeutic is instilled into the middle ear space and allowed to diffuse into the inner ear; and intracochlear delivery, where the drug is introduced directly into the inner ear via the RWM, the oval window, or a semicircular canal (**Figure 1A**). An effective method of delivery suitable for clinical translation should not require extensive surgical dissection while providing sufficient access to the organ of interest in a minimally invasive fashion. If the patient has any residual hearing, the delivery approach should try to preserve it as much as possible. While intravenous or intraperitoneal injections have been the gold standard for treatment of disease processes such as cancer or bacterial sepsis, the unique BLB surrounding the cochlea may make it difficult for drugs to reach the inner ear. Procedures for local delivery employed in animal models include cochleostomy in the lateral wall of the cochlear basal turn, canalostomy in a semicircular canal, or injection through the RWM; while recent studies have shown general safety of these procedures, they have also highlighted the risk of inner ear injury and permanent SNHL. In this section, we review various routes of application of gene therapy agents with a focus on practical applications in patients.

Intratympanic or transtympanic injections are considered generally low risk procedures to access the middle ear space. In adult patients, this can be done under topical anesthesia in the office, where a small portion of the tympanic membrane is anesthetized and up to 0.7 mL of drug can be instilled through the perforation into the middle ear. While technically simple to perform, the drug must remain in contact with the RWM for a prolonged period of time to allow enough drug to cross the RWM (Salt and Plontke, 2009). Equilibration and distribution of the drug toward other middle ear spaces or through the Eustachian tube can lead to significant losses, which can be partially overcome by either sustained release or multiple injections over time. The patient may experience minor temporary discomfort associated with the injection, and rare complications may include otorrhea or persistent TM perforation.

Another approach to access the inner ear is directly through the oval window. Normally, the stapes footplate overlies the oval window, and a mucosal epithelium similar to RWM lines the footplate facing the vestibule (King et al., 2013). In animal models, a significant but variable portion of intratympanically administered small molecule drugs were found to enter the scala vestibuli via the stapes footplate. Gadolinium contrast was found at higher levels in the vestibule than scala tympani after middle ear application. Using quantitative volumetric simulations, up to 90% of gadolinium entered the vestibule through the oval window rather than the RWM in guinea pigs (King et al., 2011). Interestingly for gentamicin, 35% of the drug entered the perilymph via the stapes and its annular ligament, which resulted in higher drug concentrations in the scala vestibuli than scala tympani due to a slower rate of elimination (Salt et al., 2016). In human cadaveric temporal bones, bisphosphonate introduced via the oval window could reach the apical turn of the cochlea (Kang et al., 2016). In patients with otosclerosis, a bone remodeling disease of the otic capsule and one of the most common causes of acquired hearing loss, access to the vestibule and scala vestibuli is possible during stapedotomy where the stapes footplate is fenestrated. Therefore, by incorporating the drug of interest into the prosthesis, the therapeutic can be released in a controlled fashion into the scala vestibuli. The U.S. gene therapy trial of Ad5.GFAP.Hath1 for the treatment of non-genetic hearing loss delivers the viral vector *via* a stapedotomy.

A direct method for accessing the RWM can be achieved through a transcanal surgical procedure. With the advent of novel surgical technologies, it is now possible to directly access the round window niche (RWN) through a transcanal approach in the vast majority of patients using an endoscope. Endoscopic ear surgery not only enables superior visualization of complex landmarks within the middle ear (**Figure 1B**) and mastoid, but also allows specialized, angled instruments to access structures through a transcanal approach (Tarabichi and Kapadia, 2016). In a recent series on round window anatomy, temporal bone studies demonstrated that there is a consistent transcanal angle to reach the RWM perpendicularly through the external auditory canal (EAC), which measured approximately 115-degrees (Fujita et al., 2016). Importantly, one of the key hurdles to reaching the true RWM is obstruction in the RWN by a pseudomembrane, as 72% of temporal bones showed partial or full obstruction, as well as bony overhangs of median length of 1.77 mm which limit the direct access to the RWM (Fujita et al., 2016). In this series, nearly a third of specimens required drilling to expose the entire RWM from the EAC. Therefore, in future studies on cochlear drug delivery, it is critical to ensure that the RWN is drilled away or filled with a drug after removal of

the pseudomembrane so that the drug is in contact with the entirety of the RWM.

The RWM is a three-layered structure lined by squamous epithelium sandwiching a connective tissue layer, which serves as a dynamic barrier that protects the inner ear. A locally administered drug must permeate through the RWM to reach the perilymph within the scala tympani. The permeability of the RWM can be influenced by particle size, charge, and concentration (Goycoolea, 2001), surgical manipulations such as air suctioning nearby (Mikulec et al., 2008), and endotoxins (Ikeda and Morizono, 1988). Conditions such as otitis media that promote middle ear inflammation could also increase RWM permeability through the regulation of cytokines and tight junction proteins (MacArthur et al., 2013). Strategies to artificially enhance transport across the RWM by prolonging the time of exposure to the drug included the use of a gelatin sponge (Jero et al., 2001), thermoreversible hydrogels (Honeder et al., 2015), partial digestion with collagenase (Wang et al., 2012), co-treatment with hyaluronic acid (Shibata et al., 2012), or microperforations (Kelso et al., 2015).

Despite improvements in surgical instrumentation and manipulation of the RWM, the bioavailability of intratympanically administered therapeutics is still remarkably low. In guinea pigs, only 2.5% of gentamicin was present in the cochlear basal turn when it was irrigated across the RWM for nearly 3 h, and only 0.17% when the bulla was instilled with the drug for 2 h (Mikulec et al., 2008). Unfortunately, it is nearly impractical to translate these protocols into clinical use due to the lengthy nature of the protocol. Furthermore, some gene vectors that are designed to efficiently transduce cells of the auditory sensory epithelium *in vitro* may need to be placed in the scala media to be effective. In CI, a growing area of investigation involves using the implant electrode as a conduit for intracochlear delivery of drugs that may rescue hair cell or neuronal damage for hearing preservation. This could be achieved either through incorporation of the drug into the electrode, or co-administration of the therapeutic at the time of cochleostomy. Implantation of electrode arrays coated with fibroblasts over-expressing brain-derived neurotrophic factor (BDNF) or neurotrophin 3 (NT3) may have a protective effect on SGNs (Rejali et al., 2007; Richardson et al., 2009; Pfingst et al., 2017). Pre-treatment with an anti-apoptotic molecule targeting the MAPK/JNK pathway shortly before electrode insertion could protect sensory epithelium in the organ of Corti from insertion trauma and preserve hearing thresholds in guinea pigs (Eshraghi et al., 2013). CI electrodes capable of eluting dexamethasone have been shown to preserve residual hearing and reduce insertion trauma in animal models (Douchement et al., 2015), which may be through reduction of cochlear fibrosis, suppression of local immune reactivity, and global changes in gene expression (Farhadi et al., 2013; Takumi et al., 2014; Wilk et al., 2016). In addition, a phase II multicenter trial in Europe was recently completed to assess the safety and efficacy of intratympanic steroids during CI (EudraCT Number: 2015-002672-25). Future implants may be optimized through the incorporation of gene delivery vectors targeting sensory cells within the scala tympani or SGNs.

TECHNICAL CONSIDERATIONS

The human middle ear and inner ear are both exquisitely well-balanced systems so that small perturbations of the microenvironment, such as the introduction of drugs and their respective delivery agents through microsurgical manipulations, could have significant effects on the homeostasis of the entire system. While animal models offer invaluable insight in predicting drug pharmacokinetics and pharmacodynamics for preclinical studies, the translation into clinical testing in patients typically presents with additional challenges owing to differences in the volume and anatomy of inner ear organs. The cochlear aqueduct, a bony channel that projects from the posterior fossa to the cochlear basal turn (**Figure 1A**), is typically obliterated in humans but widely patent in rodents. The patency of the duct has been attributed to one of the mechanisms by which drugs reach the contralateral ear in the so-called "Schreiner effect" (Stover et al., 2000). Sampling of perilymph via the RWM in rodents could lead to contamination with CSF across the cochlear aqueduct at a significant rate of 0.5–2 μL/min (Hirose et al., 2014). Rodent perilymph samples >5 μL could contain as high as 80% of CSF in guinea pigs (Salt et al., 2003). Therefore, perforation of the RWM could result in artifactual CSF flow near the basal turn, thereby displacing the drug within minutes of application. This loss can be greater if the site of injection is not completely sealed. As such, one must consider both the technique of injection and any attempts in preventing contamination when evaluating the efficacy of inner ear drug delivery agents.

In addition, the effective concentration of the drug is likely also dependent on the rate and volume of injection into the perilymph. A low rate of injection (100 nL/min) over a prolonged period of time is required to drive the drug into perilymph while minimizing traumatic perturbations to the inner ear (Salt and Rask-Andersen, 2004). In guinea pigs, without a proper seal around the injector, leakage of perilymph around the pipette resulted in wash-out of the drug by over 60% at a rate of approximately 0.09 μL/min. This loss could be mitigated by the application of hyaluronate gels over the RWM (Salt et al., 2007). Recently, Salt et al. (2017) investigated the concentration gradient along the scala tympani of a model drug (FITC-dextran) delivered via a pump incorporated into a cochlear implant in guinea pigs. A significant concentration gradient was observed despite a prolonged duration of injection of 24 h, and fluid leakage at the site of cochleostomy could lead to significant drug wash-out (Salt et al., 2017). These results highlight the importance of technical considerations when delivering drugs to the inner ear. In patients, the volume of scala tympani is significantly larger than rodents, and small volume perturbations will likely have less impact on the distribution of drugs. Furthermore, the patency of the cochlear aqueduct is reduced, and CSF pressure is typically negative when the patient is sitting when procedure is performed in the clinic. As a result, displacement of the drug either via CSF influx or leakage through cochleostomy may occur at a substantially lower rate in humans than rodents. Nevertheless, a systematic, quantitative approach is paramount when designing delivery systems for clinical applications to achieve reliable and consistent results.

FUTURE OUTLOOK

Since the first human gene therapy treatment in 1990, there have been 2930 gene therapy clinical trials that have been completed, were ongoing, or clinically approved world-wide. Over two-thirds of the trials were conducted in the United States (Hanna et al., 2016). There is also a steady increase in the number of newly approved/initiated trials over time, with 163 trials in 2015 alone and nearly 600 more trials since 2015. Adeno-associated viral vectors were utilized in 8.1% of the trials to date[2].

Currently, over 20 clinical trials for hearing loss therapies are ongoing in the United States with six potential therapeutic molecules; one of these trials involves gene therapy. There are over 80 active trials in Europe, Asia, and Australia with many more candidate drugs being actively investigated. Preliminary results should be available within the next 2 years, and other platforms are currently being tested in early clinical studies with numerous drugs on the horizon. If early results meet the specified efficacy endpoints, the inclusion criteria will likely see an expansion to other patient populations such as children with early or congenital SNHL. On the contrary, if results from these trials do not meet criteria in the treated population, meticulous follow-up studies must be carried out to determine the cause of failure, which may include patient stratification, route of delivery, and measurement of outcomes. Ultimately, the successful translation of a novel therapeutic from the laboratory bench to the otology clinic or operating room require a multidisciplinary approach through the collaboration between molecular biologists, virologists, chemists, biomedical engineers, otologic surgeons, government, and business leaders.

As treatments for hearing loss become more personalized, more gene targets that are amenable to targeting will be uncovered. Gene therapy can involve not only the insertion of a transgene through efficient viral transduction, but also silencing of a dominant negative allele through miRNA or siRNAs. Off-target effects will be minimized through enhancing the specificity of therapy. Next-generation CRISPR-Cas systems will be harnessed for precise disruption and editing of DNA or RNA for each patient.

The efficacy and specificity of the gene delivery agent will also likely improve. Engineering of the capsid proteins may further improve viral tropism so that viruses can be tuned to preferentially target the cell subpopulation in the sensory epithelium while minimizing off-target effects. Incorporating cell type-specific promoters will enable the precise targeting and gene expression in cellular subpopulations within the cochlea. Simultaneous testing in animal models and humans will highlight differences between the two, and obstacles such as viral immunogenicity can be addressed. Active, or membrane-penetrating delivery platforms may provide a method to traverse cellular tight junctions (Ruoslahti, 2017). This may significantly enhance the bioavailability of the drug if hearing is not impaired. Finally, deployment of "smart," on-demand drug delivery systems may further improve drug availability by fine-tuning the release kinetics and minimizing drug loss.

Future surgical innovations and technologies could help better detect electrophysiological changes in the inner ear associated with therapeutic interventions. Electrocochleography studies could provide insight into cochlear changes in real time during an implant and predict hearing thresholds postoperatively, and may be utilized to monitor inner ear physiology and minimize the risk of cochlear damage during electrode insertion or infusion of gene delivery vectors (Dalbert et al., 2018). More sophisticated electrodes are being developed to incorporate neuroprotective substances and drugs. The incorporation of microsurgical and robotic tools in otologic and neurotologic surgeries could make surgeries more precise, less traumatic, and customized to each patient's unique anatomy.

Current assessments of hearing levels largely rely on indirect measurements such as audiograms, otoacoustic emissions, or auditory brainstem responses. *Post mortem* temporal bone histology has been the gold standard to visualize the pathology underlying hearing loss. However, the advent of intracochlear imaging has been challenging due to the complex three-dimensional anatomy and complete encasement in the bony otic capsule. Future development of tools to non- or minimally invasively assess the function of the inner ear at a cellular resolution will likely revolutionize the way hearing loss is diagnosed and treated. Optical coherence tomography (Dong et al., 2018), micro optical coherence tomography (Iyer et al., 2016), and two photon fluorescence imaging (Yang et al., 2013) have the potential to visualize cochlear microanatomy at high resolution, thus overcoming limitations of bright field endoscopy (Chole, 2015). While synchrotron radiation phase contrast imaging reveals intracochlear microanatomy through the encased bone, future work is needed to minimize radiation energy before this technology can be translated to the clinic (Iyer et al., 2018). In the meantime, light sheet microscopy (Santi, 2011) and incorporation of calcium- or potassium-based molecular imaging markers may shed additional light on the integrity and function of hair cells and other cochlear cells in real time. Together, by taking an interdisciplinary approach and combining new genomic data, better bioengineering tools, and innovative surgical approaches, clinical success for gene therapy for SNHL and inner ear disease is not far away.

AUTHOR CONTRIBUTIONS

YR, LDL, and KMS designed the study and conducted the research and literature search. YR and KMS prepared the manuscript. All authors edited and approved the final manuscript.

[2]http://www.abedia.com/wiley/vectors.php

REFERENCES

Ahmed, H., Shubina-Oleinik, O., and Holt, J. R. (2017). Emerging gene therapies for genetic hearing loss. *J. Assoc. Res. Otolaryngol.* 18, 649–670. doi: 10.1007/s10162-017-0634-638

Akil, O., Dyka, F., Calvet, C., Emptoz, A., Lahlou, G., Nouaille, S., et al. (2019). Dual AAV-mediated gene therapy restores hearing in a DFNB9 mouse model. *Proc. Natl. Acad. Sci. U.S.A.* 116, 4496–4501. doi: 10.1073/pnas.1817537116

Akil, O., Seal, R. P., Burke, K., Wang, C., Alemi, A., During, M., et al. (2012). Restoration of hearing in the VGLUT3 knockout mouse using virally mediated gene therapy. *Neuron* 75, 283–293. doi: 10.1016/j.neuron.2012.05.019

Al-Moyed, H., Cepeda, A. P., Jung, S., Moser, T., Kügler, S., and Reisinger, E. (2019). A dual-AAV approach restores fast exocytosis and partially rescues auditory function in deaf otoferlin knock-out mice. *EMBO Mol. Med.* 11:e9396. doi: 10.15252/emmm.201809396

Askew, C., Rochat, C., Pan, B., Asai, Y., Ahmed, H., Child, E., et al. (2015). Tmc gene therapy restores auditory function in deaf mice. *Sci. Transl. Med.* 7:295ra108. doi: 10.1126/scitranslmed.aab1996

Axelsson, A. (1988). Comparative anatomy of cochlear blood vessels. *Am. J. Otolaryngol.* 9, 278–290. doi: 10.1016/s0196-0709(88)80036-x

Bainbridge, J. W. B., Mehat, M. S., Sundaram, V., Robbie, S. J., Barker, S. E., Ripamonti, C., et al. (2015). Long-term effect of gene therapy on Leber's congenital amaurosis. *N. Engl. J. Med.* 372, 1887–1897. doi: 10.1056/NEJMoa1414221

Banks, W. A. (2016). From blood–brain barrier to blood–brain interface: new opportunities for CNS drug delivery. *Nat. Rev. Drug Discov.* 15, 275–292. doi: 10.1038/nrd.2015.21

Budenz, C. L., Wong, H. T., Swiderski, D. L., Shibata, S. B., Pfingst, B. E., and Raphael, Y. (2015). Differential effects of AAV.*BDNF and AAV.Ntf*3 in the deafened adult guinea pig ear. *Sci. Rep.* 5:8619. doi: 10.1038/srep08619

Chang, K. W. (2015). Genetics of hearing loss—nonsyndromic. *Otolaryngol. Clin. North Am.* 48, 1063–1072. doi: 10.1016/j.otc.2015.06.005

Chang, Q., Wang, J., Li, Q., Kim, Y., Zhou, B., Wang, Y., et al. (2015). Virally mediated Kcnq1 gene replacement therapy in the immature scala media restores hearing in a mouse model of human Jervell and Lange-Nielsen deafness syndrome. *EMBO Mol. Med.* 7, 1077–1086. doi: 10.15252/emmm.201404929

Chien, W. W., McDougald, D. S., Roy, S., Fitzgerald, T. S., and Cunningham, L. L. (2015). Cochlear gene transfer mediated by adeno-associated virus: comparison of two surgical approaches. *Laryngoscope* 125, 2557–2564. doi: 10.1002/lary.25317

Chole, R. A. (2015). Endoscopic view of the scala tympani. *Otol. Neurotol.* 36, e97–e98. doi: 10.1097/MAO.0000000000000365

Cotanche, D. A., and Kaiser, C. L. (2010). Hair cell fate decisions in cochlear development and regeneration. *Hear. Res.* 266, 18–25. doi: 10.1016/j.heares.2010.04.012

Dai, C., Lehar, M., Sun, D. Q., Rvt, L. S., Carey, J. P., MacLachlan, T., et al. (2017). Rhesus cochlear and vestibular functions are preserved after inner ear injection of saline volume sufficient for gene therapy delivery. *J. Assoc. Res. Otolaryngol.* 18, 601–617. doi: 10.1007/s10162-017-0628-626

Dalbert, A., Pfiffner, F., Hoesli, M., Koka, K., Veraguth, D., Roosli, C., et al. (2018). Assessment of cochlear function during cochlear implantation by extra- and intracochlear electrocochleography. *Front. Neurosci.* 12:18. doi: 10.3389/fnins.2018.00018

Dalkara, D., Goureau, O., Marazova, K., and Sahel, J.-A. (2016). Let there be light: gene and cell therapy for blindness. *Hum. Gene Ther.* 27, 134–147. doi: 10.1089/hum.2015.147

Daudet, N., Gibson, R., Shang, J., Bernard, A., Lewis, J., and Stone, J. (2009). Notch regulation of progenitor cell behavior in quiescent and regenerating auditory epithelium of mature birds. *Dev. Biol.* 326, 86–100. doi: 10.1016/j.ydbio.2008.10.033

Devare, J., Gubbels, S., and Raphael, Y. (2018). Outlook and future of inner ear therapy. *Hear. Res.* 368, 127–135. doi: 10.1016/j.heares.2018.05.009

Dong, W., Xia, A., Raphael, P. D., Puria, S., Applegate, B., and Oghalai, J. S. (2018). Organ of Corti vibration within the intact gerbil cochlea measured by volumetric optical coherence tomography and vibrometry. *J. Neurophysiol.* 120, 2847–2857. doi: 10.1152/jn.00702.2017

Douchement, D., Terranti, A., Lamblin, J., Salleron, J., Siepmann, F., Siepmann, J., et al. (2015). Dexamethasone eluting electrodes for cochlear implantation: effect on residual hearing. *Cochlear Implants Int.* 16, 195–200. doi: 10.1179/1754762813Y.0000000053

Dror, A. A., and Avraham, K. B. (2010). Hearing impairment: a panoply of genes and functions. *Neuron* 68, 293–308. doi: 10.1016/j.neuron.2010.10.011

Ekdale, E. G. (2013). Comparative anatomy of the Bony Labyrinth (Inner Ear) of placental mammals. *PLoS One* 8:e66624. doi: 10.1371/journal.pone.0066624

Eshraghi, A. A., Gupta, C., Van De Water, T. R., Bohorquez, J. E., Garnham, C., Bas, E., et al. (2013). Molecular mechanisms involved in cochlear implantation trauma and the protection of hearing and auditory sensory cells by inhibition of c-jun-N-terminal kinase signaling. *Laryngoscope* 123, S1–S14. doi: 10.1002/lary.23902

Farhadi, M., Jalessi, M., Salehian, P., Ghavi, F. F., Emamjomeh, H., Mirzadeh, H., et al. (2013). Dexamethasone eluting cochlear implant: histological study in animal model. *Cochlear Implants Int.* 14, 45–50. doi: 10.1179/1754762811Y.0000000024

Fujita, T., Shin, J. E., Cunnane, M., Fujita, K., Henein, S., Psaltis, D., et al. (2016). Surgical anatomy of the human round window region: implication for cochlear endoscopy through the external auditory canal. *Otol. Neurotol.* 37, 1189–1194. doi: 10.1097/MAO.0000000000001074

Gao, X., Tao, Y., Lamas, V., Huang, M., Yeh, W.-H., Pan, B., et al. (2018). Treatment of autosomal dominant hearing loss by in vivo delivery of genome editing agents. *Nature* 553, 217–221. doi: 10.1038/nature25164

Ghosh, A., Yue, Y., Lai, Y., and Duan, D. (2008). A hybrid vector system expands adeno-associated viral vector packaging capacity in a transgene-independent manner. *Mol. Therapy* 16, 124–130. doi: 10.1038/sj.mt.6300322

Gorlin, R. J., Gorlin, R. J., Toriello, H. V., and Cohen, M. M. (1995). *Hereditary Hearing Loss and Its Syndromes*. New York, NY: Oxford University Press.

Goycoolea, M. V. (2001). Clinical aspects of round window membrane permeability under normal and pathological conditions. *Acta Oto Laryngologica* 121, 437–447. doi: 10.1080/000164801300366552

Guo, J.-Y., He, L., Qu, T.-F., Liu, Y.-Y., Liu, K., Wang, G.-P., et al. (2018). Canalostomy as a surgical approach to local drug delivery into the inner ears of adult and neonatal mice*. *J. Vis. Exp.* e57351. doi: 10.3791/57351

György, B., Meijer, E. J., Ivanchenko, M. V., Tenneson, K., Emond, F., Hanlon, K. S., et al. (2019). Gene transfer with AAV9-PHP.B rescues hearing in a mouse model of usher syndrome 3A and transduces hair cells in a non-human primate. *Mol. Ther. Methods Clin. Dev.* 13, 1–13. doi: 10.1016/j.omtm.2018.11.003

Hanna, E., Rémuzat, C., Auquier, P., and Toumi, M. (2016). Advanced therapy medicinal products: current and future perspectives. *J. Mark Access Health Policy* 4:31036. doi: 10.3402/jmahp.v4.31036

Hirose, K., Hartsock, J. J., Johnson, S., Santi, P., and Salt, A. N. (2014). Systemic lipopolysaccharide compromises the blood-labyrinth barrier and increases entry of serum fluorescein into the perilymph. *J. Assoc. Res. Otolaryngol.* 15, 707–719. doi: 10.1007/s10162-014-0476-476

Hirose, K., and Li, S.-Z. (2019). The role of monocytes and macrophages in the dynamic permeability of the blood-perilymph barrier. *Hear. Res.* 374, 49–57. doi: 10.1016/j.heares.2019.01.006

Honeder, C., Landegger, L. D., Engleder, E., Gabor, F., Plasenzotti, R., Plenk, H., et al. (2015). Effects of intraoperatively applied glucocorticoid hydrogels on residual hearing and foreign body reaction in a guinea pig model of cochlear implantation. *Acta Oto Laryngol.* 135, 313–319. doi: 10.3109/00016489.2014.986758

Husseman, J., and Raphael, Y. (2009). Gene therapy in the inner ear using adenovirus vectors. *Adv. Otorhinolaryngol.* 66, 37–51. doi: 10.1159/000218206

Ikeda, K., and Morizono, T. (1988). Changes of the permeability of round window membrane in otitis media. *Arch. Otolaryngol. Head Neck Surg.* 114, 895–897. doi: 10.1001/archotol.1988.01860200079023

Isgrig, K., McDougald, D. S., Zhu, J., Wang, H. J., Bennett, J., and Chien, W. W. (2019). AAV2.7*m*8 is a powerful viral vector for inner ear gene therapy. *Nat. Commun.* 10:427. doi: 10.1038/s41467-018-08243-8241

Isgrig, K., Shteamer, J. W., Belyantseva, I. A., Drummond, M. C., Fitzgerald, T. S., Vijayakumar, S., et al. (2017). Gene therapy restores balance and auditory functions in a mouse model of usher syndrome. *Mol. Ther.* 25, 780–791. doi: 10.1016/j.ymthe.2017.01.007

Iyer, J. S., Batts, S. A., Chu, K. K., Sahin, M. I., Leung, H. M., Tearney, G. J., et al. (2016). Micro-optical coherence tomography of the mammalian cochlea. *Sci. Rep.* 6:33288. doi: 10.1038/srep33288

Iyer, J. S., Zhu, N., Gasilov, S., Ladak, H. M., Agrawal, S. K., and Stankovic, K. M. (2018). Visualizing the 3D cytoarchitecture of the human cochlea in an intact temporal bone using synchrotron radiation phase contrast imaging. *Biomed. Opt. Express* 9, 3757–3767. doi: 10.1364/BOE.9.003757

Jawadi, Z., Applegate, B. E., and Oghalai, J. S. (2016). Optical coherence tomography to measure sound-induced motions within the mouse organ of corti in vivo. *Methods Mol. Biol.* 1427, 449–462. doi: 10.1007/978-1-4939-3615-1_24

Jero, J., Mhatre, A. N., Tseng, C. J., Stern, R. E., Coling, D. E., Goldstein, J. A., et al. (2001). Cochlear gene delivery through an intact round window membrane in mouse. *Hum. Gene Ther.* 12, 539–548. doi: 10.1089/104303401300042465

Kang, W. S., Nguyen, K., McKenna, C. E., Sewell, W. F., McKenna, M. J., and Jung, D. H. (2016). Intracochlear drug delivery through the oval window in fresh cadaveric human temporal bones. *Otol. Neurotol.* 37, 218–222. doi: 10.1097/MAO.0000000000000964

Kayyali, M. N., Wooltorton, J. R. A., Ramsey, A. J., Lin, M., Chao, T. N., Tsourkas, A., et al. (2018). A novel nanoparticle delivery system for targeted therapy of noise-induced hearing loss. *J. Control. Release* 279, 243–250. doi: 10.1016/j.jconrel.2018.04.028

Kedmi, R., Ben-Arie, N., and Peer, D. (2010). The systemic toxicity of positively charged lipid nanoparticles and the role of Toll-like receptor 4 in immune activation. *Biomaterials* 31, 6867–6875. doi: 10.1016/j.biomaterials.2010.05.027

Kelso, C. M., Watanabe, H., Wazen, J. M., Bucher, T., Qian, Z. J., Olson, E. S., et al. (2015). Microperforations significantly enhance diffusion across round window membrane. *Otol. Neurotol.* 36, 694–700. doi: 10.1097/MAO.0000000000000629

Kiernan, A. E., and Fekete, D. M. (1997). In vivo gene transfer into the embryonic inner ear using retroviral vectors. *Audiol. Neurotol.* 2, 12–24. doi: 10.1159/000259226

Kilpatrick, L. A., Li, Q., Yang, J., Goddard, J. C., Fekete, D. M., and Lang, H. (2011). Adeno-associated virus-mediated gene delivery into the scala media of the normal and deafened adult mouse ear. *Gene Ther.* 18, 569–578. doi: 10.1038/gt.2010.175

King, E. B., Salt, A. N., Eastwood, H. T., and O'Leary, S. J. (2011). Direct entry of gadolinium into the vestibule following intratympanic applications in guinea pigs and the influence of cochlear implantation. *J. Assoc. Res. Otolaryngol.* 12, 741–751. doi: 10.1007/s10162-011-0280-285

King, M. D., Alleyne, C. H. J., and Dhandapani, K. M. (2013). TNF-alpha receptor antagonist, R-7050, improves neurological outcomes following intracerebral hemorrhage in mice. *Neurosci. Lett.* 542, 92–96. doi: 10.1016/j.neulet.2013.02.051

Kopke, R., Allen, K. A., Henderson, D., Hoffer, M., Frenz, D., and Van de Water, T. (1999). A radical demise. *Toxins and trauma* share common pathways in hair cell death. *Ann. N. Y. Acad. Sci.* 884, 171–191. doi: 10.1111/j.1749-6632.1999.tb08641.x

Kwon, E. J., Skalak, M., Lo Bu, R., and Bhatia, S. N. (2016). Neuron-targeted nanoparticle for siRNA delivery to traumatic brain injuries. *ACS Nano* 10, 7926–7933. doi: 10.1021/acsnano.6b03858

Lajud, S. A., Nagda, D. A., Qiao, P., Tanaka, N., Civantos, A., Gu, R., et al. (2015). A novel chitosan-hydrogel-based nanoparticle delivery system for local inner ear application. *Otol. Neurotol.* 36, 341–347. doi: 10.1097/MAO.0000000000000445

Landegger, L. D., Pan, B., Askew, C., Wassmer, S. J., Gluck, S. D., Galvin, A., et al. (2017). A synthetic AAV vector enables safe and efficient gene transfer to the mammalian inner ear. *Nat. Biotechnol.* 35, 280–284. doi: 10.1038/nbt.3781

Lee, M. Y., Kurioka, T., Nelson, M. M., Prieskorn, D. M., Swiderski, D. L., Takada, Y., et al. (2016). Viral-mediated Ntf3 overexpression disrupts innervation and hearing in nondeafened guinea pig cochleae. *Mol. Ther. Methods Clin. Dev.* 3:16052. doi: 10.1038/mtm.2016.52

Lim, D. J., and Hussl, B. (1975). Macromolecular transport by the middle ear and its lymphatic system. *Acta Oto Laryngol.* 80, 19–31. doi: 10.3109/00016487509121296

Lin, F. R., Thorpe, R., Gordon-Salant, S., and Ferrucci, L. (2011). Hearing loss prevalence and risk factors among older adults in the United States. *J. Gerontol. A Biol. Sci. Med. Sci.* 66A, 582–590. doi: 10.1093/gerona/glr002

Liu, X., Lin, P., Perrett, I., Lin, J., Liao, Y.-P., Chang, C. H., et al. (2017). Tumor-penetrating peptide enhances transcytosis of silicasome-based chemotherapy for pancreatic cancer. *J. Clin. Invest.* 127, 2007–2018. doi: 10.1172/JCI92284

Louis Jeune, V., Joergensen, J. A., Hajjar, R. J., and Weber, T. (2013). Pre-existing anti-adeno-associated virus antibodies as a challenge in AAV gene therapy. *Hum. Gene. Ther. Methods* 24, 59–67. doi: 10.1089/hgtb.2012.243

Lustig, L., and Akil, O. (2018). Cochlear gene therapy. *Cold Spring Harb. Perspect. Med.* a033191. doi: 10.1101/cshperspect.a033191

Lv, H., Zhang, S., Wang, B., Cui, S., and Yan, J. (2006). Toxicity of cationic lipids and cationic polymers in gene delivery. *J. Control. Release* 114, 100–109. doi: 10.1016/j.jconrel.2006.04.014

MacArthur, C. J., Hausman, F., Kempton, J. B., Sautter, N., and Trune, D. R. (2013). Inner ear tissue remodeling and ion homeostasis gene alteration in murine chronic otitis media. *Otol. Neurotol.* 34, 338–346. doi: 10.1097/MAO.0b013e31827b4d0a

Manoussaki, D., Dimitriadis, E. K., and Chadwick, R. S. (2006). Cochlea's graded curvature effect on low frequency waves. *Phys. Rev. Lett.* 96:088701. doi: 10.1103/PhysRevLett.96.088701

Mikulec, A. A., Hartsock, J. J., and Salt, A. N. (2008). Permeability of the round window membrane is influenced by the composition of applied drug solutions and by common surgical procedures. *Otol. Neurotol.* 29, 1020–1026. doi: 10.1097/MAO.0b013e31818658ea

Mikulec, A. A., Plontke, S. K., Hartsock, J. J., and Salt, A. N. (2009). Entry of substances into perilymph through the bone of the otic capsule after intratympanic applications in guinea pigs: implications for local drug delivery in humans. *Otol. Neurotol.* 30, 131–138. doi: 10.1097/mao.0b013e318191bff8

Nist-Lund, C. A., Pan, B., Patterson, A., Asai, Y., Chen, T., Zhou, W., et al. (2019). Improved TMC1 gene therapy restores hearing and balance in mice with genetic inner ear disorders. *Nat. Commun.* 10:236. doi: 10.1038/s41467-018-08264-w

Pan, B., Askew, C., Galvin, A., Heman-Ackah, S., Asai, Y., Indzhykulian, A. A., et al. (2017). Gene therapy restores auditory and vestibular function in a mouse model of Usher syndrome type 1c. *Nat. Biotechnol.* 35, 264–272. doi: 10.1038/nbt.3801

Pardridge, W. M. (2016). CSF, blood-brain barrier, and brain drug delivery. *Expert. Opin. Drug Deliv.* 13, 963–975. doi: 10.1517/17425247.2016.1171315

Pfingst, B. E., Colesa, D. J., Swiderski, D. L., Hughes, A. P., Strahl, S. B., Sinan, M., et al. (2017). Neurotrophin gene therapy in deafened ears with cochlear implants: long-term effects on nerve survival and functional measures. *J. Assoc. Res. Otolaryngol.* 18, 731–750. doi: 10.1007/s10162-017-0633-639

Pietola, L., Aarnisalo, A. A., Joensuu, J., Pellinen, R., Wahlfors, J., and Jero, J. (2008). HOX-GFP and WOX-GFP lentivirus vectors for inner ear gene transfer. *Acta Oto Laryngol.* 128, 613–620. doi: 10.1080/00016480701663409

Rejali, D., Lee, V. A., Abrashkin, K. A., Humayun, N., Swiderski, D. L., and Raphael, Y. (2007). Cochlear implants and ex vivo BDNF gene therapy protect spiral ganglion neurons. *Hear. Res.* 228, 180–187. doi: 10.1016/j.heares.2007.02.010

Ren, Y., Cheung, H. W., von Maltzhan, G., Agrawal, A., Cowley, G. S., Weir, B. A., et al. (2012). Targeted tumor-penetrating siRNA nanocomplexes for credentialing the ovarian cancer oncogene ID4. *Sci. Transl. Med.* 4:147ra112. doi: 10.1126/scitranslmed.3003778

Ren, Y., Sagers, J. E., Landegger, L. D., Bhatia, S. N., and Stankovic, K. M. (2017). Tumor-penetrating delivery of siRNA against TNFα to human vestibular schwannomas. *Sci. Rep.* 7:12922. doi: 10.1038/s41598-017-13032-13039

Richardson, R. T., Wise, A. K., Thompson, B. C., Flynn, B. O., Atkinson, P. J., Fretwell, N. J., et al. (2009). Polypyrrole-coated electrodes for the delivery of charge and neurotrophins to cochlear neurons. *Biomaterials* 30, 2614–2624. doi: 10.1016/j.biomaterials.2009.01.015

Roy, S., Johnston, A. H., Newman, T. A., Glueckert, R., Dudas, J., Bitsche, M., et al. (2010). Cell-specific targeting in the mouse inner ear using nanoparticles conjugated with a neurotrophin-derived peptide ligand: potential tool for drug delivery. *Int. J. Pharm.* 390, 214–224. doi: 10.1016/j.ijpharm.2010.02.003

Rubel, E. W., and Fritzsch, B. (2002). Auditory system development: primary auditory neurons and their targets. *Annu. Rev. Neurosci.* 25, 51–101. doi: 10.1146/annurev.neuro.25.112701.142849

Ruoslahti, E. (2017). Tumor penetrating peptides for improved drug delivery. *Adv. Drug Deliv. Rev.* 110-111, 3–12. doi: 10.1016/j.addr.2016.03.008

Ruoslahti, E., Bhatia, S. N., and Sailor, M. J. (2010). Targeting of drugs and nanoparticles to tumors. *J. Cell Biol.* 188, 759–768. doi: 10.1083/jcb.200910104

Salt, A., Hartsock, J., Gill, R., Smyth, D., Kirk, J., and Verhoeven, K. (2017). Perilymph pharmacokinetics of marker applied through a cochlear implant in guinea pigs. *PLoS One* 12:e0183374. doi: 10.1371/journal.pone.0183374

Salt, A. N., Hartsock, J. J., Gill, R. M., King, E., Kraus, F. B., and Plontke, S. K. (2016). Perilymph pharmacokinetics of locally-applied gentamicin in the guinea pig. *Hear. Res.* 342, 101–111. doi: 10.1016/j.heares.2016.10.003

Salt, A. N., and Hirose, K. (2018). Communication pathways to and from the inner ear and their contributions to drug delivery. *Hear. Res.* 362, 25–37. doi: 10.1016/j.heares.2017.12.010

Salt, A. N., Kellner, C., and Hale, S. (2003). Contamination of perilymph sampled from the basal cochlear turn with cerebrospinal fluid. *Hear. Res.* 182, 24–33. doi: 10.1016/s0378-5955(03)00137-0

Salt, A. N., and Plontke, S. K. (2009). Principles of local drug delivery to the inner ear. *Audiol. Neurotol.* 14, 350–360. doi: 10.1159/000241892

Salt, A. N., and Rask-Andersen, H. (2004). Responses of the endolymphatic sac to perilymphatic injections and withdrawals: evidence for the presence of a one-way valve. *Hear. Res.* 191, 90–100. doi: 10.1016/j.heares.2003.12.018

Salt, A. N., Sirjani, D. B., Hartsock, J. J., Gill, R. M., and Plontke, S. K. (2007). Marker retention in the cochlea following injections through the round window membrane. *Hear. Res.* 232, 78–86. doi: 10.1016/j.heares.2007.06.010

Santi, P. A. (2011). Light sheet fluorescence microscopy: a review. *J. Histochem. Cytochem.* 59, 129–138. doi: 10.1369/0022155410394857

Sheffield, A. M., and Smith, R. J. H. (2018). The epidemiology of deafness. *Cold Spring Harb Perspect Med.* a033258. doi: 10.1101/cshperspect.a033258 [Epub ahead of print].

Shibata, S. B., Cortez, S. R., Wiler, J. A., Swiderski, D. L., and Raphael, Y. (2012). Hyaluronic acid enhances gene delivery into the cochlea. *Hum. Gene Ther.* 23, 302–310. doi: 10.1089/hum.2011.086

Shibata, S. B., Di Pasquale, G., Cortez, S. R., Chiorini, J. A., and Raphael, Y. (2009). Gene transfer using bovine adeno-associated virus in the guinea pig cochlea. *Gene Ther.* 16, 990–997. doi: 10.1038/gt.2009.57

Shu, Y., Tao, Y., Wang, Z., Tang, Y., Li, H., Dai, P., et al. (2016). Identification of adeno-associated viral vectors that target neonatal and adult mammalian inner ear cell subtypes. *Hum. Gene Ther.* 27, 687–699. doi: 10.1089/hum.2016.053

Smith, N. M., Gachulincova, I., Ho, D., Bailey, C., Bartlett, C. A., Norret, M., et al. (2016). An unexpected transient breakdown of the blood brain barrier triggers passage of large intravenously administered nanoparticles. *Sci. Rep.* 6:22595. doi: 10.1038/srep22595

Stamatiou, G. A., and Stankovic, K. M. (2013). A comprehensive network and pathway analysis of human deafness genes. *Otol. Neurotol.* 34, 961–970. doi: 10.1097/MAO.0b013e3182898272

Stover, T., Yagi, M., and Raphael, Y. (2000). Transduction of the contralateral ear after adenovirus-mediated cochlear gene transfer. *Gene Ther.* 7, 377–383. doi: 10.1038/sj.gt.3301108

Surovtseva, E. V., Johnston, A. H., Zhang, W., Zhang, Y., Kim, A., Murakoshi, M., et al. (2012). Prestin binding peptides as ligands for targeted polymersome mediated drug delivery to outer hair cells in the inner ear. *Int. J. Pharm.* 424, 121–127. doi: 10.1016/j.ijpharm.2011.12.042

Suzuki, J., Hashimoto, K., Xiao, R., Vandenberghe, L. H., and Liberman, M. C. (2017). Cochlear gene therapy with ancestral AAV in adult mice: complete transduction of inner hair cells without cochlear dysfunction. *Sci. Rep.* 7:45524. doi: 10.1038/srep45524

Suzuki, M., Yamasoba, T., Ishibashi, T., Miller, J. M., and Kaga, K. (2002). Effect of noise exposure on blood-labyrinth barrier in guinea pigs. *Hear. Res.* 164, 12–18. doi: 10.1016/s0378-5955(01)00397-5

Takumi, Y., Nishio, S.-Y., Mugridge, K., Oguchi, T., Hashimoto, S., Suzuki, N., et al. (2014). Gene expression pattern after insertion of dexamethasone-eluting electrode into the guinea pig cochlea. *PLoS One* 9:e110238. doi: 10.1371/journal.pone.0110238

Tao, Y., Huang, M., Shu, Y., Ruprecht, A., Wang, H., Tang, Y., et al. (2018). Delivery of adeno-associated virus vectors in adult mammalian inner-ear cell subtypes without auditory dysfunction. *Hum. Gene Ther.* 29, 492–506. doi: 10.1089/hum.2017.120

Tarabichi, M., and Kapadia, M. (2016). Principles of endoscopic ear surgery. *Curr. Opin. Otolaryngol. Head Neck Surg.* 24, 382–387. doi: 10.1097/MOO.0000000000000296

Wang, H., Murphy, R., Taaffe, D., Yin, S., Xia, L., Hauswirth, W. W., et al. (2012). Efficient cochlear gene transfection in guinea-pigs with adeno-associated viral vectors by partial digestion of round window membrane. *Gene Ther.* 19, 255–263. doi: 10.1038/gt.2011.91

Whitehead, K. A., Dorkin, J. R., Vegas, A. J., Chang, P. H., Veiseh, O., Matthews, J., et al. (2014). Degradable lipid nanoparticles with predictable in vivo siRNA delivery activity. *Nat. Commun.* 5:4277. doi: 10.1038/ncomms5277

Wilk, M., Hessler, R., Mugridge, K., Jolly, C., Fehr, M., Lenarz, T., et al. (2016). Impedance changes and fibrous tissue growth after cochlear implantation are correlated and can be reduced using a Dexamethasone eluting electrode. *PLoS One* 11:e0147552. doi: 10.1371/journal.pone.0147552

Yang, X., Pu, Y., Hsieh, C.-L., Ong, C. A., Psaltis, D., and Stankovic, K. M. (2013). Two-photon microscopy of the mouse cochlea in situ for cellular diagnosis. *J. Biomed. Opt.* 18:31104. doi: 10.1117/1.JBO.18.3.031104

Yoshimura, H., Shibata, S. B., Ranum, P. T., and Smith, R. J. H. (2018). Enhanced viral-mediated cochlear gene delivery in adult mice by combining canal fenestration with round window membrane inoculation. *Sci. Rep.* 8:2980. doi: 10.1038/s41598-018-21233-z

Zhang, H., Pan, H., Zhou, C., Wei, Y., Ying, W., Li, S., et al. (2018). Simultaneous zygotic inactivation of multiple genes in mouse through CRISPR/Cas9-mediated base editing. *Development* 145:dev168906. doi: 10.1242/dev.168906

Zhang, W., Zhang, Y., Löbler, M., Schmitz, K.-P., Ahmad, A., Pyykkö, I., et al. (2011). Nuclear entry of hyperbranched polylysine nanoparticles into cochlear cells. *Int. J. Nanomed.* 6, 535–546. doi: 10.2147/IJN.S16973

Zuris, J. A., Thompson, D. B., Shu, Y., Guilinger, J. P., Bessen, J. L., Hu, J. H., et al. (2015). Cationic lipid-mediated delivery of proteins enables efficient protein-based genome editing in vitro and in vivo. *Nat. Biotechnol.* 33, 73–80. doi: 10.1038/nbt.3081

5

Dye Tracking Following Posterior Semicircular Canal or Round Window Membrane Injections Suggests a Role for the Cochlea Aqueduct in Modulating Distribution

*Sara Talaei[1], Michael E. Schnee[1], Ksenia A. Aaron[1] and Anthony J. Ricci[1,2]**

[1] *Department of Otolaryngology-Head and Neck Surgery, Stanford University School of Medicine, Stanford, CA, United States,*
[2] *Department of Molecular and Cellular Physiology, Stanford University School of Medicine, Stanford, CA, United States*

***Correspondence:**
Anthony J. Ricci
aricci@stanford.edu

The inner ear houses the sensory epithelium responsible for vestibular and auditory function. The sensory epithelia are driven by pressure and vibration of the fluid filled structures in which they are embedded so that understanding the homeostatic mechanisms regulating fluid dynamics within these structures is critical to understanding function at the systems level. Additionally, there is a growing need for drug delivery to the inner ear for preventive and restorative treatments to the pathologies associated with hearing and balance dysfunction. We compare drug delivery to neonatal and adult inner ear by injection into the posterior semicircular canal (PSCC) or through the round window membrane (RWM). PSCC injections produced higher levels of dye delivery within the cochlea than did RWM injections. Neonatal PSCC injections produced a gradient in dye distribution; however, adult distributions were relatively uniform. RWM injections resulted in an early base to apex gradient that became more uniform over time, post injection. RWM injections lead to higher levels of dye distributions in the brain, likely demonstrating that injections can traverse the cochlea aqueduct. We hypothesize the relative position of the cochlear aqueduct between injection site and cochlea is instrumental in dictating dye distribution within the cochlea. Dye distribution is further compounded by the ability of some chemicals to cross inner ear membranes accessing the blood supply as demonstrated by the rapid distribution of gentamicin-conjugated Texas red (GTTR) throughout the body. These data allow for a direct evaluation of injection mode and age to compare strengths and weaknesses of the two approaches.

Keywords: drug delivery, cochlea aqueduct, inner ear, perilymph, endolymph, round window, posterior semicircular canal

INTRODUCTION

Inner ear end organs contain the sensory epithelium for balance and hearing. These fluid filled compartments are exquisitely sensitive to motion, particularly the fluid motion within these end organs (Hudspeth, 1989). Understanding fluid flow and compartmentalization within these systems is important at multiple levels. The ionic environment surrounding the sensory hair cells is critical to function (Wangemann and Schacht, 1996). Many pathologies associated with hearing loss and balance disorders stem from disruption of these fluid compartments or the pressure associated with these compartments [e.g., Meniere's disease (Hornibrook and Bird, 2016), Superior Semicircular Canal (SCC) Dehiscence (Minor et al., 1998), and Benign Paroxysmal Positional Vertigo (BPPV) (Vazquez-Benitez et al., 2016)]. Finally, therapies to prevent damage and to repair or replace damaged tissue will rely on our ability to deliver compounds uniformly and selectively to the inner ear compartments and end organs that require treatment. We cannot adequately design and assess therapeutics if we do not understand how the delivery system impacts drug distribution both within the ear but also to the brain and beyond.

RWM injection is a common mode of compound delivery that provides direct delivery into the perilymphatic space (Liu et al., 2005, 2007; Iizuka et al., 2008; Akil et al., 2012; Askew et al., 2015; Plontke et al., 2016; Dai et al., 2017; Landegger et al., 2017; Pan et al., 2017; Yoshimura et al., 2018). Plontke et al. (2016) showed direct intracochlear injection into the RWM of guinea pigs resulted in a basal–apical gradient in distribution of the injected markers (i.e., fluorescein or fluorescein isothiocyanate-labeled dextran). RWM injections in guinea pigs lead to compound detection in subarachnoid space, presumably traveling through the nearby cochlea aqueduct (Kaupp and Giebel, 1980). Recently, rapid detection of a biological dye in spinal cord and brain of mice after RWM injection was reported (Akil et al., 2019).

PSCC is another site for inner ear injections that offers the advantage of easy access with limited middle ear damage (Kawamoto et al., 2001; Suzuki et al., 2017; Isgrig and Chien, 2018). Data from lateral SCC (LSCC) injection of markers and dexamethasone suggest a more uniform distribution within the cochlea of guinea pigs (Salt et al., 2012a).

Here we directly compare RWM and PSCC injections at two ages in mice using similar volumes and flow rates. These experiments normalize for experimental variability as well as species and allow for direct assessment of route of entry and age. We demonstrate more uniform dye delivery using PSCC injections with less dye appearing in brain than with RWM injections. RWM injections result in more dye in the brain, implicating the cochlear aqueduct as a potential shunt to cochlear drug flow. Finally, GTTR injected in the PSCC resulted in dye appearing throughout the body, suggesting it can rapidly enter the blood supply, likely by crossing the membranous labyrinth membranes. Together these data begin to identify key parameters regulating distribution of compounds within inner ear compartments.

MATERIALS AND METHODS

Injections of trypan blue (4.6 mM, Life Technologies Corporation, United States), Methylene Blue (100 mM, ACROS Organics, United States), and GTTR [270 μM (Myrdal et al., 2005)] were made directly into the inner ear of mice. For *ex vivo* imaging, the dissected tissue was kept in Hanks' balanced salt solution (HBSS, Life Technologies Corporation, United States) buffer. C57/BL6 mice of both sexes at postnatal days of P1–P3 and P21–P23 were used for these studies. All animal procedures were approved by the Animal Care and Use Committee at Stanford University.

Injection Protocol

One microliter of compound was injected at a flow rate of 300 nl/min to five to six animals per group and the dye presence at the cochlea base, middle, and apex was monitored at different time points. Cochlear perilymphatic space for an adult mouse was previously estimated as 0.62 μl (Thorne et al., 1999). In this study, we chose a 1 μl injection volume for all experiments to provide enough dye for a complete replacement of the cochlear perilymph. No change in injection volume was used to compensate for any changes in inner ear volume with age. We tested several dyes including methylene blue, AM1-43 (100 μM, Biotium, United States), trypan blue, and GTTR. We chose to use trypan blue as the main dye for these studies because it interacted least with the tissue, it is not taken up by the cells (like AM1-43, methylene blue, or GTTR), nor does it appear to stick to the tissue (like methylene blue). 300 nl/min was selected as the fastest time that did not disrupt the tissue, we were finding a balance between going quickly to limit movement issues with the pipette placement and limiting any damage that might be caused by the fluid pressure inside the cochlea during injection. Flow rate was maintained regardless of age and injection site.

In all experiments, a 10 μl gas-tight syringe (Hamilton, United States) was mounted onto a microinjection pump [UMP3 UltraMicroPump, WPI, United States (Salt et al., 2012a)] and coupled to a glass micropipette tip. The rate and duration of injection were controlled by a microprocessor-based controller (Micro 4, WPI, United States) affixed to the microinjection pump to ensure the appropriate injection volume. The syringe and the micropipette were first filled manually with phosphate buffer saline (PBS) up to 4 μl of the syringe volume. After mounting the syringe onto the pump, using the Micro 4 controller, the pump was programmed to load a 1 μl air gap at the micropipette tip via suction, before loading the dye. Four microliters of the dye was then suctioned into the micropipette, leaving an air gap between PBS and the dye. This approach limited compression, allowing for a highly reproducible volume injection. The glass micropipettes were generated with a micropipette puller (Sutter Instrument Co., Model P-97, United States) and then scored and broken to ~25 μm inner diameter and ~45 μm outer diameter tips. Similar pipettes were used for both neonatal and adult injections. For precise localization of the micropipette tip during injections, the pump was mounted on a motorized manipulator (Exfo Burleigh, PCS-6000, United States).

Data Collection

M320 F12 ENT Microscope with a fully integrated camera (Leica, movie resolution: 720 × 480 pixels, image resolution: 2048 × 1536 pixels, Germany) was used for the surgical procedures and live imaging of the dye distribution within the cochlea. The integrated camera stored images and videos on a secure digital (SD) memory card. Example videos are presented in the **Supplementary Material S1–S4**. The injection process, starting at time 0, was video recorded in an MP4 format and converted to 8-bit JPEGs at 30 s intervals. Free Video to JPG Converter (V.5.0.101[1]) was used for converting the MP4 files. Following completion of the infusion, JPEG images (8-bit) were captured at 3-min intervals (from 4 to 34 min). SZX10 microscope (Olympus, Japan) equipped with CCD color and monochrome cameras (QIclick-F-CLR-12 and QIclick-F-M-12, 1392 × 1040 pixels, 6.45 μm^2 pixel size, Teledyne QImaging, Canada) was used for dissections and imaging of the dissected cochleae and brains at the ~5 min and 1-h time points as well as for the fluorescent images using GTTR. Images with TIFF (12-bit) and JPEG (8-bit) formats were captured.

Data Analysis

All images were analyzed similarly. Intensity was measured in 50 (*in vivo* images) and 100 μm (*ex vivo* images) diameter regions in apex, middle, and base. For all intensity measurements, Fiji software (open source image processing package[2]) was used. All statistics were performed with Origin Software using two-sample or pair-sample *t*-tests. For *in vivo* images, data from apex, middle, and base from each cochlea were pooled for group comparisons if no regional differences were observed.

Computational Modeling

Finite element method (FEM) simulation software (COMSOL Multiphysics 5.3a) was used for computing the velocity magnitude along the perilymphatic compartment, during injections via PSCC and RWM. The 2D Laminar Flow Module for incompressible flows was applied to solve Navier–Stokes equations coupled with the continuity equation for conservation of mass in the periymphatic compartment. The perilymphatic compartment was modeled as a 2D pipe with three connected sections representing scala tympani (ST), scala vestibuli (SV), and SSCs. As shown in **Figure 9C**, based on the measurements reported previously for an adult mouse (Thorne et al., 1999), 4.55 and 3.98 mm were chosen for the length of ST and SV. For simplicity, the width of each section was kept constant along the length (i.e., SV: 200 μm, ST: 140 μm). A 4 × 0.09 mm^2 section was added to represent SCCs. The cochlea aqueduct was assumed to have a 100 μm width opening in ST, at 650 μm distance from the RW. It was assumed that the injection was directly into the perilymphatic space, and no back flow was considered at the injection sites. The injection sites at PSCC and RWM were both 25 μm located in the middle length of SCC and middle width of ST, respectively. During the injection, the only inlet for the system was the injection site. In our experiments that we injected the dye at 300 nl/min through a micropipette with 25 μm diameter, the flow velocity at the micropipette tip was calculated 0.01 m/s which was chosen as the inlet velocity in our model. We first assumed that the perilymphatic space inside the inner ear is an isolated compartment with only one outlet (i.e., cochlea aqueduct) and one inlet (i.e., injection site) (**Figure 9D**). No material exchange through the walls was possible with this assumption. In our second model (**Figure 9E**), we defined a distributed leaky wall at the top of all compartments at which the fluid velocity during the injection was larger than zero (e.g., 10^{-5} m/s). This leak is meant to represent both biological and experimental leak associated with the procedure.

Neonatal Surgeries

Neonatal mice were anesthetized with hypothermia induced by placing the pups on a nitrile glove sitting on crushed ice for 3–5 min. Hypothermia was approved by Administrative Panel on Laboratory Animal Care (APLAC) and Stanford veterinary staff for use in neonatal animals. The animals were transferred to an ice water cooled aluminum block to perform the surgery. A 3–5 mm incision was made behind the ear, in the postauricular region with microscissors; muscle tissue was removed with forceps to expose the PSCC and bulla. Kimwipes (Kimtech, United States) were used for absorbing blood at the incision site. For the experiments where cochlea dye distribution was continuously recorded during and after the injection, a larger incision was made in the postauricular region (8–10 mm). The auricle, tympanic membrane, and bulla were removed while the stapes bone was left intact. This approach allowed for better viewing of the cochlea (shown in **Figure 2**). For PSCC injections, the micropipette was inserted into the PSCC using a micromanipulator. The bony labyrinth in neonatal mice was soft enough to allow micropipette tip penetration. The micropipette tip was visually assessed before and after each injection, and broken tips were not used for data collection. From this experiment it was not evident if the tip ruptured the membranous labyrinth, so it is possible that both endolymph and perilymph compartments were injected. As discussed by other groups, it is possible that the membranous labyrinth was ruptured during PSCC injections potentially causing direct access to the endolymphatic space (Kawamoto et al., 2001; Isgrig and Chien, 2018; Yoshimura et al., 2018). At the end of infusion and immediately after pulling out the injection pipette, a small droplet of 101 cyanoacrylate adhesive (Permabond, United States) was applied to the injection site, which was then covered with a muscle patch. For the RWM injections, the initial incision was made using microscissors at a position about 2 mm lower than the one in PSCC injections in order to expose the bulla. A small opening (1–2 mm) was made in the bulla to expose the RW, and the glass micropipette was inserted into the RWM. At the end of infusion, the injection pipette was removed and the RW was covered with a plug of muscle, and a droplet of cyanoacrylate was applied on the top to attach the muscle plug to the RW niche. For all neonatal surgeries, after sealing the injection site, the surgical incision was closed, and sealed with surgical glue (Suturevet Vetclose, Henry Schein Animal Health, United States). The entire procedure was accomplished within 15–20 min. For the experiments in which the cochleae were examined at 1-h post injection, pups were kept under hypothermia for the duration of the surgery and then transferred to a heating pad (37°C). Pups revived within 3–5 min. Animals were euthanized at 1-h time point for further evaluation.

Adult Surgeries

Adult mice weighing between 8.5 and 10.5 g were anesthetized with an intraperitoneal injection of a mixture of ketamine (100 mg/kg) and xylazine (10 mg/kg). While animals were

[1] https://www.dvdvideosoft.com/

[2] https://fiji.sc/

anesthetized, the surgery was performed on a heating pad at 37°C. The fur behind the left ear was removed using hair removal cream and sterilized with 10% povidone iodine followed by 70% ethanol. A postauricular skin incision of ~10 mm was made. To expose the cochlea for live imaging of the dye distribution during injection, a posterior transcanal incision was made with microscissors. Twelve and six o'clock medial cuts were then made in order to transect the remainder of the ear canal and to excise the bulla. The canal cartilage, dorsolateral surface of the auditory bulla, tympanic membrane, and ossicular chain were then removed except for the stapes bone allowing visualization of all cochlea turns (from the top view as shown in **Figure 2**), the oval window (OW), and round window (RW). All hemostasis was achieved with electrocautery (Medline, United States). After this exposure, for the PSCC injection, the sternocleidomastoid muscle was cut proximally, while the muscles covering the temporal bone were separated and retracted dorsally to expose the bony wall of the PSCC. A chemical canalostomy was achieved by applying 36.2% phosphoric acid etching gel (Young, United States) with the same caliber tip of the glass micropipette as used for injection and 20 s were allowed to take effect for bone resorption, and enough time to leave endosteum covered by a thin layer of bone (Alyono et al., 2015). A moist roll of cotton was used to remove the remaining gel. The etching treatment softened the bone enough to insert the perfusion micropipette. Using the micromanipulator, the tip of the glass micropipette was advanced (~2-3 mm) into the canal angled toward the ampulla. This assured no backflow of the injected material and a sturdy tip insertion. The injection of trypan blue was performed as above. After removing the micropipette, the hole was plugged with small pieces of muscle, and covered with 101 cyanoacrylate. For the RWM injection, after the cochlea exposure was achieved, injection was performed with a glass micropipette into the RW niche passing through the RWM. All injections were performed and recorded under the surgical microscope described earlier and the delivery site was closely monitored for leakage during all procedures. No dye leakage was observed in the neonatal and adult mice during PSCC injection. In some RWM injections (~10% of neonates and ~50% of adults) a leakage was observed from the injection site. The higher leakage rate in adult may be due to the increased intracochlear pressure compared to neonatal animals which resulted in more backflow. Those animals were not included in the study. After removing the micropipette, the RW was sealed with a plug of muscle. For the experiments where the bulla was removed and the cochlea was monitored during the injection for up to 30 min post injection, the imaging region was occasionally covered by blood or other fluids during the imaging. When removing of these fluids could not be done properly, the animal cases were removed from the data analysis. At the end of each experiment, animals were euthanized under anesthesia. Mouse temporal bones and each side of the brain were harvested and placed in HBSS after which the tissue was imaged.

RESULTS

The fluid filled inner ear consists of discreetly positioned sensory epithelium of the vestibular and auditory systems housed in a contiguous membranous compartment (Sterkers et al., 1982; Hudspeth, 1989). These end organs are located within the temporal bone and are protected by a bony capsule (Felten et al., 2016). The bony capsule is filled with perilymph, a solution very similar to cerebral spinal fluid, and surrounds a membranous labyrinth containing endolymph, a high potassium, and low calcium solution created by supporting cells within each end organ (Sterkers et al., 1988; Wangemann and Schacht, 1996). The endolymphatic compartment is located within the perilymphatic space as shown in **Figure 1** (Sterkers et al., 1988; Forge and Wright, 2002, Salt et al., 2012a; Felten et al., 2016). The perilymph and endolymph solutions are shared by the vestibular and cochlear end organs, yet the fluid composition

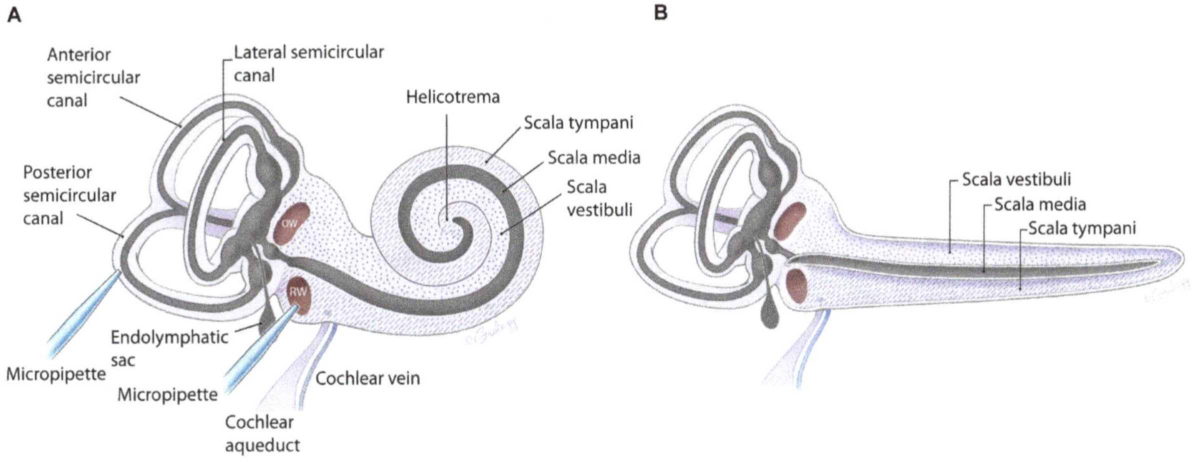

FIGURE 1 | Schematic of the mouse inner ear with coiled **(A)** and uncoiled **(B)** configurations of the cochlea. The fluidic compartments for endolymph and perilymph are depicted in gray and light purple, respectively. The cochlea compartment of scala tympani is indicated with the hatch markings and scala vestibuli with the dots. All other compartments are as labeled. The approximate location of the injection pipette is illustrated for PSCC and RWM.

is often different between end organs (Sterkers et al., 1988; Wangemann and Schacht, 1996). The mammalian cochlea has three chambers, ST and SV contain perilymph, and scala media (SM) contains endolymph (**Figure 1**). The SV contacts the OW membrane (OWM) and the ST contacts the RWM (Fernández, 1952; Salt et al., 2012a,b; Felten et al., 2016). SV is contiguous with ST, converging at the apex, at the helicotrema (Fernández, 1952; Salt et al., 1991; Felten et al., 2016; Wright and Roland, 2018). At the basal end the SV is contiguous with the vestibule while the ST ends at the RWM (**Figure 1**). The cochlear aqueduct is a small channel extending from the ST at the cochlea basal turn, adjacent to the RWM that projects into the cranial cavity (Schuknecht and Seifi, 1963; Gopen et al., 1997). The function and patency of the cochlear aqueduct remains unclear but is suggested to regulate pressure (Carlborg, 1981; Carlborg et al., 1982). The endolymphatic sac extends from the vestibule between the cochlea base and the vestibular end organs and similarly may be a reservoir for excess endolymph production (Kimura and Schuknecht, 1965; Couloigner et al., 1999). Although the inner ear contains two independent fluid compartments, flow through these compartments is complex due to the multiple routes and different resistant properties offered by the shape of the various end organ components. The potential for ion transport between compartments further complicates our understanding of compound delivery (Salt et al., 1991; Salt et al., 2012b).

In the present work, flow within the inner ear was visualized by injecting trypan blue at two independent sites indicated in **Figure 1A**. The impact of age on the dye distribution within the cochlea after a PSCC or RWM injection was studied by applying similar injection protocols to neonatal and adult mice and comparing the results.

Figure 2 presents *in vivo* images used for analysis of the dye distribution within cochlea for each experimental group. The images show dye progression within the cochlea at different time points during the injection. From the imaging angle shown in these pictures, the distribution of the dye upon PSCC injection was visible in the cochleae of both neonatal and adult mice. The dye first appeared at the OW region (see **Figure 2** PSCC neonate time 30 s as example), continued to the cochlea base, and then migrated toward the apex. Although we did not have the resolution to differentiate migration in ST and SV, the later appearance of the dye at RW region (after reaching the apex) suggests that the dye had first entered the SV and then continued into the ST compartment as was reported in the literature (Salt et al., 2012a). The dye distribution pathway in the cochlea upon RWM injection was not as clearly visible at this imaging angle (see alternate *ex vivo* images in **Figure 5**). Despite this difficulty we could track dye in each configuration but cannot compare absolute intensity values between ages for this experiment. In contrast to PSCC injections, visual inspection of RWM injections, *ex vivo*, show dye accumulation at the cochlea base with less dye found in middle turn and virtually no dye seen at the apex.

Data from **Figure 2** were analyzed by measuring the average intensity values of pixels within each region of interest (ROI, 50 μm diameter) for each animal. ROIs are demarcated in the last column of **Figure 2**. Average intensities in the apex, middle, and base were measured from time 0 (starting the injection) until 34 min after starting the infusion. Video examples for each condition are presented in the **Supplementary Material S1–S4**. The graphs in **Figures 3A–L** present data analyzed from the movies (**Supplementary Videos**) for individual animals selected

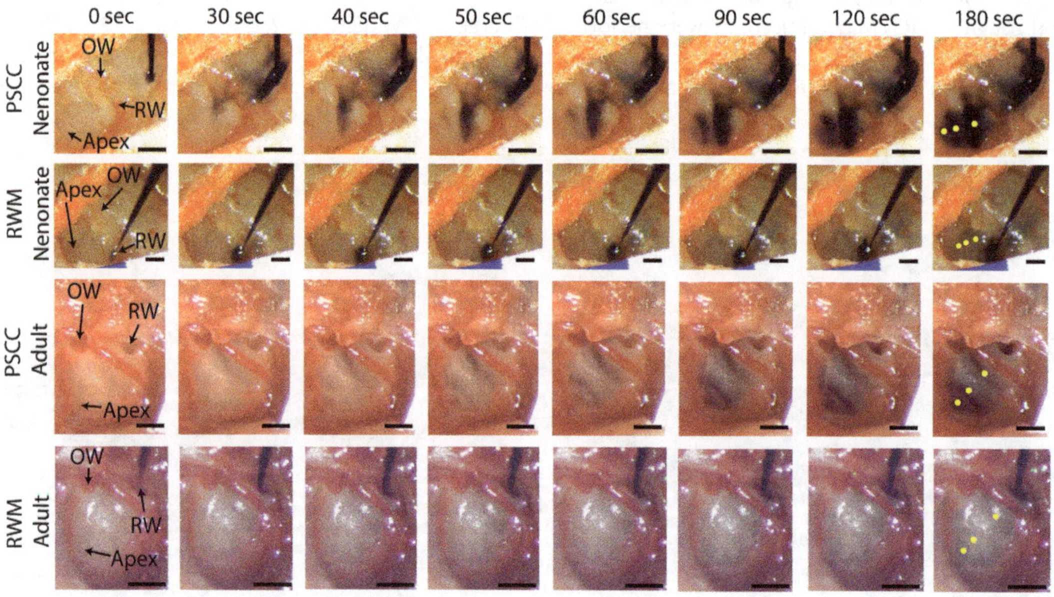

FIGURE 2 | *In vivo* monitoring of trypan blue dye distribution along the cochlea during PSCC and RWM injection in neonatal and adult mice. In all experiments, the microinjection pump was turned on at 0 s injecting 1 μl of the dye at 300 nl/min. The regions of interest where the intensity was measured at **apex**, **middle**, and **base** for each experiment are shown in yellow in the last picture of each row (180 s). Scale bar is 500 μm. The *X*-axis provides time snapshots and the *Y*-axis the specific group being injected.

as those with parameters closest to the mean values (presented in **Figure 4**). **Figures 3A,D,G,J** show the intensity value decreased significantly for the first 3 min, during dye injection through the PSCC or RWM (**Figure 3M**). Lower intensity (I) values indicate darker regions, meaning the dye is reaching that area. The intensity changes relative to time 0 (ΔI) are plotted (as $-\Delta I$ to more intuitively reflect an increase in dye concentration) for apex, middle, and base in **Figures 3B,E,H,K**. I_{max} was defined as the intensity change (ΔI) at 3 min after starting the injection. We interpret intensity changes as equivalent to changes in dye levels. In PSCC injected mice (n = 5 for each group of adults and neonates), dye increased at each location for both ages during the entirety of the injection (**Figures 3A,B,D,E**). In RWM injected neonatal animals (n = 6, **Figures 3G,H**), there was an increase in dye in basal regions with a modest change for mid and very little change for apical regions. Adult RWM (n = 5) showed a similar pattern to neonatal, though there was a measurable change in the apical region (**Figures 3J,K**). These data suggest more dye

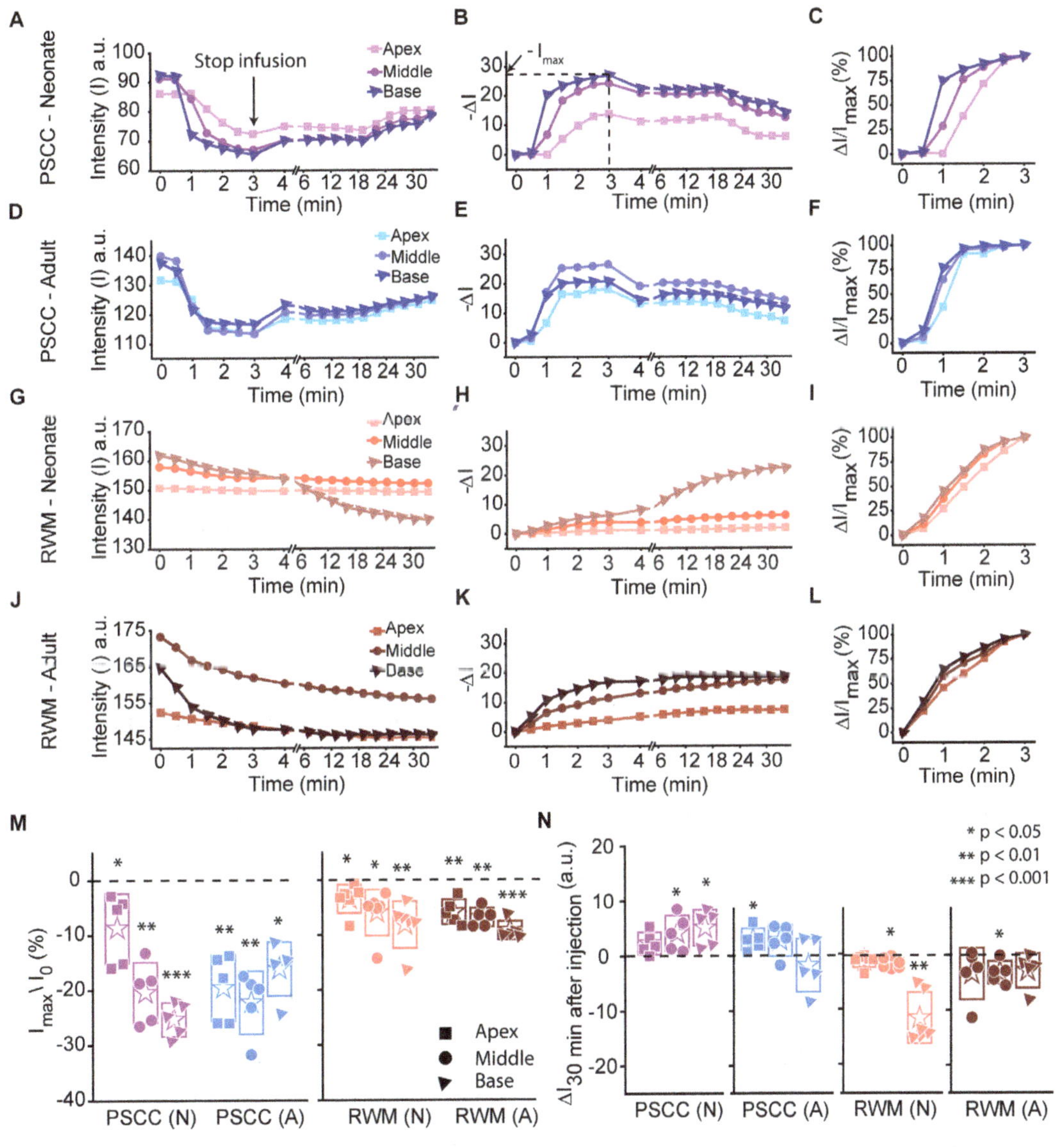

FIGURE 3 | Representative plots obtained from one animal in each experimental group (n = 5, 6 in each group) showing dye distribution along the cochlea during PSCC and RWM injection in neonatal and adult mice from starting the pump up to 34 min. Injection time was from 0 to 3 min. Graphs **(A,D,G,J)** show the raw intensity measurements in the apex (squares), middle (circles), and base (triangles). Graphs **(B,E,H,K)** present intensity changes in the same regions at each time point with respect to the initial values at 0 min. ΔI is plotted with a reversed sign ($-\Delta I$) so that larger numbers indicate increased dye. I_{max} was defined as the intensity change (ΔI) at 3 min. Graphs **(C,F,I,L)** show the percentage of intensity change at each time point, in respect to I_{max}, during injection. **(M)** Intensity changes 3 min after starting the pump in respect to the intensity values at 0 min (I_0). Asterisks indicate levels of significant change in intensity values between 3 and 0 min at each cochlear region. **(N)** Intensity changes from 4 min (time point when the micropipette was removed) until 30 min later. Asterisks indicate levels of significant change in intensity values between 34 and 4 min at each cochlear region. Boxes represent standard deviations of the mean. Pair-sample t-test in panels **(M,N)** were used for calculating the p-values.

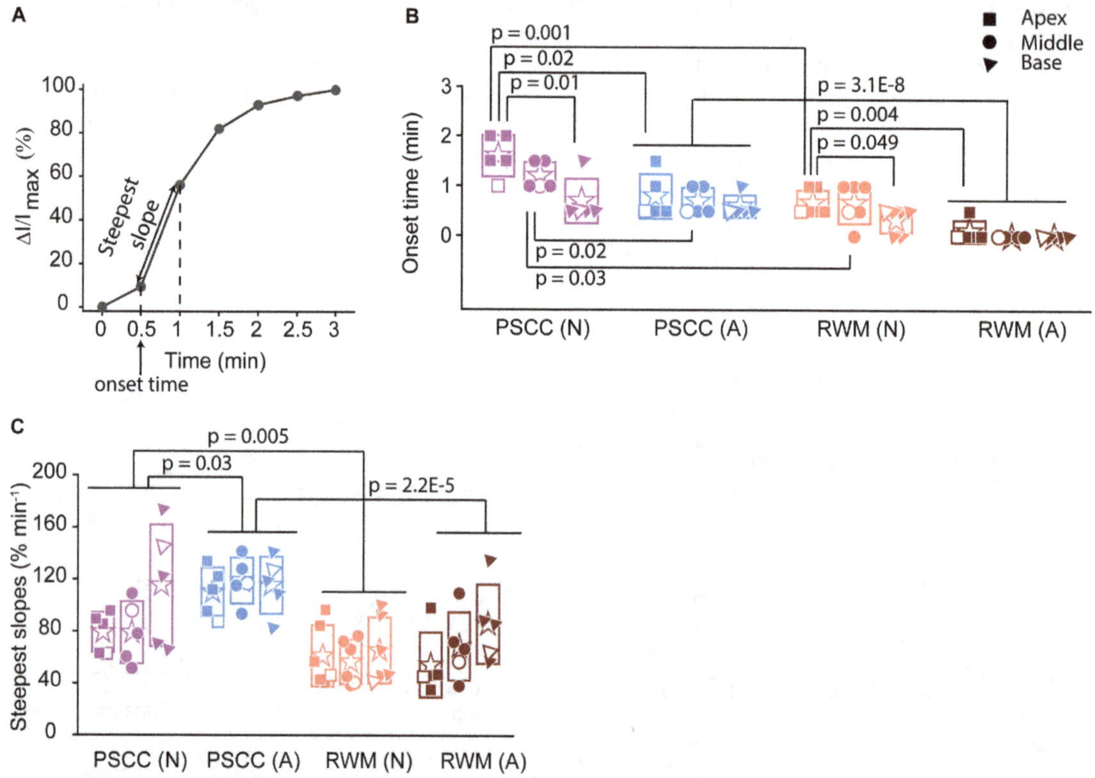

FIGURE 4 | Analysis of normalized intensity changes in the cochlea during the injection period (0–3 min) (summary from data in **Figure 3**). In each plot N is neonatal and A is adult. Apical is represented by squares, middle by the circles, and base by triangles. Open symbols represent data from the individual examples presented in **Figures 3A–L**. Graph **(A)** describes the measured parameters presented in panels **(B,C)**. **(B)** Onset time and **(C)** steepest slope obtained from individual animals as shown in the third column of **Figure 3**. Boxes represent standard deviations of the mean. In panels **(B)** and **(C)** statistical comparisons are done on pooled data showed with horizontal lines. Two-sample *t*-test in panels **(B,C)** were used for calculating the *p*-values.

entry for adult compared to neonatal animals for both injection sites and also that dye reaches the apex more readily for PSCC injections than for RWM injections.

A slight increase in the intensity value was observed at the end of infusion (indicated by the arrow in **Figure 3A**), correlating with the time when the glass micropipette was removed from the injection site. This increase was not observed in RWM injected animals, likely because the limited amount of dye present at apex and middle ROIs did not allow for the dye reduction detection. The lack of change in the basal region is not due to a lack of dye and perhaps suggests a difference due to injection site.

In PSCC injected animals, the dye level reduced slowly after stopping the infusion (**Figures 3A,B,D,E,N**). In RWM injected neonatal mice ($n = 6$), after stopping the infusion, apex dye levels were unchanged, there was an increase in dye levels for mid regions and a more robust change at the basal turns, likely indicating a continued progression of dye from the base toward the apex (**Figures 3G,H,N**). In RWM injected adults ($n = 5$), dye levels increased in all turns within 30 min post injection again suggesting continued dye progression after the perfusion (**Figures 3J,K,N**).

A summary of maximal changes monitored at the end of the injection (from the imaging angle shown in **Figure 2**) shows a base to apex gradient for PSCC injected neonates and RWM injected animals (**Figure 3M**). PSCC data lose this gradient in adult, while RWM injections are not different between ages. The relative changes associated with PSCC injection were greater than RWM injections (**Figure 3M**); however, the orientation of cochlea during *in vivo* imaging provides a better view for monitoring the dye progression in PSCC injection compared to the RWM so we performed additional experiments to obtain more equivalent views (see **Figures 5, 6** for more direct comparisons at different orientations).

Dye distribution was evaluated 30 min after stopping the infusion relative to the time immediately after removing the pipette (ΔI_{30min}). The majority of PSCC mice showed a reduction in dye accumulation, as indicated by positive values at 30 min post injection (**Figure 3N**). RWM injected mice showed a continued increase in dye accumulation as indicated by negative values meaning more dye present (**Figure 3N**). These data support the idea that PSCC had uniform distribution early with later time points reflecting diffusion out of the cochlea. In contrast, RWM injections showed less dye within the cochlea; the existing dye distributed more uniformly over the following 30 min.

To evaluate the kinetic differences between modes of injection independent of absolute concentrations we normalized data to the time point immediately before termination of the injection

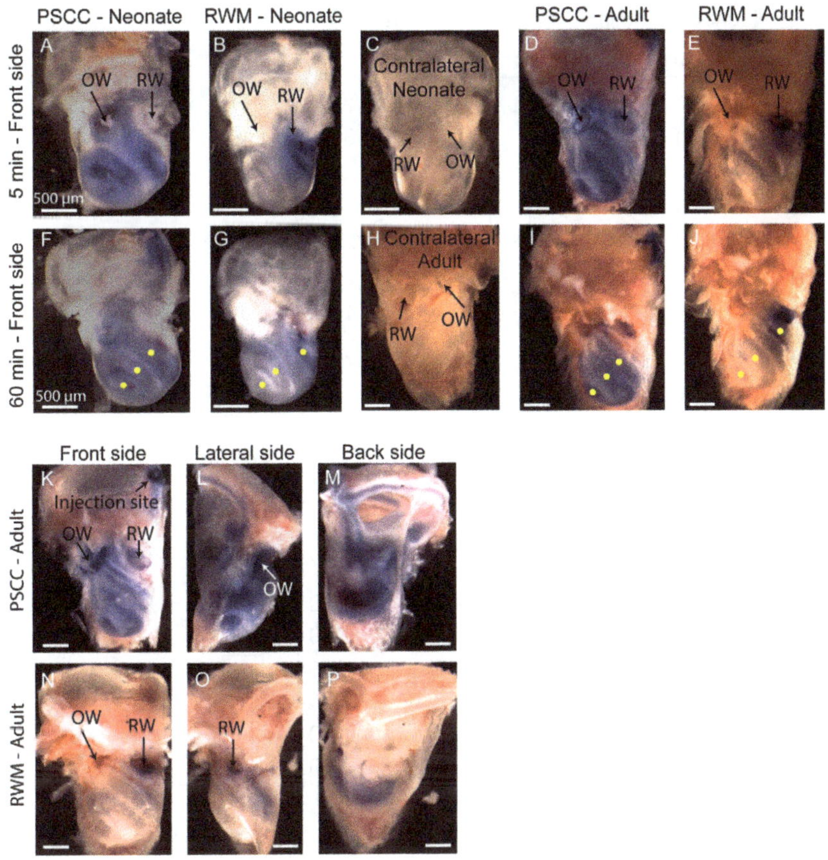

FIGURE 5 | Representative pictures of the mouse cochleae, after injecting trypan blue through RWM and PSCC, at 5- **(A–E)** and 60-min **(F–J)** post injection. The contralateral cochleae of neonatal and adult mice are also presented for comparisons **(C,H)**. Regions of interest (100 µm diameter) where the average intensity values were measured are shown with yellow dots in **(F,G,I,J)**. Front, lateral, and back side of adult mice, 5 min after injecting through PSCC **(K–M)** and RWM **(N–P)**.

(**Figures 3C,F,I,L**). The presented examples demonstrate time delays and rate differences in dye progression between modes of delivery and age. The dramatic differences in dye level are not included in these plots but rather simply an indication of the timing differences, summaries of which are presented in **Figure 4**. The measured parameters are depicted in **Figure 4A**. Data from the individual examples shown in **Figures 3A–L**, are indicated with open symbols in **Figures 4B,C**. The onset time is defined as the first time point where the steepest rate of change for dye accumulation occurs (**Figure 4A**). **Figure 4B** summarizes changes in onset time between groups. A delay in onset time was observed between regions for neonatal animals, being most delayed in the apex, regardless of delivery mode. Adult animals did not show intracochlear differences in onset time. PSCC injections were more delayed than RWM injections in all groups as might be predicted from the longer distance between the injection site and cochlea in PSCC compared to RWM delivery. The age difference may simply represent the change in size of the inner ear reducing resistance to flow in adult mice.

The intensity change over time was not linear for any age or delivery mode (**Figures 3C,F,I,L**). To compare rates of change we simply used the steepest slope as described in **Figure 4A**, for each experimental group. Given that these measurements are during perfusion a common slope is predicted that basically relates injection rate to cochlea properties. Reductions in this rate suggest that flow is bifurcating or that different resistances are encountered. That is, if the dye splits into flow in multiple directions the rate will be reduced for either pathway. Results of this analysis are shown in **Figure 4C**. The steepest slope had larger values in the PSCC injected animals (both neonates and adults) compared to the RWM injected ones. The PSCC injected adult mice had steeper slopes compared to the neonatal ones; but no significant difference in the slope was observed between the neonatal and adult mice injected through the RWM. The slope difference between ages is likely a result of a reduced resistance to flow in the adult animal. The steeper slope with PSCC injections suggests higher levels of dye are entering the cochlea from this site of injection at each time unit. All biological paths from the PSCC injection lead through the cochlea while the RWM injection can bifurcate to the cochlea aqueduct prior to distributing through the entire cochlea. This simple difference likely accounts for the difference in dye distributions for the two injection sites.

A problem with the *in vivo* imaging is that orientation of the cochlea makes it more difficult to assess distribution with RWM injections. To further assess diffusion post injection and to better visualize dye distributions throughout the cochlea a

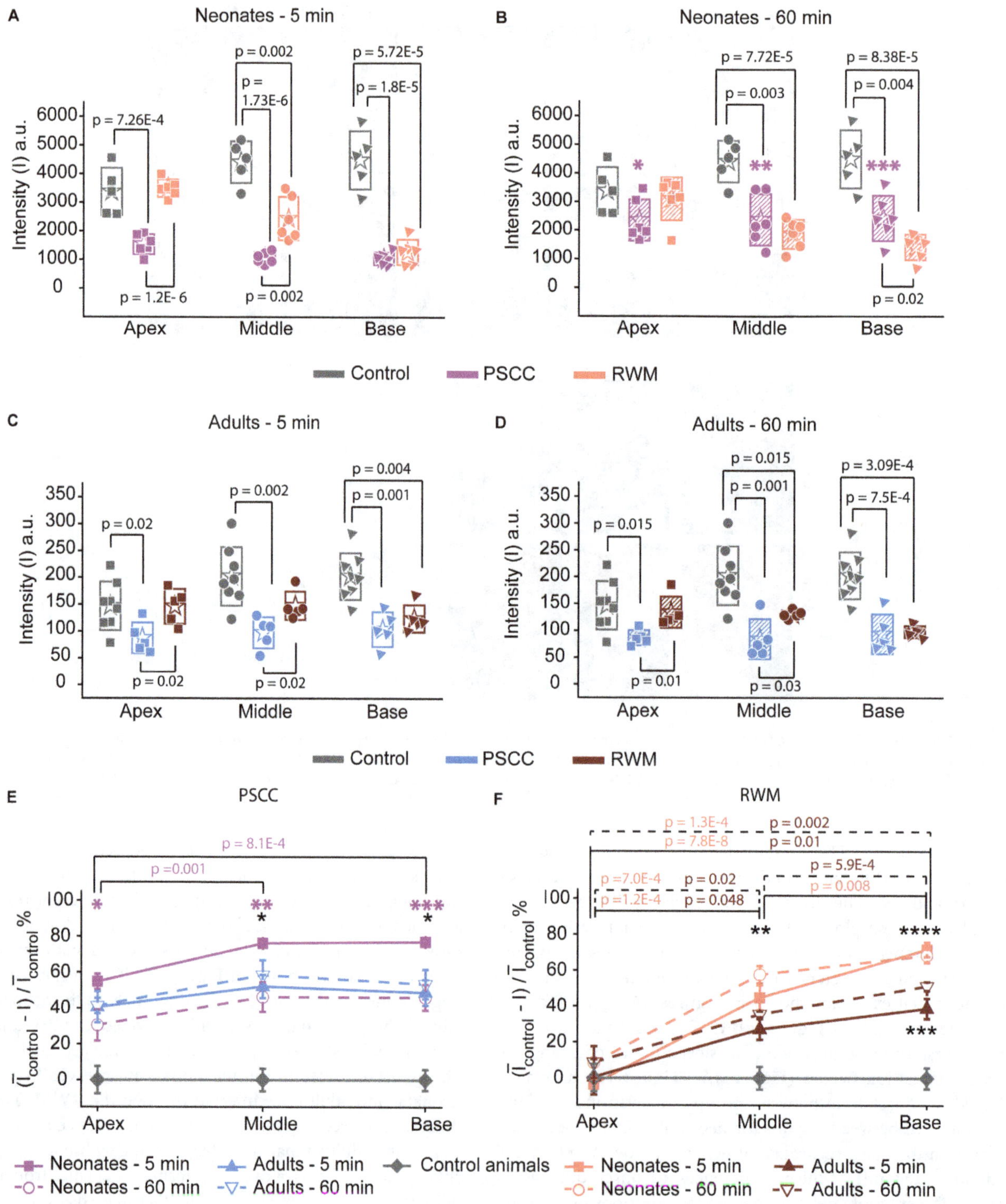

FIGURE 6 | *Ex vivo* assessment of the presence of trypan blue in the PSCC and RWM injected and contralateral cochleae of neonatal mice at 5 **(A)** and 60 min **(B)**, and adult mice, at 5- **(C)** and 60-min **(D)** post injection. The contralateral cochleae of neonatal and adult mice were used as control (non-injected) cochleae. Average intensity values measured within 100 μm regions (shown with yellow dots in **Figures 5F,G,I,J**) in apex, middle, and base. Measurements in panels **(A,B)** were taken from pictures with TIFF formats (12 bit) and panels **(C,D)** from the ones with JPEG (8 bit). Boxes represent standard deviations of the mean. Percentage of intensity change at each region of cochlea in respect to the control values at both time points for PSCC **(E)** and RWM **(F)** injected animals. Error bars represent standard errors. Purple asterisks in panels **(B)** and **(E)** indicate significant differences between data values at 60 min compared to 5 min at each cochlear region of PSCC injected neonates (*p = 0.03, **p = 0.006, ***p = 0.002). Black asterisks in panels **(E,F)** indicate significant differences between the data values for neonatal and adult mice (*p = 0.006 at 5 min, **p = 0.003 at 60 min, ***p = 8.3E–4 at 5 min, ****p = 0.007 at 60 min). Two-sample t-test was used for calculating the p-values between groups.

separate set of experiments was performed where the brains and both cochleae were obtained at 5- and 60-min post injection for each experimental group. This approach allows us to evaluate dye distribution *ex vivo* within the cochlea from angles that were not accessible in the *in vivo* images. A representative cochlea from each group of experiments (n = 6 and n = 5 in each group of neonatal and adult cochleae, respectively) is shown in **Figure 5**. No dye was detected in any contralateral cochleae. It is clear from the images that the PSCC injections achieved more uniformly distributed dye than did the RMW injections. To better assess the dye pathway with RWM injections and to investigate uniformity of distribution, images were obtained from three perspectives at 5 min post injection (**Figures 5K–P**). These data demonstrate that PSCC has high dye levels throughout the cochlea and even SCCs. In contrast, RWM injections show dye in the basal areas with less distribution to apical regions. In addition, these data suggest that dye intensity differences may in part be due to the dye going elsewhere. This conclusion is supported also by the reduced steepest slopes described in **Figure 4**.

The intensity values from regions with 100 μm diameter at apex, middle, and base were measured for each cochlea as indicated by yellow dots in **Figures 5F,G,I,J**. Immediate dissection and inspection of cochlea following the end of PSCC injection (about 5 min post injection) show all cochlea regions were significantly darker than non-injected ones, at both ages (**Figures 6A,C**). In contrast, RWM injected animals showed a steep gradient where only base in adults and base and middle in neonates were significantly darker than the non-injected cochleae at the 5-min time point (**Figures 6A,C**).

As shown in **Figures 6A,C**, the dye was highest at the basal turn of PSCC or RWM injected cochlea, ~5 min after injection, and values did not differ from each other at either age (p = 0.3). In contrast, apical measurements in neonates show dye levels higher for PSCC injected cochleae than RWM injected cochleae (p = 1.2E−6) while neonatal RWM injected cochleae were not different from control (p = 0.7). In adults, apical values in PSCC remained different from RWM injected values (p = 0.02) but apical values in RWM are again not different from control (p = 0.98).

One hour after injection, dye levels in the PSCC injected neonatal cochleae were significantly reduced in all regions compared to 5 min after injection (**Figures 6B,E**, see asterisks). Adult animals showed no difference in the dye levels for PSCC injections for any region compared to the 5 min time point (**Figures 6C–E**). No significant difference in the cochlear dye levels was observed in RWM injected neonatal (**Figures 6A,B,F**) or adult (**Figures 6C,D,F**) for 1 h compared to 5 min after injection, suggesting dilution was not happening with this mode of injection at either age.

The percentage of intensity change at each ROI in respect to the control values is summarized at early (**Figure 6E**) and late (**Figure 6F**) time points for PSCC and RWM injected animals, respectively. For simplicity, the control data from neonatal and adult mice are combined. The dye distribution in neonatal animals presented a gradient from base to apex, after PSCC injection at the 5-min time point (**Figure 6E**) but not at the 60-min time point. This gradient did not exist in the PSCC injected adults at either time points. A steep gradient in dye distribution at both 5 and 60 min was observed after RWM injection in both neonatal and adult mice (**Figure 6F**).

One possibility is that part of the dye injected through the RWM travels through the cochlea aqueduct which is located very close to the injection site. In contrast, the PSCC injection site is at the opposite end of the cochlear perilymphatic space, so that during the injection perilymph will be pushed through the cochlea aqueduct while dye enters the cochlea. We inspected the brains of injected animals as a proxy for dye traveling through the cochlea aqueduct. Brain images from each group of injected animals are shown in **Figure 7**. No dye was detected in the brain of the neonatal mice injected through PSCC (at 5 or 60 min, n = 6 per group). However, trypan blue was detected in 5/6 neonatal mice brains injected through RWM at both 5 and 60 min supporting the idea of dye travel through the cochlea aqueduct. In PSCC injected adult mice, no dye was detected in the brain 5 min after injection, but small traces of trypan

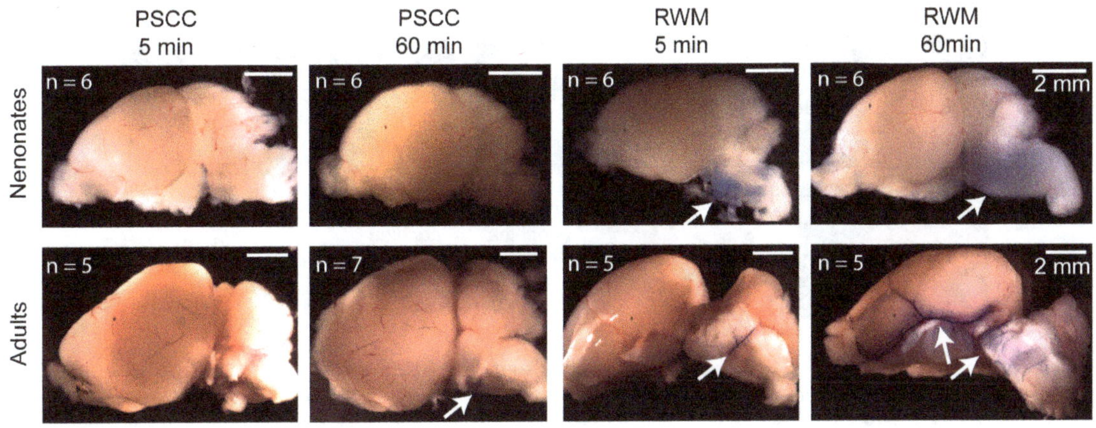

FIGURE 7 | Representative brain pictures of the neonatal and adult mice injected with trypan blue through PSCC or RWM, 5 and 60 min after injection. Number of evaluated brains in each group of experiments is indicated. The arrows point to the regions where the dye was observed.

blue were observed in four out of seven adult mice 1 h after injection, suggesting travel through the cochlea aqueduct post injection. The dye was also detected in all adult mice brains injected through RWM at both time points (n = 5 for each). Thus, these data are consistent with the hypothesis that RWM injections lose dye through the cochlea aqueduct more readily than PSCC injections.

Different Substances Have Different Distributions After PSCC Injection

It has previously been suggested that the chemical composition of the injected compound can affect distribution within the ear (Nomura, 1961; Salt and Plontke, 2018). In order to investigate the potential variations in compounds progression in the cochlea following the same mode of delivery and using the same injection parameters, two other compounds were tested. We injected GTTR and methylene blue via PSCC in neonatal animals as described above. The results are shown in **Figure 8**. Methylene blue presented very similar to trypan blue. One hour after injecting methylene blue into the PSCC of P1 mice, no dye was visible through the skin, and after dissection, no trace of dye was detected in the brain or contralateral cochlea (**Figure 8F**). However, GTTR distribution was starkly different. One hour after injecting GTTR into the left PSCC of mice at P1, it was detected through the skin of the animals (**Figure 8A**). Three hours after the injection, the drug was still visible in different parts of the body through the skin (**Figure 8B**). The fluorescent pictures of a mouse's paws and tail, 1 h after PSCC injection of GTTR is shown in **Figure 8C**, in comparison with the non-injected pup. GTTR was also injected to P5 mice through PSCC. One hour after the injection, the drug was visible through the whole cochlea, and most of the inner and outer hair cells (**Figure 8D**). **Figure 8E** shows that GTTR was also detected in the brain of the P5 injected pups, 1 day after PSCC injection. For this level of distribution, the GTTR must be able to access the blood supply by crossing membranes within the inner ear. These experiments highlighted the fact that in addition to the injection parameters (e.g., volume, flow rate), mode of delivery (e.g., PSCC, RWM), and resistance to the flow within the cochlea that can influence the distribution patterns within the inner ear, under the same conditions, different molecules can propagate differently within the cochlea and whole body.

DISCUSSION

Over the past decade, RWM and PSCC injections are more commonly used for delivering compounds into the inner ear delivering viral vectors for genetic manipulations. Our data set

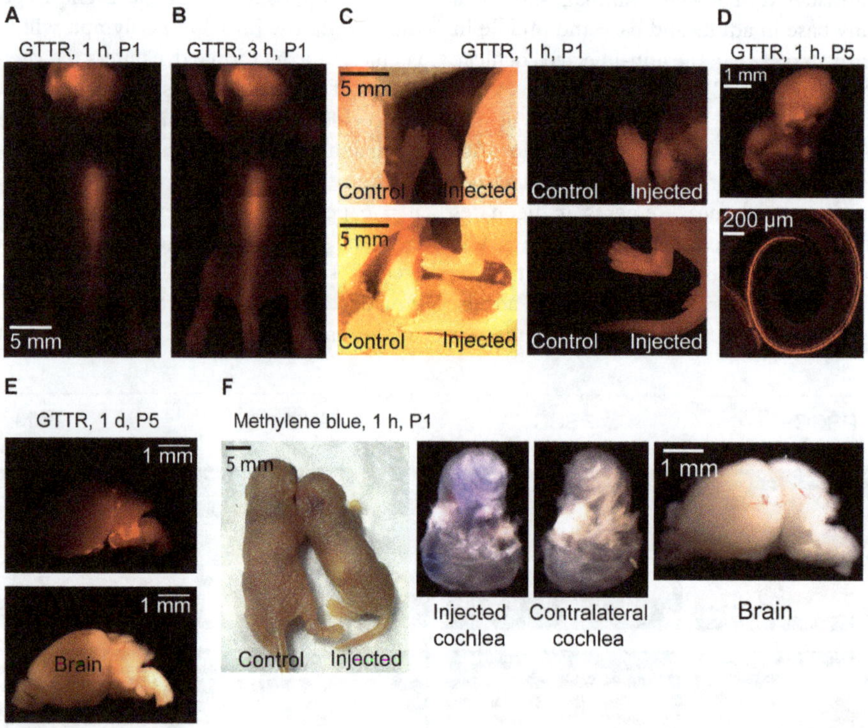

FIGURE 8 | Representative pictures of GTTR and methylene blue distribution in neonatal mice after 1 μl injection into the left PSCC. n = 3 for all experiments except GTTR injection to P5 mice and evaluation at 1-h time point (n = 4). GTTR was observed through the skin of the animal, 1 **(A)** and 3 h **(B)** after injection. **(C)** Comparing injected and non-injected pups, 1 h after GTTR injection. The bright field and fluorescent images are shown in left and right panels, respectively. **(D)** GTTR in the injected cochlea, 1 h after injection to a P5 pup. Otic capsule and SCCs are shown in the top. Organ of corti is shown in the bottom. **(E)** Brain of the GTTR injected pup, 1 day after injection at P5. The bright field and fluorescent images are shown on the top and bottom images, respectively **(F)** 1 h after methylene blue injection to P1 pup.

compares PSCC and RWM delivery in neonatal and adult mice using comparable technologies. Identifying and characterizing parameters that modulate drug distribution in the cochlea could help better understand fluid regulation within the inner ear and aid in developing more effective delivery methods for research and therapeutic purposes. Our data provide information on the route of dye flow upon RWM and PSCC injections (**Figure 9**), the resistance to the dye flow at different ages, and the spread of the dye inside the injected cochlea, to the contralateral cochlea and brain within the first hour after injection.

Our data suggest that PSCC is a better route for drug delivery to the cochlea compared to RWM delivery for several reasons. First, at least in mice, the surgical approach is simpler and the likelihood of damage to middle ear is reduced compared to RWM injection. Second, higher levels of dye reached the cochlea. Third, the dye was more uniformly distributed throughout the cochlea with PSCC injections. And fourth, the dye was more restricted to the inner ear where the injection took place and under these conditions did not reach the brain within the first hour after injection. Our hypothesis for the differences is that the cochlea aqueduct position relative to the injection site is regulating how much dye reaches the cochlea.

Figures 9A,B summarize the hypothesis generated from the data collected in this study. In PSCC injections (**Figure 9A**), the dye first traveled through the SCC and then entered the basal turn of the cochlea via the SV consistent with previous reports (Salt et al., 2012a). Therefore, the compounds first flow through the SV toward the helicotrema, and then continue through the ST toward the cochlea aqueduct/RWM region. In this direction, the cochlear aqueduct can act as a release valve allowing perilymph to flow and be replaced by the injected volume. Our data support a previous report from guinea pig data suggesting PSCC injection provides a more uniform cochlea distribution of drugs (Salt et al., 2012a). In RWM injection (**Figure 9B**), the dye directly entered the cochlea through ST. At the end of infusion, a sharp gradient in the dye distribution from base to apex was observed at both ages. This is also in agreement with the results reported by Plontke et al. (2016) who showed a basal-apical gradient in the concentration of fluorescein after RWM injection to guinea pigs, and other groups who tested gene expression in mice cochlea by injecting viral vectors through the RWM, observing lower gene expression in the apex compared to the base (Askew et al., 2015; Chien et al., 2015; Yoshimura et al., 2018). We also measured a lower level of dye intensity changes 1-h after injection within the cochleae of RWM injected neonatal animals compared to the PSCC injected ones.

RWM injection has flow direction from the vestibule end of the ST, where the cochlea aqueduct may act to shunt flow (dye) away from the cochlea, toward the brain, thus reducing dye entry into the cochlea. The presence of dye in the brain of animals injected through RWM supports this hypothesis. Transduction in the contralateral ear and brain after RWM injection of viral vectors has been reported in the literature (Landegger et al., 2017), while no gene expression in the contralateral ear was reported after PSCC injection of viral vectors into the cochlea (Kawamoto et al., 2001) also consistent with the above hypothesis.

Monitoring of dye progression within the cochlea provides a direct investigation of fluid dynamics but it is not without limitations. One limitation is that the bony capsule in adult mice is thicker than the cartilaginous otic capsule in neonates, making absolute comparisons of intensity between ages untenable. Evaluating dye distributions *ex vivo* did provide the needed resolution to probe adult cochlea dye distributions more directly. The dye intensity was large enough to be detected through the bone so relative changes and timing in dye distribution were compared within each age group. A second major limitation is that the imaging plane provides different volumes for apex, middle, and base so that data can be misleading regarding absolute differences between regions. This problem is compounded by the injection sites being on opposite ends of the perilymphatic space so that imaging orientation can bias dye tracking depending on injection site. The *ex vivo* experiments allowed viewing of cochlea from multiple orientations and so allowed us to interpret dye changes more convincingly. A third limitation in these comparisons is the difference in anesthesia. Hypothermia as an anesthetic in neonatal mice could affect dye distribution indirectly for neonatal animals. It is possible that the difference in apparent resistance is in part due to the temperature difference, in addition to the size difference between adult and neonatal. However, the expected change in viscosity is about threefold which when investigated in the model described below had little effect on the results. Our measurements occur either during perfusion or for at most 1-h post perfusion which does not allow enough time for diffusion to be effective. It is possible that changes in volume or wall mechanics alter the resistance to flow in a temperature dependent way that we cannot account for and so some caution should be taken in comparing across modes of anesthesia. In general, though the major findings happen within groups. The sampling rate due to the small changes in intensity were relatively slow and so it is possible that subtle differences in dye kinetics could be missed. Overall the fundamental conclusions presented are consistent with previous studies and well supported by the data presented here.

Using a FEM simulation, we generated a simplified model to demonstrate the feasibility of our hypothesis that the nearness of the injection site to the cochlea aqueduct dictates the pattern of dye distribution within the cochlea. **Figure 9C** presents the model geometries which represent an unrolled perilymphatic space including the ST and SV and SCCs. The color gradient in **Figure 9C** is also represented in **Figure 9B** as a tool to understand how the cochlea was unrolled. Also included in the model structure are the cochlear aqueduct and the two injection sites. The simulation was run on two models with the same geometry but different boundary conditions. The first model assumed that the perilymphatic space is an isolated compartment with no permeability or leak. The only flow inlet was the injection site, and the only outlet was the cochlea aqueduct (**Figure 9D**). The second model assumed that in addition to the cochlea aqueduct acting as an outlet, a distributed leakage occurred within the perilymphatic space during the injection (**Figure 9E**). The figure presents velocity as an indicator of flow and is expected to be a correlate of the dye distributions measured during the injection. The direction of the flow was from injection site to the cochlea

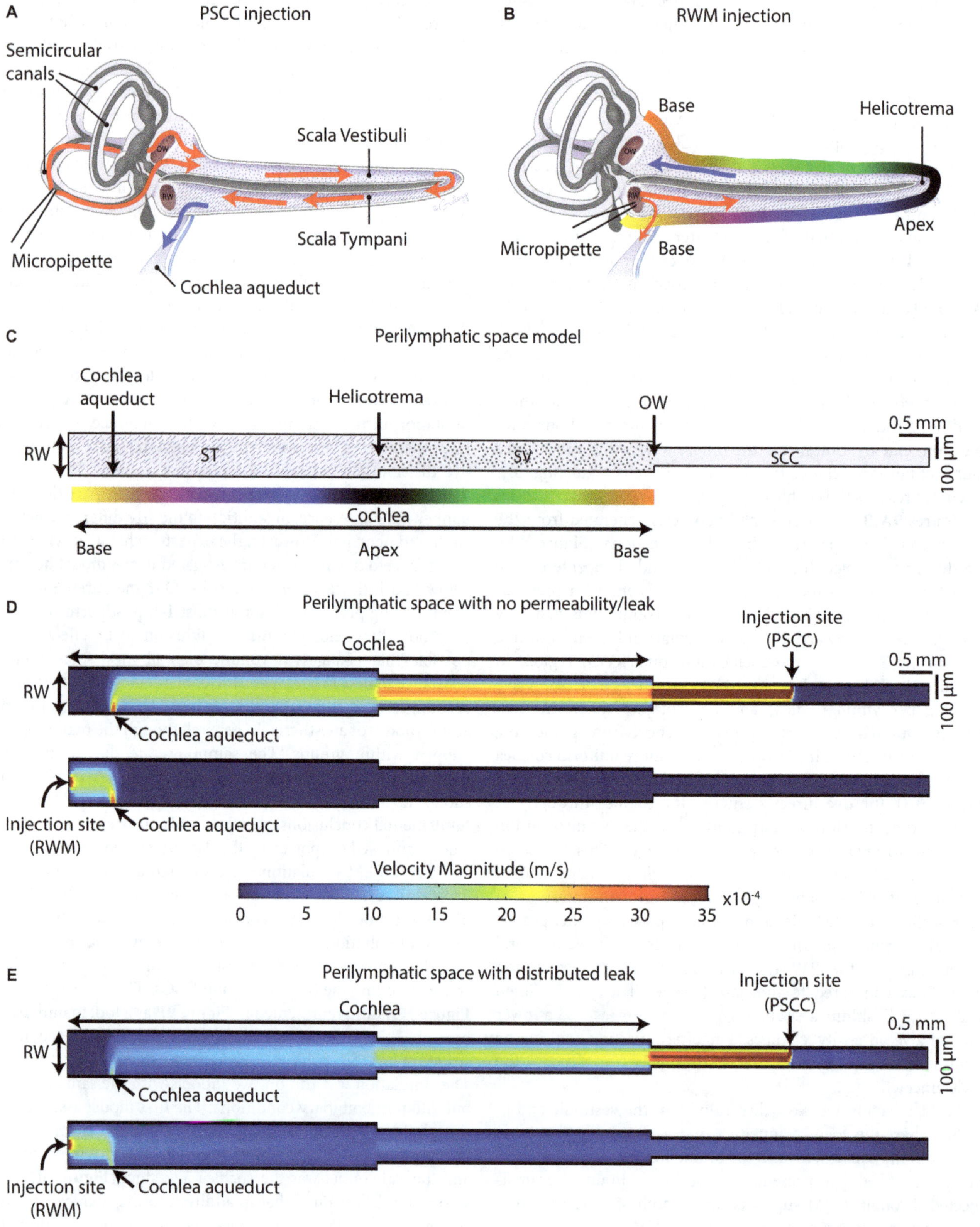

FIGURE 9 | Schematic of mouse cochlea in uncoiled configuration. Pathways of dye distribution in PSCC **(A)** and RWM **(B)** injections are shown in red. Blue arrows show the flow direction of perilymph during injection. **(C)** 2D geometry of the perilymphatic compartment applied for computational modeling of the flow during injections. Results of computing velocity magnitude along the perilymphatic compartment with **(D)** and without **(E)** permeability or leak in the walls. Injection sites (PSCC on the top and RWM on the bottom) were the fluid inlets and cochlea aqueduct was defined as the outlet.

aqueduct, no intrinsic cochlea flow was included. Unrolling the cochlea shows the clear difference in location of the injection sites with the RWM injection reaching the cochlea aqueduct before the cochlea and the PSCC injection reaching the cochlea before the cochlea aqueduct. This fundamental difference is postulated to explain the difference in dye distribution. In PSCC injection (**Figure 9D**, top), a relatively uniform high velocity is distributed along the SV and ST during the injection. In contrast in RWM injection (**Figure 9D**, bottom), the high resistance within the cochlea, due to it being a closed system, the velocity distribution is limited to the area between the RW and the cochlea aqueduct. This example is meant to show the importance of the outlet position relative to the cochlea and injection site. In the second model where a perilymphatic leak was included, the velocity pattern was more like the dye patterns observed experimentally. The basal to apex gradient with RWM injection as well as the lower velocity values in the cochlea due to the bifurcation with the cochlea aqueduct were observed. The PSCC injection resulted in higher average cochlear velocities and more uniformity throughout the cochlea than did RWM injections. This model is used simply to illustrate the validity of our hypothesis and a great deal more detailed information is needed to make it more physiologically realistic.

Our hypothesis supports a significant role for the cochlea aqueduct in dictating flow through the cochlea. As patency of the cochlea aqueduct is potentially variable, particularly between species, it will be important to assess cochlea aqueduct in human if therapeutic approaches are being considered. Gopen et al. (1997) examined temporal bones in human and showed that 93% of the cochlea aqueducts in 101 samples were not completely obstructed (i.e., in 34% the central lumen was patent throughout the length of aqueduct and in 59% the lumen was filled with loose connective tissue). The similarity of data between guinea pig and mouse supports a similar role in fluid regulation for the cochlea aqueduct. The functional role of the cochlear aqueduct is unclear but is postulated to serve as a pressure regulator for the inner ear (Carlborg et al., 1982) and its role in modulating drug delivery must be considered.

Despite providing a uniform distribution of the compounds with PSCC injections, gene expression within the cochlea induced by delivering viral vectors through the PSCC has resulted in higher rates of transduction in the apex compared to the base (Isgrig et al., 2019). This discrepancy between uniformity of the viral vector's distribution and level of gene expression along the cochlea prompted further investigations to search for factors other than the viral vector distribution that can be responsible for gene expression non-uniformity. We found no difference in elimination times along the cochlea for dyes when compared between injection sites within 1-h after injection. Since we do not know the time frame of elimination, it remains plausible that the transduction gradient is a result of exposure time to the virus. It is also possible that like GTTR, the viral vectors' distribution is influenced by permeability properties and not driven by accessibility via the injected flow. Another possibility though is that there are tonotopic differences in how the virus interacts with sensory and supporting cells. Our data simply show that dye distribution patterns do not directly mimic expression patterns from viral transduction.

Our experiments suggest a higher resistance to fluid flow within the cochlea of younger animals. A longer onset time to steepest rate of change in dye concentration and smaller rate of intensity change in neonatal animals compared to the adults during injection are observations supporting this conclusion. The higher resistance is likely due to the fluid pathways with smaller dimensions in younger animals. It might also be a function of cochlea aqueduct patency with reduced patency modulating total resistance to flow. Thus, animal age can also influence the rate of delivery.

In RWM injections, where the injection site is near the opening of the cochlea aqueduct into the ST, more dye was observed in the brain of animals compared to PSCC injections. Our results are in agreement with the observations of Akil et al. (2019) who injected a biological dye into the RWM of neonatal mice, and within a few minutes detected the dye in the brain and spinal cord of the mice (Akil et al., 2019). Kaupp and Giebel (1980) also reported the appearance of lyophilized rhodamine in the subarachnoidal space after direct application of the substance into the tympanic perilymph near the RW (Kaupp and Giebel, 1980). Gene expression was also observed in the brain after RWM delivery of viral vectors into the cochlea (Landegger et al., 2017). These data support the idea that the cochlear aqueduct can provide a pressure sensitive pathway to the brain. Compounds shunting to the brain, which happens more in older animals and with RWM injections, reduces the dose of injected compounds received by the cochlea. This shunting can also explain the difference in steepest slopes obtained between injection sites. Together these data support the idea that the cochlear aqueduct serves as a pressure release valve and must be taken into account when trying to deliver compounds to the cochlea. Recent data (Yoshimura et al., 2018) demonstrated uniform delivery to the cochlea with RWM injection if a hole was first created in the PSCC. This hole likely provides an additional outlet for the flow that directs more fluid toward the apex, OW, and SCCs successively. Thus, this is very much in accord with a release valve role for the cochlea aqueduct.

Contrary to the trypan blue and methylene blue experiments, injection of GTTR into the PSCC of neonatal mice resulted in distribution of the compound throughout the body within 1 h. This supports the idea of Nomura that cochlear capillaries have different permeabilities based on chemical structure (Nomura, 1961). It also suggests that the chemical structure of compounds may dictate their permeation across the inner ear membranes in order to access the blood supply. Careful consideration of the chemical properties of a given compound will be needed when local inner ear drug delivery is the goal.

CONCLUSION

Data presented here are in good agreement with work from others suggesting that the mode of drug delivery (i.e., RWM or PSCC injection) will alter the distribution of compounds within the cochlea. PSCC injection provides a more uniform distribution throughout the cochlea regardless of age. PSCC injections also result in less dye accessing brain. Flow resistance decreases with age but remains an impediment to distribution.

Data are consistent with the cochlear aqueduct serving as a pressure release valve that can help to uniformly distribute drugs when injected through the PSCC but can inhibit drug delivery to the cochlea by diverting flow (drug) when injected via the RWM. And finally, the chemical nature of the delivered compound will affect the drug spread based on its ability to cross membranes and potentially enter the blood stream.

ETHICS STATEMENT

The animal study was reviewed and approved by the Stanford APLAC.

AUTHOR CONTRIBUTIONS

ST, MS, and KA: data collection. ST, MS, and AR: data analysis, interpretation, and figure production. ST and AR: method development and writing – original draft. ST: surgical approach, injection technique, anesthesia and recovery for neonatal animals. ST: computational modeling. MS: method development including micropipette production, dye selection, and injection technique. KA: surgical approach, injection technique, anesthesia and recovery for adult animals. AR: resources, supervision, and funding acquisition. ST, MS, KA, and AR: writing – review and editing.

ACKNOWLEDGMENTS

We thank C. Gralapp for assistance in preparation of the coiled and uncoiled inner ear diagrams. Our thanks for core support from the Stanford Initiative to Cure Hearing Loss through generous gifts from the Bill and Susan Oberndorf Foundation.

REFERENCES

Akil, O., Blits, B., Lustig, L. R., and Leake, P. A. (2019). Virally mediated overexpression of glial-derived neurotrophic factor elicits age- and dose-dependent neuronal toxicity and hearing loss. *Hum. Gene Ther.* 30, 88–105. doi: 10.1089/hum.2018.028

Akil, O., Rebecca Seal, P., Burke, K., Wang, C., Alemi, A., During, M., et al. (2012). Restoration of hearing in the vglut3 knockout mouse using virally mediated gene therapy. *Neuron* 75, 283–293. doi: 10.1016/j.neuron.2012.05.019

Alyono, J. C., Corrales, C. E., Huth, M. E., Blevins, N. H., and Ricci, A. J. (2015). Development and characterization of chemical cochleostomy in the guinea pig. *Otolaryngol. Head Neck Surg.* 152, 1113–1118. doi: 10.1177/0194599815573703

Askew, C., Rochat, C., Pan, B., Asai, Y., Ahmed, H., Child, E., et al. (2015). Tmc gene therapy restores auditory function in deaf mice. *Sci. Trans. Med.* 7:295ra108. doi: 10.1126/scitranslmed.aab1996

Carlborg, B. (1981). On physiological and experimental variation of the perilymphatic pressure in the cat. *Acta Otolaryngol.* 91, 19–28. doi: 10.3109/00016488109138478

Carlborg, B., Densert, B., and Densert, O. (1982). Functional patency of the cochlear aqueduct. *Ann. Otol. Rhinol. Laryngol.* 91, 209–215. doi: 10.1177/000348948209100219

Chien, W. W., McDougald, D. S., Roy, S., Fitzgerald, T. S., and Cunningham, L. L. (2015). Cochlear gene transfer mediated by adeno-associated virus: comparison of two surgical approaches. *Laryngoscope* 125, 2557–2564. doi: 10.1002/lary.25317

Couloigner, V., Teixeira, M., Sterkers, O., and Ferrary, E. (1999). In vivo study of the electrochemical composition of luminal fluid in the guinea pig endolymphatic sac. *Acta Oto Laryngol.* 119, 200–202. doi: 10.1080/00016489950181666

Dai, C., Lehar, M., Sun, D. Q., Rvt, L. S., Carey, J. P., MacLachlan, T., et al. (2017). Rhesus cochlear and vestibular functions are preserved after inner ear injection of saline volume sufficient for gene therapy delivery. *J. Assoc. Res. Otolaryngol* 18, 601–617. doi: 10.1007/s10162-017-0628-6

Felten, D. L., O'Banion, M. K., and Maida, M. S. (2016). "14 - sensory systems," in *Netter's Atlas of Neuroscience*, 3edn Edn, eds D. L. Felten, M. K. O'Banion, and M. S. Maida, (Philadelphia: Elsevier), 353–389.

Fernández, C. (1952). Dimensions of the cochlea (guinea pig). *J. Acoust. Soc. Am.* 24, 519–523. doi: 10.1121/1.1906929

Forge, A., and Wright, T. (2002). The molecular architecture of the inner ear. *Br. Med. Bull.* 63, 5–24. doi: 10.1093/bmb/63.1.5

Gopen, Q., Rosowski, J. J., and Merchant, S. N. (1997). Anatomy of the normal human cochlear aqueduct with functional implications. *Hear. Res.* 107, 9–22. doi: 10.1016/s0378-5955(97)00017-8

Hornibrook, J. and Bird, P. (2016). A new theory for ménière's disease: Detached saccular otoconia. *Otolaryngol. Head. Neck. Surg.* 156, 350–352. doi: 10.1177/0194599816675843

Hudspeth, A. J. (1989). How the ear's works work. *Nature* 341, 397–404. doi: 10.1038/341397a0

Iizuka, T., Kanzaki, S., Mochizuki, H., Inoshita, A., Narui, Y., Furukawa, M., et al. (2008). Noninvasive in vivo delivery of transgene via adeno-associated virus into supporting cells of the neonatal mouse cochlea. *Hum. Gene Ther.* 19, 384–390. doi: 10.1089/hum.2007.167

Isgrig, K., and Chien, W. W. (2018). Posterior semicircular canal approach for inner ear gene delivery in neonatal mouse. *J. Vis. Exp.* 2:56648.

Isgrig, K., McDougald, D. S., Zhu, J., Wang, H. J., Bennett, J., and Chien, W. W. (2019). AAV2.7m8 is a powerful viral vector for inner ear gene therapy. *Nat. Commun.* 10:427. doi: 10.1038/s41467-018-08243-1

Kaupp, H., and Giebel, W. (1980). Distribution of marked perilymph to the subarachnoidal space. *Arch. Oto Rhino Laryngol.* 229, 245–253. doi: 10.1007/bf02565527

Kawamoto, K., Oh, S. H., Kanzaki, S., Brown, N., and Raphael, Y. (2001). The functional and structural outcome of inner ear gene transfer via the vestibular and cochlear fluids in mice. *Mol. Ther.* 4, 575–585. doi: 10.1006/mthe.2001.0490

Kimura, R. S., and Schuknecht, H. F. (1965). Membranous hydrops in the inner ear of the guinea pig after obliteration of the endolymphatic sac. *ORL* 27, 343–354. doi: 10.1159/000274693

Landegger, L. D., Pan, B., Askew, C., Wassmer, S. J., Gluck, S. D., Galvin, A., et al. (2017). A synthetic AAV vector enables safe and efficient gene transfer to the mammalian inner ear. *Nat. Biotechnol.* 35, 280–284. doi: 10.1038/nbt.3781

Liu, Y., Okada, T., Nomoto, T., Ke, X., Kume, A., Ozawa, K., et al. (2007). Promoter effects of adeno-associated viral vector for transgene expression in the cochlea in vivo. *Exp. Amp Mol. Med.* 39, 170–175. doi: 10.1038/emm.2007.19

Liu, Y., Okada, T., Sheykholeslami, K., Shimazaki, K., Nomoto, T., Muramatsu, S., et al. (2005). Specific and efficient transduction of cochlear inner hair cells with recombinant adeno-associated virus type 3 vector. *Mol. Ther.* 12, 725–733. doi: 10.1016/j.ymthe.2005.03.021

Minor, L. B., Solomon, D., Zinreich, J. S., and Zee, D. S. (1998). Sound- and/or pressure-induced vertigo due to bone dehiscence of the superior semicircular canal. *JAMA Otolaryngol. Head Neck Surg.* 124, 249–258.

Myrdal, S. E., Johnson, K. C., and Steyger, P. S. (2005). Cytoplasmic and intra-nuclear binding of gentamicin does not require endocytosis. *Hear. Res.* 204, 156–169. doi: 10.1016/j.heares.2005.02.002

Nomura, Y. (1961). Capillary permeability of the cochlea: an experimental study. *Ann. Otol. Rhinol. Laryngol.* 70, 81–101. doi: 10.1177/000348946107000106

Pan, B., Askew, C., Galvin, A., Heman-Ackah, S., Asai, Y., Indzhykulian, A. A., et al. (2017). Gene therapy restores auditory and vestibular function in a mouse model of usher syndrome type 1c. *Nat. Biotechnol.* 35, 264–272. doi: 10.1038/nbt.3801

Plontke, S. K., Hartsock, J. J., Gill, R. M., and Salt, A. N. (2016). Intracochlear drug injections through the round window membrane: measures to improve drug retention. *Audiol. Neurotol.* 21, 72–79. doi: 10.1159/000442514

Salt, A. N., Hartsock, J. J., Gill, R. M., Piu, F., and Plontke, S. K. (2012a). Perilymph pharmacokinetics of markers and dexamethasone applied and sampled at the lateral semi-circular canal. *J. Assoc. Res. Otolaryngol* 13, 771–783. doi: 10.1007/s10162-012-0347-y

Salt, A. N., King, E. B., Hartsock, J. J., Gill, R. M., and O'Leary, S. J. (2012b). Marker entry into vestibular perilymph via the stapes following applications to the round window niche of guinea pigs. *Hear. Res.* 283, 14–23. doi: 10.1016/j.heares.2011.11.012

Salt, A. N., Ohyama, K., and Thalmann, R. (1991). Radial communication between the perilymphatic scalae of the cochlea. I: estimation by tracer perfusion. *Hear. Res.* 56, 29–36. doi: 10.1016/0378-5955(91)90150-8

Salt, A. N., and Plontke, S. K. (2018). Pharmacokinetic principles in the inner ear: influence of drug properties on intratympanic applications. *Hear. Res.* 368, 28–40. doi: 10.1016/j.heares.2018.03.002

Schuknecht, H. F., and Seifi, A. E. (1963). Experimental observations on the fluid physiology of the inner ear. *Ann. Otol. Rhinol. Laryngol.* 72, 687–712. doi: 10.1177/000348946307200308

Sterkers, O., Ferrary, E., and Amiel, C. (1988). Production of inner ear fluids. *Physiol. Rev.* 68, 1083–1128. doi: 10.1152/physrev.1988.68.4.1083

Sterkers, O., Saumon, G., Tran Ba Huy, P., and Amiel, C. (1982). K, Cl, and H2O entry in endolymph, perilymph, and cerebrospinal fluid of the rat. *Am. J. Physiol.* 243, F173–F180. doi: 10.1152/ajprenal.1982.243.2.F173

Suzuki, J., Hashimoto, K., Xiao, R., Vandenberghe, L. H., and Liberman, M. C. (2017). Cochlear gene therapy with ancestral AAV in adult mice: complete transduction of inner hair cells without cochlear dysfunction. *Sci. Rep.* 7:45524. doi: 10.1038/srep45524

Thorne, M., Salt, A. N., DeMott, J. E., Henson, M. M., Henson, O. W., and Gewalt, S. L. (1999). Cochlear fluid space dimensions for six species derived from reconstructions of three–dimensional magnetic resonance images. *Laryngoscope* 109, 1661–1668. doi: 10.1097/00005537-199910000-00021

Vazquez-Benitez, G., Perez-Campos, A., Masgrau, N. A., and Perez-Barrios, A. (2016). Unexpected tumor: primary asymptomatic schwannoma in thyroid gland. *Endocr. Pathol.* 27, 46–49. doi: 10.1007/s12022-015-9409-0

Wangemann, P. and Schacht, J. (1996). "Homeostatic mechanisms in the cochlea," in *The Cochlea*, eds P. Dallos, A. N. Popper, and R. R. Fay (New York: NY, Springer), 130–185.

Wright, C. G., and Roland, P. S. (2018). "Anatomy of the helicotrema and cochlear apex," in *Cochlear Anatomy via Microdissection with Clinical Implications: An Atlas*, eds C. G. Wright, and P. S. Roland, (Cham: Springer International Publishing), 27–43. doi: 10.1007/978-3-319-71222-2_2

Yoshimura, H., Shibata, S. B., Ranum, P. T., and Smith, R. J. H. (2018). Enhanced viral-mediated cochlear gene delivery in adult mice by combining canal fenestration with round window membrane inoculation. *Sci. Rep.* 8:2980. doi: 10.1038/s41598-018-21233-z

6

Use of Gases to Treat Cochlear Conditions

Jay C. Buckey*

Space Medicine Innovations Laboratory, Center for Hyperbaric Medicine, Department of Medicine, Geisel School of Medicine at Dartmouth, Lebanon, NH, United States

Correspondence:
Jay C. Buckey
jay.buckey@dartmouth.edu

Although the cochlear vascular supply (stria vascularis) is designed to block to certain compounds and molecules, it must enable gas exchange to survive. The inner ear capillaries must deliver oxygen and remove carbon dioxide for the cochlea to function. These gases diffuse through tissues across a concentration gradient to reach the desired target. Tight junctions or the endothelial basement membrane do not impede them. Therefore, gases that can diffuse into the inner ear are attractive as therapeutic agents. The two gases most often used in this way are oxygen and hydrogen, although carbon dioxide, ozone, and argon have also been investigated. Typically, oxygen is delivered as hyperbaric oxygen (HBO) (oxygen at pressure higher than atmospheric) to provide increased oxygen levels to the inner ear. This not only relieves hypoxia, but also has anti-inflammatory and other biochemical effects. HBO is used clinically to treat idiopathic sudden sensorineural hearing loss, and both animal and human studies suggest it may also assist recovery after acute acoustic trauma. Laboratory studies suggest hydrogen works as a free radical scavenger and reduces the strong oxidants hydroxyl radicals and peroxynitrite. It also has anti-apoptotic effects. Because of its anti-oxidant and anti-inflammatory effects, it has been studied as a treatment for ototoxicity and shows benefit in an animal model of cisplatinum toxicity. Gas diffusion offers an effective way to provide therapy to the inner ear, particularly since some gases (oxygen, hydrogen, carbon dioxide, ozone, argon) have important therapeutic effects for minimizing cochlear damage.

Keywords: hyperbaric, oxygen, hydrogen, cochlea, inner ear

USING GASES TO GET POTENTIALLY THERAPEUTIC INTERVENTIONS TO THE COCHLEA

Hyperbaric oxygen (HBO) treatment is the most common example of using gas diffusion to deliver a therapeutic agent to the cochlea. HBO is oxygen provided at levels above atmospheric pressure and is dosed in ATA (atmospheres absolute). One hundred percent oxygen given at normal atmospheric pressure is 1 ATA of oxygen. Most hyperbaric treatments are provided within a pressurized chamber with oxygen at 2.0–2.5 ATA. At these pressures, HBO increases oxygen dissolved in plasma dramatically, which elevates the oxygen content of blood reaching tissues. The driving force for this gas uptake is the basic physics of gases. The partial pressure of a gas in a liquid will match the partial pressure of the gas in the atmosphere around it (Henry's law). The partial pressure of nitrogen in the body, for example, matches that in the atmosphere. Gases dissolve into tissue throughout the body (blood, muscle, fat) based on their solubility and the inner ear is no exception.

The amount of oxygen that can be delivered under pressure is striking. The partial pressure of oxygen in room air is approximately 150 mmHg. The partial pressure of 100% oxygen is 760 mmHg. HBO at 2.0 atmospheres absolute provides an oxygen partial pressure of 1520 mmHg to the lung, or approximately 10 times the partial pressure in room air. Early studies showed that HBO at sufficient pressure provides enough oxygen to meet all the body's oxygen needs solely from oxygen dissolved in plasma. For example, the classic study by Boerema et al. demonstrated that when essentially all red blood cells were removed from a pig (i.e., the hematocrit was basically zero) the pig could survive without any signs of ischemia when given 100% oxygen at 3.0 ATA (Boerema et al., 1960; Boerema, 1964). Similarly, Lambertsen et al. (1953) showed that oxygen saturations in venous blood of humans exposed to 3.5 ATA was at arterial levels measured with air at normal atmospheric pressure. The high concentration of oxygen in the plasma created by HBO creates a strong gradient for diffusion into hypoxic tissue.

This same diffusion effect occurs with other gases. For example, divers take on large amounts of the gases they breath at depth. When breathing air, the deeper the diver goes (i.e., the higher the pressure) the greater the amount of nitrogen that dissolves in tissues. At these higher pressures, nitrogen gas has a narcotic effect due to the effect of the dissolved nitrogen on nerve transmission. This produces the hazardous "rapture of the deep," or nitrogen narcosis, characterized by diminished brain function, and an inability to think clearly. When divers ascend they are at risk for decompression sickness as the gas that was dissolved in tissue starts the process of elimination from the body. If the ascent is too fast, bubbles of the gas may form leading to the characteristic symptoms of the "bends" (e.g., pain in joints, embolic stroke). Although decompression sickness usually results from nitrogen, divers using special gas mixes containing hydrogen can also get decompression sickness as the hydrogen which dissolved in tissue during the dive leaves the tissue as the diver ascends and the pressure around the diver is reduced. Individuals don't need to dive, however, to increase the amount of a particular gas in the body. Just increasing the concentration of a gas in the atmosphere at normal atmospheric pressure (say 2% hydrogen or 20% argon in air) will increase the uptake of that gas into tissue. Also, hydrogen can be delivered to tissues by ingesting or injecting water or saline saturated with hydrogen.

OXYGEN AS A COCHLEAR THERAPEUTIC

The cochlea has a high oxygen requirement and so is sensitive to disruptions of its blood supply (Thalmann et al., 1972). As described above, the hypoxia-relieving effect of HBO is well known and has been considered its primary mechanism of action for many conditions. In the setting of acute ischemia, HBO creates a large oxygen concentration gradient between well-perfused and poorly perfused areas. The high oxygen tension in the inspired air increases the oxygen dissolved in the blood, which in turn increases tissue oxygen levels and promotes oxygen diffusion into the poorly perfused tissue. This immediate hypoxia relieving effect is the rationale behind the use of HBO for conditions associated with acute interruption of the blood supply (e.g., compromised flaps and grafts, crush injuries).

For the cochlea, hypoxia can result from various insults. Acoustic trauma, for example, can lead to reduced cochlear blood flow and inner ear hypoxia (Lamm and Arnold, 1999). Acoustic trauma can disrupt the microcirculation in the cochlea and lead to local ischemia (Shi, 2016). This may be more of an issue in older individuals since there is atrophy of the stria vascularis over time (Shi, 2016) and so disruption of this atrophic stria could lead to more extensive damage. HBO has been shown to be effective in treating acoustic trauma possibly due to relief of cochlear hypoxia (Kuokkanen et al., 1997; Lamm et al., 1998a,b; Lamm and Arnold, 1999; Fakhry et al., 2007; Bayoumy et al., 2019). Another condition where hypoxia may also play an important role is idiopathic sudden sensorineural hearing loss (ISSNHL). As the name implies, the reason for this hearing loss is not known, but it may well result from the sudden loss or compromise of the cochlear circulation. Another possibility is that inflammation in the cochlea may compromise the stria vascularis and lead to hypoxia. The Undersea and Hyperbaric Medical Society lists ISSNL as an approved indication for HBO treatment, and it is often used successfully for this (Stachler et al., 2012; Ajduk et al., 2017; Cho et al., 2018).

One continuing controversy surrounding the use of HBO to relieve hypoxia is whether it might be detrimental by creating oxidative stress in the compromised region. The high levels of oxygen that HBO provides could increase reactive oxygen species (ROS) within the tissue. ROS are thought to be important factors in causing cochlear damage in both acoustic trauma and cisplatinum toxicity (Kamogashira et al., 2015). Since ROS may underlie some of the cochlear damage resulting from acoustic insults, increasing ROS might be harmful. One rodent study suggests this might be true. Cakir et al. (2006) showed that giving HBO shortly after acoustic trauma due to noise led to worse outcomes. This has not been a universal finding, however. In the study by Kuokkanen et al. (2000) rats were exposed to impulse noise and HBO was given daily for 10 days. Hair cell survival was improved in the HBO treatment group compared to controls (Kuokkanen et al., 2000). Recent studies in humans suggest benefit from HBO after acute acoustic trauma (Bayoumy et al., 2019). **Table 1** summarizes some of the main results when HBO has been used in acute acoustic trauma. Overall the results have been positive. This issue of ROS damage from HBO is also a consideration for cisplatinum toxicity, since increased ROS are thought to be an important factor in cisplatinum-induced damage. Cobanoglu et al. (2019) recently reported that HBO treatment of rats after receiving cisplatinum led to improved recovery after the insult compared to the untreated control group. Interestingly, in a study of cisplatinum-induced nephrotoxicity, Aydinoz et al. (2007) showed that once-daily HBO provided benefit, while twice-daily HBO seemed to potentiate the damage.

One possible reason for the different outcomes is that HBO may have competing effects. While the extra oxygen may increase ROS production, HBO may also reduce neutrophil adhesion (Atochin et al., 2000; Miljkovic-Lolic et al., 2003; Francis et al., 2017) which is a key step in the initiation of inflammation. HBO may also downregulate the expression of COX-2, which could also reduce inflammation and potentially improve outcomes (Yin et al., 2002). A growing body of evidence shows that HBO can affect both inflammation and proteases [e.g., matrix metalloproteases (MMPs)]. For example, in ischemic wounds HBO decreases many MMP levels and increases some tissue inhibitors of MMPs (TIMPs), and so seems to influence proteolytic activity (Zhang and Gould, 2014). Zhang et al. (2008) showed (also in ischemic wounds) that HBO reduced neutrophil infiltration, inflammation, and cell apoptosis. HBO has anti-inflammatory effects in other settings. Sumen et al. (2001) showed that HBO reduced inflammation caused by carrageenan to the same degree as diclofenac. Similar results were found by Wilson et al. (2007) also in a rodent model. In a traumatic brain injury model, Vlodavsky et al. (2006) showed that HBO reduced inflammation in the injured animals treated with HBO compared to controls. Several studies have shown the HBO reduces inflammation and improves outcomes in acute pancreatitis (Christophi et al., 2007; Nikfarjam et al., 2007; Bai et al., 2009). The reactive oxygen and nitrogen species generated by brief HBO exposures may serve as signaling intermediates in several cellular pathways including nitric oxide synthase, HIF-1, VEGF, and heme-oxygenase (HO-1) (Gu et al., 2008). HBO can increase wound growth factor synthesis, mobilize stem cell progenitors from bone marrow, and reduce monocyte chemokine and inflammatory cytokine production (Thom, 2011). Recently, HBO has been shown to be effective in moderately severe ulcerative colitis, another condition in which both inflammation and hypoxia are important contributors to the disease (Dulai et al., 2018). Taken together, the data suggest that HBO is more often beneficial than harmful in acute ischemia, although questions remain.

Another potentially interesting effect of HBO is that it up-regulates anti-oxidant enzymes (superoxide dismutase, catalase, glutathione peroxidase). A growing body of evidence shows that hyperoxia (HBO exposure) prior to hypoxia improves ischemic tolerance. Peng et al. (2008) showed that mice exposed to HBO survived longer in a 10% oxygen environment than mice who had received sham treatments. The pre-treated mice also showed longer swimming times when exposed to a hypoxic environment. Li et al. (2008) showed that antioxidant enzymes were upregulated in rats exposed to hyperoxia, and that they were also able to tolerate ischemia better than controls. Gu et al. (2008) showed upregulation of hypoxia inducible factor-1 alpha and erythropoietin in rats exposed to hyperoxia. These studies also support observations in humans that pretreatment with HBO prior to cardiopulmonary bypass improves outcomes, which may be related to an improved ability to tolerate ischemic stress (Alex et al., 2005; Yogaratnam et al., 2010). These data suggest that HBO might be able to prevent or minimize damage due to acoustic trauma if used prior to exposure. While this may not be a practical approach to preventing acoustic trauma in many settings, research in this area could help reveal the mechanisms underlying cochlear damage with noise or other insults.

HYDROGEN AS A COCHLEAR THERAPEUTIC

Like oxygen, hydrogen also can easily move into the cochlea from the bloodstream. Huang et al. (2010) and Ohta (2014) reviewed the use of hydrogen as a therapeutic gas. Evidence

TABLE 1 | Summary of results from studies using hyperbaric oxygen in acute acoustic trauma.

Author	Subjects	Intervention	Outcome measure	Results
Kuokkanen et al., 1997	39 rats, 15 treatment, 24 control	2.5 ATA for 90 min daily for 10 days	ABR thresholds	HBO showed less threshold shift than control $p = 0.07$
Lamm and Arnold, 1999	Multiple groups of 16 guinea pigs compared to 22 controls	2.6 ATA for 60 min, 60 min after noise exposure	Cochlear microphonic, compound action potential, ABR	HBO+ prednisolone provided best recovery compared to other therapies tested
Kuokkanen et al., 2000	3 groups of rats. 14 HBO, 24 exposed no HBO, 10 non-exposed controls	2.5 ATA for 90 min daily for 10 days starting 2–3 h after exposure	ABR, histology	Improved thresholds and less hair cell loss in HBO group
Cakir et al., 2006	4 groups of 6 rats	2.4 ATA for 90 min. Group 1 treated 1 h post-exposure, groups 2,3,4 treated 2, 6, 24, 46 h post-exposure	DPOAEs	Worse recovery in animals given HBO 1 h post-exposure. Possible faster recovery in 2 and 6 h groups
Bayoumy et al., 2019	23 noise exposed humans compared to 18 controls. All received oral steroids	Oral steroids plus 2.5 ATA for 90 min daily for 10 sessions starting 4.4 ± 2.7 days after injury	Audiometry	Significantly better improvement in thresholds in HBO group

ATA, atmospheres absolute; HBO, hyperbaric oxygen; ABR, auditory brainstem response; DPOAE, distortion product otoacoustic emission.

suggests that hydrogen serves as a free radical scavenger and can reduce the strong oxidants hydroxyl radical and peroxynitrite (Kikkawa et al., 2014). Both antioxidant and anti-inflammatory effects have been seen with hydrogen administration in animal models (Huang et al., 2010, 2011). Animals receiving hydrogen in experimentally induced ischemia-reperfusion injury showed less organ damage than controls and studies on the central nervous system, liver, and kidney suggest hydrogen can protect tissue from oxidative stress. Also, hydrogen may affect gene expression, and this may contribute to its anti-apoptotic and anti-inflammatory effects (Ohta, 2014). Overall, these properties suggest that hydrogen may be useful in situations where ROS produce damage.

Since cisplatinum toxicity and acoustic trauma both involve oxidative stress to the cochlea, hydrogen may prove useful in these conditions. Kikkawa et al. (2014) studied cultured mouse cochlear explants exposed to cisplatinum both with and without hydrogen in the culture medium. As expected, cisplatinum caused hair cell loss but hydrogen significantly increased the survival of auditory hair cells. They were also able to show that significantly fewer hydroxyl radicals were produced in the hydrogen-treated cochleae. Fransson et al. (2017) studied the use of hydrogen to protect against cisplatinum induced ototoxicity in a guinea pig model. The guinea pigs breathed hydrogen (2% in air) for 60 min immediately after receiving an injection of cisplatinum. The hydrogen reduced the threshold shifts, prevented inner hair cell loss, and reduced damage to outer hair cells. Chen et al. (2017) examined the use of an abdominal injection of hydrogen-saturated saline on noise-induced hearing loss in a guinea pig model. The guinea pigs that received pre treatment with hydrogen-saturated saline had less hearing loss and the authors concluded this was related to anti-oxidant and anti-inflammatory activity (Chen et al., 2017). Kurioka et al. (2014) had guinea pigs inhale various concentrations of hydrogen for 5 h a day for 5 days after noise exposure. Compared to controls, the hydrogen-treated guinea pigs had better recovery in auditory brainstem response thresholds, less outer hair cell damage, and reduced oxidative DNA damage.

OTHER GASES

Carbon dioxide dilates cerebral blood vessels and so perhaps offers a way to increase blood flow to the cochlea after its blood supply has been disrupted after an insult. Carbon dioxide is often given with oxygen (5% carbon dioxide mixed with 95% oxygen). This mixture, called Carbogen, is designed to complement the vasodilating effect of the carbon dioxide with a high level of oxygen to increase oxygen delivery to hypoxic tissues. Dengerink et al. (1984) showed that Carbogen increased cochlear blood flow after it had been reduced by noise exposure. Hatch et al. (1991) studied the relative contributions of carbon dioxide and Carbogen on noise-induced hearing loss in guinea pig model. Carbon dioxide alone (5% carbon dioxide in air) did not provide benefit, while Carbogen and oxygen did, suggesting that the oxygen was more important than the carbon dioxide in reducing noise-induced damage.

Data also suggest that ozone may be useful in preventing or mitigating cochlear damage. Onal et al. (2017) gave ozone for several days to guinea pigs prior to reversible cochlear ischemia, which produced reperfusion injury. The guinea pigs pretreated with ozone had less cochlear damage as well as elevated levels of antioxidant enzymes compared to the control group. The authors concluded that ozone might stimulate endogenous antioxidant defenses leading to these favorable outcomes. Ozone has also been given after a cochlear insult. Kocak et al. (2016) treated rats with intratympanic and rectal ozone for 7 days 1 week after receiving cisplatinum for 3 days to produce ototoxicity. The rats that received ozone showed less outer hair cell and stria vascularis damage and had improved DPOAEs compared to the control rats. The mechanism for this response remains unclear.

Hollig et al. (2014) reviewed the protective effects of argon. Although argon is typically viewed as being inert and non-reactive, a growing body of evidence shows that it can be neuroprotective and organoprotective for tissues exposed to oxygen and glucose deprivation. A human study evaluated argon (24% Ar, 60% N2, 16% O2) in volunteers exposed to 85 dB of white noise for an hour and reported better outcomes with the argon containing mix (Matsnev et al., 2007). The mechanism underlying the neuroprotective and organoprotective effects of argon, however, is not known.

CONCLUSION

Although the cochlea has barriers to many molecules and drugs, gases can diffuse readily into the cochlea. If a gas with therapeutic properties can be introduced into the bloodstream it can diffuse into the inner ear and have the desired effect. The two most commonly used gases for treating the cochlear are oxygen and hydrogen, both of which have shown benefit for conditions such as acute acoustic trauma, although many questions remain about the optimal timing, correct dosing, and mechanism of action. Gases such as ozone and argon may also have benefit and deserve further study.

AUTHOR CONTRIBUTIONS

JB was responsible for researching and writing the manuscript.

REFERENCES

Ajduk, J., Ries, M., Trotic, R., Marinac, I., Vlatka, K., and Bedekovic, V. (2017). Hyperbaric oxygen therapy as salvage therapy for sudden sensorineural hearing loss. *J. Int. Adv. Otol.* 13, 61–64. doi: 10.5152/iao.2017.3185

Alex, J., Laden, G., Cale, A. R., Bennett, S., Flowers, K., Madden, L., et al. (2005). Pretreatment with hyperbaric oxygen and its effect on neuropsychometric dysfunction and systemic inflammatory response after cardiopulmonary bypass: a prospective randomized double-blind trial. *J. Thorac. Cardiovasc. Surg.* 130, 1623–1630. doi: 10.1016/j.jtcvs.2005.08.018

Atochin, D. N., Fisher, D., Demchenko, I. T., and Thom, S. R. (2000). Neutrophil sequestration and the effect of hyperbaric oxygen in a rat model of temporary middle cerebral artery occlusion. *Undersea Hyperb. Med.* 27, 185–190.

Aydinoz, S., Uzun, G., Cermik, H., Atasoyu, E. M., Yildiz, S., Karagoz, B., et al. (2007). Effects of different doses of hyperbaric oxygen on cisplatin-induced nephrotoxicity. *Ren. Fail.* 29, 257–263. doi: 10.1080/08860220601166487

Bai, X., Sun, B., Pan, S., Jiang, H., Wang, F., Krissansen, G. W., et al. (2009). Down-regulation of hypoxia-inducible factor-1alpha by hyperbaric oxygen attenuates the severity of acute pancreatitis in rats. *Pancreas* 38, 515–522. doi: 10.1097/MPA.0b013e31819cac24

Bayoumy, A. B., van der Veen, E. L., van Ooij, P. A. M., Besseling-Hansen, F. S., Koch, D. A. A., Stegeman, I., et al. (2019). Effect of hyperbaric oxygen therapy and corticosteroid therapy in military personnel with acute acoustic trauma. *J. R. Army Med. Corps.* doi: 10.1080/00016480801901634 [Epub ahead of print].

Boerema, I. (1964). The value of hyperbaric oxygen in thoracic surgery. *J. Thorac. Cardiovasc. Surg.* 48, 177–184.

Boerema, I., Meyne, N. G., Brummelkamp, W. H., Bouma, S., Mensch, M. H., Kamermans, F., et al. (1960). Life without blood. *Ned. Tijdschr. Geneeskd.* 104, 949–954.

Cakir, B. O., Ercan, I., Civelek, S., Korpinar, S., Toklu, A. S., Gedik, O., et al. (2006). Negative effect of immediate hyperbaric oxygen therapy in acute acoustic trauma. *Otol. Neurotol.* 27, 478–483. doi: 10.1097/01.mao.0000224080.77849.3d

Chen, L., Han, M., Lu, Y., Chen, D., Sun, X., Yang, S., et al. (2017). Molecular mechanisms underlying the protective effects of hydrogen-saturated saline on noise-induced hearing loss. *Acta Otolaryngol.* 137, 1063–1068. doi: 10.1080/00016489.2017.1328743

Cho, I., Lee, H. M., Choi, S. W., Kong, S. K., Lee, I. W., Goh, E. K., et al. (2018). Comparison of two different treatment protocols using systemic and intratympanic steroids with and without hyperbaric oxygen therapy in patients with severe to profound idiopathic sudden sensorineural hearing loss: a randomized controlled trial. *Audiol. Neurootol.* 23, 199–207. doi: 10.1159/000493558

Christophi, C., Millar, I., Nikfarjam, M., Muralidharan, V., and Malcontenti-Wilson, C. (2007). Hyperbaric oxygen therapy for severe acute pancreatitis. *J. Gastroenterol. Hepatol.* 22, 2042–2046. doi: 10.1111/j.1440-1746.2006.03380.x

Cobanoglu, H. B., Vuralkan, E., Arslan, A., Mirasoglu, B., and Toklu, A. S. (2019). Is hyperbaric oxygen therapy effective in cisplatin-induced ototoxicity in rats? *Clin. Exp. Otorhinolaryngol.* 12, 66–71. doi: 10.21053/ceo.2017.01704

Dengerink, H. A., Axelsson, A., Miller, J. M., and Wright, J. W. (1984). The effect of noise and carbogen on cochlear vasculature. *Acta Otolaryngol.* 98, 81–88. doi: 10.3109/00016488409107537

Dulai, P. S., Buckey, J. C. Jr., Raffals, L. E., Swoger, J. M., Claus, P. L., O'Toole, K., et al. (2018). Hyperbaric oxygen therapy is well tolerated and effective for ulcerative colitis patients hospitalized for moderate-severe flares: a phase 2A pilot multi-center, randomized, double-blind, sham-controlled trial. *Am. J. Gastroenterol.* 113, 1516–1523. doi: 10.1038/s41395-018-0005-z

Fakhry, N., Rostain, J. C., and Cazals, Y. (2007). Hyperbaric oxygenation with corticoid in experimental acoustic trauma. *Hear. Res.* 230, 88–92. doi: 10.1016/j.heares.2007.05.005

Francis, A., Kleban, S. R., Stephenson, L. L., Murphy, P. S., Letourneau, P. R., Fang, X. H., et al. (2017). Hyperbaric oxygen inhibits reperfusion-induced neutrophil polarization and adhesion via plasmin-mediated VEGF release. *Plast. Reconstr. Surg. Glob. Open* 5:e1497. doi: 10.1097/GOX.0000000000001497

Fransson, A. E., Kisiel, M., Pirttila, K., Pettersson, C., Videhult Pierre, P., and Laurell, G. F. E. (2017). Hydrogen Inhalation protects against ototoxicity induced by intravenous cisplatin in the guinea pig. *Front. Cell. Neurosci.* 11:280. doi: 10.3389/fncel.2017.00280

Gu, G. J., Li, Y. P., Peng, Z. Y., Xu, J. J., Kang, Z. M., Xu, W. G., et al. (2008). Mechanism of ischemic tolerance induced by hyperbaric oxygen preconditioning involves upregulation of hypoxia-inducible factor-1alpha and erythropoietin in rats. *J. Appl. Physiol.* 104, 1185–1191. doi: 10.1152/japplphysiol.00323.2007

Hatch, M., Tsai, M., LaRouere, M. J., Nuttall, A. L., and Miller, J. M. (1991). The effects of Carbogen, carbon dioxide, and oxygen on noise-induced hearing loss. *Hear. Res.* 56, 265–272. doi: 10.1016/0378-5955(91)90176-a

Hollig, A., Schug, A., Fahlenkamp, A. V., Rossaint, R., Coburn, M., and Argon Organo-Protective, N. (2014). Argon: systematic review on neuro- and organoprotective properties of an "inert" gas. *Int. J. Mol. Sci.* 15, 18175–18196. doi: 10.3390/ijms151018175

Huang, C. S., Kawamura, T., Toyoda, Y., and Nakao, A. (2010). Recent advances in hydrogen research as a therapeutic medical gas. *Free Radic. Res.* 44, 971–982. doi: 10.3109/10715762.2010.500328

Huang, Y., Xie, K., Li, J., Xu, N., Gong, G., Wang, G., et al. (2011). Beneficial effects of hydrogen gas against spinal cord ischemia-reperfusion injury in rabbits. *Brain Res.* 1378, 125–136. doi: 10.1016/j.brainres.2010.12.071

Kamogashira, T., Fujimoto, C., and Yamasoba, T. (2015). Reactive oxygen species, apoptosis, and mitochondrial dysfunction in hearing loss. *Biomed Res. Int.* 2015:617207. doi: 10.1155/2015/617207

Kikkawa, Y. S., Nakagawa, T., Taniguchi, M., and Ito, J. (2014). Hydrogen protects auditory hair cells from cisplatin-induced free radicals. *Neurosci. Lett.* 579, 125–129. doi: 10.1016/j.neulet.2014.07.025

Kocak, H. E., Taskin, U., Aydin, S., Oktay, M. F., Altinay, S., Celik, D. S., et al. (2016). Effects of ozone (O3) therapy on cisplatin-induced ototoxicity in rats. *Eur. Arch. Otorhinolaryngol.* 273, 4153–4159. doi: 10.1007/s00405-016-4104-4

Kuokkanen, J., Aarnisalo, A. A., and Ylikoski, J. (2000). Efficiency of hyperbaric oxygen therapy in experimental acute acoustic trauma from firearms. *Acta Otolaryngol. Suppl.* 543, 132–134. doi: 10.1080/000164800454206

Kuokkanen, J., Virkkala, J., Zhai, S., and Ylikoski, J. (1997). Effect of hyperbaric oxygen treatment on permanent threshold shift in acoustic trauma among rats. *Acta Otolaryngol. Suppl.* 117, 80–82. doi: 10.3109/00016489709124088

Kurioka, T., Matsunobu, T., Satoh, Y., Niwa, K., and Shiotani, A. (2014). Inhaled hydrogen gas therapy for prevention of noise-induced hearing loss through reducing reactive oxygen species. *Neurosci. Res.* 89, 69–74. doi: 10.1016/j.neures.2014.08.009

Lambertsen, C. J., Dough, R. H., Cooper, D. Y., Emmel, G. L., Loeschcke, H. H., and Schmidt, C. F. (1953). Oxygen toxicity; effects in man of oxygen inhalation at 1 and 3.5 atmospheres upon blood gas transport, cerebral circulation and cerebral metabolism. *J. Appl. Physiol.* 5, 471–486.

Lamm, K., and Arnold, W. (1999). Successful treatment of noise-induced cochlear ischemia, hypoxia, and hearing loss. *Ann. N. Y. Acad. Sci.* 884, 233–248. doi: 10.1111/j.1749-6632.1999.tb08645.x

Lamm, K., Lamm, C., and Arnold, W. (1998a). Effect of isobaric oxygen versus hyperbaric oxygen on the normal and noise-damaged hypoxic and ischemic guinea pig inner ear. *Adv. Otorhinolaryngol.* 54, 59–85. doi: 10.1159/000059054

Lamm, K., Lamm, H., and Arnold, W. (1998b). Effect of hyperbaric oxygen therapy in comparison to conventional or placebo therapy or no treatment in idiopathic sudden hearing loss, acoustic trauma, noise-induced hearing loss and tinnitus. A literature survey. *Adv. Otorhinolaryngol.* 54, 86–99. doi: 10.1159/000059055

Li, J., Liu, W., Ding, S., Xu, W., Guan, Y., Zhang, J. H., et al. (2008). Hyperbaric oxygen preconditioning induces tolerance against brain ischemia-reperfusion injury by upregulation of antioxidant enzymes in rats. *Brain Res.* 1210, 223–229. doi: 10.1016/j.brainres.2008.03.007

Matsnev, E. I., Sigaleva, E. E., Tikhonova, G. A., and Buravkova, L. B. (2007). Otoprotective effect of argon in exposure to noise. *Vestn. Otorinolaringol.* 3, 22–26.

Miljkovic-Lolic, M., Silbergleit, R., Fiskum, G., and Rosenthal, R. E. (2003). Neuroprotective effects of hyperbaric oxygen treatment in experimental focal cerebral ischemia are associated with reduced brain leukocyte myeloperoxidase activity. *Brain Res.* 971, 90–94. doi: 10.1016/s0006-8993(03)02364-3

Nikfarjam, M., Cuthbertson, C. M., Malcontenti-Wilson, C., Muralidharan, V., Millar, I., and Christophi, C. (2007). Hyperbaric oxygen therapy reduces severity and improves survival in severe acute pancreatitis. *J. Gastrointest. Surg.* 11, 1008–1015. doi: 10.1007/s11605-007-0175-2

Ohta, S. (2014). Molecular hydrogen as a preventive and therapeutic medical gas: initiation, development and potential of hydrogen medicine. *Pharmacol. Ther.* 144, 1–11. doi: 10.1016/j.pharmthera.2014.04.006

Onal, M., Elsurer, C., Selimoglu, N., Yilmaz, M., Erdogan, E., Bengi Celik, J., et al. (2017). Ozone prevents cochlear damage from ischemia-reperfusion injury in guinea pigs. *Artif. Organs* 41, 744–752. doi: 10.1111/aor.12863

Peng, Z., Ren, P., Kang, Z., Du, J., Lian, Q., Liu, Y., et al. (2008). Up-regulated HIF-1alpha is involved in the hypoxic tolerance induced by hyperbaric oxygen preconditioning. *Brain Res.* 1212, 71–78. doi: 10.1016/j.brainres.2008.03.027

Shi, X. (2016). Pathophysiology of the cochlear intrastrial fluid-blood barrier (review). *Hear. Res.* 338, 52–63. doi: 10.1016/j.heares.2016.01.010

Stachler, R. J., Chandrasekhar, S. S., Archer, S. M., Rosenfeld, R. M., Schwartz, S. R., Barrs, D. M., et al. (2012). Clinical practice guideline: sudden hearing loss. *Otolaryngol. Head Neck Surg.* 146(3 Suppl.), S1–S35. doi: 10.1177/0194599812436449

Sumen, G., Cimsit, M., and Eroglu, L. (2001). Hyperbaric oxygen treatment reduces carrageenan-induced acute inflammation in rats. *Eur. J. Pharmacol.* 431, 265–268. doi: 10.1016/s0014-2999(01)01446-7

Thalmann, R., Miyoshi, T., and Thalmann, I. (1972). The influence of ischemia upon the energy reserves of inner ear tissues. *Laryngoscope* 82, 2249–2272. doi: 10.1288/00005537-197212000-00013

Thom, S. R. (2011). Hyperbaric oxygen: its mechanisms and efficacy. *Plast. Reconstr. Surg.* 127(Suppl. 1), 131S–141S. doi: 10.1097/PRS.0b013e3181fbe2bf

Vlodavsky, E., Palzur, E., and Soustiel, J. F. (2006). Hyperbaric oxygen therapy reduces neuroinflammation and expression of matrix metalloproteinase-9 in the rat model of traumatic brain injury. *Neuropathol. Appl. Neurobiol.* 32, 40–50. doi: 10.1111/j.1365-2990.2005.00698.x

Wilson, H. D., Toepfer, V. E., Senapati, A. K., Wilson, J. R., and Fuchs, P. N. (2007). Hyperbaric oxygen treatment is comparable to acetylsalicylic acid treatment in an animal model of arthritis. *J. Pain* 8, 924–930. doi: 10.1016/j.jpain.2007.06.005

Yin, W., Badr, A. E., Mychaskiw, G., and Zhang, J. H. (2002). Down regulation of COX-2 is involved in hyperbaric oxygen treatment in a rat transient focal cerebral ischemia model. *Brain Res.* 926, 165–171. doi: 10.1016/s0006-8993(01)03304-2

Yogaratnam, J. Z., Laden, G., Guvendik, L., Cowen, M., Cale, A., and Griffin, S. (2010). Hyperbaric oxygen preconditioning improves myocardial function, reduces length of intensive care stay, and limits complications post coronary artery bypass graft surgery. *Cardiovasc. Revasc. Med.* 11, 8–19. doi: 10.1016/j.carrev.2009.03.004

Zhang, Q., Chang, Q., Cox, R. A., Gong, X., and Gould, L. J. (2008). Hyperbaric oxygen attenuates apoptosis and decreases inflammation in an ischemic wound model. *J. Invest. Dermatol.* 128, 2102–2112. doi: 10.1038/jid.2008.53

Zhang, Q., and Gould, L. J. (2014). Hyperbaric oxygen reduces matrix metalloproteinases in ischemic wounds through a redox-dependent mechanism. *J. Invest. Dermatol.* 134, 237–246. doi: 10.1038/jid.2013.301

7

Extracellular Vesicles from Auditory Cells as Nanocarriers for Anti-Inflammatory Drugs and Pro-Resolving Mediators

*Gilda M. Kalinec[1], Lucy Gao[2], Whitaker Cohn[2], Julian P. Whitelegge[2], Kym F. Faull[2] and Federico Kalinec[1]**

[1]*Department of Head and Neck Surgery, David Geffen School of Medicine, University of California, Los Angeles, Los Angeles, CA, United States,*
[2]*Pasarow Mass Spectrometry Laboratory, Department of Psychiatry and Biobehavioral Sciences, Jane and Terry Semel Institute for Neuroscience and Human Behavior, David Geffen School of Medicine, University of California, Los Angeles, Los Angeles, CA, United States*

***Correspondence:**
Federico Kalinec
fkalinec@mednet.ucla.edu

Drug- and noise-related hearing loss are both associated with inflammatory responses in the inner ear. We propose that intracochlear delivery of a combination of pro-resolving mediators, specialized proteins and lipids that accelerate the return to homeostasis by modifying the immune response rather than by inhibiting inflammation, might have a profound effect on the prevention of sensorineural hearing loss. However, intracochlear delivery of such agents requires a reliable and effective method to convey them, fully active, directly to the target cells. The present study provides evidence that extracellular vesicles (EVs) from auditory HEI-OC1 cells may incorporate significant quantities of anti-inflammatory drugs, pro-resolving mediators and their polyunsaturated fatty acid precursors as cargo, and potentially could work as carriers for their intracochlear delivery. EVs generated by HEI-OC1 cells were divided by size into two fractions, small (≤150 nm diameter) and large (>150 nm diameter), and loaded with aspirin, lipoxin A4, resolvin D1, and the polyunsaturated fatty acids (PUFA) arachidonic, eicosapentaenoic, docosahexanoic, and linoleic. Bottom-up proteomics revealed a differential distribution of selected proteins between small and large vesicles. Only 17.4% of these proteins were present in both fractions, whereas 61.5% were unique to smaller vesicles and only 3.7% were exclusively found in the larger ones. Importantly, the pro-resolving protein mediators Annexin A1 and Galectins 1 and 3 were only detected in small vesicles. Lipidomic studies, on the other hand, showed that small vesicles contained higher levels of eicosanoids than large ones and, although all of them incorporated the drugs and molecules investigated, small vesicles were more efficiently loaded with PUFA and the large ones with aspirin, LXA4 and resolvin D1. Importantly, our data indicate that the vesicles contain all necessary enzymatic components for the *de novo* generation of eicosanoids from fatty acid precursors, including pro-inflammatory agents, suggesting that their cargo should be carefully tailored to avoid interference with their therapeutic purpose. Altogether, these results support the idea that both small and large EVs from auditory HEI-OC1 cells could be used as nanocarriers for anti-inflammatory drugs and pro-resolving mediators.

Keywords: extracellular vesicles, HEI-OC1 cells, cochlear inflammation, pro-resolving mediators, drug nanocarriers, intracochlear drug delivery

INTRODUCTION

Drug- and noise-related hearing loss (DRHL and NRHL, respectively) are intimately associated with inflammatory responses in the inner ear (Kaur et al., 2016; Lowthian et al., 2016; Kalinec et al., 2017; Keithley, 2018). Inflammation, a normal biological reaction aimed at restoring tissue and organ functionality and homeostasis, is usually divided into two phases: initiation and resolution (Kumar et al., 2014). The initiation of inflammation is characterized by the up-regulation of pro-inflammatory mediators such as leukotrienes, prostaglandins, and thromboxanes. When the inflammatory response peaks, the resolution phase starts. Inflammatory resolution is an active process achieved mostly by the action of specialized protein and lipid pro-resolving mediators (Perretti, 2015; Perretti et al., 2015; Kalinec et al., 2017). We have recently proposed that stimulation of pro-resolving pathways associated with cochlear inflammatory processes could be an important new therapeutic approach for preventing or ameliorating DRHL and NRHL (Kalinec et al., 2017), with pro-resolving mediators accelerating the return to homeostasis by modifying the immune response rather than by inhibiting inflammation (Dalli and Serhan, 2019). The successful implementation of this clinical strategy, however, has several challenges. It requires, for instance, identifying safe and efficient ways to deliver a combination of pro-resolving mediators into the cochlea in clinically significant amounts, without compromising their pharmacokinetics and therapeutic efficacy and with minimal adverse effects to the host. Thus, this study was aimed at evaluating whether extracellular vesicles (EVs) from auditory HEI-OC1 cells could be adequate carriers for these agents.

Recent studies have shown that packaging drugs into nanoscale synthetic particles can improve pharmacokinetic efficiency and therapeutic efficacy (Li et al., 2017; Hao and Li, 2019). Nonetheless, the use of these drug-loaded artificial nanoparticles has several disadvantages. For example, microparticles are usually toxic, they are not stable in biological environments, assembling them is usually expensive, and they are not well suited to carry several different drugs simultaneously (Tang et al., 2012). EVs, in contrast, are naturally adapted for conveying molecular products from cells that generate and/or store them to cells that need them. After dexamethasone treatment, for example, Hensen cells in the guinea pig organ of Corti accumulate Annexin A1 in their cytoplasm and release it to the external milieu inside EVs (Kalinec et al., 2009). EVs have demonstrated promise as a natural delivery system for combinations of small molecules, proteins, oligonucleotides, and pharmacological drugs (Robbins and Morelli, 2014; Armstrong and Stevens, 2018).

EVs have unique advantages as carriers to deliver drugs, such as their ability to overcome natural biological barriers and their intrinsic cell targeting properties. Besides, since EVs are formed from cellular membranes, they are not toxic and they can be easily manipulated for drug-packaging without restrictions associated with the physicochemical properties of drugs. Furthermore, since EVs do not self-replicate, they lack endogenous tumor-formation potential. Importantly, EVs are known to be effective for gene and drug delivery, and their surface and cargo can be engineered to target specific cell types and to deliver specific components (Marcus and Leonard, 2013). Moreover, encapsulating some pharmacological drugs into EVs reduce their toxicity (Tang et al., 2012). Finally, EVs can be produced in a scaled manner more easily than other therapeutics (Lai et al., 2019), and because of their small size and scarce presence of membrane histocompatibility molecules, they carry a reduced possibility for immune rejection (Reis et al., 2016). Not less important, intracochlear delivery of EVs loaded with adeno-associated virus has been already successfully used for rescuing hearing in a mouse model for hereditary deafness (György et al., 2017).

EVs are released by cells as self-contained vesicles encapsulating a small portion of the parent cell cytoplasm. Cells naturally produce a diverse spectrum of EVs, spanning from small vesicles of about 50 nm diameter, to large vesicles up to 10 μm diameter (Mathieu et al., 2019). In the 1980s the smallest EV, between 50 and 150 nm in diameter, were called "exosomes," and this term rapidly became the most frequently used in the EV field (Tkach et al., 2018); the bigger EVs are known as "ectosomes" or microvesicles. This categorization is also associated with the specific origin of the vesicles, with exosomes deriving from the fusion of multivesicular endosomes with the plasma membrane and microvesicles shedding directly from the plasma membrane (Colombo et al., 2014). Independently of their origin, EVs consist of a lipid bilayer, with integral and surface proteins, and containing in the core cytoplasmic proteins, lipids, RNAs (including messenger RNA and microRNAs), DNA, and metabolites (Pinheiro et al., 2018). They are usually enriched in proteins involved in vesicle genesis and trafficking, signal transduction, cytoskeleton organization, antigen presentation and transport, and vesicle targeting to acceptor cells or to the extracellular matrix (Robbins and Morelli, 2014). Typically, they also contain proteins belonging to the tetraspanin protein family such as CD9, CD63 and CD81. The lipid components of EVs include ceramide (sometimes used to differentiate them from lysosomes), cholesterol, sphingolipids, and phosphoglycerides with long and saturated fatty-acyl chains (Skotland et al., 2017). Importantly, it has been reported that EVs naturally contain lipid mediators such as arachidonic and 12-hydroxyeicosatetraenoic (12-HETE) acids, leukotriene B4, leukotriene C4, and prostaglandins E2 and J2 (PGE2 and 15d-PGJ2, respectively), as well as lipid-related proteins (Record, 2018). The outer surface of EVs, in turn, is rich in mannose, polylactosamine, α-2,6 sialic acid, N-linked glycans, lectins, and galectins (Laulagnier et al., 2004; Yanez-Mo et al., 2015). Nonetheless, each type of EV has a unique molecular signature that depends on the parent cell lineage and status (for example, healthy or pathological), and the stimulus that elicited their generation and release.

There is no actual proof yet that small EVs have a function different to that of larger EVs (Tkach et al., 2018; Vagner et al., 2019), although there is agreement in that these different EV populations may have different composition even when released by the same cell type (Mathivanan et al., 2010; Bobrie et al., 2012; Romancino et al., 2013; Zaborowski et al., 2015; Kowal et al., 2016; Xu et al., 2016; Vagner et al., 2019). A recent "consensus" publication, co-authored by several prominent scientists in the field of EVs, stated that "EVs in the small size range likely represent vesicles heterogeneous in origin" with unknown portions of exosomes and ectosomes (Mateescu et al., 2017). The definition of larger EVs is even less precise, with these vesicles comprising a wide range of membrane-enclosed entities. Indeed, it is not yet clear how to divide EVs into their relevant subtypes, or even how many functionally distinct subtypes there are (Mateescu et al., 2017). In addition, increasing evidence suggests that different classes of EVs, and different populations within each class, may harbor unique molecular cargos and have specific functions (Kowal et al., 2016; Willms et al., 2016; Jeppesen et al., 2019), clearly indicating the limitations of the size-based classification. Thus, looking for a better characterization, EVs have been divided by size into small and large (Tkach et al., 2018; Vagner et al., 2019). A similar approach was followed in the present study, with HEI-OC1 EVs divided into two fractions: small EVs (S-EVs, ≤150 nm in diameter, mostly exosomes), and large EVs (L-EVs, >150 nm in diameter, mostly microvesicles).

In summary, endogenously produced EVs are an attractive drug delivery system mainly because of their small size, low immunogenicity, absence of toxic effects, and stability in biological environments (Akao et al., 2011; Fuhrmann et al., 2015; Wong et al., 2016). In addition, EVs can be loaded with a designed combination of therapeutic agents and engineered to target specific cell types (Marcus and Leonard, 2013). Although the actual suitability of EVs for intracochlear delivery of anti-inflammatory and pro-resolving agents, as well as its true potential for preventing or alleviating DRHL and NRHL, will require additional research, confirming them as a possible safe and efficient nanocarrier for these agents is a crucial initial step. In the present study, we investigate the production of EVs by auditory HEI-OC1 cells, characterize them by proteomics and targeted lipidomics, and evaluate their capability to incorporate simultaneously anti-inflammatory and pro-resolving agents in clinically significant quantities. Our results support the idea that EVs from HEI-OC1 cells could, indeed, be used as nanocarriers for intracochlear delivery of drugs and molecular mediators aimed at facilitating the resolution of inflammatory processes.

MATERIALS AND METHODS

HEI-OC1 Cells

Immortomouse™-derived HEI-OC1 cells were grown in polystyrene cell culture dishes (CellStar™, Greiner Bio-One, NC, USA) using DMEM (Gibco, Gaithersburg, MD, USA) supplemented with 10% FBS (HyClone, Thermo Fisher Scientific, Waltham, MA, USA), at 33°C and 10% CO_2 as previously described (Kalinec et al., 2003). At approximately 80% confluence, cells were washed with PBS and fresh cell culture media supplemented with 10% exosome-depleted FBS (Cat. #A2720801, Thermo Fisher Scientific, Waltham, MA, USA) was added. After a further 24 h under the same incubation conditions, the cell culture media was removed and processed for EV isolation and characterization.

EVs Isolation and Physical Characterization

EVs were isolated from the cell culture media using the commercially available exoEasy™ isolation kit (Qiagen) following the manufacturer-suggested procedure. Two cell culture dishes of 100 mm diameter were used per condition, yielding 16 ml (8 ml/dish) of medium; this medium was pre-filtered to exclude particles larger than 800 nm, and the filtrate loaded onto the exoEasy™ spin columns (4 ml per column, total four columns per condition). After centrifugation (500× *g*, 5 min) to remove the residual liquid, 1 ml of elution buffer was added to each column, and then centrifuged again for 5 min at 500× *g* to collect the eluate. Isolated EV samples (1 ml each in elution buffer per column) were pooled, PBS was added to obtain a final volume of 200 ml, and then this EV suspension was filtered by tangential flow with a Sartorious Vivaflow 50 device with a 200 nm pore size (Cat. #VF05P7. Sartorious GmbH, Göttingen, Germany). This device allows the recovery of two fractions: the retained one (L-EVs) with particles of diameter greater than 200 nm, and the filtrate (S-EVs) with particles smaller than 200 nm diameter. The L-EVs fraction was further ultra-filtered and concentrated using Sartorious Vivaspin 2 with 200 nm pore size (Cat. #VS0271), and the second filtrate incorporated to the S-EVs fraction. Next, this combined S-EVs fraction was further ultra-filtered and concentrated using Sartorious Vivaspin 2 with 100 kDa pore size (Cat. #VS0241). Using this procedure, the original EVs obtained from HEI-OC1 cells were separated by size into two fractions, S-EVs (diameter ≤150 nm) and L-EVs (diameter >150 nm).

The counting and sizing of EVs in the L-EVs and S-EVs fractions was accomplished with the Microfluidic Resistive Pulse Sensing (MRPS™) technique using a Spectradyne nCS1™ instrument (Spectradyne LLC, Torrance, CA, USA; Cleland et al., 2016; Grabarek et al., 2019). This method is based on monitoring transient changes in electric current, also known as the Coulter principle, caused by particles passing through a narrow orifice (Song et al., 2017). When a nanoparticle passes through the constriction, it blocks some of the electrical sensing current, increasing the electrical resistance of the constriction by an amount proportional to the nanoparticle volume. Monitoring the electrical resistance as a function of time thus yields a number of short pulses, each corresponding to the passage of a nanoparticle, with the pulse amplitude yielding the nanoparticle volume, and the duration corresponding to the particle dwell time and thus the particle velocity. As the particles are entrained in the suspending fluid, the pulse duration yields the volumetric flow rate. One can thus obtain measurements of the concentration of nanoparticles as a function of nanoparticle size, directly from the temporal record of electrical resistance. This is a well-established technique, with the Coulter counter being the most commonly-used automated instrument for particle analysis (Vaclavek et al., 2019). At present, there are two commercially-available RPS instruments for counting and sizing EVs, the qNano (Izon Science Limited, New Zealand) and the nCS1™ (Spectradyne LLC, Torrance, CA, USA; Vaclavek et al., 2019). The qNano instrument expands RPS technique to a broader range of particle diameters by using an elastic pore that can be stretched, an approach known as Tunable Resistive Pulse Sensing (TRPS; Weatherall and Willmott, 2015). This instrument, however, requires user-dependent manual settings that reduce data reproducibility (Tkach et al., 2018). Rather than a single elastic pore, the MRPS™ technique in the nCS1™ instrument uses disposable polydimethylsiloxane cartridges, each with a constriction of a particular size in a microfluidic channel acting as a sensing gate (Cleland et al., 2016).

In the present study, we used two different disposable polydimethylsiloxane cartridges, TS-400 and TS-900. TS-400 cartridges were utilized in experiments with S-EVs (range 65–400 nm particle size) and TS-900 cartridges in those with L-EVs (range 130–900 nm particle size; Cleland et al., 2016; Grabarek et al., 2019). Samples were first diluted with PBS (1:10) and then supplemented with 0.1% BSA as recommended by the instrument manufacturer, and counting and sizing determined as the average of triplicate measurements on two independent samples. Since the instrument does not discriminate between EVs generated by HEI-OC1 cells from those contributed by the FBS used in cell culture or the abundant silicate particles present in BSA solutions, the values for the number of particles per diameter were background-corrected by subtracting bin-by-bin the numbers obtained in matched control samples of both culture media containing exosome-depleted FBS (CM+ED-FBS) and PBS+0.1% BSA. Particle concentration is depicted in the figures provided by the instrument in the form of Concentration Spectral Density (CSD), which corresponds to the density of particles per ml of solution per nm of particle diameter (particles/ml.nm). The use of CSD allows the comparison of measurements made with different cartridges since the CSD is independent of the cartridge parameters and bin widths. The data, however, can be exported in either CSD or in absolute concentration (particles/ml), which is obtained by multiplying

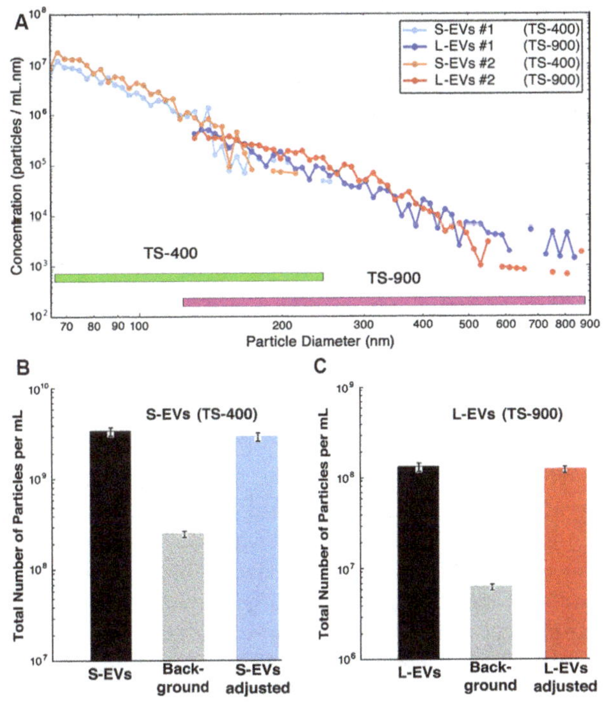

FIGURE 1 | Counting and sizing HEI-OC1 extracellular vesicles (HEI-OC1 EVs). **(A)** Computer-generated concentration spectral density (CSD) vs. particle size for two independent samples (S1 and S2) in the whole size range. Values for S1 and S2 are already corrected by bin-by-bin background subtraction of the values obtained from matched CM+ED-FBS and PBS+0.1% BSA (see **Supplementary Figure S1**). Note that the TS-400 and TS-900 cartridges have an overlapping region. **(B)** Bar graphic depicting the total number of particles in the small-EVs (S-EVs) fraction [average of S1 and S2 = $(3.3 \pm 0.1) \times 10^9$ particles/ml], the total background [$(1.30 \pm 0.04) \times 10^8$ particles/ml for CM+ED-FBS plus $(1.35 \pm 0.08) \times 10^8$ particles/ml for PBS+0.1% BSA = $(2.65 \pm 0.12) \times 10^8$ particles/ml], and average of adjusted values [$(3.3 \pm 0.1) \times 10^9$ – $(2.65 \pm 0.12) \times 10^8$ = $(3.0 \pm 0.2) \times 10^9$ particles/ml]. **(C)** Bar graphs depicting the total number of particles in the large-EVs (L-EVs) fraction [average of S1 and S2 = $(1.39 \pm 0.07) \times 10^8$ particles/ml], the total background [$(4.8 \pm 0.2) \times 10^5$ particles/ml for CM+ED-FBS plus $(5.3 \pm 0.4) \times 10^6$ particles/ml for PBS+0.1% BSA = $(5.8 \pm 0.6) \times 10^6$ particles/ml], and average of adjusted values [$(1.39 \pm 0.69) \times 10^8$ – $(5.8 \pm 0.6) \times 10^6$ = $(1.3 \pm 0.7) \times 10^8$ particles/ml]. Note that in all panels the scale of the Y-axis is logarithmic, but panel **(A)** is in CSD units (particles/ml.nm) whereas panels **(B,C)** are in absolute concentration units (particles/ml).

the CSD values by the width of the respective bins. In the present study, **Figure 1A**, **Supplementary Figure S1** display CSD plots, but **Figures 1B,C** as well as numerical values in the text are provided in absolute concentration.

Proteomic Studies

Bottom-up proteomics was performed using well-established protocols as recently described (Kalinec et al., 2019). Briefly, peptide samples were desalted using a modified version of Rappsilber's protocol (Rappsilber et al., 2007) and fractionated *via* high pH reverse phase chromatography (Agilent Poroshell 120). The fractions were then analyzed by in-line nanobore reversed-phase chromatography coupled to nanospray ionization on a hybrid quadrupole-Orbitrap mass spectrometer (nLC-MS/MS; QE-Plus, Thermo Fisher Scientific, Waltham, MA, USA; Capri and Whitelegge, 2017). The data were processed using Proteome Discoverer 2.2 (Thermo Fisher Scientific, Waltham, MA, USA), which provides measurements of relative abundance for the identified peptides, and mined using mouse protein databases (Kanehisa and Goto, 2000; Kanehisa et al., 2014).

Loading of EVs and Targeted Lipidomic Analysis

HEI-OC1 EVs were loaded with 10 mM aspirin (ASP; Catalog No. A5376, Sigma-Aldrich, St. Louis, MO, USA), arachidonic (AA), eicosapentaenoic (EPA), docosahexaenoic (DHA), and linoleic (LA) acids (Sigma-Aldrich, St. Louis, MO, USA), lipoxin A4 (LXA_4) and resolvin D1 (RvD1; CAS No. 89663-86-5 and CAS No. 872993-05-0, respectively, Cayman Chemical, Ann Arbor, MI, USA), alone or combined. Loading was performed by co-incubation for 1 h at 25°C with sonication for 5 min (Kalinec et al., 2019), a procedure favored by the hydrophobic nature of the molecules selected as cargo (Armstrong et al., 2017). These particular molecules were chosen because they are either pro-resolving mediators (ASP, LXA4, RvD1) or precursors of pro-resolving mediators (AA, EPA, DHA, and LA). Unloaded drug was removed by tangential flow filtration followed by ultrafiltration and concentration as already described in "EVs Isolation and Physical Characterization" section. This procedure increases more than 20-fold the PBS washing volume, rendering a more thorough wash-out of any unincorporated drug than the second purification step with exoEasy^{TM} columns performed in our previous study (Kalinec et al., 2019).

For confirming ASP incorporation by S-EVs and L-EVs, dried samples were treated with *N,O*-bis(trimethylsilyl)trifluoroacetamide reagent (Pierce, 50 μl of reagent, 60°C, 60 min), and aliquots (1 μl) of the solution were analyzed by GC/MS (Thermo Q Exactive GC) for detection of the trimethylsilyl ASP derivative. Peak areas from the reconstructed ion chromatograms (m/z 195.04622-195.04818) for the fragment ion corresponding to the loss of a methyl and acetyl group from the molecular ion (observed m/z 195.04713, calculated 195.04720 for $C_9H_{11}O_3Si$) were compared to those obtained from known amounts of ASP treated in the same way.

For targeted lipidomics, S-EVs and L-EVs were divided into 10 groups: S-Control: S-EVs untreated; S-EVs #2: S-EVs incubated with 10 mM ASP; S-EVs #3: S-EVs incubated with 10 mM LXA4 + 10 mM RvD1; S-EVs #4: S-EVs incubated with 10 mM AA+EPA+DHA+LA; S-EVs #5: S-EVs incubated with 10 mM AA+EPA+DHA+LA+ASP; L-Control: L-EVs untreated; L-EVs #2: L-EVs incubated with 10 mM ASP; L-EVs #3: L-EVs incubated with 10 mM LXA4+RvD1; L-EVs #4: L-EVs incubated with 10 mM AA+EPA+DHA+LA; L-EVs #5: L-EVs incubated with 10 mM AA+EPA+DHA+LA+ASP. Samples of each of these groups were sent to the UC San Diego Lipidomic Core for fatty acid and eicosanoid analysis[1]. As previously described (Eguchi et al., 2016), samples were supplemented with 26 deuterated internal standards and brought to a volume of 1 ml with PBS containing 10% methanol. They were then partially purified by solid-phase extraction on Strata-X columns (Phenomenex, Torrance, CA, USA) following the procedure outlined by the manufacturer. The columns were eluted with methanol (1 ml), the eluent was dried under vacuum and redissolved in 50 μl of buffer A (water/acetonitrile/acetic acid, 60:40:0.02 (v/v/v) and immediately used for LC-MS analysis. Eicosanoids were analyzed as previously described (Quehenberger et al., 2010, 2011). Briefly, eicosanoids were separated by reverse-phase chromatography using a 1.7-μM 2.1 × 100-mm BEH Shield Column (Waters, Milford, MA, USA) and an Acquity UPLC system (Waters, Milford, MA, USA). The column was equilibrated with buffer A and 5 μl of sample was injected *via* the autosampler. Samples were eluted with a step gradient to 100% buffer B consisting of acetonitrile/isopropanol = 50:50 (v/v). The liquid chromatography effluent was interfaced with a mass spectrometer, and mass spectral analysis was performed on an AB SCIEX 6500 QTrap mass spectrometer equipped with an IonDrive Turbo V source (AB SCIEX, Framingham, MA, USA). Eicosanoids and polyunsaturated fatty acids (PUFA) were measured using multiple reaction monitoring (MRM) transitions with the instrument operating in the negative ion mode (Wang et al., 2014). Collisional activation of the eicosanoid precursor ions was achieved with nitrogen as the collision gas, and eicosanoids were identified by matching their MRM signals and chromatographic retention times with those of pure identical standards. Detailed instrument settings are summarized elsewhere (Quehenberger et al., 2018). Eicosanoids were quantified by the stable isotope dilution method. Briefly, identical amounts of deuterated internal standards were added to each sample and to all the primary standards used to generate standard curves. To calculate the amounts of eicosanoids in a sample, ratios of peak areas between endogenous eicosanoids and matching deuterated internal eicosanoids were calculated. Ratios were converted to absolute amounts by linear regression analysis of standard curves generated under identical conditions.

RESULTS

Counting and Sizing EVs

Previous studies of our laboratory showed that auditory HEI-OC1 cells generate abundant EVs (Kalinec et al., 2019). This earlier study, however, suggested that they were mostly L-EVs, with a significant lower number of S-EVs. This was an unexpected result that, if confirmed, would indicate that the mechanism of EV generation could be different in HEI-OC1 than in other cell populations. Thus, the first goal of the present study was to evaluate the number of S-EVs and L-EVs generated by HEI-OC1 cells. Since the nanotracking technique used in our previous study is dependent on the optical properties of the particles, which vary with their size, we switched to a different technique, Microfluidic Resistive Pulse Sensing (MRPS).

The data provided by the nCS1^{TM} MRPS instrument, using TS-400 and TS-900 cartridges, is summarized in **Figure 1**. The number of particles vs. diameter of particle curves corresponding

[1] http://www.ucsd-lipidmaps.org

to S-EVs and L-EVs from two independent samples (#1 and #2) are depicted in **Figure 1A**, with values expressed in CSD units (particles/ml.nm). Each point of these curves represents the average of three measurements per sample, and they are already adjusted by bin-by-bin background subtraction of the values obtained from matched CM+ED-FBS and PBS+0.1% BSA control samples (confidence intervals are depicted by the diameter of the graphic points corresponding to every value; for background values, also in CSD units, see **Supplementary Figure S1**). The data shows that the number of EVs varies in inverse proportion to their size, with a maximum of around 1×10^7 particles/ml and a minimum of about 1×10^5 particles/ml for S-EVs, and a range of around 1×10^6 to 1×10^3 particles/ml for L-EVs (note that these values are expressed in absolute concentration units). When the areas under the size distribution plots were summed, and background subtracted, the S-EVs samples contained an adjusted average of $(3.0 \pm 0.2) \times 10^9$ particles/ml, corresponding to a total of $(3.3 \pm 0.1) \times 10^9$ particles/ml minus $(2.65 \pm 0.08) \times 10^8$ particles/ml for background (**Figure 1B**). L-EVs samples, in turn, contained an adjusted average of $(1.3 \pm 0.7) \times 10^8$ particles/ml, as a consequence of a total value of $(1.39 \pm 0.69) \times 10^8$ particles/ml in experimental samples and $(5.8 \pm 0.4) \times 10^6$ particles/ml for background (**Figure 1C**). Thus, in contrast to the results using the nanotracking technique (Kalinec et al., 2019), our present data indicate that HEI-OC1 cells generate more S-EVs than L-EVs. Other information apparent from these figures is that the fractions are not absolutely "pure," since the S-EVs one still contains a certain number of particles with diameters larger than 150 nm and, vice-versa, the L-EVs fraction contains vesicles with diameters smaller than 150 nm (**Figure 1A**).

Interestingly, using the formulas $V = 4/3\ (\pi r^3)$ and $S = 4\pi r^2$, the particle diameters provided by the nCS1™ instrument to estimate the EVs' radius, and assuming the EVs are perfectly spherical, the calculated total volumes (S-EVs = 3.1×10^{14} nm^3; L-EVs = 6.4×10^{14} nm^3) and surface (membrane) areas (S-EVs = 1.8×10^{13} nm^2; L-EVs = 1.2×10^{13} nm^2) of the vesicles present in each fraction are of the same order of magnitude.

Protein Profiling of HEI-OC1 EVs

Next, we wonder whether S-EVs and L-EVs shared a similar protein profile or, instead, they contain some unique protein markers that could be used for identification or classification. To investigate this issue, we performed bottom-up proteomics.

A total of 620 *bona fide* EV proteins were detected in our proteomic studies, 489 of them in the S-EVs fraction and 131 in the L-EVs fraction (**Supplementary Tables S1, S2**). From them, 381 (61.5%) were unique for S-EVs, 23 (3.7%) were specific for the L-EVs, and 108 (17.4%) were found in both fractions. Interestingly, 86.7% (26 out of 30) of the proteins listed in the ExoCarta exosome database as those more frequently identified in exosomes (Keerthikumar et al., 2016) were detected in S-EVs; in contrast, only 15 out of these 30 (50%) were detected in the L-EVs fraction. CD63, CD81, and PDCD6IP (*aka* Alix), all considered exosome biomarkers, were identified only in S-EVs (**Table 1**).

TABLE 1 | Expression in small extracellular vesicles (S-EVs) and large EVs (L-EVs) fractions of the proteins more frequently identified in exosomes.

Score ExoCarta	Gene symbol	Present in S-EVs?	Present in L-EVs?
1	CD9	-	-
2	HSPA8	YES	YES
3	PDCD6IP	YES	-
4	GAPDH	YES	YES
5	ACTB	YES	YES
6	ANXA2	YES	-
7	CD63	YES	-
8	SDCBP	-	-
9	ENO1	YES	YES
10	HSP90AA1	YES	YES
11	TSG101	-	-
12	PKM	YES	YES
13	LDHA	YES	-
14	EEF1A1	YES	YES
15	YWHAZ	YES	YES
16	PGK1	YES	YES
17	EEF2	YES	YES
18	ALDOA	YES	-
19	HSP90AB1	YES	YES
20	ANXA5	YES	-
21	FASN	-	-
22	YWHAE	YES	YES
23	CLTC	YES	-
24	CD81	YES	-
25	ALB	YES	YES
26	VCP	YES	YES
27	TPI1	YES	-
28	PPIA	YES	-
29	MSN	YES	-
30	CFL1	YES	YES

ExoCarta: http://exocarta.org/Archive/ExoCarta_top100_protein_details_5.txt. Accessed January 29, 2019. Twenty-six out of the 30 (86.7%) proteins more frequently identified in exosomes were found in S-EVs, but only 15 (50%) of them were found in L-EVs.

More importantly, the protein mediators of inflammatory resolution Annexin A1 (ANXA1) and Galectins 1 and 3 (Gal-1 and Gal-3) were only detected in the S-EVs fraction too (**Supplementary Tables S1, S2**). On the other hand, only one cytokine (CSF1, colony-stimulating factor 1) was detected in HEI-OC1 EVs, but it was present in both fractions S-EVs and L-EVs.

Except for the difference in the total number of proteins in each fraction, the distribution profiles by cellular origin, biological and molecular functions were quite similar in S-EVs and L-EVs (**Figures 2–4**). Most of the proteins detected in both fractions originated from cell membranes, cytoplasm, nucleus, or cytosol, with minor percentages of extracellular origin or from organoids (mitochondria, endoplasmic reticulum) and the cytoskeleton (**Figure 2**). They were mostly involved in metabolism or regulation of other biological processes, as well as in response to stimuli, cell organization and biogenesis, and transport (**Figure 3**). The most common function was molecular binding, either to other proteins, RNA, metal ions or nucleotides, but proteins with catalytic or structural function were also significantly represented (**Figure 4**). In every case, the proteins identified as "Others" include all those belonging to groups with less than 5% of the total.

In summary, we found that the S-EVs fraction contains a larger number and greater diversity of proteins than the

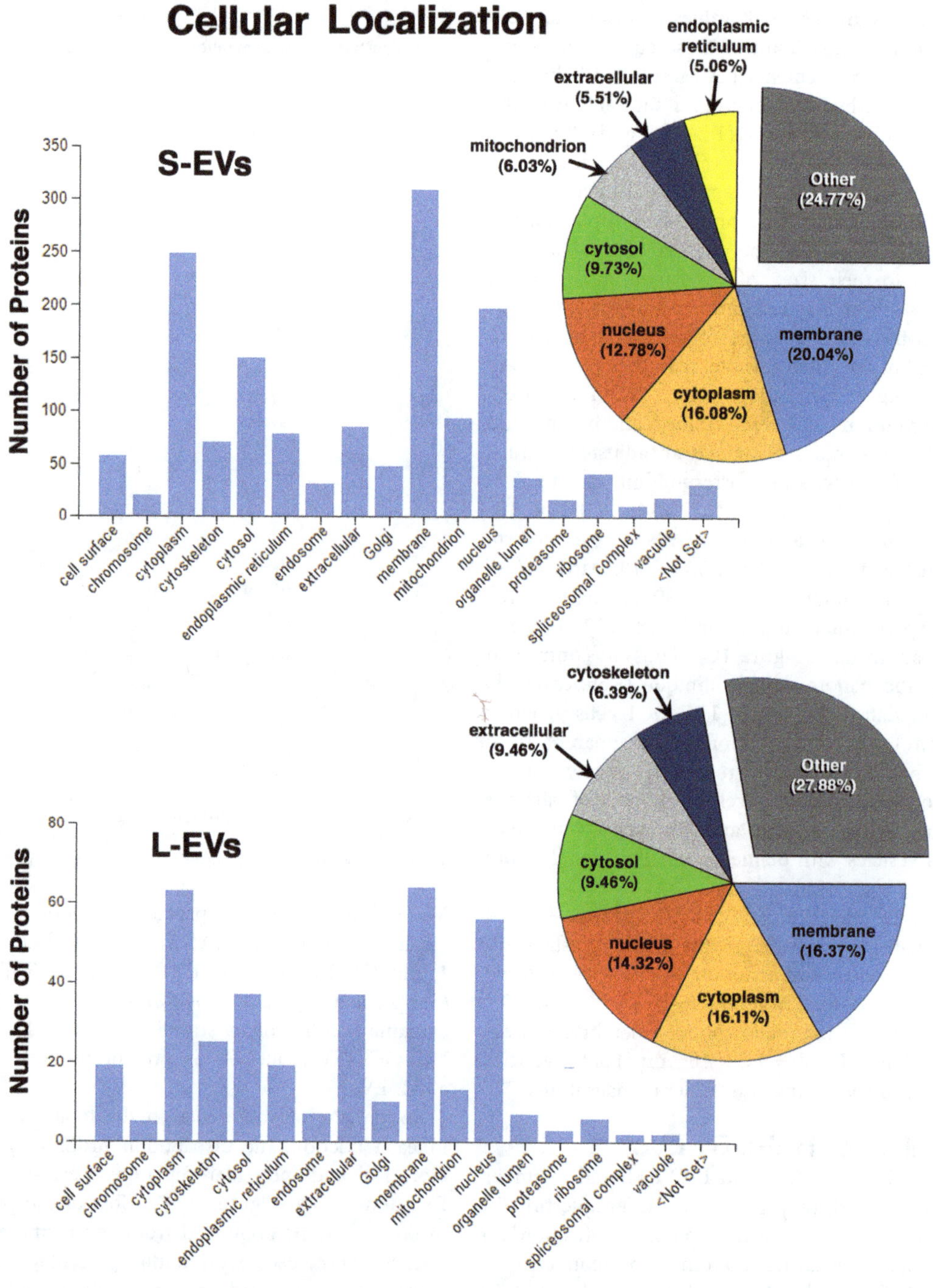

FIGURE 2 | Proteomic analysis. Characterization of proteins from HEI-OC1 EVs by cellular localization.

L-EVs, but the similarities observed in their distribution profiles (**Figures 2–4**) suggest that this difference could be associated with the involvement of a more efficient cellular mechanism of protein sorting and/or loading into S-EVs from a single pool of molecules rather than the existence of two different pools, one for S-EVs and other for L-EVs. The presence of ANXA1, Gal-1, and Gal-3 makes S-EVs more attractive as potential nanocarriers in pro-resolving therapies.

EVs' Loading and Target Lipidomic Analysis

The absence of toxic effects and the ability to incorporate as cargo the drugs and molecules of interest are crucial requirements for a useful drug carrier. As already mentioned, EVs are not toxic, lack endogenous tumor-formation potential, and they show very low immunogenicity. In addition, they can be easily loaded with pharmacological agents using simple procedures. Therefore, we decided to investigate the loading of S-EVs and L-EVs from HEI-OC1 cells with ASP, the eicosanoids LXA4, RvD1, and the PUFA AA, DHA, EPA, and LA, all of them recognized anti-inflammatory and pro-resolving agents. While ASP incorporation was evaluated by GC/MS, eicosanoids were identified and quantified by targeted lipidomics using LC/MS/MS-MRM. Importantly, in addition to revealing the identity and concentration of around 150 eicosanoids, PUFA, and related compounds, the lipidomic profiles revealed the presence and amounts of endogenous pro-inflammatory components that could counter the pro-resolving effects of the cargo.

Co-incubation of HEI-OC1 EVs (10 ml, with 1 × 10^8 S-EVs and L-EVs per ml) with ASP (10 mM) resulted in the incorporation of 6.9 ± 0.1 µg/ml (~38 µM) of ASP in S-EVs samples, and 61.8 ± 0.6 µg/ml (~0.34 mM) ASP in L-EVs samples. These results suggest that EVs, particularly L-EVs could be loaded with pharmacologically effective quantities of this drug.

Of the 150 components of the lipidomic profiles, only 19 were detected in untreated (Control) samples, with four of them detected only in S-Control, six only in L-Control, and nine found in both fractions (**Figure 5**, **Supplementary Table S3**). In addition, while free AA, DHA, and EPA were found in untreated EVs, LXA4, ATL-LXA4, Resolvins, Maresins, and Protectins were not detected (**Table 2**, **Supplementary Table S3**).

As shown in **Table 2** both, S-EVs #3 and #4 and L-EVs #3 and #4, were able to simultaneously incorporate AA, EPA, and DHA in amounts between 5 and 6 nmol per ml of suspension (about 1.5–2.0 ng/ml). Importantly, in EVs loaded with these PUFA, all 19 metabolites originally detected in S-Control and L-Control samples (**Figure 5**) showed an increased concentration in both fractions. Moreover, 50 other metabolites previously undetected were found in these EVs, making a total of 69 eicosanoids identified in the samples (**Supplementary Table S3**). Inflammatory agents were not detected in Control and ASP-loaded EVs, but those loaded with PUFAs generate several prostaglandins [e.g., PGD_2(189.18 pmol/ml], PGE_2(48.94 pmol/ml), PGF_{2a} (15.64 pmol/ml), leukotriene B4 (LTB_4, 3.84 pmol/ml), and thromboxane B2 (TXB2, 1.18 pmol/ml), among others (**Supplementary Table S3**). The generation of PUFA derivatives suggests the existence of an active biosynthetic mechanism within HEI-OC1 EVs. LXA4 and AT-LXA4 (ASP triggered-LXA4) were also detected in these groups in amounts varying roughly between 3 and 10 pmol/ml (about 0.35 ng/ml). Since the limit of detection of the lipidomic experiments was around 0.002 pmol/ml, the measured values represent increases of at least 3–4 orders of magnitude (1,000-fold to 10,000-fold) relative to the control conditions. As expected, S-EVs and L-EVs also incorporated LXA4 and RvD1, although in lower amounts than their precursors AA, EPA, and DHA. It should be noted, however, that the amounts of LXA4 and RvD1 incorporated by HEI-OC1 EVs ranged from 15 to 210 pmol/ml (roughly 5–70 µg/ml), six orders of magnitude higher than the normal concentrations of these pro-resolving mediators in human serum [2–120 pg/ml (Colas et al., 2014; Dalli et al., 2017)]. Curiously, AT-LXA4 was not found in ASP-loaded EVs (S-EVs #2 and #5, and L-EVs #2, and #5), but was detected in EVs loaded with LXA4 (S-EVs #3 and L-EVs#3) and AA, its fatty acid precursor (S-EVs #4 and #5, and L-EVs #4, and #5).

DISCUSSION

The present study provides evidence that auditory HEI-OC1 cells generate abundant EVs, both small (<150 nm diameter) and larger (>150 nm diameter), which can be loaded with anti-inflammatory drugs, PUFA, and pro-resolving mediators, either alone or combined, in amounts significantly higher than those normally found in human serum. Proteomic studies detected a differential presence of selected proteins in S-EVs and L-EVs fractions. In particular, S-EVs contained a larger variety of proteins, including the pro-resolving mediators ANXA1, Gal-1 and Gal-3, than L-EVs. Targeted lipidomic studies, in turn, identified eicosanoids that were present in one of the EV fractions and not in the other. These results support the idea that HEI-OC1 EVs could be advantageously used as nanocarriers for delivery of drugs and molecular mediators aimed at facilitating the resolution of inflammatory processes. In particular, they could potentially be useful as vehicles for the intracochlear delivery of pro-resolving agents aimed at preventing or alleviating DRHL and NRHL.

Counting and Sizing EVs

The present results indicate that HEI-OC1 cells secrete near two orders of magnitude more S-EVs than L-EVs, with the number of EVs decreasing monotonically with their increase in diameter (**Figure 1A**). Since the instrument used for the measurements counts individual particles and estimates their diameter, arithmetic calculations from the data (assuming that all the EVs were perfect spheres) indicated that the total volume and total membrane area of the vesicles present in each fraction were of the same order of magnitude, suggesting that the drug-loading capability of both fractions should be roughly similar.

The abundance of S-EVs is in contradiction to the data we reported in a recent publication, where the counting and sizing of HEI-OC1 EVs were based on light-scattering technology (Kalinec et al., 2019). The distribution of EVs by size as estimated with that technique showed a low concentration of particles with diameters below 200 nm, suggesting that HEI-OC1 EVs consisted mostly of L-EVs. However, as already discussed in that publication, although currently considered as reliable, light-scattering techniques are not exempt from problems (Witwer et al., 2013; Koritzinsky et al., 2017; Grabarek et al., 2019). In particular, particles with an optical index close to that of the suspension medium or with high curvature radius (small diameter) scatter much less light than those with a significantly different index or larger diameter. This sensitivity dependence makes small biological particles essentially undetectable (Cleland et al., 2016; Grabarek et al., 2019), a fact that could explain the difference between our preliminary results and those reported here.

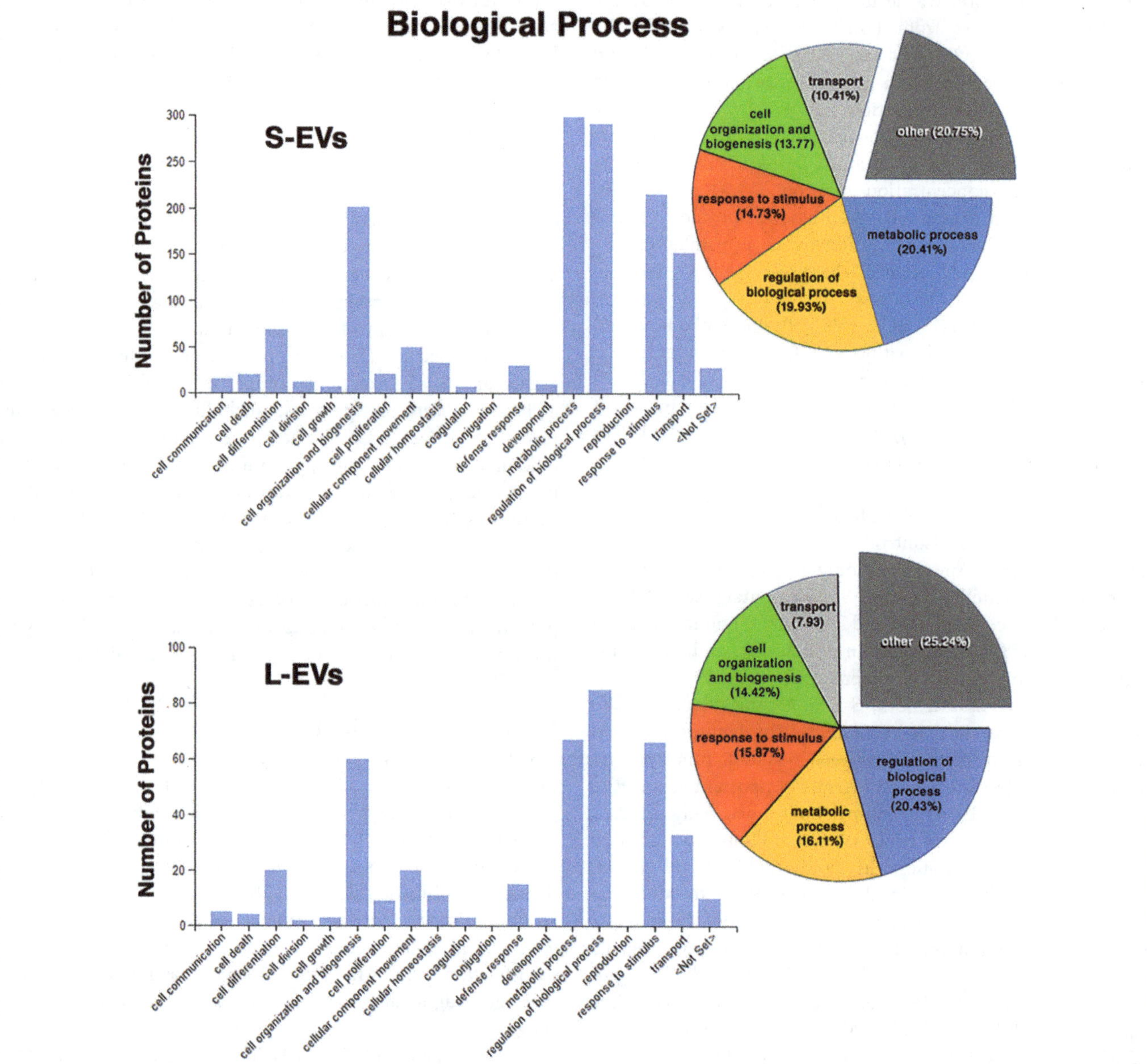

FIGURE 3 | Proteomic analysis. Characterization of proteins from HEI-OC1 EVs by associated biological process.

In the present study, HEI-OC1 EVs were counted and sized with an instrument (Spectradyne nCS1^{TM}) based on a completely different technique, Microfluidic Resistive Pulse Sensing (MRPS^{TM}; Cleland et al., 2016; Grabarek et al., 2019). MRPS is based on monitoring transient changes in electric current, also known as the Coulter principle, caused by particles passing through a narrow orifice (Song et al., 2017). Using the nCS1^{TM} for counting and sizing, EVs have some important advantages. The nCS1^{TM} is capable of measuring the size distribution of EVs with diameters ranging from 35 nm up to 10 μm over concentrations ranging from 10^7 to 10^{12} particles/ml, and statistically significant data sets can be acquired rapidly (minutes). Because the nCS1^{TM} uses electrical sensing, not optical detection, measurements are independent of the material properties of the particles. Importantly, the small sample volume required for analysis (3 μl) is set by the size of the analyte reservoir in the disposable cartridge. Moreover, the measurement does not rely on user-adjustable parameters, rendering more reproducible results. Although not completely free of limitations (analysis of particles with diameters <55 nm with this technique is still complicated, and the use of different cartridges makes cumbersome the evaluation of samples with a big range of particle's diameters), MRPS is probably the best currently available technique for analyzing particles in the nanometer range (Grabarek et al., 2019).

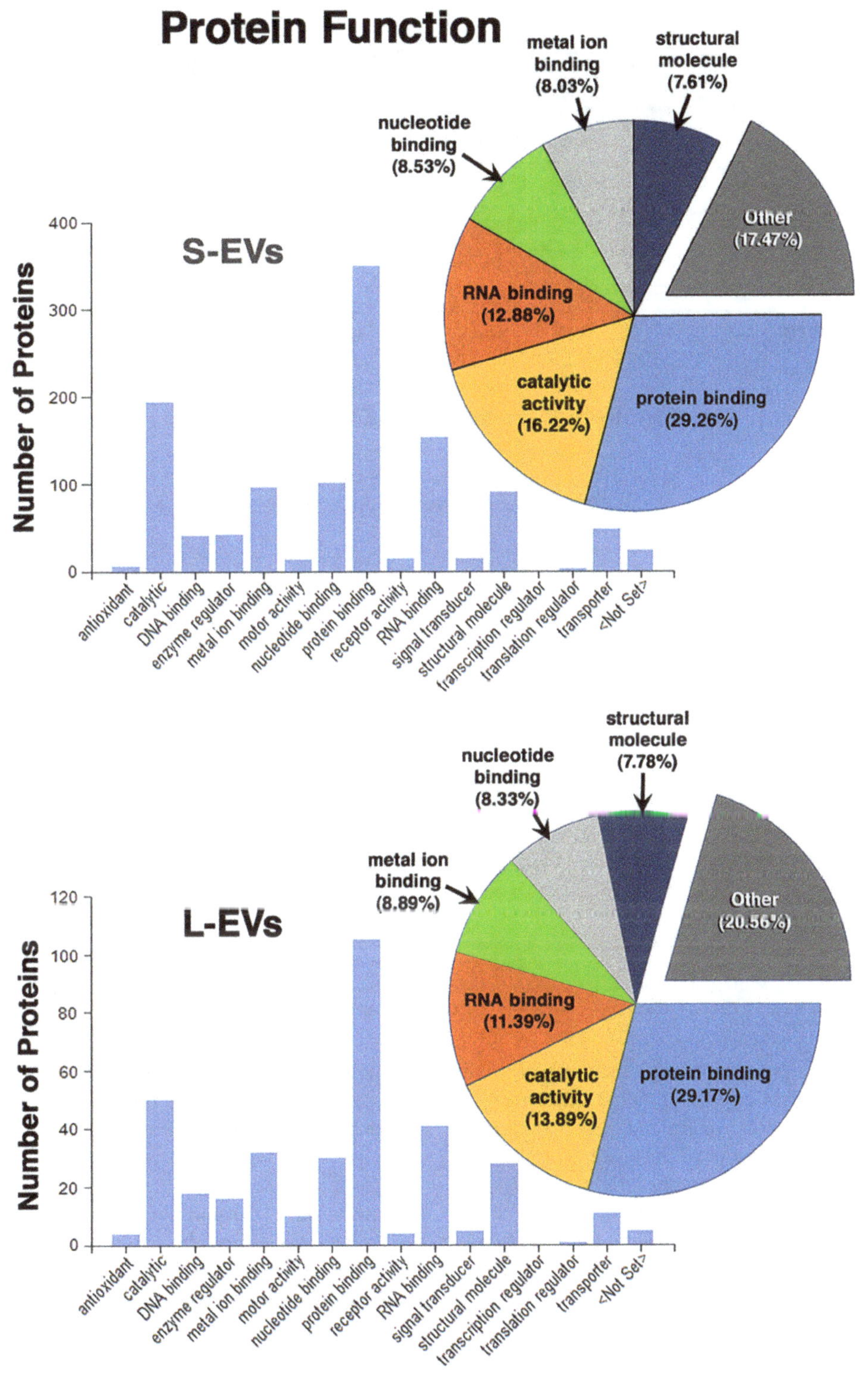

FIGURE 4 | Proteomic analysis. Characterization of proteins from HEI-OC1 EVs by molecular function.

Protein Profiles of S-EVs and L-EVs

A recent "consensus" publication, co-authored by several prominent scientists in the field of EVs, stated that "EVs in the small size range likely represent vesicles heterogeneous in origin" with unknown portions of exosomes and ectosomes (Mateescu et al., 2017). The definition of larger EVs is even less precise, with these vesicles comprising a wide range of membrane-enclosed entities. Indeed, it is not yet clear how to divide EVs into

Metabolites Unique to S-EVs

	16-HDoHE	15-HETE	8-HETE	8-HETrE
S-Control	0.02	0.10	0.08	0.20
L-Control	ND	ND	ND	ND

Metabolites Unique to L-EVs

	PGD2	dhk PGE2	15-oxoETE	14(15)-EpETE	9(10)-EpOME	12(13)-EpOME
S-Control	ND	ND	ND	ND	ND	ND
L-Control	0.02	0.24	1.06	0.56	0.56	1.30

	11-HETE	5-HETE	13-HODE	12-HETE	12-HEPE	14-HDoHE	9-HODE	9-oxoODE	9,10-diHOME
S-Control	0.06	0.14	0.44	2.52	0.06	0.22	0.80	0.18	0.02
L-Control	0.80	0.32	1.22	4.30	0.22	0.54	1.62	2.10	0.04

Metabolites Detected in S-EVs *and* L-EVs

FIGURE 5 | Lipidomic analysis. Only 19 out of 150 metabolites investigated were detected in Control HEI-OC1 EVs, four of them in S-EVs, six in L-EVs, and nine in both fractions. Values expressed in pmol/ml. ND, Not Detected.

TABLE 2 | Lipidomic analysis.

Group	Free AA	Free EPA	Free DHA	AT-LXA$_4$	LXA$_4$	RvD1
S-Control	17.84	0.52	6.02	ND	ND	ND
S-EVs #2	28.86	0.72	10.34	ND	ND	ND
S-EVs #3	50.02	2.20	19.62	1.56	55.40	15.44
S-EVs #4	6,370.88	4,764.42	5,149.18	20.26	24.46	ND
S-EVs #5	5,872.28	4,633.08	5,625.40	13.36	15.94	ND
L-Control	154.54	94.24	110.38	ND	ND	ND
L-EVs #2	73.98	38.58	47.52	ND	ND	ND
L-EVs #3	25.28	12.64	13.92	6.26	207.34	70.70
L-EVs #4	3,596.42	2,707.80	3,438.06	8.00	9.14	ND
L-EVs #5	2,183.12	2,387.16	2,393.28	7.36	9.24	ND

Incorporation of fatty acids and pro-resolving mediators by HEI-OC1 EVs. S-Control: S-EVs untreated; S-EVs #2: S-EVs incubated with 10 mM ASP; S-EVs #3: S-EVs incubated with 10 mM LXA4 + 10 mM RvD1; S-EVs #4: S-EVs incubated with 10 mM AA+EPA+DHA+LA; S-EVs #5: S-EVs incubated with 10 mM AA+EPA+DHA+LA+ASP; L-Control: L-EVs untreated; L-EVs #2: L-EVs incubated with 10 mM ASP; L-EVs #3: L-EVs incubated with 10 mM LXA4+RvD1; L-EVs #4: L-EVs incubated with 10 mM AA+EPA+DHA+LA; L-EVs #5: L-EVs incubated with 10 mM AA+EPA+DHA+LA+ASP. Results are expressed in pmol/ml. ND, Not Detected.

their relevant subtypes, or even how many functionally distinct subtypes are there (Mateescu et al., 2017). In addition, every EV subtype could have different protein and lipid composition and, consequently, a different function (Kowal et al., 2016; Willms et al., 2016). Thus, recent studies have searched for a better characterization of different EV subtypes, and one of the common classifications is division by size into small and large (Vagner et al., 2019). A similar approach was followed in the present study.

Our results show that S-EVs and L-EVs do not contain the same repertoire of proteins. In fact, only 17.4% (108 out of the 620) proteins identified as belonging to HEI-OC1 EVs are common to both fractions, whereas 61.5% (381 out of 620) are unique to S-EVs and 3.7% (23 out of 620) were found only in L-EVs. As shown in **Table 1**, 86.7% of the proteins more frequently found in exosomes were present in S-EVs from HEI-OC1 cells, whereas only 50% were also present in the L-EVs fraction. Two proteins (SDCBP, an adapter protein involved in exosome biogenesis, and FASN, a fatty acid synthase) frequently identified in exosomes and previously reported in HEI-OC1 EVs (Kalinec et al., 2019) were not detected in the present study. Interestingly, the protein most frequently found in exosomes from other cell populations, tetraspanin CD9, was also absent in EVs from HEI-OC1 cells. This confirmed our preliminary results (Kalinec et al., 2019), and those of others, suggesting that not all S-EVs have the same tetraspanin profile (Vagner et al., 2019). For instance, CD9 and CD63 were variably detected in S-EVs and L-EVs, whereas CD81 was exclusively detected in S-EVs. However, only the co-localization of CD81 with CD63 qualifies an S-EV as an exosome (Kowal et al., 2016; Tkach et al., 2018). Thus, we can conclude that our S-EVs samples probably contain classical exosomes since CD63 and CD81 were abundant in this fraction (**Table 1**).

Other difference between our current and earlier preliminary results was the finding of ANXA1 and ANXA5 in S-EVs (**Supplementary Tables S1, S2**). We commented in our previous work the oddity that "two of the most common annexins found in exosomes (ANXA1 and ANXA5) were either found at low levels or not appeared at all" in our samples (Kalinec et al., 2019). The fact that both of them were now found only in the S-EVs fraction suggests that they were probably present in our preliminary samples, but in non-detectable levels. The presence of ANXA1, in particular, provides important support to our idea of using HEI-OC1 EVs as nanocarriers of drugs and molecular mediators aimed at the resolution of inflammatory responses in the cochlea. ANXA1 (Annexin A1) is a potent anti-inflammatory and pro-resolving protein (see Kalinec et al., 2017 and references therein). Many of the cellular and molecular processes associated with the anti-inflammatory properties of glucocorticoids are modulated by ANXA1, and it is considered an important modulator of both the innate and adaptive immune systems.

Interestingly, the authors of a recent publication (Jeppesen et al., 2019) proposed that ANXA1 would be a specific marker of microvesicles shed from the plasma membrane, and ANXA5 a component of apoptotic vesicles. The subcellular distribution of ANXA1 is unusual (for instance see Buckingham and Flower, 2017); it is abundant in the cytoplasm of some cell populations, but a small proportion is also found on the external surface of the plasma membrane or attached to their inner leaflet. Sometimes, even a single membrane pool of ANXA1 has been detected in particular cells. In guinea pig Hensen cells (Kalinec et al., 2009) and HEI-OC1 cells, ANXA1 was found in the cytoplasm, with membrane localization observed only after stimulation with glucocorticoids; in contrast, Jeppesen et al. (2019) localized ANXA1 only in the plasma membrane of DKO-1 and Gli36 human cancer cells, which they used in the reported study. Therefore, while Jeppesen et al. (2019) detected only membrane-bound ANXA1 in microvesicles from human cancer cells, cytoplasmic ANXA1 could be abundant in exosomes from auditory HEI-OC1 cells. Likewise, although ANXA5 is prominent in apoptotic vesicles, its presence in exosomes or microvesicles from some cell populations cannot be discarded.

We also confirmed the presence in S-EVs of Gal-1 and Gal-3 (**Supplementary Tables S1, S2**), a family of glycan-binding proteins that regulate the initiation, amplification and resolution of acute and chronic inflammatory responses (see Kalinec et al., 2017 and references therein). Gal-1 has been associated with a range of anti-inflammatory effects on various cell types, whereas Gal-3 enhances the phagocytic capabilities of neutrophils, a property that may in part account for its protective role in infections. On the other hand, the only pro-inflammatory cytokine detected in HEI-OC1 EVs, the Colony Stimulating Factor 1 (CSF-1), was found in both fractions. CSF-1 is known to be involved in the proliferation, differentiation, and survival of monocytes and macrophages, and it has been implicated in promoting tissue repair following injury (Zhang et al., 2012). Recently, however, it was proposed that CSF-1 has a dual role as pro-inflammatory and anti-inflammatory/regulatory cytokine dependent on the particular immune response (Bhattacharya et al., 2015).

Lipids in S-EVs and L-EVs

Lipids are involved in a number of crucial cellular functions. For instance, in addition to be essential components of cellular membranes, lipid mediators play important roles in cell signaling, including inflammation and immunity (Poorani et al., 2016). It is well known that specific lipids are enriched in EVs compared to their parent cells (Skotland et al., 2017), and there are several possible explanations for these dissimilarities. The composition of the cell medium is important for the lipid composition of the cells and most probably for EVs lipid profile too (Stoll and Spector, 1984). Different growth conditions may also contribute, since different cell densities may change the lipid composition of a cell and intracellular trafficking pathways (Kavaliauskiene et al., 2014). However, since in our experiments all these factors were identical for S-EVs and L-EVs, any difference should be associated with the precise origin of the particles.

LXA4, AT-LXA4, Resolvins, Maresins, and Protectins, in contrast to free AA, DHA, and EPA, were not detected in S-Control and L-Control (**Table 2**, **Supplementary Table S3**). On the other hand, four eicosanoids unique to S-EVs and six unique to L-EVs were detected in Control samples, while another nine were common to both fractions (**Figure 5**). Those unique to S-Control were the HydroxyEicosaTetraEnoic acids 8-HETE, 15-HETE, and 8-HETrE, which derive from AA, and 16-HDoHE (HydroxyDocosaHexaEnoic acid), an autoxidation product of DHA (Poorani et al., 2016; for a complete list of eicosanoid abbreviations see **Supplementary Table S3**, worksheet 3). These products of PUFAs are pre-dominantly pro-inflammatory, but they are also intermediaries in the generation of lipoxins and epi-lipoxins and enhance the generation of nitric oxide (NO), another pro-resolving mediator (Kalinec et al., 2017). Interestingly, two pro-inflammatory eicosanoids, prostaglandin D2 (PGD2) and 13,14-dihydro-15-keto-PGE2 (DHK-PGE2), were detected in L-Control but not in S-Control (**Figure 5**). In mammals, large amounts of PGD2 are found only in mast cells and the brain; in fact, PGD2 is the most abundant prostaglandin in the brain and the one that changes the most under pathological conditions (Figueiredo-Pereira et al., 2015). While prostaglandin E2 (PGE2) and 15-deoxy-Δ12,14-prostaglandin J2 (15-d-PGJ2) are frequently found in EVs (Subra et al., 2010), to our knowledge the literature only reports the presence of PGD2 in EVs in one study performed on exosomes from RBL-2H3 cells, a mast cell model (Subra et al., 2010). Other eicosanoids only detected in L-Control were 15-oxoETE (oxo EicosaTetraEnoic acid, an oxylipin produced by oxidation of 15-HETE), 14(15)-EpETE [a cytochrome P450 (CYP)-metabolite of EPA], 9(10)-EpOME and 12(13)-EpOME (products of the metabolism of linoleic acid by CYP enzymes). Just like all those detected in both fractions, these metabolites participate in pro-inflammatory and pro-resolving pathways, suggesting they are part of a delicate physiological balance.

An important piece of information provided by our lipidomic studies was the significant increase in the variety and amount of lipid metabolites present in EVs loaded with AA, EPA, and DHA (see below). More than 50 metabolites undetected in S-Control or L-Control were found in these EVs, making a total of 69 eicosanoids identified in our samples (**Supplementary Table S3**). For instance, in the absence of exogenously added

PUFAs few pro-inflammatory eicosanoids were detected, and those that were detected were present at trace levels. In contrast, prostaglandins PGD2, DHK-PGE2, PGF2α, PGE2, PGE1, PGD1, PGE3, PGD3, 15K PGF2α, 15K PGE2, DHK-PGD2, 11β PGE2, Thromboxane B2 (TXB2), and other pro-inflammatory agents were detected in both S-EVs and L-EVs loaded with PUFAs (**Supplementary Table S3**). The data suggest that all pathways, including those mediated by COX (cyclooxygenase), 5-LOX (lipooxygenase), 12-15 LOX and CYP (cytochrome P450), are endogenously present in the HEI-OC1 EVs, and are sufficiently active to produce abundant molecular products when supplied with substrates. It should be emphasized that, since EVs were loaded exogenously in the absence of cells, we can confidently assume that all these molecular products were generated in the EVs, suggesting the existence in EVs of an active metabolic mechanism.

Most of these AA, EPA and DHA metabolites are part of pathways that give rise not only to potent pro-resolving mediators but also to pro-inflammation agents. Many of the prostaglandins, including the highly induced PGD2, are considered pro-inflammatory. In general, under steady-state physiological conditions, one would expect a balance between pro- and anti-inflammatory molecules so that homeostasis is preserved. When this balance is altered, depending on the side to which it is tilted, either there will be suppression or exaggeration of inflammation. Our results suggest that incorporation of PUFAs as cargo induces the generation of pro-inflammatory agents in the HEI-OC1 EVs, which could interfere with the goal of accelerating the resolution of inflammatory processes. Thus, if HEI-OC1 EVs are used as nanocarriers, their cargo should be carefully tailored to ensure that it will promote the return to the normal balance.

Loading of S-EVs and L-EVs

EVs are able to incorporate as cargo different types of molecules, such as miRNAs, messenger RNAs, siRNAs, proteins, and even drugs like doxorubicin and curcumin (Sun et al., 2010; Lai et al., 2013; Yang et al., 2015). Moreover, EVs can be loaded exogenously or endogenously. In the first approach, the molecule of interest is included in EVs after isolation, while the endogenous approach is based on active encapsulation, particularly during EV biogenesis, *via* transforming the producing cells with the selected molecule (Pinheiro et al., 2018). EVs loading, however, depends on different factors, including the cellular origin of the EVs, which dictates their molecular composition, and the physical-chemical properties of the intended cargo (e.g., hydrophobicity). In the case of hydrophilic drugs, for instance, special strategies such as hydrophobic insertion, covalent surface chemistry, and membrane permeabilization, may be necessary to facilitate loading (Armstrong et al., 2017). Incorporation of drugs like dexamethasone and aspirin inside EVs, on the other hand, should not be a surprise, since they are hydrophobic. Likewise, fatty acids and lipid mediators should be easily incorporated. However, the loading of other drugs and molecules of interest by HEI-OC1 EVs must be demonstrated before serious consideration of their use as nanocarriers.

Incorporation of dexamethasone by HEI-OC1 EVs was already reported in our preliminary study (Kalinec et al., 2019), and here we present proof that they can be loaded with ASP, LXA4, RvD1, and the eicosanoid precursors AA, EPA, and DHA. These results support the idea that HEI-OC1 EVs could be ideal vehicles for intracochlear delivery of drugs and molecular mediators aimed at facilitating the resolution of cochlear inflammatory processes.

The amount of ASP incorporated by HEI-OC1 EVs was surprisingly high, with significantly more loading by L-EVs (61.8 ± 0.6 μg/ml) than by S-EVs (6.9 ± 0.1 μg/ml). Since the volume of L-EVs per ml is only about twice the volume of S-EVs per ml (6.4×10^{14} nm^3 vs. 3.1×10^{14} nm^3), we speculate that could be some structural problem limiting ASP incorporation in S-EVs. For instance, the different loading of ASP by S-EVs and L-EVS could be related to differences in the curvature of the EV membrane and/or surface charge (Zhou and Raphael, 2007). It has been shown that ASP interacts with membrane lipids, being incorporated first to the external layer and translocating to the internal by flip-flop before being internalized. During this process, the physical properties of the full structure, including their thickness, bending elasticity, and permeability, are affected (Zhou and Raphael, 2005; Sharma et al., 2017). These changes could be more significant in small EVs, hindering the incorporation of ASP, while L-EVs could more readily accommodate the salicylate molecules (Zhou and Raphael, 2007).

ASP, in addition to its proven anti-inflammatory, pro-resolving, and anti-oxidant properties, is the only drug to date that has shown beneficial effects for the mitigation of sensorineural hearing loss in clinical trials (see Kalinec et al., 2017 and references therein). ASP not only blocks the biosynthesis of prostaglandins but also stimulates the endogenous production of pro-resolving mediators, such as ASP-triggered lipoxins (AT-LXs) and resolvins (AT-RVs), which promote the resolution of inflammation by stimulating phagocytosis of cellular debris and counter-regulate pro-inflammatory cytokines without being immunosuppressive (Serhan, 2014). ASP-triggered pro-resolving mediators are generated by the activity of ASP-acetylated cyclooxygenase on PUFA substrates, including AA, EPA, and DHA (Clària and Serhan, 1995; Clària et al., 1996; Serhan et al., 2002; Dalli et al., 2013; Serhan, 2014). In addition to exhibiting similar anti-inflammatory and pro-resolving characteristics of native mediators, the ASP-triggered forms (R epimers) resist rapid inactivation by oxido-reductases and have longer *in vivo* half-lives (Serhan, 2014). Intriguingly, our present results indicate that incorporation of ASP as cargo did not produce detectable amounts of AT-LXA4 in HEI-OC1 EVs in contrast to the significant amounts found in EVs loaded with AA, EPA and DHA (**Table 2**: compare groups S-EVs #2 and L-EVs #2 with S-EVs #4 and #5, and L-EVs #4 and #5). These results present a puzzle: how is an ASP-triggered mediator produced in the absence of ASP, and why the generation of an ASP-triggered mediator is not affected by the presence of ASP? Since ASP-acetylated COX-2 generates ATLs from PUFA, we can speculate that minimum amounts of acetylated COX-2 could be naturally present in EVs and the process triggered by an excess of substrate even in absence of ASP. Conversely, if no PUFAs are present, even incorporation of abundant ASP will not trigger the production of ATLs because of the absence of substrate. However, without specific data, this is only guesswork and, clearly, finding answers to these questions require further investigation.

Whereas the incorporation of lipid precursors and pro-resolving mediators by HEI-OC1 EVs was not unexpected given their hydrophobic nature, the amounts were surprisingly high. All these agents were found in concentrations roughly six to seven orders of magnitude higher than the normal values present in human serum [micrograms/ml in HEI-OC1 EVs vs. picograms/ml in human serum (Colas et al., 2014; Dalli et al., 2017)]. Therefore, delivery of very small volumes of EV suspension would be sufficient to reach clinically significant amounts of these pro-resolving mediators in specific organs and tissues. This is particularly important for their intracochlear delivery, given the small size of the auditory organ.

Other very important result is the demonstration that EVs can be loaded simultaneously with different precursors and drugs and that this can be accomplished by simple co-incubation of the EVs with the different agents. As abundantly described in the literature, EVs have been loaded with different molecules either endogenously or exogenously. For instance, mesenchymal and tumor cells incubated with chemotherapeutic drugs, subsequently produced EVs loaded with these drugs (Tang et al., 2012; Pascucci et al., 2014). The main disadvantage of this endogenous approach, however, is that drug incorporation into the cells and into the EVs depends on the particular cells and the mechanisms involved in molecular sorting into EVs, which largely remain to be elucidated. The exogenous approach, which involves loading of EVs after their isolation as described here, is simpler, but not exempt of potential complications. For example, incorporation of hydrophilic agents may be problematic, but even in these situations high loading efficiencies can be obtained with sonication, extrusion or following saponin treatments (Vader et al., 2016).

S-EVs or L-EVs?

As known from the literature (Mathivanan et al., 2010; Bobrie et al., 2012; Romancino et al., 2013; Zaborowski et al., 2015; Kowal et al., 2016; Xu et al., 2016; Vagner et al., 2019) and confirmed by our results, S-EVs and L-EVs have different composition and, probably, different functions. Since we are interested in using them as nanocarriers of pre-defined molecular cargoes to play specific functions, we wonder whether one of these fractions could be more qualified than the other to be exploited for our therapeutic goal.

One important parameter, the potential amount of cargo able to be incorporated by one fraction or the other, provided some interesting hints. As reported in "Results" section, the total volume and surface (membrane) area of the vesicles present in each fraction are of the same order of magnitude, suggesting that they should be able to incorporate nearly similar amounts of exogenous cargo. However, the already discussed issue of ASP incorporation indicates that this is not necessarily true.

Proteomic results suggest that HEI-OC1 S-EVs, but not L-EVs, contain ANXA1, Gal-1 and Gal-3, known regulators and mediators of inflammation resolution (Kalinec et al., 2017). This result makes S-EVs more attractive as potential nanocarriers in pro-resolving therapies. In addition, they contain many unique proteins that are probably part of the proteome of the parent cells and could perhaps be associated with the function and/or protection of the hearing organ (Kowal et al., 2016; Kalinec et al., 2019). However, dexamethasone can be incorporated as cargo in any EV, and it is already known that this glucocorticoid induces the release of ANXA1 (Kalinec et al., 2009), galectins and other proteins from Hensen cells of the organ of Corti (Kalinec et al., unpublished). Thus, the differences in the proteome of S-EVs and L-EVs could be compensated, at least partially, by the judicious choice of their cargo to include the right molecules and/or pharmacological agents.

Our lipidomic studies showed only small differences between S-Control and L-Control. Most importantly, they showed a huge increase in the variety and amount of lipid metabolites present in EVs of both fractions loaded with AA, EPA, and DHA, erasing any potential difference between S-Control and L-Control (**Supplementary Table S3**). Although the idea of loading EVs with precursors of pro-resolving mediators, expecting their transformation into lipoxins, resolvins, protectins and/or maresins in the target organ, was very attractive, the observed generation of a number of pro-inflammatory agents inside the EVs makes it inconvenient. In contrast, the fact that L-EVs showed a more efficient incorporation of ASP, LXA4, and RvD1 than S-EVs suggests that larger vesicles could be more effective carriers for anti-inflammatory and pro-resolving agents than smaller ones. Nevertheless, experiments aimed specifically at comparing S-EVs and L-EVs drug delivery to particular organ or cell targets must be performed before arriving at a definitive conclusion. Studies pursuing this goal are currently being performed in our laboratory.

CONCLUSION

In the present study, we provide evidence that auditory HEI-OC1 cells generate abundant EVs that can be loaded with combinations of anti-inflammatory drugs and pro-resolving agents in significantly higher concentrations than those normally required for clinical significance. Proteomic and lipidomic studies detected a differential distribution of selected proteins and lipids between small (S-EVs) and large (L-EVS) vesicles. For instance, the S-EVs fraction contains a larger number and diversity of proteins than the L-EVs that could be associated with the involvement of a more efficient cellular mechanism of protein sorting and/or loading. In particular, S-EVs contain the pro-resolving protein mediators ANXA1, Gal-1 and Gal-3 as well as a variety of other molecules that were not found in the larger vesicles. EVs from both fractions can be loaded with anti-inflammatory drugs and pro-resolving mediators, either alone or mixed, making possible the generation of particles with cargoes containing a cocktail of molecules aimed at accelerating inflammation resolution and improving the organ response to inflammation damage. Importantly, since incorporation of PUFAs induces the generation of pro-inflammatory agents in the EVs, which could interfere with the resolution of inflammatory processes, these precursors should not be included as cargo when planning a therapeutic intervention. Therefore, altogether, these results provide support to the idea that EVs from auditory HEI-OC1 cells could be useful nanocarriers for the delivery of anti-inflammatory drugs and pro-resolving mediators, but their cargo should be carefully tailored to ensure that it will indeed promote the successful resolution of inflammatory processes.

AUTHOR CONTRIBUTIONS

GK cultured the cells, isolated EVs, and prepared all the experimental samples. LG, JW, and KF performed proteomic analyses and aspirin incorporation measurements. WC contributed significantly to proteomic analysis and data interpretation. FK designed the study and wrote the manuscript. JW and particularly KF helped edit the manuscript.

ACKNOWLEDGMENTS

We thank Dr. Franklin Monzon and Ms. Ngoc Do (Spectradyne LLC, Torrance, CA, USA) for access to the Spectradyne nCS1^{TM} instrument and their help with EV measurements. Erdim Sertoğlu, M.D., helped with the aspirin measurements.

REFERENCES

Akao, Y., Iio, A., Itoh, T., Noguchi, S., Itoh, Y., Ohtsuki, Y., et al. (2011). Microvesicle-mediated RNA molecule delivery system using monocytes/macrophages. *Mol. Ther.* 19, 395-399. doi: 10.1038/mt.2010.254

Armstrong, J. P., Holme, M. N., and Stevens, M. M. (2017). Re-engineering extracellular vesicles as smart nanoscale therapeutics. *ACS Nano* 11, 69–83. doi: 10.1021/acsnano.6b07607

Armstrong, J. P. K., and Stevens, M. M. (2018). Strategic design of extracellular vesicle drug delivery systems. *Adv. Drug Deliv. Rev.* 130, 12–16. doi: 10.1016/j.addr.2018.06.017

Bhattacharya, P., Budnick, I., Singh, M., Thiruppathi, M., Alharshawi, K., Elshabrawy, H., et al. (2015). Dual role of GM-CSF as a pro-inflammatory and a regulatory cytokine: implications for immune therapy. *J. Interferon Cytokine Res.* 35, 585–599. doi: 10.1089/jir.2014.0149

Bobrie, A., Colombo, M., Krumeich, S., Raposo, G., and Thery, C. (2012). Diverse subpopulations of vesicles secreted by different intracellular mechanisms are present in exosome preparations obtained by differential ultracentrifugation. *J. Extracell. Vesicles* 1:18397. doi: 10.3402/jev.v1i0.18397

Buckingham, J. C., and Flower, R. J. (2017). "Chapter 25-Annexin A1," in *Stress: Neuroendocrinology and Neurobiology*, ed. G. Fink (Academic Press), 257–263. doi: 10.1016/B978-0-12-802175-0.00025-5

Capri, J., and Whitelegge, J. P. (2017). Full membrane protein coverage digestion and quantitative bottom-up mass spectrometry proteomics. *Methods Mol. Biol.* 1550, 61–67. doi: 10.1007/978-1-4939-6747-6_6

Clària, J., Lee, M. H., and Serhan, C. N. (1996). Aspirin-triggered lipoxins (15-epi-LX) are generated by the human lung adenocarcinoma cell line (A549)-neutrophil interactions and are potent inhibitors of cell proliferation. *Mol. Med.* 2, 583–596. doi: 10.1007/bf03401642

Clària, J., and Serhan, C. N. (1995). Aspirin triggers previously undescribed bioactive eicosanoids by human endothelial cell-leukocyte interactions. *Proc. Natl. Acad. Sci. U S A* 92, 9475–9479. doi: 10.1073/pnas.92.21.9475

Cleland, A. N., Fraikin, J.-L., Meinhold, P., and Monzon, F. (2016). Nanoparticle characterization—one size does not fit all: nanoparticle size analysis for nanomedicine applications. *Drug Dev. Deliv.* 6:20.

Colas, R. A., Shinohara, M., Dalli, J., Chiang, N., and Serhan, C. N. (2014). Identification and signature profiles for pro-resolving and inflammatory lipid mediators in human tissue. *Am. J. Physiol. Cell Physiol.* 307, C39–C54. doi: 10.1152/ajpcell.00024.2014

Colombo, M., Raposo, G., and Thery, C. (2014). Biogenesis, secretion, and intercellular interactions of exosomes and other extracellular vesicles. *Annu. Rev. Cell Dev. Biol.* 30, 255–289. doi: 10.1146/annurev-cellbio-101512-122326

Dalli, J., Colas, R. A., Quintana, C., Barragan-Bradford, D., Hurwitz, S., Levy, B. D., et al. (2017). Human sepsis eicosanoid and proresolving lipid mediator temporal profiles: correlations with survival and clinical outcomes. *Crit. Care Med.* 45, 58–68. doi: 10.1097/ccm.0000000000002014

Dalli, J., and Serhan, C. N. (2019). Identification and structure elucidation of the pro-resolving mediators provides novel leads for resolution pharmacology. *Br. J. Pharmacol.* 176, 1024–1037. doi: 10.1111/bph.14336

Dalli, J., Winkler, J. W., Colas, R. A., Arnardottir, H., Cheng, C. Y., Chiang, N., et al. (2013). Resolvin D3 and aspirin-triggered resolvin D3 are potent immunoresolvents. *Chem. Biol.* 20, 188–201. doi: 10.1016/j.chembiol.2012.11.010

Eguchi, A., Lazic, M., Armando, A. M., Phillips, S. A., Katebian, R., Maraka, S., et al. (2016). Circulating adipocyte-derived extracellular vesicles are novel markers of metabolic stress. *J. Mol. Med.* 94, 1241–1253. doi: 10.1007/s00109-016-1446-8

Figueiredo-Pereira, M. E., Rockwell, P., Schmidt-Glenewinkel, T., and Serrano, P. (2015). Neuroinflammation and J2 prostaglandins: linking impairment of the ubiquitin-proteasome pathway and mitochondria to neurodegeneration. *Front. Mol. Neurosci.* 7:104. doi: 10.3389/fnmol.2014.00104

Fuhrmann, G., Serio, A., Mazo, M., Nair, R., and Stevens, M. M. (2015). Active loading into extracellular vesicles significantly improves the cellular uptake and photodynamic effect of porphyrins. *J. Control. Release* 205, 35–44. doi: 10.1016/j.jconrel.2014.11.029

Grabarek, A. D., Weinbuch, D., Jiskoot, W., and Hawe, A. (2019). Critical evaluation of microfluidic resistive pulse sensing for quantification and sizing of nanometer- and micrometer-sized particles in biopharmaceutical products. *J. Pharm. Sci.* 108, 563–573. doi: 10.1016/j.xphs.2018.08.020

György, B., Sage, C., Indzhykulian, A. A., Scheffer, D. I., Brisson, A. R., Tan, S., et al. (2017). Rescue of hearing by gene delivery to inner-ear hair cells using exosome-associated AAV. *Mol. Ther.* 25, 379–391. doi: 10.1016/j.ymthe.2016.12.010

Hao, J., and Li, S. K. (2019). Inner ear drug delivery: recent advances, challenges, and perspective. *Eur. J. Pharm. Sci.* 126, 82–92. doi: 10.1016/j.ejps.2018.05.020

Jeppesen, D. K., Fenix, A. M., Franklin, J. L., Higginbotham, J. N., Zhang, Q., Zimmerman, L. J., et al. (2019). Reassessment of exosome composition. *Cell* 177, 428.e18–445.e18. doi: 10.1016/j.cell.2019.02.029

Kalinec, G. M., Cohn, W., Whitelegge, J. P., Faull, K. F., and Kalinec, F. (2019). Preliminary characterization of extracellular vesicles from auditory HEI-OC1 cells. *Ann. Otol. Rhinol. Laryngol.* 128, 52S–60S. doi: 10.1177/0003489419836226

Kalinec, G. M., Lomberk, G., Urrutia, R. A., and Kalinec, F. (2017). Resolution of cochlear inflammation: novel target for preventing or ameliorating drug-, noise- and age-related hearing loss. *Front. Cell. Neurosci.* 11:192. doi: 10.3389/fncel.2017.00192

Kalinec, G. M., Webster, P., Lim, D. J., and Kalinec, F. (2003). A cochlear cell line as an *in vitro* system for drug ototoxicity screening. *Audiol. Neurootol.* 8, 177–189. doi: 10.1159/000071059

Kalinec, F., Webster, P., Maricle, A., Guerrero, D., Chakravarti, D. N., Chakravarti, B., et al. (2009). Glucocorticoid-stimulated, transcription-independent release of annexin A1 by cochlear Hensen cells. *Br. J. Pharmacol.* 158, 1820–1834. doi: 10.1111/j.1476-5381.2009.00473.x

Kanehisa, M., and Goto, S. (2000). KEGG: kyoto encyclopedia of genes and genomes. *Nucleic Acids Res.* 28, 27–30. doi: 10.1093/nar/28.1.27

Kanehisa, M., Goto, S., Sato, Y., Kawashima, M., Furumichi, M., and Tanabe, M. (2014). Data, information, knowledge and principle: back to metabolism in KEGG. *Nucleic Acids Res.* 42, D199–D205. doi: 10.1093/nar/gkt1076

Kaur, T., Borse, V., Sheth, S., Sheehan, K., Ghosh, S., Tupal, S., et al. (2016). Adenosine A1 receptor protects against cisplatin ototoxicity by suppressing the NOX3/STAT1 inflammatory pathway in the cochlea. *J. Neurosci.* 36, 3962–3977. doi: 10.1523/JNEUROSCI.3111-15.2016

Kavaliauskiene, S., Nymark, C. M., Bergan, J., Simm, R., Sylvänne, T., Simolin, H., et al. (2014). Cell density-induced changes in lipid composition and intracellular trafficking. *Cell. Mol. Life Sci.* 71, 1097–1116. doi: 10.1007/s00018-013-1441-y

Keerthikumar, S., Chisanga, D., Ariyaratne, D., Al Saffar, H., Anand, S., Zhao, K., et al. (2016). ExoCarta: a web-based compendium of exosomal cargo. *J. Mol. Biol.* 428, 688–692. doi: 10.1016/j.jmb.2015.09.019

Keithley, E. M. (2018). "Cochlear inflammation associated with noise exposure," in *Inflammatory Mechanisms in Mediating Hearing Loss*, eds V. Ramkumar and L. Rybak (Cham: Springer), 91–114.

Koritzinsky, E. H., Street, J. M., Star, R. A., and Yuen, P. S. (2017). Quantification of exosomes. *J. Cell. Physiol.* 232, 1587–1590. doi: 10.1002/jcp.25387

Kowal, J., Arras, G., Colombo, M., Jouve, M., Morath, J. P., Primdal-Bengtson, B., et al. (2016). Proteomic comparison defines novel markers to characterize heterogeneous populations of extracellular vesicle subtypes. *Proc. Natl. Acad. Sci. U S A* 113, E968–E977. doi: 10.1073/pnas.1521230113

Kumar, V., Abbas, A. K., and Aster, J. C. (2014). *Robbins and Cotran Pathological Basis of Disease.* Philadelphia, PA: Elsevier.

Lai, P., Weng, J., Guo, L., Chen, X., and Du, X. (2019). Novel insights into MSC-EVs therapy for immune diseases. *Biomark. Res.* 7:6. doi: 10.1186/s40364-019-0156-0

Lai, R. C., Yeo, R. W., Tan, K. H., and Lim, S. K. (2013). Exosomes for drug delivery—a novel application for the mesenchymal stem cell. *Biotechnol. Adv.* 31, 543–551. doi: 10.1016/j.biotechadv.2012.08.008

Laulagnier, K., Motta, C., Hamdi, S., Roy, S., Fauvelle, F., Pageaux, J. F., et al. (2004). Mast cell- and dendritic cell-derived exosomes display a specific lipid composition and an unusual membrane organization. *Biochem. J.* 380, 161–171. doi: 10.1042/bj20031594

Li, L., Chao, T., Brant, J., O'Malley, B. Jr., Tsourkas, A., and Li, D. (2017). Advances in nano-based inner ear delivery systems for the treatment of sensorineural hearing loss. *Adv. Drug Deliv. Rev.* 108, 2–12. doi: 10.1016/j.addr.2016.01.004

Lowthian, J. A., Britt, C. J., Rance, G., Lin, F. R., Woods, R. L., Wolfe, R., et al. (2016). Slowing the progression of age-related hearing loss: rationale and study design of the ASPIRIN in HEARING, retinal vessels imaging and neurocognition in older generations (ASPREE-HEARING) trial. *Contemp. Clin. Trials* 46, 60–66. doi: 10.1016/j.cct.2015.11.014

Marcus, M. E., and Leonard, J. N. (2013). FedExosomes: engineering therapeutic biological nanoparticles that truly deliver. *Pharmaceuticals* 6, 659–680. doi: 10.3390/ph6050659

Mateescu, B., Kowal, E. J., van Balkom, B. W., Bartel, S., Bhattacharyya, S. N., Buzas, E. I., et al. (2017). Obstacles and opportunities in the functional analysis of extracellular vesicle RNA—an ISEV position paper. *J. Extracell. Vesicles* 6:1286095. doi: 10.1080/20013078.2017.1286095

Mathieu, M., Martin-Jaular, L., Lavieu, G., and Théry, C. (2019). Specificities of secretion and uptake of exosomes and other extracellular vesicles for cell-to-cell communication. *Nat. Cell Biol.* 21, 9–17. doi: 10.1038/s41556-018-0250-9

Mathivanan, S., Lim, J. W., Tauro, B. J., Ji, H., Moritz, R. L., and Simpson, R. J. (2010). Proteomics analysis of A33 immunoaffinity-purified exosomes released from the human colon tumor cell line LIM1215 reveals a tissue-specific protein signature. *Mol. Cell. Proteomics* 9, 197–208. doi: 10.1074/mcp.m900152-mcp200

Pascucci, L., Cocce, V., Bonomi, A., Ami, D., Ceccarelli, P., Ciusani, E., et al. (2014). Paclitaxel is incorporated by mesenchymal stromal cells and released in exosomes that inhibit *in vitro* tumor growth: a new approach for drug delivery. *J. Control. Release* 192, 262–270. doi: 10.1016/j.jconrel.2014.07.042

Perretti, M. (2015). The resolution of inflammation: new mechanisms in patho-physiology open opportunities for pharmacology. *Semin. Immunol.* 27, 145–148. doi: 10.1016/j.smim.2015.06.001

Perretti, M., Leroy, X., Bland, E. J., and Montero-Melendez, T. (2015). Resolution pharmacology: opportunities for therapeutic innovation in inflammation. *Trends Pharmacol. Sci.* 36, 737–755. doi: 10.1016/j.tips.2015.07.007

Pinheiro, A., Silva, A. M., Teixeira, J. H., Goncalves, R. M., Almeida, M. I., Barbosa, M. A., et al. (2018). Extracellular vesicles: intelligent delivery strategies for therapeutic applications. *J. Control. Release* 289, 56–69. doi: 10.1016/j.jconrel.2018.09.019

Poorani, R., Bhatt, A. N., Dwarakanath, B. S., and Das, U. N. (2016). COX-2, aspirin and metabolism of arachidonic, eicosapentaenoic and docosahexaenoic acids and their physiological and clinical significance. *Eur. J. Pharmacol.* 785, 116–132. doi: 10.1016/j.ejphar.2015.08.049

Quehenberger, O., Armando, A. M., Brown, A. H., Milne, S. B., Myers, D. S., Merrill, A. H., et al. (2010). Lipidomics reveals a remarkable diversity of lipids in human plasma. *J. Lipid Res.* 51, 3299–3305. doi: 10.1194/jlr.M009449

Quehenberger, O., Dahlberg-Wright, S., Jiang, J., Armando, A. M., and Dennis, E. A. (2018). Quantitative determination of esterified eicosanoids and related oxygenated metabolites after base hydrolysis. *J. Lipid Res.* 59, 2436–2445. doi: 10.1194/jlr.d089516

Quehenberger, O., Yamashita, T., Armando, A. M., Dennis, E. A., and Palinski, W. (2011). Effect of gestational hypercholesterolemia and maternal immunization on offspring plasma eicosanoids. *Am. J. Obstet. Gynecol.* 205, 156.e15–156.e25. doi: 10.1016/j.ajog.2011.03.044

Rappsilber, J., Mann, M., and Ishihama, Y. (2007). Protocol for micro-purification, enrichment, pre-fractionation and storage of peptides for proteomics using StageTips. *Nat. Protoc.* 2, 1896–1906. doi: 10.1038/nprot.2007.261

Record, M. (2018). Introduction to the Thematic Review Series on Extracellular Vesicles: a focus on the role of lipids. *J. Lipid Res.* 59, 1313–1315. doi: 10.1194/jlr.e086132

Reis, M., Ogonek, J., Qesari, M., Borges, N. M., Nicholson, L., Preußner, L., et al. (2016). Recent developments in cellular immunotherapy for HSCT-associated complications. *Front. Immunol.* 7:500. doi: 10.3389/fimmu.2016.00500

Robbins, P. D., and Morelli, A. E. (2014). Regulation of immune responses by extracellular vesicles. *Nat. Rev. Immunol.* 14, 195–208. doi: 10.1038/nri3622

Romancino, D. P., Paterniti, G., Campos, Y., De Luca, A., Di Felice, V., d'Azzo, A., et al. (2013). Identification and characterization of the nano-sized vesicles released by muscle cells. *FEBS Lett.* 587, 1379–1384. doi: 10.1016/j.febslet.2013.03.012

Serhan, C. N. (2014). Pro-resolving lipid mediators are leads for resolution physiology. *Nature* 510, 92–101. doi: 10.1038/nature13479

Serhan, C. N., Hong, S., Gronert, K., Colgan, S. P., Devchand, P. R., Mirick, G., et al. (2002). Resolvins: a family of bioactive products of omega-3 fatty acid transformation circuits initiated by aspirin treatment that counter proinflammation signals. *J. Exp. Med.* 196, 1025–1037. doi: 10.1084/jem.20020760

Sharma, V. K., Mamontov, E., Ohl, M., and Tyagi, M. (2017). Incorporation of aspirin modulates the dynamical and phase behavior of the phospholipid membrane. *Phys. Chem. Chem. Phys.* 19, 2514–2524. doi: 10.1039/c6cp06202d

Skotland, T., Sandvig, K., and Llorente, A. (2017). Lipids in exosomes: current knowledge and the way forward. *Prog. Lipid Res.* 66, 30–41. doi: 10.1016/j.plipres.2017.03.001

Song, Y., Zhang, J., and Li, D. (2017). Microfluidic and nanofluidic resistive pulse sensing: a review. *Micromachines* 8:E204. doi: 10.3390/mi8070204

Stoll, L. L., and Spector, A. A. (1984). Changes in serum influence the fatty acid composition of established cell lines. *in vitro* 20, 732–738. doi: 10.1007/bf02618879

Subra, C., Grand, D., Laulagnier, K., Stella, A., Lambeau, G., Paillasse, M., et al. (2010). Exosomes account for vesicle-mediated transcellular transport of activatable phospholipases and prostaglandins. *J. Lipid Res.* 51, 2105–2120. doi: 10.1194/jlr.m003657

Sun, D., Zhuang, X., Xiang, X., Liu, Y., Zhang, S., Liu, C., et al. (2010). A novel nanoparticle drug delivery system: the anti-inflammatory activity of curcumin is enhanced when encapsulated in exosomes. *Mol. Ther.* 18, 1606–1614. doi: 10.1038/mt.2010.105

Tang, K., Zhang, Y., Zhang, H., Xu, P., Liu, J., Ma, J., et al. (2012). Delivery of chemotherapeutic drugs in tumour cell-derived microparticles. *Nat. Commun.* 3:1282. doi: 10.1038/ncomms2282

Tkach, M., Kowal, J., and Théry, C. (2018). Why the need and how to approach the functional diversity of extracellular vesicles. *Philos. Trans. R. Soc. Lond. B Biol. Sci.* 373:20160479. doi: 10.1098/rstb.2016.0479

Vaclavek, T., Prikryl, J., and Foret, F. (2019). Resistive pulse sensing as particle counting and sizing method in microfluidic systems: designs and applications review. *J. Sep. Sci.* 42, 445–457. doi: 10.1002/jssc.201800978

Vader, P., Mol, E. A., Pasterkamp, G., and Schiffelers, R. M. (2016). Extracellular vesicles for drug delivery. *Adv. Drug Deliv. Rev.* 106, 148–156. doi: 10.1016/j.addr.2016.02.006

Vagner, T., Chin, A., Mariscal, J., Bannykh, S., Engman, D., and Vizio, D. D. (2019). Protein composition reflects extracellular vesicle heterogeneity. *Proteomics* 19:e1800167. doi: 10.1002/pmic.201800167

Wang, Y., Armando, A. M., Quehenberger, O., Yan, C., and Dennis, E. A. (2014). Comprehensive ultra-performance liquid chromatographic separation and mass spectrometric analysis of eicosanoid metabolites in human samples. *J. Chromatogr. A* 1359, 60–69. doi: 10.1016/j.chroma.2014.07.006

Weatherall, E., and Willmott, G. R. (2015). Applications of tunable resistive pulse sensing. *Analyst* 140, 3318–3334. doi: 10.1039/c4an02270j

Willms, E., Johansson, H. J., Mager, I., Lee, Y., Blomberg, K. E., Sadik, M., et al. (2016). Cells release subpopulations of exosomes with distinct molecular and biological properties. *Sci. Rep.* 6:22519. doi: 10.1038/srep22519

Witwer, K. W., Buzas, E. I., Bemis, L. T., Bora, A., Lasser, C., Lotvall, J., et al. (2013). Standardization of sample collection, isolation and analysis methods in extracellular vesicle research. *J. Extracell. Vesicles* 2:20360. doi: 10.3402/jev.v2i0.20360

Wong, W. Y., Lee, M. M., Chan, B. D., Kam, R. K., Zhang, G., Lu, A. P., et al. (2016). Proteomic profiling of dextran sulfate sodium induced acute ulcerative colitis mice serum exosomes and their immunomodulatory impact on macrophages. *Proteomics* 16, 1131–1145. doi: 10.1002/pmic.201500174

Xu, R., Greening, D. W., Zhu, H. J., Takahashi, N., and Simpson, R. J. (2016). Extracellular vesicle isolation and characterization: toward clinical application. *J. Clin. Invest.* 126, 1152–1162. doi: 10.1172/jci81129

Yanez-Mo, M., Siljander, P. R., Andreu, Z., Zavec, A. B., Borras, F. E., Buzas, E. I., et al. (2015). Biological properties of extracellular vesicles and their physiological functions. *J. Extracell. Vesicles* 4:27066. doi: 10.3402/jev.v4.27066

Yang, T., Martin, P., Fogarty, B., Brown, A., Schurman, K., Phipps, R., et al. (2015). Exosome delivered anticancer drugsacross the blood-brain barrier for brain cancer therapy in *Danio rerio*. *Pharm. Res.* 32, 2003–2014. doi: 10.1007/s11095-014-1593-y

Zaborowski, M. P., Balaj, L., Breakefield, X. O., and Lai, C. P. (2015). Extracellular vesicles: composition, biological relevance, and methods of study. *Bioscience* 65, 783–797. doi: 10.1093/biosci/biv084

Zhang, M. Z., Yao, B., Yang, S., Jiang, L., Wang, S., Fan, X., et al. (2012). CSF-1 signaling mediates recovery from acute kidney injury. *J. Clin. Invest.* 122, 4519–4532. doi: 10.1172/JCI60363

Zhou, Y., and Raphael, R. M. (2005). Effect of salicylate on the elasticity, bending stiffness, and strength of SOPC membranes. *Biophys. J.* 89, 1789–1801. doi: 10.1529/biophysj.104.054510

Zhou, Y., and Raphael, R. M. (2007). Solution pH alters mechanical and electrical properties of phosphatidylcholine membranes: relation between interfacial electrostatics, intramembrane potential, and bending elasticity. *Biophys. J.* 92, 2451–2462. doi: 10.1529/biophysj.106.096362

8

Targeting Inflammatory Processes Mediated by TRPVI and TNF-α for Treating Noise-Induced Hearing Loss

Asmita Dhukhwa[1], Puspanjali Bhatta[1], Sandeep Sheth[2], Krishi Korrapati[3], Coral Tieu[3], Chaitanya Mamillapalli[4], Vickram Ramkumar[1] and Debashree Mukherjea[3]*

[1] Department of Pharmacology, Southern Illinois University School of Medicine, Springfield, IL, United States, [2] Department of Pharmaceutical Sciences, College of Pharmacy, Larkin University, Miami, FL, United States, [3] Department of Otolaryngology, Southern Illinois University School of Medicine, Springfield, IL, United States, [4] Department of Internal Medicine, Southern Illinois University School of Medicine, Springfield, IL, United States

***Correspondence:**
Debashree Mukherjea
dmukherjea@siumed.edu

Noise trauma is the most common cause of hearing loss in adults. There are no known FDA approved drugs for prevention or rescue of noise-induced hearing loss (NIHL). In this study, we provide evidence that implicates stress signaling molecules (TRPV1, NOX3, and TNF-α) in NIHL. Furthermore, we provide evidence that inhibiting any one of these moieties can prevent and treat NIHL when administered within a window period. Hearing loss induced by loud noise is associated with the generation of reactive oxygen species (ROS), increased calcium (Ca^{2+}) in the endolymph and hair cells, and increased inflammation in the cochlea. Increased (Ca^{2+}) and ROS activity persists for several days after traumatic noise exposure (NE). Chronic increases in (Ca^{2+}) and ROS have been shown to increase inflammation and apoptosis in various tissue. However, the precise role of Ca^{2+} up-regulation and the resulting inflammation causing a positive feedback loop in the noise-exposed cochlea to generate sustained toxic amounts of Ca^{2+} are unknown. Here we show cochlear TRPV1 dysregulation is a key step in NIHL, and that inflammatory TNF-α cytokine-mediated potentiation of TRPV1 induced Ca^{2+} entry is an essential mechanism of NIHL. In the Wistar rat model, noise produces an acute (within 48 h) and a chronic (within 21 days) increase in cochlear gene expression of TRPV1, NADPH oxidase 3 (NOX3) and pro-inflammatory mediators such as tumor necrosis factor-α (TNF-α) and cyclooxygenase-2 (COX2). Additionally, we also show that H_2O_2 (100 μM) produces a robust increase in Ca^{2+} entry in cell cultures which is enhanced by TNF-α via the TRPV1 channel and which involves ERK1/2 phosphorylation. Mitigation of NIHL could be achieved by using capsaicin (TRPV1 agonist that rapidly desensitizes TRPV1. This mechanism is used in the treatment of pain in diabetic peripheral neuropathy) pretreatment or by inhibition of TNF-α with Etanercept (ETA), administered up to 7 days prior to NE or within 24 h of noise. Our results demonstrate the importance of the synergistic interaction between TNF-α and TRPV1 in the cochlea and suggest that these are important therapeutic targets for treating NIHL.

Keywords: noise exposure, inflammation, TRPV1, TNF-α, capsaicin, Etanercept, cochlea, hearing loss

INTRODUCTION

Noise exposure is the most common cause of hearing loss in adults globally. It is associated with the generation of ROS in the cochlea by increasing its metabolic activity. NE decreases cochlear blood flow (CBF) (Thorne and Nuttall, 1987) and decreases cochlear oxygen tension (Hawkins, 1971). This stresses the highly metabolically active cochlea leading to increased ROS production in the cochlea (Yamane et al., 1995a; Ohlemiller et al., 1999; Yamashita et al., 2004). Yamane et al. (1995b) found that noise trauma results in an increase in superoxide anion at the luminal surface of marginal cells in the stria vascularis (SV). A secondary peak of superoxide radicals occurs hours later as a result of cochlear reperfusion and persists 7–10 days post NE. Subsequent studies confirmed that ROS increases in the cochlea following noise trauma (Henderson et al., 1999; Ohlemiller et al., 1999) and persists for several days after NE (Hu et al., 2002; Yamashita et al., 2005). This eventually leads to hair cell death that continues for days after NE (Bohne, 1976). Latest studies by Haryuna et al. (2016) report cochlear levels of H_2O_2 14 days post NE (69 $\pm$ 32.99 pmol/ml) being significantly higher, compared to H_2O_2 levels in control unexposed rat cochlea (7.08 $\pm$ 0.96 pmol/ml), thus confirming earlier studies.

The generation of ROS by noise trauma is considered to be a critical event which initiates damage to the outer hair cells (OHCs), SV and spiral ganglion cells (SGCs), leading to hearing loss (Bohne et al., 2007; Murai et al., 2008). However, the mechanisms mediating the toxicity of ROS generation are less clearly defined. The primary source of ROS is a cochlear-specific NADPH oxidase isoform, NOX3 (Banfi et al., 2004). We previously reported that one source of ROS generation in the cochlea triggered by noise is the NADPH oxidase enzyme (Ramkumar et al., 2004). Oxidative stress in the cochlea induces the expression of NOX3 along with the non-specific cation channel, TRPV1. We have previously shown that NOX3 up-regulates TRPV1, leading to enhanced Ca^{2+} influx and inflammation in the cochlear tissues (Mukherjea et al., 2011) and that TRPV1 activation can generate ROS via NOX3 by increasing intracellular Ca^{2+} release, thus forming a feedback loop. TRPV1 has been shown to be increased in a noise-induced tinnitus model (Bauer et al., 2007). However, noise-induced increase in TRPV1 causing sustained increased calcium (Ca^{2+}) in the cochlea has not been shown.

Abbreviations: ABR, auditory brainstem response; ANOVA, analysis of variance; COX-2, Cyclooxygenase-2; dB, decibel; DRG, dorsal root ganglion; EDTA, ethylenediaminetetraacetic acid; ERK1/2, extracellular signal-regulated kinase 1 and 2; ETA, Etanercept; FDA, Food and Drug Administration; GAPDH, glyceraldehyde-3 phosphate dehydrogenase; HEK, human embryonic kidney; H_2O_2, hydrogen peroxide; iNOS, inducible nitric oxide synthase; ICAM, intercellular adhesion molecules; IL, interleukin; JNK, c-Jun N-terminal kinase; MAPK, mitogen activated protein kinase; NE, noise exposure; NGF, nerve growth factor; NIHL, noise-induced hearing loss; NOX-3, NADPH oxidase 3; OC, Organ of Corti; OHC, outer hair cell; PBS, phosphatase buffer saline; ROS, reactive oxygen species; S.E.M., standard error of mean; SEM, scanning electron microscopy; s.c, sub-cutaneous; SGC, spiral ganglion cell; SL, spiral ligament; SPL, sound pressure level; SV, stria vascularis; TNF-α, tumor necrosis factor alpha; TRPV1, transient receptor potential vanilloid 1; TT, trans-tympanic; UB/OC-1, University Bristol/Organ of Corti-1; VR, vanilloid receptor.

Excessive NE has been associated with increased Ca^{2+} in the endolymph and hair cells (Ikeda and Morizono, 1988; Fridberger et al., 1998; Chan and Rouse, 2016). Increased Ca^{2+} and ROS activity persisting for several days after traumatic NE are well documented (Li et al., 1997; Hu et al., 2002; Yamashita et al., 2005). Interestingly, chronic increases in Ca^{2+} and ROS has been shown to increase inflammation and apoptosis in various tissues (Nicotera and Orrenius, 1992; Orrenius et al., 1992a,b; Vass et al., 1995; Sinha et al., 2013). However, the precise role of Ca^{2+} in mediating persistent cochlear inflammation and hearing loss is not clear.

The role of inflammation in the development of hearing loss was suggested by a study showing that the administration of a corticosteroid, an anti-inflammatory agent, protected against sensorineural hearing loss (Kanzaki and Ouchi, 1981). It has been demonstrated that the cochlea itself produced these pro-inflammatory cytokines which could increase migration of inflammatory cells from the circulation to the cochlea (Hirose et al., 2005; Kim H.J. et al., 2008). ROS also activates a series of downstream events, including the activation of mitogen-activated protein kinase (MAPK), such as JNK, leading to the formation of pro-inflammatory cytokines in the cochlea and eventual apoptosis of OHCs (So et al., 2007; Bas et al., 2009). Our interest in TRPV1 was based on our early studies with freshly isolated DRG neurons. In these studies, NGF increased the expression of TRPV1 in DRG neurons by increasing ROS generation (Puntambekar et al., 2005). Increases in TRPV1 activity has been linked to inflammation in several pathological conditions (Basu and Srivastava, 2005; Razavi et al., 2006; Bertin et al., 2014; Brito et al., 2014; Liu et al., 2014) and knockdown of TRPV1 reduces cisplatin-mediated inflammation and ototoxicity (Mukherjea et al., 2008). We have also shown the synergy between TRPV1 and NOX3 in the cochlea (Mukherjea et al., 2011). Trans-tympanic (TT) administration of capsaicin (TRPV1 agonist) in the rat cochlea mediates an acute and transient increase in inflammatory markers such as TNF-α, COX2, and iNOS at 24 h, which returned to baseline values by 72 h and did not involve loss of OHC's or apoptotic molecules (Mukherjea et al., 2011). This acute TRPV1 activation and subsequent desensitization were accompanied with a temporary threshold shift at 24 h which returned to baseline values within 72 h. Thus transient inflammation of the cochlea was associated with transient hearing loss. These findings suggest a coordinated action of TRPV1, NOX3, TNF-α and other inflammatory cytokines in mediating hearing loss, and thus are potential targets for otoprotective therapies.

Noise exposure increases the production of pro-inflammatory cytokines such as TNF-α, IL-1β, and IL6 in the cochleae (Fujioka et al., 2006; Bas et al., 2009). TNF-α, the master regulator of inflammatory cytokine cascade, is produced by spiral ligament (SL) fibrocytes, OHCs and supporting cells in the organ of Corti after NE (Zou et al., 2005; Fujioka et al., 2006). Noise exposed cochlear level of TNF-α cytokine (191.07 pg/mg) has been reported to be significantly higher when compared to untreated control levels (58.28 pg/mg) in the rat cochlea by Arslan et al. (2017). Additionally, infusion of TNF-α into the guinea pig cochlea leads to the infiltration of inflammatory cells, such as leukocytes, causing cochlear damage (Keithley et al., 2008). Organ of Corti explants exposed to TNF-α demonstrated apoptosis associated with increased expression of phosphorylated c-Jun N terminal kinase, cleaved caspase-3, apoptosis-inducing factor cluster formation, and translocation of the apoptotic marker endonuclease G to the nuclei of hair cells (Infante et al., 2012). Interestingly, the auditory protection afforded by certain antioxidants like melatonin have been linked to regulation of TNF-α in rats exposed to traumatic noise (Bas et al., 2009). Thus, homeostatic regulation of TNF-α in the cochlea is essential for normal physiological hearing.

In the present study, we show that NE initiates a cascade of events involving both acute and chronic induction of TRPV1, NOX3, and TNF-α, leading to permanent hearing loss. We show that the induction of both TRPV1 and TNF-α and the resulting synergy between these two molecules could promote intracellular Ca^{2+} overload, thus predisposing the cochlea to permanent hearing loss. In this study, we show that desensitization of TRPV1 (capsaicin) or inhibition of TNF-α (Etanercept, an FDA approved inhibitor of TNF-α) protected against NIHL in a rat model. This study, for the first time, shows that inhibition of inflammation either as pre-treatment or within a window of opportunity post noise insult can protect and treat NIHL.

MATERIALS AND METHODS

Drugs, Reagents and Antibodies

H_2O_2, capsaicin, protease inhibitor, and phosphatase inhibitor cocktails 2 and 3 were purchased from Sigma-Aldrich (St. Louis, MO, United States). TNF-α cytokine was purchased from Sigma-Aldrich (St. Louis, MO, United States). Etanercept or Enbrel was purchased from Walgreens pharmacy for animal use. Various primary antibodies used were as follows: p-ERK1/2, ERK1/2, NOX3, β-actin from Santa Cruz Biotechnology (Dallas, TX, United States); TNF-α, Cox2 and iNOS from Cell Signaling Technology (Danvers, MA, United States); Alexa Fluor 488 Phalloidin from Thermo Fisher Scientific (Waltham, MA, United States). Secondary antibodies used were as follows: donkey anti-rabbit IRDye 680RD, goat anti-mouse IRDye 800RD (no. 926-32214) from LI-COR Biosciences (Lincoln, NE, United States); Alexa Fluor 488 goat anti-rabbit (no. A11008) and RNA Later were purchased from Thermo Fisher Scientific (Berkeley, MO, United States); Alexa Fluor 647 goat anti-mouse IgG1 (no. A-21240) from Molecular Probes (Eugene, OR, United States). Apoptosis was measured using ApopTag® Red *In Situ* Apoptosis Detection Kit (Millipore Sigma, United States). Prolong gold anti-fade (Invitrogen) was used to mount immunohistochemistry samples for imaging.

Cell Culture

Immortalized mouse organ of Corti cells, UB/OC-1, were kindly provided by Dr. Matthew Holley (The University of Sheffield, United Kingdom). These cells were cultured in RPMI-1640 media (HyClone) supplemented with 10% FetalClone® II serum (HyClone). UB/OC-1 cells were kept at 33°C in a humidified incubator with 10% CO2. Cells were cultured thrice a week for passaging and the sub-confluent monolayer of cells was used for experiments. HEK-VR1 (HEK cells stably transfected with TRPV1 also known as VR1) cells (Puntambekar et al., 2005) were grown in growth medium consisted of 90% DMEM, 10% fetal bovine serum (Invitrogen, Grand Island, NY, United States), and 0.2 mg/ml G418 sulfate (Calbiochem, La Jolla, CA, United States) for selection of resistance. Cells were cultured at 37°C, in the presence of 5% CO2 and 95% ambient air.

Calcium Assay

UB/OC-1 or HEK-VR1 cells were grown on glass coverslips to detect Ca^{2+} entry induced by TRPV1 activation. Five μm Fluo-4 AM was added to the cells for 20 min, followed by 3 rinses in the physiological buffer (HEPES:10 mM, NaCl: 130 mM, KCl 4 mM, glucose 4 mM, pH 7.3). Timed baseline fluorescent imaging was performed in calcium buffer by confocal microscopy using an argon laser at 488 nm. Live fluorescent images were recorded every 3 s for 10 min. Baseline (F0) fluorescent images were collected for the first 10 scans and then the drug was added at 30 s to obtain the relative F1 values. Data were analyzed using the Leica software as the ratio of fluorescence/baseline fluorescence and reported as the percentage of relative fluorescence compared to the baseline.

Apoptosis Assay

Apoptosis was detected by TUNEL assay using ApopTag® Red *In Situ* Apoptosis Detection Kit. Briefly, UB/OC-1 cells were fixed with 4% paraformaldehyde, for 10 min and washed thrice with PBS. Cells were then permeabilized using proteinase K (1:100 dilution) (provided in the kit) for 20 min at room temperature. At the end of incubation, the coverslips were rinsed with 1 × Tris-buffered saline (TBS) and incubated with 1 × terminal deoxynucleotidyl transferase (TdT) equilibration buffer for 30 min. TdT labeling reaction mixture (60 μl/coverslip) was added and incubated for 1 h at 37°C. Next, the cover-slips were rinsed twice with 1 × TBS, stained with DAPI and mounted using Prolong gold anti-fade (Invitrogen) mounting medium. Excess mounting media was wiped off and the edges were sealed using nail polish. Slides were then imaged using a Leica confocal microscope.

Western Blotting

UB/OC-1 cells were homogenized in ice-cold lysis buffer (50 mM Tris-HCL, 10 mM Magnesium chloride and 1 mM EDTA) in the presence of protease inhibitor and phosphatase inhibitor cocktail 2 and 3. The whole-cell lysates were then used for Western blotting. After transfer to nitrocellulose membranes, blots were probed with different primary antibodies, followed by a fluorescent-tagged secondary antibody, and visualized by imaging using LICOR odyssey image. Licor Odyssey software was used to analyze the bands. The individual bands were normalized with total proteins for ERK1/2 and these were then further normalized as % of controls to 100%.

Animal Procedures and Sample Collection

Male Wistar rats (175–200 gm) were used for this study under an animal care protocol approved by the Laboratory and Animal

Care and Use Committee (SIU School of Medicine). Pretreatment ABRs were performed. Animals were then treated according to the experimental paradigm.

Oral capsaicin (20 mg/kg) as a preventive strategy: was delivered starting 24 h prior to NE, on the day of NE, and 24 h post NE (3 consecutive treatments), and post-treatment ABR's were collected 21 days post NE.

ETA as Prevention strategy: consisted of a single administration of ETA either trans-tympanicaly (TT) (5 μg/μl) or s.c (3 mg/kg) or PBS (TT-50 μl or s.c ~100–200 μl) either 3 or 7 days prior to NE.

ETA as Treatment: consisted of NE followed by a single ETA treatment either TT or SC administration at either 2 h or 24 h post noise injury. Post-treatment ABR thresholds were determined at 21 days post NE and cochleae were excised for morphological, molecular and biochemical studies. Cochleae used for RNA preparations were flushed immediately with RNA Later solution and stored in RNA Later for 24 h at 4°C. Those used for immunohistochemical studies were perfused and fixed with 4% paraformaldehyde, while those used for SEM were perfused and fixed with 2.5% glutaraldehyde. Cochleae used for whole mounts were decalcified for 14–20 days in 100 mM EDTA at room temperature.

Noise Exposure (NE)

Male Wistar rats were exposed to octave band noise at 122 dB centered at 16 kHz for 1 h under isofluorane anesthesia, with the 3-inch silicon tubes attached to the high-frequency transducer resting in the external auditory canal. This exposure typically results in a 30–50 dB temporary threshold shift (measured as an immediate pre-to-post NE shift in ABR thresholds) across all frequencies; with slightly more elevation at those frequencies around 16 kHz and 20–40 dB permanent threshold shift measured at 21 days post NE at all frequencies. Acoustic stimuli are calibrated using a cloth model rat and a Bruel & Kjaer Pulse System with a 1/2 inch free-field microphone (B&K model 4191). Baseline noise levels in the test chamber (with background test noise turned off) are typically measured below 20 dB SPL in the 4–40 kHz range.

Intra-Tympanic Injections

Male rats were anesthetized with ketamine/xylazine. A 30 gauge insulin needle (5/8 inch in length) was used to puncture the tympanic membrane in the anteroinferior region. A volume of 30 μl of saline or ETA (5 μg/μl) was injected through the tympanic membrane. Rats remained undisturbed for 15 min and the procedure was repeated in the other ear (Sheehan et al., 2018).

Auditory Brainstem Evoked Responses (ABRs)

Pretreatment ABR thresholds were determined using the high-frequency Intelligent Hearing Systems (IHS) on naive rats prior to any treatment or NE for each ear. Animals were tested with a stimulus intensity series that was initiated at 90 dB SPL and reached a minimum of 10 dB SPL. The stimulus intensity levels were decreased in 10 dB increments, and the evoked ABR waveforms were observed on a video monitor. Threshold was analyzed by readers blinded to condition and defined as the lowest intensity capable of eliciting a replicable, visually detectable response at the ABR waveforms II and III. The auditory stimuli included tone bursts at 8, 16, and 32 kHz with a 10 ms plateau and a 1 ms rise/fall time presented at a rate of 5/s. The threshold was defined as the lowest intensity capable of evoking a reproducible, visually detectable response with two distinct waveforms and minimum amplitude of 0.5 μV.

Scanning Electron Microscopy (SEM)

Cochleae were carefully dissected out and sample preparation was performed as stated in Huang et al. (2007). Briefly, the round and oval windows and the apex of the cochlea were perforated with a small pick. The perilymphatic space was perfused with 2.5% glutaraldehyde in 0.1M sodium cacodylate (Cac) buffer pH 7.2, by placing a 1-mL syringe with a modified butterfly catheter over the apex. Each specimen was then placed in the glutaraldehyde solution overnight and refrigerated. Cochlear surface and perilymphatic space were rinsed three times with Cac buffer the next day. The specimen was then perfused with 1% osmium tetroxide and placed on a tissue rotator for 15 min. The sample was then rinsed in 0.1M of Cac buffer three times. Under the dissecting microscope, the bony capsule of the cochlea was carefully removed, and the lateral wall was cut away to reveal the organ of Corti over the middle turn, basal turn and hook regions. The tissue was serially dehydrated in 2 × 50%, 70%, 85%, 95%, and 3 × 100% ethyl alcohol. Each specimen was critical point dried using hexamethyldisilazane (HMDS) and placed on a stub for sputter coating with approximately 10 nm of gold/palladium alloy. The tissue was then viewed, and photographs were taken with a Hitachi S-3000N scanning electron microscope.

For each region of the cochlea, at least two representative samples of 33 OHCs (or 11 OHCs per row) was examined. The number of missing OHCs within each sample was then counted. These SEM techniques allow for a descriptive analysis of cellular scarring and stereocilia bundles. The results are presented as the percent hair cell damage per cochlear turn (Kamimura et al., 1999). OHC data were collected and counted by an experimenter blind to the treatment group.

Immunohistochemistry (IHC)

Cochleae used for whole mounts or mid modiolar sections were decalcified for 14–20 days in 100 mM EDTA at room temperature and either microdissected or mounted into OCT and cryosectioned. For IHC processing, primary antibody (1:100 titer) and secondary fluorescent-labeled antibodies (1:200 titer) were used. Slides were imaged by Leica confocal microscope (Leica America).

RNA Isolation

Cochleae were pared down to the bone to remove all extraneous tissue, crushed in liquid nitrogen followed by extraction in 500 μl of TRI reagent. 0.1 ml of chloroform was added, and the tube was shaken vigorously for 15 s and centrifuged at 12,000 × *g* for 15 min. RNA was extracted by washing the pellet with 0.5 ml ice-cold isopropanol followed by cold 75% treated ethanol. The ethanol was removed and the tube was air-dried briefly. The RNA pellet was resuspended in nuclease-free water and RNA levels were determined using optical density readings corresponding to wavelengths of 260, 280, and 230 nm using a spectrophotometer (Eppendorf BioPhotometer, Hamburg, Germany).

Real-Time RT-PCR

Five hundred nanogram of total RNA was converted to cDNA using the iScript cDNA Synthesis Kit (Bio-Rad, Hercules, CA, United States). The reaction mixture was set up as follows: 500 ng of total RNA, 4 μl of iScript reaction mix, 1 μl of iScript reverse transcriptase, nuclease-free water to bring the total volume to 20 μl. The reaction mix was incubated at 25°C for 5 min, 42°C for 30 min and 85°C for 5 min. This cDNA reaction mix was used for real-time PCR, as described previously (Mukherjea et al., 2011). Gene-specific primer pairs were used for the various reactions and mRNA expression levels were normalized to the levels of GAPDH. The primer sets were purchased from Sigma Genosys (St. Louis, MO, United States), and were as follows:

Rodent-GAPDH (sense): 5′-ATGGTGAAGGTCGGTGTG AAC-3′
(antisense): 5′-TGTAGTTGAGGTCAATGAAGG-3′
Rodent TRPV1 (sense): 5′-CAAGGCTGTCTTCATCA TC-3′
(antisense): 5′-AGTCCAGTTTACCTCGTCCA-3′
Rodent NOX3 (sense): 5′-GTGAACAAGGGAAGGCT CAT-3′
(antisense): 5′-GACCCACAGAAGAACACGC-3′
Rodent-TNF-α (sense): 5′-CAGACCCTCACACTCAGA TCA-3′
(antisense): 5′-TGAAGAGAACCTGGGAGTAGA-3′
Rodent-COX2 (sense): 5′-TGATCGAAGACTACGTGCA AC-3′
(antisense): 5′-GTACTCCTGGTCTTCAATGTT-3′
Rodent iNOS (sense): 5′-AAGTACGAGTGGTTCCA GGA-3′
(antisense): 5′-GCACAGCTGCATTGATCTCG-3′

Statistical Analysis

Statistical significance differences among groups were performed using either student's *t*-Test or ANOVA, followed by Tukey's *post hoc* test. $p < 0.05$ was considered to be statistically significant.

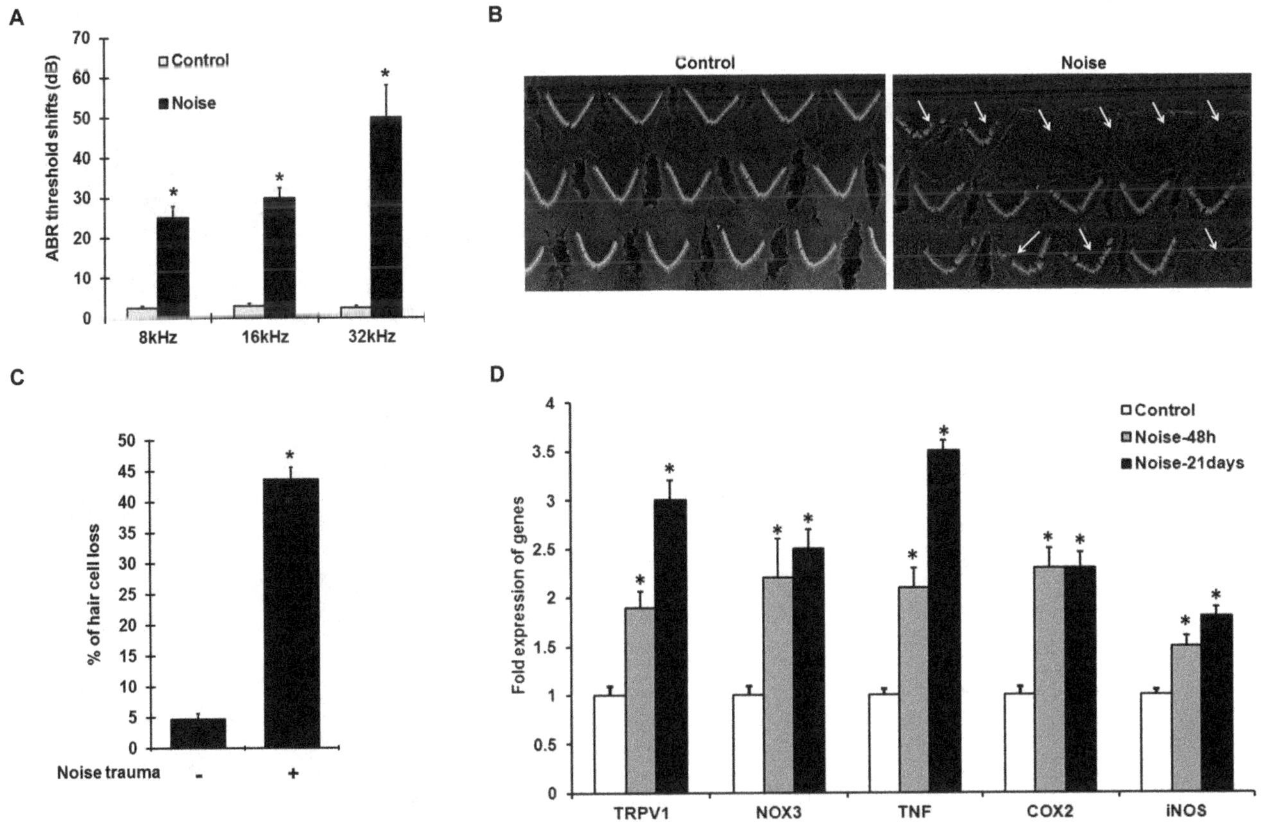

FIGURE 1 | NIHL is associated with persistent increases in gene expression of pro-inflammatory mediators. **(A)** Pre-treatment ABR's were performed and rats were noise exposed. Post treatment ABR thresholds shifts, recorded 21 days after noise exposure were 25 ± 4, 30 ± 3, and 52 ± 7 dB at 8, 16, and 32 kHz respectively. **(B)** SEM of the basal turn of cochlea showing damage/loss OHCs (see arrows) after 21 days. **(C)** Graphical representation showing damage/loss of 43 ± 4% of OHCs ($n = 6$), compared to controls. **(D)** Noise increased the expression of stress-responsive and inflammatory genes at 48 h and 21 days post noise exposure. Significant increases in all the genes (normalized to *GAPDH*) were observed compared to control cochleae. Asterisk (*) denotes statistically significant difference between noise-exposed and control cochlea. Statistical significance was analyzed using student's *t*-Test or ANOVA and Tukey's *post hoc* analysis.

RESULTS

Noise Exposure Increases Cochlear Inflammatory Genes

Noise exposure induces ABR threshold shifts of 25–50 ± 8 dB in rats at 8, 16, and 32 kHz tested (**Figure 1A**), and is associated with increased cochlear TRPV1 and TNF-α expression. Scanning electron microscopic (SEM) images of the organ of Corti show ~40–50% damage/loss of OHCs (**Figures 1B,C**) in the noise-exposed animals. The expression of cochlear stress and inflammatory genes measured by qPCR at 48 h and 21 days following NE were elevated in a time-dependent manner. Interestingly, the increases for TRPV1 and TNF-α were significantly greater at 21 days than at 48 h. TRPV1 expression was increased to 2.0 ± 0.2 fold at 48 h and further increased to 3 ± 0.2 fold by 21 days while TNF-α expression increased from 2.1 ± 0.2 to 3.5 ± 0.2 fold over the same time period. NOX3, iNOS, and COX2 expression increased significantly at 48 h to 2.2 ± 0.4, 1.5 ± 0.2, and 2.3 ± 0.2 fold, respectively, with no significant changes at 21 days post-NE (**Figure 1D**). These findings demonstrate the induction of TRPV1, TNF-α, and NOX3 as early and persistent markers of NIHL.

ROS Increases TRPV1-Dependent Ca^{2+} Entry Which Is Potentiated by TNF-α

To establish the role of TRPV1 channel in NIHL in, *in vitro* studies and examine whether TNF-α potentiates TRPV1-induced Ca^{2+} influx, H_2O_2 was used to mimic ROS produced following NE. HEKVR1 and immortalized organ of Corti (UB/OC-1) cells were used. The cells were loaded with Ca^{2+} dye - Fluo-4AM washed and imaged every 3 s for 300 s. Basal fluorescence was captured for 10 scans and 100μM H_2O_2 was added at 30 s and the resulting fluorescence captured. H_2O_2 treatment elicited a rapid robust Ca^{2+} response within 10 s which returned to

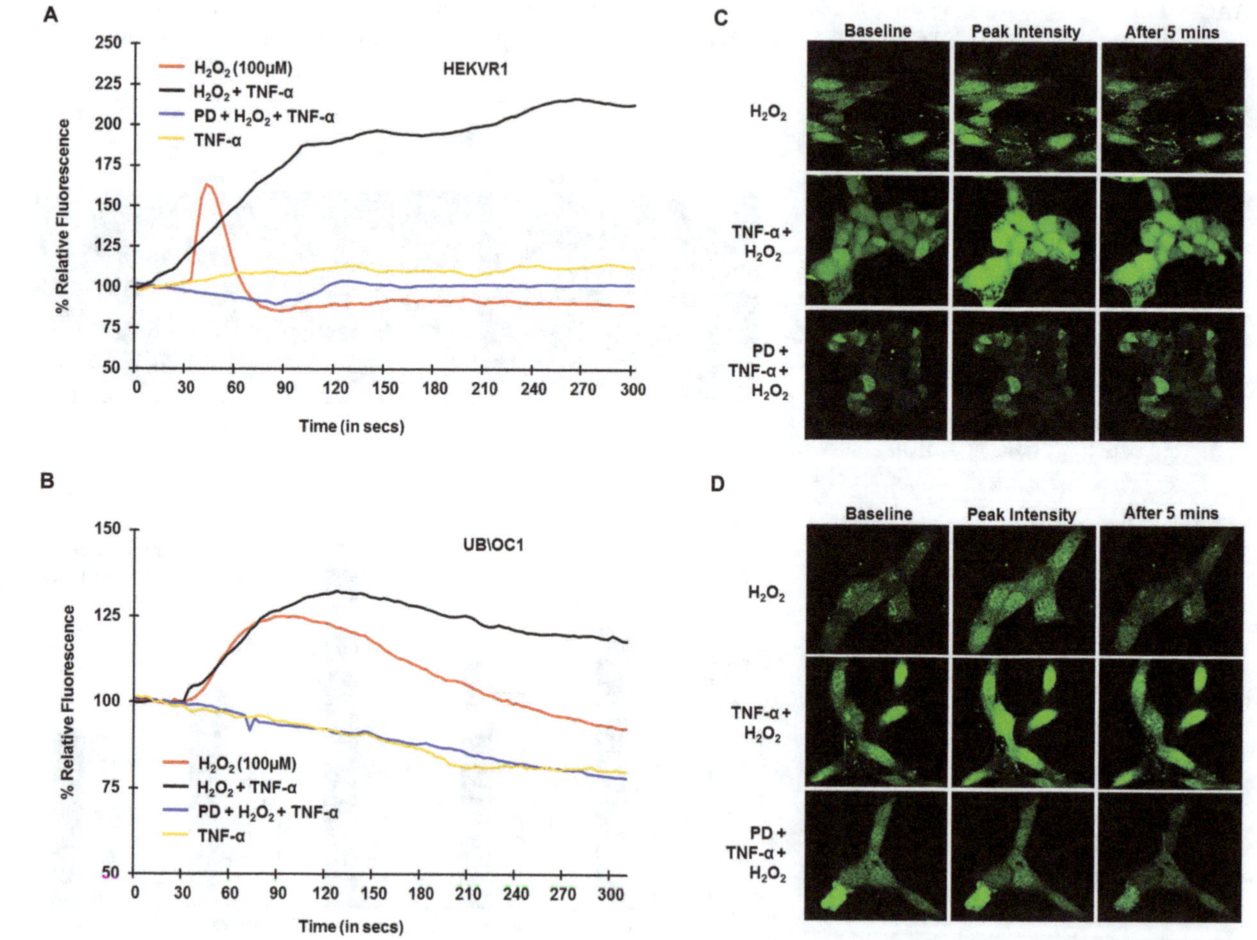

FIGURE 2 | TRPV1 mediated Ca^{2+} release by ROS is potentiated by TNF-α and requires ERK activation. HEKVR1 or UB/OC-1 cells were loaded with Fluo-4AM dye and baseline fluorescence was recorded every 3 s by confocal microscopy. Graphical representations of % relative fluorescence was calculated using F/F0 ratios. For TNF-α studies, 0.1 ng/ml of this cytokine was added, followed by addition of 100 μM H_2O_2 after 60 s and fluorescence recorded for 5 min. **(A,B)** H_2O_2 elicits a rapid robust Ca^{2+} response in HEKVR1 **(A)** as well as UB/OC-1 cells **(B)** and this was potentiated by pretreatment with TNF-α. Pretreatment with ERK inhibitor-PD98059 (10 μM) for 30 min inhibits ROS mediated Ca^{2+} response completely, confirming the role of *ERK activation* in both cell lines. **(C,D)** Are representative images of the Ca^{2+} response of the two cell lines (**C**: HEKVR1 cells, **D**: UB/OC-1 cells) used in the study.

baseline by 60 s. Similar robust Ca^{2+} response was seen in UB/OC-1 cells starting at 30 s that returned to baseline by 3 min. The differences in temporal profile are due to fewer TRPV1 channels in UB/OC-1 cells (data not shown) compared to HEKVR1 cells. Pretreatment with TNF-α (0.1 μg/ml) for 10 min prior to treatment with H_2O_2 resulted in a prolonged and sustained Ca^{2+} fluorescence in both HEKVR1 and UB/OC-1 cells which is observed until 5 min (**Figures 2A,B**). Pictorial representation of baseline, maximal and fluorescence after 5 min is shown in HEKVR1 cells (**Figure 2C**) and in UB/OC-1 cells (**Figure 2D**). Since extracellular signal-regulated kinase (ERK) activation contributes to the pathology of NIHL (Meltser et al., 2010; Maeda et al., 2013), we tested the involvement of this kinase in TRPV1-mediated Ca^{2+} influx by pre-treating the ERK inhibitor, PD98059. Our data indicate that TRPV1-mediated Ca^{2+} entry is ERK1/2 dependent, as pretreatment of the cells with 10 μM PD98059 blunted the Ca^{2+} release in both HEKVR1 as well as UB/OC-1 cells (**Figures 2A,B**).

To further confirm the involvement of TRPV1 in H_2O_2 mediated Ca^{2+} entry, knockdown of TRPV1 was achieved by transfecting the UB/OC-1 cells with siRNA for TRPV1 (Mukherjea et al., 2008). Knockdown of TRPV1 by siTRPV1 abolished the Ca^{2+} response in UB/OC-1 cells by H_2O_2 and pretreatment with TNF-α did not have any effect, suggesting that H_2O_2-stimulated Ca^{2+} entry was mediated via TRPV1 (**Figure 3A**). Furthermore, inhibition of TRPV1 by transfection

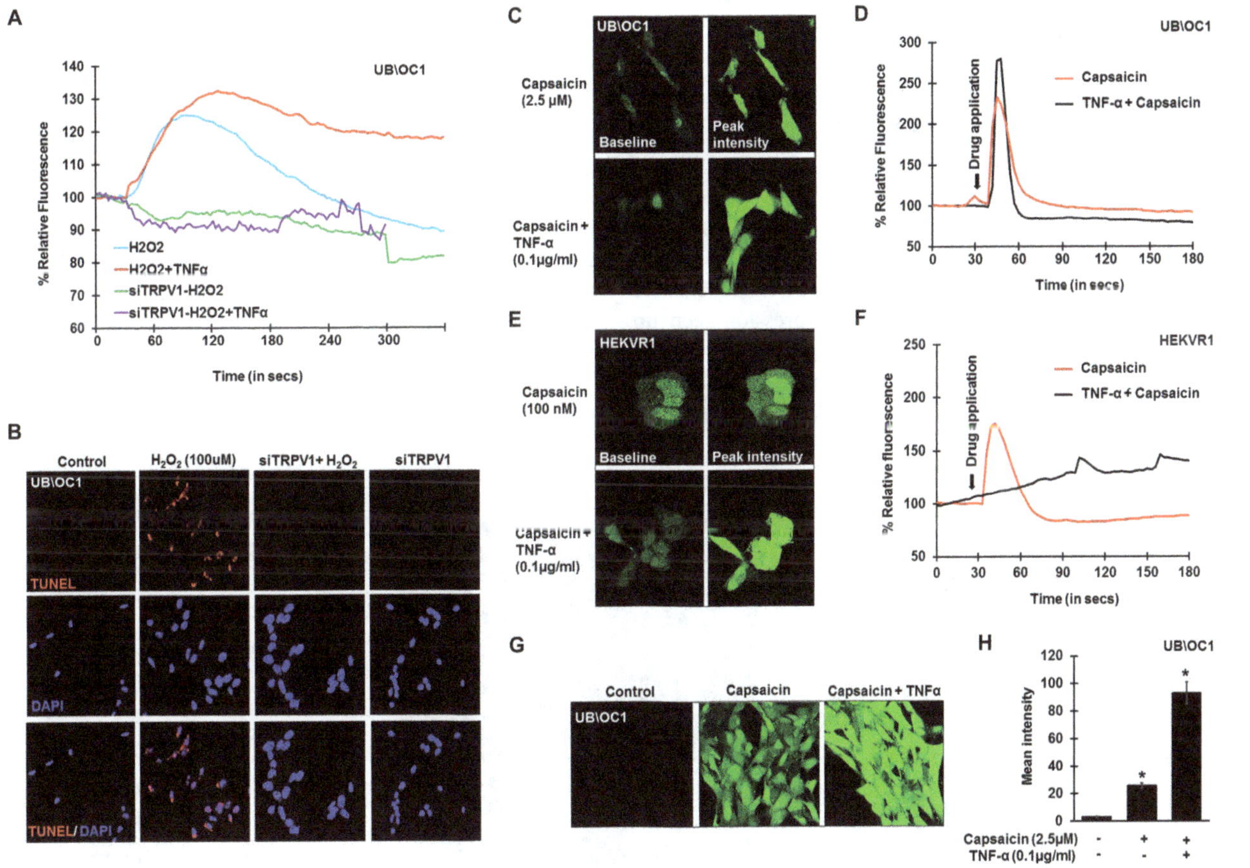

FIGURE 3 | TNF-α potentiates direct TRPV1 activation. UB/OC-1 or HEKVR1 cells were plated on cover slips for these experiments. **(A)** UB/OC-1 cells were treated with siTRPV1 (10 nM) or siScramble (5 nM) for 48 h, loaded with Fluo-4AM dye and treated with 100 μM H_2O_2 and imaged every 3 s for 5 min. siTRPV1 treatment completely abolishes H_2O_2 mediated Ca^{2+} release, while siScramble had no effect on H_2O_2 mediated Ca^{2+} release. Pre-treatment with TNF-α (0.1 ng/ml) for 10 min followed by 100 μM H_2O_2 did not elicit any Ca^{2+} response, indicating that TRPV1 is essential in ROS mediated Ca^{2+} release. **(B)** Knockdown of TRPV1 by siRNA inhibits H_2O_2 mediated apoptosis in UB/OC-1 cells. UB/OC-1 cells were treated with siTRPV1 (10 nM) or siScramble (5 nM) for 48 h prior to H_2O_2 (100 μM) for another 48 h. The reaction was then stopped and cells fixed with freshly prepared 4% paraformaldehyde and apoptosis was detected by TUNEL staining. H_2O_2 treatment for 48 h shows 74 ± 7% cell death which was abolished by knockdown of TRPV1. **(C–F)** UB/OC-1 or HEKVR1 cells loaded with Fluo-4AM were either pre-treated with TNF-α 0.1 ng/ml or PBS for 10 min, and baseline scanned for fluorescence for 10 scans, treated with TRPV1 direct agonist capsaicin (2.5 μM for UB/OC-1 or 100 nM for HEKVR1) and imaged every 3 s for 3 min. Capsaicin elicits a sharp and robust Ca^{2+}response which was further potentiated by addition of TNF-α cytokine. **(C)** Pictorial representation of UB/OC-1 cells eliciting a sharp and robust response to capsaicin (2.5 μM) which was further induced by TNF-α pretreatment. **(D)** Graphical representation of Ca^{2+}response in UB/OC-1 cells. **(E)** Pictorial representation of HEKVR1 cells eliciting a sharp and robust response to capsaicin (100 nM). Interestingly, TNF-α pretreatment, elicits a persistant Ca^{2+}response in HEKVR1 cells. **(F)** Graphical representation of Ca^{2+}response in HEKVR1 cells. **(G,H)** Pictorial and graphical representation of UB/OC-1 cells showing a tremendous increase in Ca^{2+} release with capsaicin treatment over basal fluorescence, which was further increased with the addition of TNF-α. Asterisk (*) denotes statistically significant difference compared to untreated control.

of UB/OC-1 cells with siRNA inhibited apoptosis induced by 100 μM H_2O_2 as seen by TUNEL staining (**Figure 3B**). To further confirm the role of TNF-α in potentiating the Ca^{2+} response via the TRPV1 channel, UB/OC-1, and HEKVR1 cells were loaded with Fluo-4AM dye and pretreated with either PBS or TNF-α (0.1 μg/ml) for 10 min. Addition of capsaicin (2.5 μM for UB/OC-1 cells and 100 nM for HEKVR1 cells) produced a robust increase in Ca^{2+} uptake in both UB/OC-1 and HEKVR1 cells compared to capsaicin alone (**Figures 3C,D** for UB/OC-1 and **Figures 3E,F** for HEKVR1). More prolonged exposure of UB/OC-1 cells to the capsaicin + TNF-α combination for 30 min increased baseline fluorescence from 100 ± 2% to 741 ± 22% with capsaicin treatment to 3,146 ± 532% increase with capsaicin + TNF-α (**Figures 3G,H**). These data indicate that ROS (such as H_2O_2) can activate TRPV1 to increase intracellular Ca^{2+} accumulation and that this action is potentiated by TNF-α via an ERK 1/2 dependent pathway in the cochlea.

ERK Activation Is Essential for ROS Mediated Apoptosis and in TNF-α Mediated Inflammation

To establish the role of ROS activation of ERK phosphorylation, UB/OC-1 cells were treated with H_2O_2 (100 μM). Increase in ERK1/2 phosphorylation in UB/OC-1 cells treated with 100 μM H_2O_2 was observed in a time-dependent manner (**Figures 4A,B**), with significantly elevated expression seen up to 120 min post-treatment. Additionally, inhibition of ERK activation by PD98059 prior to treatment with 100 μM H_2O_2 showed significantly decreased cell death by TUNEL (**Figure 4C**). Interestingly, TNF-α (0.1 μg/ml) treatment alone significantly activates ERK 1/2 phosphorylation and elicited a bell-shaped curve with the highest expression seen at 15 min post-treatment (**Figures 4D,E**).

Desensitization of TRPV1 by Capsaicin Administration Prevents NIHL

In these studies, pre-treatment ABRs from naïve rats were recorded and rats were then treated with daily oral PBS or capsaicin starting 24 h prior to noise, on the day of NE, and at 24 h post NE. The final ABRs were recorded 21 days post NE. Schematic representation of the treatment paradigm has been depicted in **Figure 5A**. The noise produced ABR threshold shifts of 21.6 ± 1.7, 35.5 ± 1.9, and 43.9 ± 2.3 dB at 8, 16, and 32 kHz, respectively. Oral capsaicin reduced threshold shifts to 3.9 ± 1.4, 6.1 ± 1.8, and 8.9 ± 2.1 dB at 8, 16, and 32 kHz respectively. Oral capsaicin administration did not show any significant ABR threshold shift compared to control (1 ± 1.1, 1 ± 1.1, 3 ± 1.6 dB threshold shift at 8, 16, and 32 kHz respectively). Statistical significance was calculated using one way ANOVA with Tukey's *post hoc* analyses, $p < 0.05$, $N = 6$ (**Figure 5B**). Gene expression analyses of the various stress response, inflammatory and apoptotic markers by qPCR of the rat cochleae showed that oral capsaicin inhibits the upregulation of all the stress markers by noise (**Figure 5C**). Fold increases in gene expressions by noise over oral PBS treated control rat cochleae were 4.4 ± 0.7 fold for TRPV1, 4.7 ± 0.6 for TNF-α, 4.6 ± 0.7 for NOX3, 3 ± 0.2 for COX2 and 3 ± 0.1 for Bax, while the cochleae

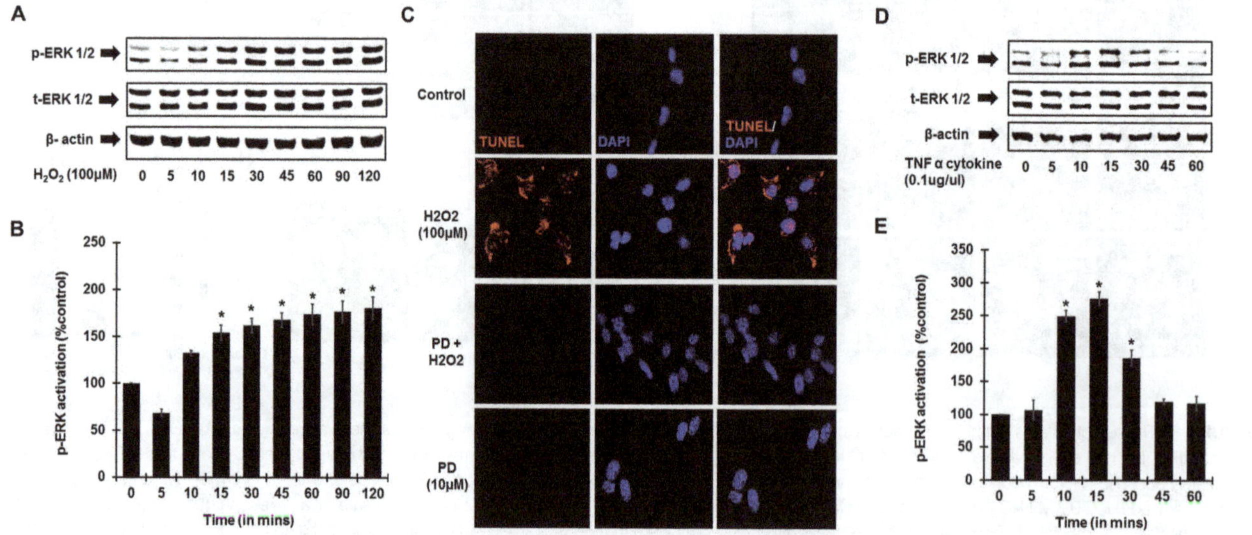

FIGURE 4 | ROS and TNF-α activate ERK phosphorylation. UB/OC-1 cells were used for these assays. **(A)** ROS activates ERK phosphorylation in UB/OC-1 cells. UB/OC-1 cells were treated with 100 μM H_2O_2 and probed for phospho-ERK1/2 activation by western blotting and normalized to total ERK, with β-actin acting as loading control. Phospho-ERK activation was elicited in a time dependent manner, with significantly increased expression seen up to 120 min post treatment. **(B)** Graphical representation of ROS mediated ERK activation in UB/OC-1 cells. **(C)** ROS induced apoptosis is ERK dependent. UB/OC-1 cells were pre-treated with vehicle or ERK inhibitor PD98059 (10 μM) for 45 min prior to treatment with 100 μM H_2O_2 for 48 h. H_2O_2 treatment showed 80 ± 8% cell death, which was significantly decreased by pretreatment with ERK inhibitor PD98059 as observed by TUNEL staining. **(D,E)** TNF-α (0.1 μg/ml) treatment elicits ERK activation in UB/OC-1 cells. ERK activation by TNF-α (0.1 μg/ml) treatment elicited a bell shape curve with highest expression seen at 15 min post treatment in UB/OC-1 cells ($p < 0.05$, * indicates statistically significant compared to control).

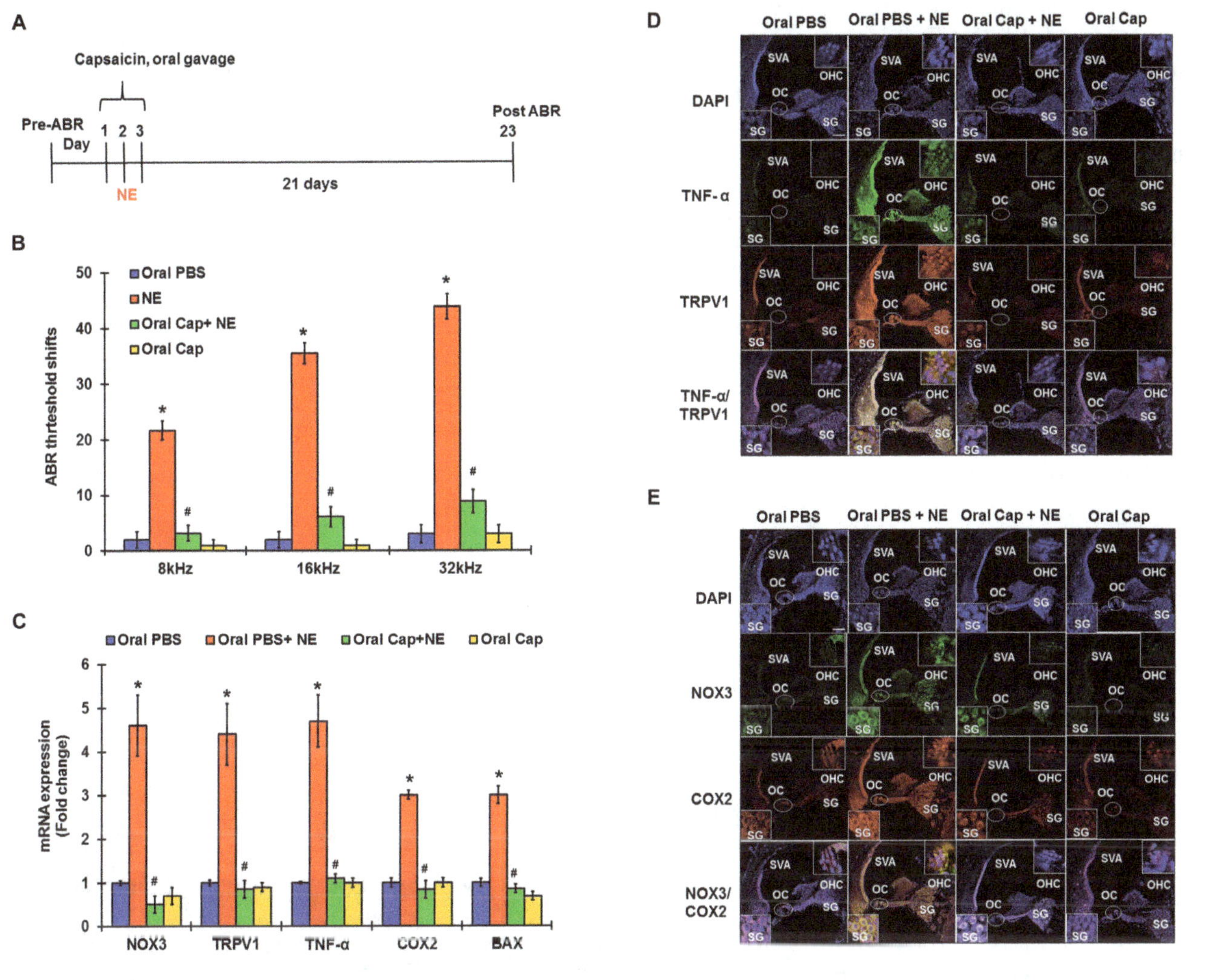

FIGURE 5 | Desensitization of TRPV1 by capsaicin pretreatment abrogates NIHL. Pretreatment ABRs were performed, followed by oral capsaicin and noise exposure. Post treatment ABR threshold were recorded 21 days after noise exposure. **(A)** Schematic diagram of animal treatments. **(B)** Noise exposure showed 25–45 dB threshold shift at 8, 16, and 32 kHz, which was abrogated by oral capsaicin. Asterisk (*) denotes statistically significant difference from the noise + vehicle group. Statistics were performed using ANOVA and Tukey's *post hoc* analysis, $N = 6$. **(C)** Gene expression analyses of the various stress response, inflammatory and apoptotic markers by qPCR of the rat cochleae showed that oral capsaicin treatment inhibits the upregulation of all the stress markers by NE. Fold increases in gene expressions by NE over oral PBS treated control rat cochleae were as follows: TRPV1 (4.4 ± 0.7), TNF-α (4.7 ± 0.6), NOX3 (4.6 ± 0.7), COX2 (3 ± 0.2), Bax (3 ± 0.1), while the oral Cap + NE group showed basal levels of gene expression where TRPV1 (0.85 ± 0.2), TNF-α (0.9 ± 0.1), NOX3 (0.5 ± 0.2), COX2 (0.84 ± 0.2) and Bax (0.86 ± 0.1). Oral Capsaicin treatment alone showed basal levels of all genes namely: TRPV1 (0.9 ± 0.1), TNF-α (1 ± 0.15), NOX3 (0.7 ± 0.2), COX2 (1 ± 0.1) and Bax (0.69 ± 0.1). **(D,E)** Immunolabelling of rat cochlear mid-modiolar sections was performed 21 days post noise exposure. Noise exposure increased TRPV1, TNF-α, NOX3 and COX2 immunoreactivity, which was significantly decreased by oral capsaicin pretreatment. Scale bars represent 50 μm (* shows significant difference compared to oral PBS group, # shows significant difference compared to NE).

from rats administered oral capsaicin + noise group showed basal levels of gene expression and oral capsaicin treatment alone showed basal levels of all genes tested (**Figure 5C**). Fluorescent immunolabelling of the mid-modiolar sections of the rat cochleae with TRPV1 and TNF-α antibody shows a robust increase in fluorescence in cochleae from noise-exposed rats but not in cochleae from rats administered oral capsaicin followed by noise (**Figure 5D**). Additionally, immunofluorescent staining of inflammatory mediators such as NOX3 and COX2 also show a similar decrease in expression in rat cochleae pre-treated with oral capsaicin (**Figure 5E**). Thus, capsaicin protects against NIHL and associated cochlear inflammatory markers.

TNF-α Inhibition Can Prevent and Treat NIHL

To determine whether inhibition of the inflammatory TNF-α signaling could ameliorate NIHL, we administered ETA by either TT or s.c injections. The drug treatment was administered either as a single preventive pretreatment given prior to noise or as a single rescue treatment administered after noise. Schematic representation of the 4 different treatment paradigms have been shown in **Figure 6A**. We hypothesized that sequestering TNF-α by ETA pretreatment either 3 days or 7 days prior to NE should diminish TNF-α-mediated inflammation in the cochlea. Further, in the event of unanticipated NE, rescue ETA treatment if given within a window period of either 2 or 24 h post-NE, would alleviate the TNF-α induced inflammation and ameliorate NIHL.

Single ETA administration (TT-150 μg/30 μl, or s.c: 3 mg/kg) or sterile PBS (TT-30 μl, s.c:1 ml) was performed either before or after NE according to the experimental design. Post-treatment ABR assessments were performed 21 days following NE. The cochleae were collected and processed for various biochemical and immunohistochemical assays. At least four animals were used per treatment group. Noise produced 36.25 ± 3, 45 ± 3, and 48.75 ± 2.5 dB threshold shifts, recorded at 8, 16, and 32 kHz. Gene expression analyses by real-time RT-PCR showed that noise increased the expression of cochlear TRPV1, NOX3, TNF-α, iNOS and COX2 by ~2–5 fold. ETA was administered either 7 or 3 days prior to NE by either TT or s.c administration. The 7 days pretreatment paradigm showed significant protection from NIHL with threshold shifts measuring at s.c ETA being 12.5 ± 3.6, 15 ± 5, and 16.25 ± 5.3 dB at 8, 16, and 32 kHz, respectively. The TT ETA produced threshold shifts of 16.3 ± 3.3, 16.3 ± 3.8, and 16.3 ± 4.6 dB at 8, 16, and 32 kHz, respectively (**Figures 6B,C**). Immunohistochemistry of mid-modiolar sections of treated animals show decreased TNF-α and NOX3 staining by both routes of administration compared to NE group alone (**Figure 6D**). Similar otoprotection was achieved by ETA administered 3 days prior to NE (**Figures 6B,C**).

To determine whether ETA treatment could be used to alleviate or lessen the extent of NIHL due to unanticipated NE and provide a window of opportunity for treatment, we administered a single dose of ETA 2 h or 24 h after noise by either TT or s.c routes. The treatment paradigms are depicted

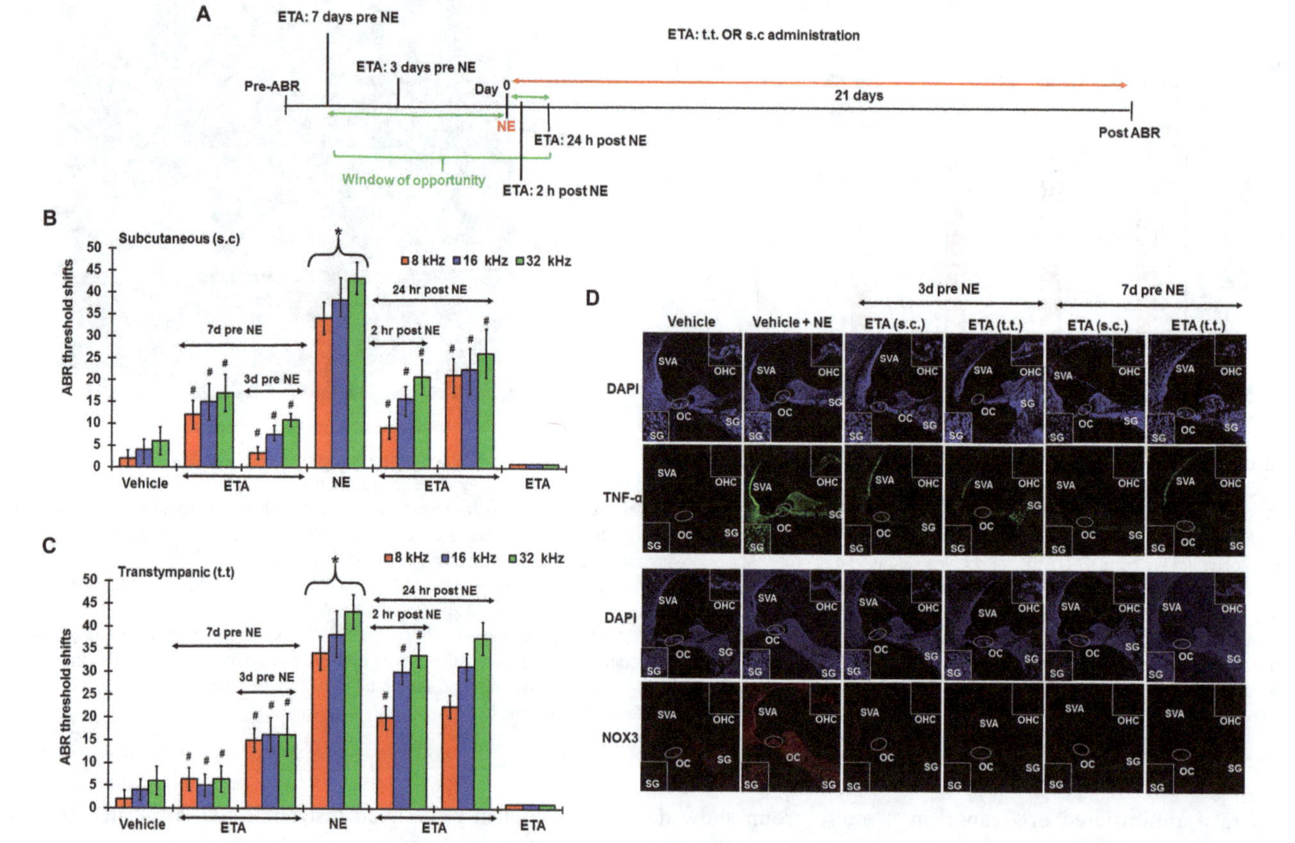

FIGURE 6 | Etanercept can prevent and treat unanticipated NIHL. Pretreatment ABRs were performed in naïve Wistar rats. Treatment were performed either according to the prevention paradigm or the rescue paradigm. Post treatment ABR thresholds were recorded 21 days after noise exposure for both paradigms. ABR threshold shift was measured. Noise trauma demonstrates a 25–60 dB elevation in hearing threshold. **(A)** Schematic diagram of animal treatments. **(B,C)** Graphical representation of ABR threshold shifts measured at 21 days post NE and were grouped according to route of administration (**B**: s.c administration, and **C**: TT administration). Pretreatments with either route of administration show similar degree of prevention from NIHL when administered at either 7 or 3 days before NE. Rescue treatments indicate better protection via the sub-cutaneous route when administered within 24 h post NE. Rescue treatment with transtympanic administration of ETA at 2 h also elicits significant protection from NIHL, though the protection is not as strong as the s.c treatment administered at the same time point. Rescue treatment with TT ETA at 24 h post NE elicits ABR threshold shifts that are lower than NE alone, however, significance is only seen at 8 kHz frequency. **(D)** ETA pretreatment down regulates noise exposure induced TNF-α and NOX3 protein expression in the cochleae as seen by immunolabelling of mid-modiolar sections (* shows significant difference compared to oral PBS group, # shows significant difference compared to NE).

schematically in **Figure 6A**. We show that ETA administered within 2 h of noise by the s.c route provides significantly better protection from NIHL compared to the TT route (s.c. ETA: 9.16 ± 2.6, 15.8 ± 2.8 and 20.8 ± 4.0 dB threshold shifts) compared to TT route of administration (20 ± 2.6, 30 ± 2.7 and 33.75 ± 2.7 dB threshold shifts) at 8, 16, and 32 kHz respectively (**Figures 6B,C**). Immunolabelling of the mid-modiolar sections of the rat cochleae for TNF α and NOX3 indicate that ETA treatment decreases the expression of these proteins in the cochlea. Gene expression analyses of the stress response genes also show decreased expression of TNF-α and NOX3 compared to noise. Interestingly, TRPV1 gene expression though lower than NE are still high. Initiation of ETA 24 h post NE by the s.c route provided significantly greater protection from NIHL with threshold shifts of (s.c. ETA: 21.25 ± 3.9, 22.5 ± 4.9, and 26.25 ± 5.6 dB) compared to trans-tympanic administration (TT ETA: 22.5 ± 2.5, 31.25 ± 2.9, and 37.5 ± 3.6 dB) at 8, 16, and 32 kHz respectively (**Figures 6B,C**). Immunolabelling of the cochlear sections for TNF-α and NOX3 indicate decreased expression of these two proteins (**Figure 7A**). Gene expression studies also show decreased cochlear TNF-α and NOX3, however, the levels of TRPV1 and COX2 are not significantly different than NE (**Figure 7B**). We believe that the increased TRPV1 and COX2 gene expression levels signify that the cochlea is severely compromised and TNF-α sequestration at 24 h (especially for the TT administration) is too late to reverse/significantly decrease the chronic inflammatory cascade.

DISCUSSION

The goal of this study was to determine the salient mechanism of NE mediated NIHL and to identify tangible targets for otoprotective therapy. NE has historically been associated with increased ROS generation (Yamane et al., 1995a; Ohlemiller et al., 1999), increased Ca^{2+} in the endolymph and hair cells (Ikeda and Morizono, 1988; Fridberger et al., 1998; Chan and Rouse, 2016), and increased inflammation (Zou et al., 2005; Fujioka et al., 2006) in the cochlea in several different animal models. Increased Ca^{2+} and ROS activity have been reported to persist for several days after traumatic NE (Li et al., 1997; Hu et al., 2002; Yamashita et al., 2005). However, a direct link between ROS, Ca^{2+}, and inflammation has not yet been established. In this present study, we proposed that development of NIHL is associated with an acute as well as a chronic increase in ROS, Ca^{2+}, and inflammation and that inhibition of any one arm of this triad of events by repurposing FDA approved drugs is a viable translatable solution.

Our hypotheses were based on observation of a cascade of events occurring early after NE. NE produces an early increase

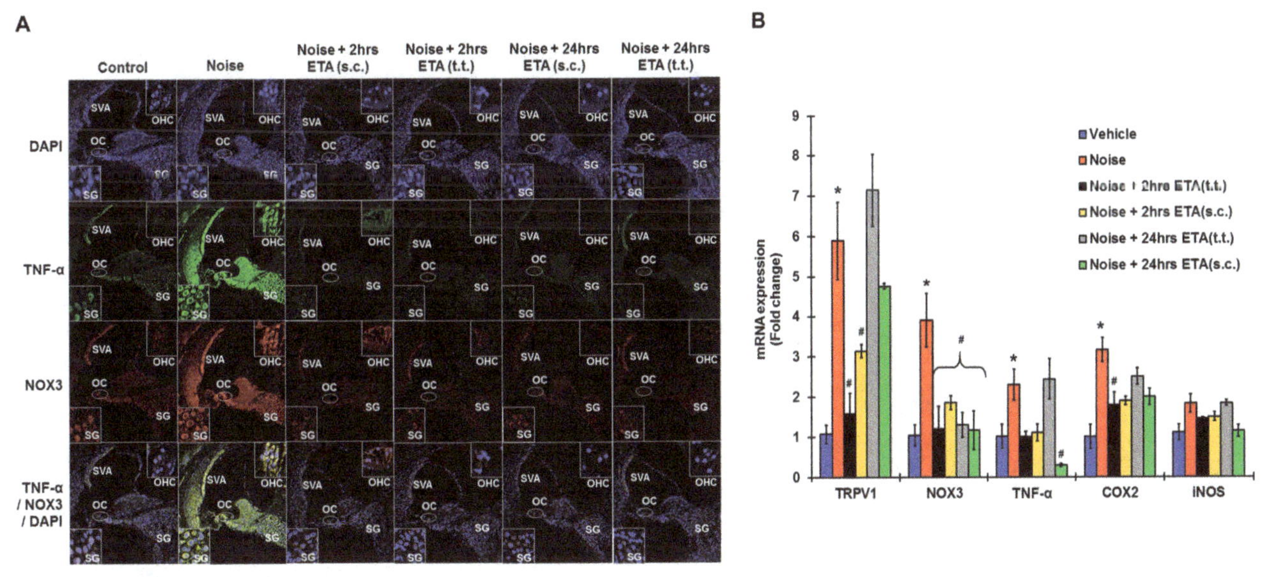

FIGURE 7 | Etanercept rescue treatment down regulates noise induced inflammation in a time dependent manner. Rescue paradigm: Noise exposure (OBN 122 dB, centered at 16 kHz for 1 h) was performed, and ETA treatment was rendered at 2 or 24 h post NE (by either sc. or TT injections). Cochleae were collected 21 days after noise exposure and processed for immunohistochemistry or gene expression studies by qPCR. **(A)** Mid-modiolar sections were immunolabelled for TNF-α (green) and NOX3 (red). Noise exposure increased the expression of these proteins in spiral ligament, stria vascularis, organ of Corti and in the spiral ganglion cells. Etanercept treatment down regulates the expression of TNF-α and NOX3 in all treatment groups. **(B)** Cochlear gene expression studies by qPCR were conducted for TRPV1, NOX3, TNF-α, COX2, and iNOS. GAPDH was used as the housekeeping gene. Noise exposure increased the expression of these genes to (5.9 ± 0.96, 3.9 ± 0.66, 2.3 ± 0.38, 3.2 ± 0.3, 1.83 ± 0.23) for TRPV1, NOX3, TNF, COX2, and iNOS respectively. TT-ETA treatment when administered at 2 h post NE elicits (1.6 ± 0.4, 1.2 ± 0.57, 1 ± 0.13, 1.45 ± 0.03, 1.8 ± 0.30), s.c-ETA treatment at 2 h post NE elicits (3.13 ± 0.16, 1.9 ± 0.17, 1.1 ± 0.21, 1.5 ± 0.11, 1.9 ± 0.2), TT-ETA treatment when administered at 24 h post NE elicits (7.14 ± 0.89, 1.3 ± 0.32, 2.44 ± 0.5, 1.84 ± 0.07, 2.5 ± 0.2), while s.c-ETA treatment at 24 h post NE elicits (4.75 ± 0.07, 1.2 ± 0.48, 0.3 ± 0.04, 1.14 ± 0.15, 2 ± 0.20) for TRPV1, NOX3, TNF, COX2 and iNOS respectively. It was interesting to note that ETA treatment abolishes the TNF-α and NOX3 gene expression in all groups except for the TT-ETA at 24 h, which reflects ABR threshold shifts and the degree of protection established or lack thereof (* shows significant difference compared to oral PBS group, # shows significant difference compared to NE).

in cochlear NOX3, TRPV1 and inflammatory mediators (TNF-α, iNOS, and COX2) in the rat at 48 h that persisted for at least 21 days. The expression of TRPV1 and TNF-α were significantly higher at 21 days compared to 48 h post NE and led us to speculate that these genes, along with NOX3 were an essential part of a positive feedback loop for the development of NIHL.

Proposed Mechanism of Action

Cochlear injury induced by noise trauma activates and increases NOX3 and TRPV1 expression which contributes to increases in TNF-α production, ERK activation, and inflammation. Unresolved chronic inflammation results in damage or death of cells in the cochlea and hearing loss. Blocking any one of these moieties of the pathway will prevent and treat NIHL (**Figure 8**).

Chronic TRPV1 channel activation leads to chronic increases in intracellular Ca^{2+} accumulation. Thus, induction of TRPV1 by noise could lead to Ca^{2+} overload in cochlear structures expressing these channels. Interestingly, chronic increases in Ca^{2+} and ROS have been shown to increase inflammation and apoptosis in various tissues (Nicotera and Orrenius, 1992; Orrenius et al., 1992a,b; Vass et al., 1995; Sinha et al., 2013). Our studies of cisplatin-induced hearing loss have implicated TRPV1 activation in the generation of ROS via NOX3, inflammation, and apoptosis in the cochlea (Mukherjea et al., 2008; Mukherjea et al., 2011). In the present study, we have shown that noise-induced ROS mimicked by H_2O_2 *in vitro*, can activate TRPV1 channel and increase Ca^{2+} influx in an immortalized organ of Corti cell line UB/OC-1 as well as in HEKVR1 cells. However, when these cell lines were pretreated with TNF-α for 10 min, the addition of H_2O_2 elicited a strong persistent opening of the TRPV1 channel. Thus, we show that NE not only dysregulates the TRPV1 channel expression but that the accompanying inflammation as mediated by TNF-α (and possibly other cytokines) will further potentiate this action, eventually leading to cell death. The novelty of this observation is that this is the first time TNF-α mediated potentiation of TRPV1 mediated Ca^{2+} entry has been implicated in hearing loss. Similar phenomenon of TNF-α induced potentiation of Ca^{2+} current evoked by TRPV1 has been reported in rat pulmonary sensory neurons in asthma (Hu et al., 2010), in cultured trigeminal ganglions isolated from neonatal rats (Meng et al., 2016), in human synoviocytes (Kochukov et al., 2009) and in sensitization of the spinal cord in the pain model (Spicarova and Palecek, 2010).

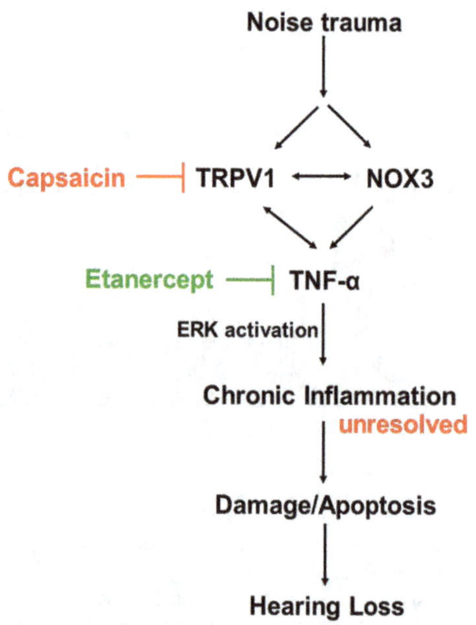

FIGURE 8 | Proposed mechanism of prevention and treatment of NIHL. Noise exposure increases stress response molecules TRPV1, cochlear specific NADPH oxidase NOX3 and inflammatory mediators such as TNF-α, iNOS and COX2, acutely (within 48 h) and chronically (21 days post noise exposure). Inhibition of either TRPV1 by desensitization with oral capsaicin or inhibition of TNF-α with Etanercept (TNF-α inhibitor) show amelioration of noise induced hearing loss.

Direct TRPV1 agonist capsaicin can activate and subsequently desensitize the TRPV1 receptor rapidly. Interestingly, our data indicate that rats pre-treated with oral capsaicin prior to noise, show complete protection from ABR threshold shifts. Protein, as well as gene expression studies of the cochleae of these animals, indicate that pretreatment with capsaicin not only abolishes the noise-induced increases in TRPV1 but also inhibits NOX3, TNF-α, COX2, and iNOS. It was interesting to note that capsaicin administered prior to noise suppresses ROS generation as well as inflammation.

Our next hypothesis was that if inflammation due to TNF-α were to be inhibited prior to NE, the degree of NIHL will be ameliorated. We further hypothesized that in the event of unanticipated NE, TNF-α sequestration within a limited time window will afford some degree of protection from NIHL. We used ETA, a fusion protein consisting of two p75 TNF receptors bound to human IgG1receptor (Mohler et al., 1993) and currently used to treat autoimmune diseases like plaque psoriasis, psoriatic arthritis, ankylosing spondylitis among others. Prophylactic treatment with ETA performed either 3 or 7 days prior to noise, significantly protected from the ABR threshold shift measured at 21 days post NE. It appears that either systemic administration by subcutaneous injections or local delivery by TT injection were equally effective at protecting from NIHL when given 7 days prior to noise. Similarly, both routes of administration are equally effective in preventing NIHL when given 3 days prior to NE. The 3 days ETA pre-treatment regimen shows stronger protection than the 7 days pre-treatment regimen. This is a very interesting observation that inhibition of inflammation either systemically or locally prior to noise would ameliorate noise-induced ABR threshold shift. This implies that when used prophylactically in an uninjured body with basal levels of inflammation, the availability of a TNF-α antagonist can reduce the local levels of TNF-α and this prevents subsequent up regulation of TRPV1, thus lessening the impact of traumatic noise on the cochlea. It also indicates that lower levels of TNF-α in systemic circulation prevent recruitment of immune-competent cells by the cochlea. Lower levels of circulating TNF-α would also modulate the expression of adhesion molecules such as ICAM-1 in the cochlea (Kim H. et al., 2008) which have been shown to be upregulated by noise (Tan et al., 2016). Additionally, local inhibition of

TNF-α is equally relevant as this lowers the cochlear ability to ramp up inflammation in response to traumatic noise. Most importantly, the effectiveness of trans-tympanic ETA indicates that in an uninjured cochlea, this large molecule (~150 kD) can cross the round window and protect against permanent NIHL. Furthermore, the *trans*-tympanic administration of ETA would avoid the global suppression of immunity associated with the systemic route.

In unanticipated NEs, we show that systemic ETA can decrease hearing loss when administered within a 2–24 h time period following NE. An interesting observation is that while post noise administration of ETA reduces the cochlear expression of TNF-α and NOX3, the high levels of TRPV1 persists and could contribute to the residual hearing loss observed in these animals. This finding could also indicate a slower turnover of TRPV1 mRNA or to differential regulation of TRPV1 and TNF-α by noise. ETA administered by the localized TT injection show a significant lowering of ABR threshold shifts when administered within 2 h of noise but not at 24 h of noise. This could reflect a slower onset of action of ETA via the TT route post injury (probably due to slower/decreased entry into the endolymph following TT injections) to prevent irreversible changes in the cochlea which are initiated within 24 h following noise. We hypothesize that systemic (peripheral) administration of the drug could enable rapid delivery to the SV via the blood stream while dampening the systemic inflammation and possibly decreasing the recruitment of immune-competent cells from systemic circulation. This would enable the cochlea to mount the resolution phase of the inflammatory cascade, which is reflected as decreased threshold shifts or amelioration of hearing loss. Thus, as a rescue treatment, the subcutaneous route provides a wider window of opportunity than the TT route.

ETA has been shown to inhibit cochlear inflammation caused by immunologic stimulation (Satoh et al., 2003; Wang et al., 2003) and cochlear electrode insertion trauma (Ihler et al., 2014). ETA has also been studied in the treatment of immune-mediated cochlea-vestibular disorders as well as autoimmune inner ear diseases in humans with varying successes (Cohen et al., 2005; Matteson et al., 2005; Van Wijk et al., 2006). Subcutaneous administration of ETA in noise-exposed guinea pigs showed hearing preservation at 8 kHz, when determined at 3 h post noise, due to the preservation of cochlear blood flow (Arpornchayanon et al., 2013). This study complements our data which indicates a window of opportunity for subcutaneous treatment from 7 days prior to NE to within 24 h post NE.

CONCLUSION

This study shows that NE causes an acute phase of stress and inflammation in the cochlea, which progress to a chronic inflammatory phase that leads to damage or death of the various sensorineural cells in the cochlea. TRPV1 and TNF-α (and their subsequent synergy) are important components of this inflammatory response. Accordingly, we show that inhibition of TRPV1 or TNF-α can successfully protect and even rescue from NIHL. The translation potential of these data is significant, as it gives the physicians a window of opportunity to treat patients exposed to traumatic noise.

ETHICS STATEMENT

The animal study was reviewed and approved by Southern Illinois University School of Medicine Laboratory Animal Care and Use Committee (LACUC).

AUTHOR CONTRIBUTIONS

DM developed the idea for the research mentioned in this manuscript. AD, DM, and PB performed the experiments and data analysis. AD and DM wrote the manuscript and edited the figures. KK helped with gene expression analyses. VR, SS, CM, and CT critiqued and revised the manuscript.

REFERENCES

Arpornchayanon, W., Canis, M., Ihler, F., Settevendemie, C., and Strieth, S. (2013). TNF-α inhibition using etanercept prevents noise-induced hearing loss by improvement of cochlear blood flow in vivo. *Int. J. Audiol.* 52, 545–552. doi: 10.3109/14992027.2013.790564

Arslan, H. H., Satar, B., Serdar, M., and Yilmaz, E. (2017). Changes in proinflammatory cytokines in the cochlea in relation to hearing thresholds in noise-exposed rats. *J. Int. Adv. Otol.* 13, 308–312. doi: 10.5152/iao.2017.1674

Banfi, B., Malgrange, B., Knisz, J., Steger, K., Dubois-Dauphin, M., and Krause, K. H. (2004). NOX3, a superoxide-generating NADPH oxidase of the inner ear. *J. Biol. Chem.* 279, 46065–46072. doi: 10.1074/jbc.m403046200

Bas, E., Martinez-Soriano, F., Lainez, J. M., and Marco, J. (2009). An experimental comparative study of dexamethasone, melatonin and tacrolimus in noise-induced hearing loss. *Acta Otolaryngol.* 129, 385–389. doi: 10.1080/00016480802566279

Basu, S., and Srivastava, P. (2005). Immunological role of neuronal receptor vanilloid receptor 1 expressed on dendritic cells. *Proc. Natl. Acad. Sci. U.S.A.* 102, 5120–5125. doi: 10.1073/pnas.0407780102

Bauer, C. A., Brozoski, T. J., and Myers, K. S. (2007). Acoustic injury and TRPV1 expression in the cochlear spiral ganglion. *Int. Tinnitus J.* 13, 21–28.

Bertin, S., Aoki-Nonaka, Y., de Jong, P. R., Nohara, L. L., Xu, H., Stanwood, S. R., et al. (2014). The ion channel TRPV1 regulates the activation and proinflammatory properties of CD4(+) T cells. *Nat. Immunol.* 15, 1055–1063. doi: 10.1038/ni.3009

Bohne, B. A. (1976). Safe level for noise exposure? *Ann. Otol. Rhinol. Laryngol.* 85(6 PT. 1), 711–724. doi: 10.1177/000348947608500602

Bohne, B. A., Harding, G. W., and Lee, S. C. (2007). Death pathways in noise-damaged outer hair cells. *Hear. Res.* 223, 61–70. doi: 10.1016/j.heares.2006.10.004

Brito, R., Sheth, S., Mukherjea, D., Rybak, L. P., and Ramkumar, V. (2014). TRPV1: a potential drug target for treating various diseases. *Cells* 3, 517–545. doi: 10.3390/cells3020517

Chan, D. K., and Rouse, S. L. (2016). Sound-induced intracellular Ca2+ dynamics in the adult hearing cochlea. *PLoS one* 11:e0167850. doi: 10.1371/journal.pone.0167850

Cohen, S., Shoup, A., Weisman, M. H., and Harris, J. (2005). Etanercept treatment for autoimmune inner ear disease: results of a pilot placebo-controlled study. *Otol. Neurotol.* 26, 903–907. doi: 10.1097/01.mao.0000185082.28598.87

Fridberger, A., Flock, A., Ulfendahl, M., and Flock, B. (1998). Acoustic overstimulation increases outer hair cell Ca2+ concentrations and causes dynamic contractions of the hearing organ. *Proc. Natl. Acad. Sci. U.S.A.* 95, 7127–7132. doi: 10.1073/pnas.95.12.7127

Fujioka, M., Kanzaki, S., Okano, H. J., Masuda, M., Ogawa, K., and Okano, H. (2006). Proinflammatory cytokines expression in noise-induced damaged cochlea. *J. Neurosci. Res.* 83, 575–583. doi: 10.1002/jnr.20764

Haryuna, T. S. H., Riawan, W., Reza, M., Purnami, N., and Adnan, A. (2016). Curcumin prevents cochlear oxidative damage after noise exposure. *Int. J. Pharm. Pharm. Sci.* 8, 175–178.

Hawkins, J. E. Jr. (1971). The role of vasoconstriction in noise-induced hearing loss. *Ann. Otol. Rhinol. Laryngol.* 80, 903–913. doi: 10.1177/000348947108000617

Henderson, D., McFadden, S. L., Liu, C. C., Hight, N., and Zheng, X. Y. (1999). The role of antioxidants in protection from impulse noise. *Ann. N. Y. Acad. Sci.* 884, 368–380. doi: 10.1111/j.1749-6632.1999.tb08655.x

Hirose, K., Discolo, C. M., Keasler, J. R., and Ransohoff, R. (2005). Mononuclear phagocytes migrate into the murine cochlea after acoustic trauma. *J. Comp. Neurol.* 489, 180–194. doi: 10.1002/cne.20619

Hu, B. H., Henderson, D., and Nicotera, T. M. (2002). Involvement of apoptosis in progression of cochlear lesion following exposure to intense noise. *Hear. Res.* 166, 62–71. doi: 10.1016/s0378-5955(02)00286-1

Hu, Y., Gu, Q., Lin, R. L., Kryscio, R., and Lee, L. Y. (2010). Calcium transient evoked by TRPV1 activators is enhanced by tumor necrosis factor-{alpha} in rat pulmonary sensory neurons. *Am. J. Physiol. Lung. Cell Mol. Physiol.* 299, L483–L492. doi: 10.1152/ajplung.00111.2010

Huang, X., Whitworth, C. A., and Rybak, L. P. (2007). Ginkgo biloba extract (EGb 761) protects against cisplatin-induced ototoxicity in rats. *Otol. Neurotol.* 28, 828–833. doi: 10.1097/mao.0b013e3180430163

Ihler, F., Pelz, S., Coors, M., Matthias, C., and Canis, M. (2014). Application of a TNF-alpha-inhibitor into the scala tympany after cochlear electrode insertion trauma in guinea pigs: preliminary audiologic results. *Int. J. Audiol.* 53, 810–816. doi: 10.3109/14992027.2014.938369

Ikeda, K., and Morizono, T. (1988). Calcium transport mechanism in the endolymph of the chinchilla. *Hear. Res.* 34, 307–311. doi: 10.1016/0378-5955(88)90010-x

Infante, E. B., Channer, G. A., Telischi, F. F., Gupta, C., Dinh, J. T., Vu, L., et al. (2012). Mannitol protects hair cells against tumor necrosis factor α-induced loss. *Otol. Neurotol.* 33, 1656–1663. doi: 10.1097/MAO.0b013e31826bedd9

Kamimura, T., Whitworth, C. A., and Rybak, L. P. (1999). Effect of 4-methylthiobenzoic acid on cisplatin-induced ototoxicity in the rat. *Hear. Res.* 131, 117–127. doi: 10.1016/s0378-5955(99)00017-9

Kanzaki, J., and Ouchi, T. (1981). Steroid-responsive bilateral sensorineural hearing loss and immune complexes. *Arch. Otorhinolaryngol.* 230, 5–9. doi: 10.1007/bf00665374

Keithley, E. M., Wang, X., and Barkdull, G. C. (2008). Tumor necrosis factor alpha can induce recruitment of inflammatory cells to the cochlea. *Otol. Neurotol.* 29, 854–859. doi: 10.1097/MAO.0b013e31818256a9

Kim, H., Hwang, J.-S., Woo, C.-H., Kim, E.-Y., Kim, T.-H., Cho, K. J., et al. (2008). TNF-α-induced up-regulation of intercellular adhesion molecule-1 is regulated by a Rac-ROS-dependent cascade in human airway epithelial cells. *Exp. Mol. Med.* 40:167. doi: 10.3858/emm.2008.40.2.167

Kim, H. J., So, H. S., Lee, J. H., Park, C., Lee, J. B., Youn, M. J., et al. (2008). Role of proinflammatory cytokines in cisplatin-induced vestibular hair cell damage. *Head Neck* 30, 1445–1456. doi: 10.1002/hed.20892

Kochukov, M. Y., McNearney, T. A., Yin, H., Zhang, L., Ma, F., Ponomareva, L., et al. (2009). Tumor necrosis factor-alpha (TNF-alpha) enhances functional thermal and chemical responses of TRP cation channels in human synoviocytes. *Mol. Pain* 5:49. doi: 10.1186/1744-8069-5-49

Li, W., Zhao, L., Jiang, S., and Gu, R. (1997). Effects of high intensity impulse noise on ionic concentrations in cochlear endolymph of the guinea pig. *Chin. Med. J.* 110, 883–886.

Liu, B., Yang, F., Zhan, H., Feng, Z.-Y., Zhang, Z.-G., Li, W.-B., et al. (2014). Increased severity of inflammation correlates with elevated expression of TRPV1 nerve fibers and nerve growth factor on interstitial cystitis/bladder pain syndrome. *Urol Int.* 92, 202–208. doi: 10.1159/000355175

Maeda, Y., Fukushima, K., Omichi, R., Kariya, S., and Nishizaki, K. (2013). Time courses of changes in phospho- and total- MAP kinases in the cochlea after intense noise exposure. *PLoS one* 8:e58775. doi: 10.1371/journal.pone.0058775

Matteson, E. L., Choi, H. K., Poe, D. S., Wise, C., Lowe, V. J., McDonald, T. J., et al. (2005). Etanercept therapy for immune-mediated cochleovestibular disorders: a multi-center, open-label, pilot study. *Arth. Rheum.* 53, 337–342. doi: 10.1002/art.21179

Meltser, I., Tahera, Y., and Canlon, B. (2010). Differential activation of mitogen-activated protein kinases and brain-derived neurotrophic factor after temporary or permanent damage to a sensory system. *Neuroscience* 165, 1439–1446. doi: 10.1016/j.neuroscience.2009.11.025

Meng, J., Wang, J., Steinhoff, M., and Dolly, J. O. (2016). TNFalpha induces co-trafficking of TRPV1/TRPA1 in VAMP1-containing vesicles to the plasmalemma via Munc18-1/syntaxin1/SNAP-25 mediated fusion. *Sci. Rep.* 6:21226. doi: 10.1038/srep21226

Mohler, K. M., Torrance, D. S., Smith, C. A., Goodwin, R. G., Stremler, K. E., Fung, V. P., et al. (1993). Soluble tumor necrosis factor (TNF) receptors are effective therapeutic agents in lethal endotoxemia and function simultaneously as both TNF carriers and TNF antagonists. *J. Immunol.* 151, 1548–1561.

Mukherjea, D., Jajoo, S., Sheehan, K., Kaur, T., Sheth, S., Bunch, J., et al. (2011). NOX3 NADPH oxidase couples transient receptor potential vanilloid 1 to signal transducer and activator of transcription 1-mediated inflammation and hearing loss. *Antioxid. Redox. Signal* 14, 999–1010. doi: 10.1089/ars.2010.3497

Mukherjea, D., Jajoo, S., Whitworth, C., Bunch, J. R., Turner, J. G., Rybak, L. P., et al. (2008). Short interfering RNA against transient receptor potential vanilloid 1 attenuates cisplatin-induced hearing loss in the rat. *J. Neurosci.* 28, 13056–13065. doi: 10.1523/JNEUROSCI.1307-08.2008

Murai, N., Kirkegaard, M., Jarlebark, L., Risling, M., Suneson, A., and Ulfendahl, M. (2008). Activation of JNK in the inner ear following impulse noise exposure. *J. Neuro.* 25, 72–77. doi: 10.1089/neu.2007.0346

Nicotera, P., and Orrenius, S. (1992). Ca2+ and cell death. *Ann. N. Y. Acad. Sci.* 648, 17–27.

Ohlemiller, K. K., Wright, J. S., and Dugan, L. L. (1999). Early elevation of cochlear reactive oxygen species following noise exposure. *Audiol. Neurootol.* 4, 229–236. doi: 10.1159/000013846

Orrenius, S., Burkitt, M. J., Kass, G. E., Dypbukt, J. M., and Nicotera, P. (1992a). Calcium ions and oxidative cell injury. *Ann. Neurol.* 32(Suppl.), S33–S42.

Orrenius, S., McCabe, M. J. Jr., and Nicotera, P. (1992b). Ca(2+)-dependent mechanisms of cytotoxicity and programmed cell death. *Toxicol Lett.* 64-65, 357–364. doi: 10.1016/0378-4274(92)90208-2

Puntambekar, P., Mukherjea, D., Jajoo, S., and Ramkumar, V. (2005). Essential role of Rac1/NADPH oxidase in nerve growth factor induction of TRPV1 expression. *J. Neurochem.* 95, 1689–1703. doi: 10.1111/j.1471-4159.2005.03518.x

Ramkumar, V., Whitworth, C. A., Pingle, S. C., Hughes, L. F., and Rybak, L. P. (2004). Noise induces A1 adenosine receptor expression in the chinchilla cochlea. *Hear. Res.* 188, 47–56. doi: 10.1016/s0378-5955(03)00344-7

Razavi, R., Chan, Y., Afifiyan, F. N., Liu, X. J., Wan, X., Yantha, J., et al. (2006). TRPV1+ sensory neurons control beta cell stress and islet inflammation in autoimmune diabetes. *Cell* 127, 1123–1135. doi: 10.1016/j.cell.2006.10.038

Satoh, H., Firestein, G. S., Billings, P. B., Harris, J. P., and Keithley, E. M. (2003). Proinflammatory cytokine expression in the endolymphatic sac during inner ear inflammation. *J. Assoc. Res. Otolaryngol.* 4, 139–147. doi: 10.1007/s10162-002-3025-7

Sheehan, K., Sheth, S., Mukherjea, D., Rybak, L. P., and Ramkumar, V. (2018). Trans "-tympanic drug delivery for the treatment of ototoxicity. *J. Vis. Exp.* 133, e56564. doi: 10.3791/56564

Sinha, K., Das, J., Pal, P. B., and Sil, P. C. (2013). Oxidative stress: the mitochondria-dependent and mitochondria-independent pathways of apoptosis. *Arch. Toxicol.* 87, 1157–1180. doi: 10.1007/s00204-013-1034-4

So, H., Kim, H., Lee, J.-H., Park, C., Kim, Y., Kim, E., et al. (2007). Cisplatin cytotoxicity of auditory cells requires secretions of proinflammatory cytokines via activation of ERK and NF-kappaB. *J. Assoc. Res. Otolaryngol.* 8, 338–355. doi: 10.1007/s10162-007-0084-9

Spicarova, D., and Palecek, J. (2010). Tumor necrosis factor alpha sensitizes spinal cord TRPV1 receptors to the endogenous agonist N-oleoyldopamine. *J Neuroinflamm.* 7:49. doi: 10.1186/1742-2094-7-49

Tan, W. J., Thorne, P. R., and Vlajkovic, S. M. (2016). Characterisation of cochlear inflammation in mice following acute and chronic noise exposure. *Histochem. Cell Biol.* 146, 219–230. doi: 10.1007/s00418-016-1436-5

Thorne, P. R., and Nuttall, A. L. (1987). Laser doppler measurements of cochlear blood flow during loud sound exposure in the guinea pig. *Hear. Res.* 27, 1–10. doi: 10.1016/0378-5955(87)90021-9

Van Wijk, F., Staecker, H., Keithley, E., and Lefebvre, P. P. (2006). Local perfusion of the tumor necrosis factor alpha blocker infliximab to the inner ear improves autoimmune neurosensory hearing loss. *Audiol. Neurootol.* 11, 357–365. doi: 10.1159/000095897

Vass, Z., Nuttall, A. L., Coleman, J. K., and Miller, J. M. (1995). Capsaicin-induced release of substance P increases cochlear blood flow in the guinea pig. *Hear. Res.* 89, 86–92. doi: 10.1016/0378-5955(95)00127-4

Wang, X., Truong, T., Billings, P. B., Harris, J. P., and Keithley, E. M. (2003). Blockage of immune-mediated inner ear damage by etanercept. *Otol. Neurotol.* 24, 52–57. doi: 10.1097/00129492-200301000-00012

Yamane, H., Nakai, Y., Takayama, M., Iguchi, H., Nakagawa, T., and Kojima, A. (1995a). Appearance of free radicals in the guinea pig inner ear after noise-induced acoustic trauma. *Eur. Arch. Otorhinolaryngol.* 252, 504–508. doi: 10.1007/bf02114761

Yamane, H., Nakai, Y., Takayama, M., Konishi, K., Iguchi, H., Nakagawa, T., et al. (1995b). The emergence of free radicals after acoustic trauma and strial blood flow. *Acta Otolaryngol. Suppl.* 519, 87–92. doi: 10.3109/00016489509121877

Yamashita, D., Jiang, H. Y., Le Prell, C. G., Schacht, J., and Miller, J. M. (2005). Post-exposure treatment attenuates noise-induced hearing loss. *Neuroscience* 134, 633–642. doi: 10.1016/j.neuroscience.2005.04.015

Yamashita, D., Jiang, H. Y., Schacht, J., and Miller, J. M. (2004). Delayed production of free radicals following noise exposure. *Brain Res.* 1019, 201–209. doi: 10.1016/j.brainres.2004.05.104

Zou, J., Pyykko, I., Sutinen, P., and Toppila, E. (2005). Vibration induced hearing loss in guinea pig cochlea: expression of TNF-alpha and VEGF. *Hear. Res.* 202, 13–20. doi: 10.1016/j.heares.2004.10.008

9

Delivering Therapeutics to the Cochlea: The Importance of the Patient's Perspective

Marie-Josée Duran[1]* and Ralph Holme[2]

[1] Fondation Pour l'Audition, Paris, France, [2] Action on Hearing Loss, London, United Kingdom

****Correspondence:***
Marie-Josée Duran
mj.duran@pourlaudition.org

Hearing loss represents a major sensory impairment in humans with a strong impact on quality of life. The current standard of care for chronic sensorineural hearing loss is limited to hearing aids and implantable devices like cochlear implants. Treatments for acute hearing loss consist of systemic or intratympanic corticosteroids. Emerging therapies are being developed to prevent hearing loss or to restore it at the cellular level. Many challenges and questions remain as to the delivery of these therapeutics into the inner ear. Scientists, clinicians, and industry stakeholders should always consider the treatment burden from the patient's perspective when designing new drug delivery approaches. This article highlights key issues to consider.

Keywords: drug delivery, systemic, intratympanic, intracochlear, treatment burden, compliance

INTRODUCTION

Worldwide, 466 million individuals suffer from disabling hearing loss and untreated hearing loss is estimated to cost $750bn according to the World Health Organization (WHO) making it a major public health issue (World Health Organization [WHO], 2019). Hearing loss can have a devastating impact on quality of life cutting people off from friends and family leading to isolation and loneliness. Hearing loss is also linked to an increased risk of dementia (Livingston et al., 2017). Besides hearing aids and cochlear implants for chronic hearing loss, and corticosteroids for sudden sensorineural hearing loss (Chandrasekhar et al., 2019), no therapies have been approved by regulatory agencies to prevent or treat hearing loss. Such treatments have the potential to address a growing unmet clinical need and transform the lives of millions of people. The most common form of hearing loss is sensorineural hearing loss, which accounts for 90% of all hearing loss (Cruickshanks et al., 2003). Treating this type of hearing loss will require finding safe and effective methods of delivering drug, gene and cell-based therapies to the inner ear - a complex organ, not easily accessible making it a challenge for drug delivery.

Emerging Therapeutics for Inner Ear Disorders

A recent review of emerging therapies by Schilder et al. (2019) identified 43 biotech and pharmaceutical companies that are, or have been, engaged in developing over 80 different therapies. Over 20 have already reached clinical trials. Most aim to prevent hearing loss caused by exposure to loud noise, medications that are toxic to the ear, such as aminoglycoside antibiotics or cisplatin, or to treat sudden sensorineural hearing loss. A smaller number aim to restore hearing by triggering the regeneration of damaged cell types or correcting genetic causes of hearing loss by gene therapy. Cell therapies to replace damaged inner ear cells are also under development.

The success of these approaches will require the therapeutic to reach its site of action at the right dose, over the right time course and without causing unwanted side effects. Research into developing techniques to efficiently deliver therapeutics into the inner ear is therefore timely and of the upmost importance. It is also vital to consider what patients want and need from new treatments.

Therapeutic Delivery: Considerations From the Patient's Perspective

Systemic

The most desirable treatment from the patient's perspective would be a drug taken orally with no adverse side effects. This will be particularly important for prophylactic treatments targeting age-related hearing loss that may require frequent dosing or for otoprotective drugs designed to be administered before exposure to noise. An oral tablet that can be self-administered would have minimal impact on everyday life and would be the ideal solution for prevention of noise-induced hearing loss amongst military personnel.

Intravenous (IV) delivery of prophylactic treatments may be acceptable to patients if the frequency of dosing is low, for treating acute or sudden onset hearing loss where a patient may be actively seeking medical help, or is already under medical care if being treated with IV aminoglycosides or cisplatin. Regular dosing might require time off work and disruption to everyday life making such treatments less acceptable to patients.

Although systemic delivery of therapeutics to the cochlea is most desirable it may not always be possible. Challenges can include unwanted side effects and, depending on the drug's chemical properties and pharmacokinetics, insufficient amounts crossing the blood-labyrinth barrier and reaching the cochlea (Salt and Plontke, 2018).

Intratympanic

Injection of a therapeutic through the tympanic membrane may overcome some of the challenges faced with systemic delivery of inner ear therapeutics. It may reduce the risk of unwanted side effects and increase the availability of the therapeutic at the side of action, particularly if used in conjunction with polymers to control drug release over a period of time. Although minimally invasive, patients are unlikely to tolerate repeated administration and may become uncompliant. This is because the procedure can be painful, requires patients to take time from their daily activities to visit a clinic and requires them to avoid water entering the ear while the tympanic membrane heals. This could become burdensome. This route of administration is therefore most suited to the treatment of acute forms of hearing loss or the delivery of therapeutics to trigger regeneration of hearing which may be associated with significant improvement in hearing and infrequent administration. Advances in technologies able to reduce the discomfort and pain associated with intratympanic injection could make this approach more acceptable in the future for frequent administration of therapeutics. One such example uses magnetic forces to drive iron nanoparticles that can be linked to a therapeutic into the middle ear and cochlea (Mittal et al., 2019). It is currently in preclinical development. Another way to decrease repeated drug delivery is by prolonging the time the drug is in contact with the round window through the use of hydrogels able to sustain drug release, reviewed by Patel et al. (2019).

Intracochlear

Not all therapeutics injected into the middle ear will reach the cochlea at the required concentration, and for cell and gene therapies direct delivery to cochlea via a cochleostomy maybe the only option. This approach requires surgery under a general anesthesia requiring patients to spend time in hospital and recovering from the surgery. Therefore this approach is unlikely to be acceptable to patients for treatments that need frequent administration or for those that provide only modest improvements in hearing. The approach is also associated with the risk of causing permanent damage to any residual hearing, so is unlikely be acceptable to patients with milder forms of hearing loss. The exception may be people with genetic forms of hearing loss that are predicted to lead to a rapid loss of hearing. Intracochlear administration is therefore most suited to the delivery of "single shot" treatments to restore hearing or correct a genetic fault. Some are considering implantable intracochlear drug delivery devices for regular drug infusions to the inner ear. This alternative could be adopted by patients provided the refill chamber is easily accessible without surgery and the time between refills is acceptable.

Finally, cochlear implants are being designed to deliver drugs to the cochlea. Approaches include coating the electrode in biodegradable eluting polymers or cells to release factors that reduce trauma and promote spiral ganglion survival (Roemer et al., 2016; Scheper et al., 2019). These technologies aim to enhance the benefit gained from cochlear implants, so are likely to be acceptable to patients already undergoing cochlear implant surgery.

CONCLUSION

A new generation of therapeutics is emerging. It is vital that the field develops safe and efficient methods to deliver these to the inner ear. Disruptive technologies requiring expertise from different fields (pharmacology, formulation, engineering...) are needed. A collaborative and international effort promoting such multidisciplinary research recently emerged with the launch of the International Society of Inner Ear Therapeutics (Schilder et al., 2018). This will benefit from patients' input.

Depending on the nature of the treatment and expected outcome, different patient populations are likely to tolerate different levels of risk and invasiveness. It is therefore important to seek the target patient population's view at the early stages of developing a therapeutic to ensure its planned method of delivery is acceptable.

AUTHOR CONTRIBUTIONS

Both authors wrote the manuscript.

REFERENCES

Chandrasekhar, S. S., Tsai Do, B. S., Schwartz, S. R., Bontempo, L. J., Faucett, E. A., Finestone, S. A., et al. (2019). Clinical practice guideline: sudden hearing loss (Update). *Otolaryngol. Head Neck Surg.* 161, S1–S45.

Cruickshanks, K. J., Tweed, T. S., Wiley, T. L., Klein, B. E., Klein, R., Chappell, R., et al. (2003). The 5-year incidence and progression of hearing loss: the epidemiology of hearing loss study. *Arch. Otolaryngol. Head Neck Surg.* 129, 1041–1046.

Livingston, G., Sommerlad, A., Orgeta, V., Costafreda, S. G., Huntley, J., Ames, D., et al. (2017). Dementia prevention, intervention, and care. *Lancet* 390, 2673–2734.

Mittal, R., Pena, S. A., Zhu, A., Eshraghi, N., Fesharaki, A., Horesh, E. J., et al. (2019). Nanoparticle-based drug delivery in the inner ear: current challenges, limitations and opportunities. *Artif. Cells Nanomed. Biotechnol.* 47, 1312–1320. doi: 10.1080/21691401.2019.1573182

Patel, J., Szczupak, M., Rajguru, S., Balaban, C., and Hoffer, M. (2019). Inner ear therapeutics: an overview of middle ear delivery. *Front. Cell Neurosci.* 13:261. doi: 10.3389/fncel.2019.00261

Roemer, A., Köhl, U., Majdani, O., Klöß, S., Falk, C., Haumann, S., et al. (2016). Biohybrid cochlear implants in human neurosensory restoration. *Stem Cell Res. Ther.* 7:148.

Salt, A. N., and Plontke, S. K. (2018). Pharmacokinetic principles in the inner ear: influence of drug properties on intratympanic applications. *Hear Res.* 368, 28–40. doi: 10.1016/j.heares.2018.03.002

Scheper, V., Hoffmann, A., Gepp, M. M., Schulz, A., Hamm, A., Pannier, C., et al. (2019). Stem cell based drug delivery for protection of auditory neurons in a guinea pig model of cochlear implantation. *Front. Cell Neurosci.* 13:177. doi: 10.3389/fncel.2019.00177

Schilder, A. G. M., Blackshaw, H., Lenarz, T., Warnecke, A., Lustig, L. R., and Staecker, H. (2018). Biological therapies of the inner ear: what otologists need to consider. *Otol. Neurotol.* 39, 135–137. doi: 10.1097/mao.0000000000001689

Schilder, A. G. M., Su, M. P., Blackshaw, H., Lustig, L., Staecker, H., Lenarz, T., et al. (2019). Hearing protection, restoration, and regeneration: an overview of emerging therapeutics for inner ear and central hearing disorders. *Otol. Neurotol.* 40, 559–570. doi: 10.1097/MAO.0000000000002194

World Health Organization [WHO] (2019). Available at: http://www.who.int/deafness/en/ (Accessed May 30, 2019).

10

Local Drug Delivery for the Treatment of Neurotology Disorders

Fabrice Piu and Kathie M. Bishop*

Otonomy Inc., San Diego, CA, United States

***Correspondence:**
Fabrice Piu
fpiu@otonomy.com

Neurotology disorders such as vertigo, tinnitus, and hearing loss affect a significant proportion of the population (estimated 39 million in the United States with moderate to severe symptoms). Yet no pharmacological treatments have been developed, in part due to limitations in effective drug delivery to the anatomically protected inner ear compartment. Intratympanic delivery, a minimally invasive injection performed in the office setting, offers a potential direct route of administration. Currently, off-label use of therapeutics approved to treat disorders via systemic administration are being injected intratympanically, mostly in the form of aqueous solutions, but provide variable levels of drug exposure for a limited time requiring repeated injections. Hence, current drug delivery approaches for neurotology disorders are sub-optimal. This review, following a description of pharmacokinetic considerations of the inner ear, explores the merits of novel delivery approaches toward the treatment of neurotology disorders. Methodologies employing local delivery to the inner ear are described, including direct intracochlear delivery as well as intratympanic methods of infusion and injection. Intratympanic injection delivery formulation strategies including hydrogels, polymers and nanoparticulate systems are explored. These approaches represent progress toward more effective delivery options for the clinical treatment of a variety of neurotology disorders.

Keywords: drug delivery, local, inner ear, neurotology disorders, intratympanic administration

INTRODUCTION

Neurotology disorders of the inner ear such as hearing loss, vertigo, and tinnitus affect a large proportion of the population with significant impact on patient's quality of life (National Institute of Health, 2000). It is estimated that, in the United States alone, 1 in 8 individual (or about 39 million) suffers from moderate to severe hearing loss, tinnitus or vertigo (Neitzel et al., 2017). Inner ear disorders of cochlear origin most commonly manifest themselves clinically as hearing loss due to a number of factors such as age-related hearing loss (presbycusis), ototoxicity-related hearing loss (i.e., due to certain classes of chemotherapeutics or antibiotics), noise induced hearing loss (NIHL), sudden sensorineural hearing loss (SSNHL), and genetic forms of hearing loss. The most commonly diagnosed vestibular disorders include benign paroxysmal positional vertigo (BPPV), labyrinthitis or vestibular neuritis. In addition, a confluence of symptoms is evident in disorders such as Meniere's disease where patients experience vertigo, hearing loss, tinnitus, and aural fullness, and tinnitus itself is a debilitating symptom accompanying many forms of hearing loss (D'aldin et al., 1999; Gupta and Sataloff, 2003; Swartz and Longwell, 2005; Harris and Salt, 2007;

Liu and Yan, 2007; Panda et al., 2008; Chan, 2009). The medical management of these disorders has largely focused on systemic delivery of drugs, surgical intervention, device use (e.g., hearing aids and cochlear implants) and behavioral therapy (Barritt, 2008). However, these approaches vary in their effectiveness and thus significant unmet need for the treatment of inner ear disorders exists.

Pharmacologic treatment of inner ear disorders such as hearing loss, tinnitus, and vertigo disorders has been challenging due to poor drug availability to this protected compartment with systemic administration. A shift is occurring toward the implementation of novel technologies and local routes of administration (Barritt, 2008; Swan et al., 2008; Hu and Parnes, 2009; McCall et al., 2009). Primarily, it is the result of the recognition that systemic routes of administration for inner ear therapy are severely limited due to poor drug exposure to the otic compartment due to the blood-labyrinth barrier, and significant risks of undesirable side effects with systemic delivery. This review explores and discusses novel approaches being developed for the therapeutic management of otic disorders. These technologies focus on local delivery directly to the middle ear, via passive absorbption through the round window membrane (intratympanic) or through other minor routes (diffusion through the oval window, bony channels, fissula and fenestrum) to the inner ear, or directly to the inner ear (intracochlear). A special emphasis is given to intratympanic injection, a minimally invasive drug delivery approach, and formulation strategies for intratympanic injection including hydrogels, polymers and nanoparticulate systems because of their convenience of use and potential to deliver therapeutic levels of drug over an extended period of time.

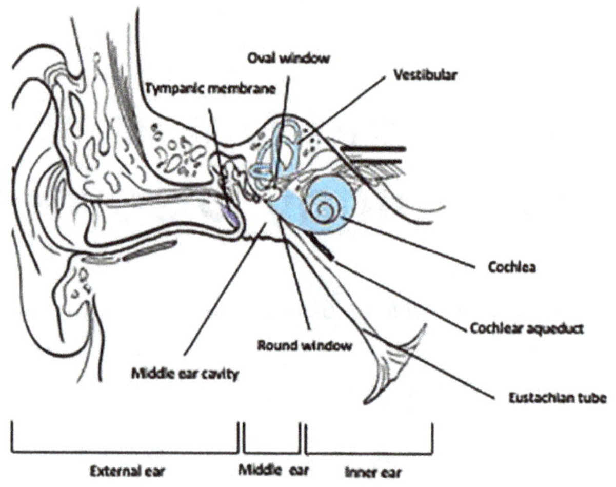

FIGURE 1 | Anatomy of the ear.

TABLE 1 | Pharmacokinetics of the inner ear.

	Systemic delivery	Local delivery
Absorption	Via stria vascularis and blood labyrinth barrier	Via round window, oval window and bony otic capsule
Distribution	Into inner ear fluid spaces, inner ear tissues; driven by passive diffusion	
Metabolism	Via protein binding, enzymatic processes	
Excretion	Via loss to fluid spaces in the cochlea, uptake into intercellular spaces, loss to cochlear bloodstream, loss to the cerebrospinal fluid via the cochlear aqueduct, and to the middle ear via the round window and oval window membranes	

PHARMACOKINETIC CONSIDERATIONS OF THE INNER EAR

The ear, the sensory organ comprising the auditory system (sound processing) and the vestibular system (balance and equilibrium) is anatomically and functionally divided into three regions: the outer ear, middle ear and the inner ear (**Figure 1**). The external ear is the external portion of the organ whose function is to collect and direct sound waves toward the tympanic membrane and the middle ear. The middle ear, an air-filled hollow called the tympanic cavity, is located behind the tympanic membrane and comprised of bony and ligament structures (auditory ossicles and stapes) providing a mechanical linkage between the tympanum and the inner ear for the transmission of sound waves. The inner ear is a fluid-filled compartment and the core organ for auditory signal transduction. It consists of two major compartments: the cochlea where auditory signal processing takes place and the vestibular where balance is modulated. The inner ear is a complex network of fluid-filled tubes known as the bony otic capsule and composed of two compartments with membranous barriers, one filled with perilymph, the other with endolymph. The bony otic capsule is the major anatomic and physiological barrier to inner ear drug delivery. The cochlea comprises a highly specialized structure, the organ of Corti, that contains the mechano-sensory cells of the inner ear (hair cells). Two structures separate the middle ear and the inner ear. The round window membrane (RWM) is a semi permeable membrane composed of three layers: outer epithelial layer facing the middle ear, a middle connective layer, and an inner cellular layer. Its permeability is known to be affected by many factors under normal and pathological conditions (Goycoolea, 1992). The other structure is the oval window, which is covered by the footplate of the stapes in the middle ear.

Because of its anatomical complexity, the pharmacokinetics of the inner ear are multifaceted. The large fluid-filled extracellular spaces that comprise it have multiple interconnections, in addition to interfacing with outside compartments such as the systemic blood circulation, the cerebrospinal fluid, and the middle ear cavity (via the oval and round window membranes). In general, the pharmacokinetic processes in the inner ear follow the established ADME principles but are centered on inner ear fluids rather than blood circulation (**Table 1**; Plontke and Zenner, 2002; Salt and Plontke, 2005, 2009; Salt, 2006).

Absorption of drug substances in the inner ear is largely dependent of the route of administration (**Figure 2**). Following systemic administration, pharmacological agents enter the inner ear via the stria vascularis, an area of capillary loops and small blood vessels located at the upper portion of the cochlear

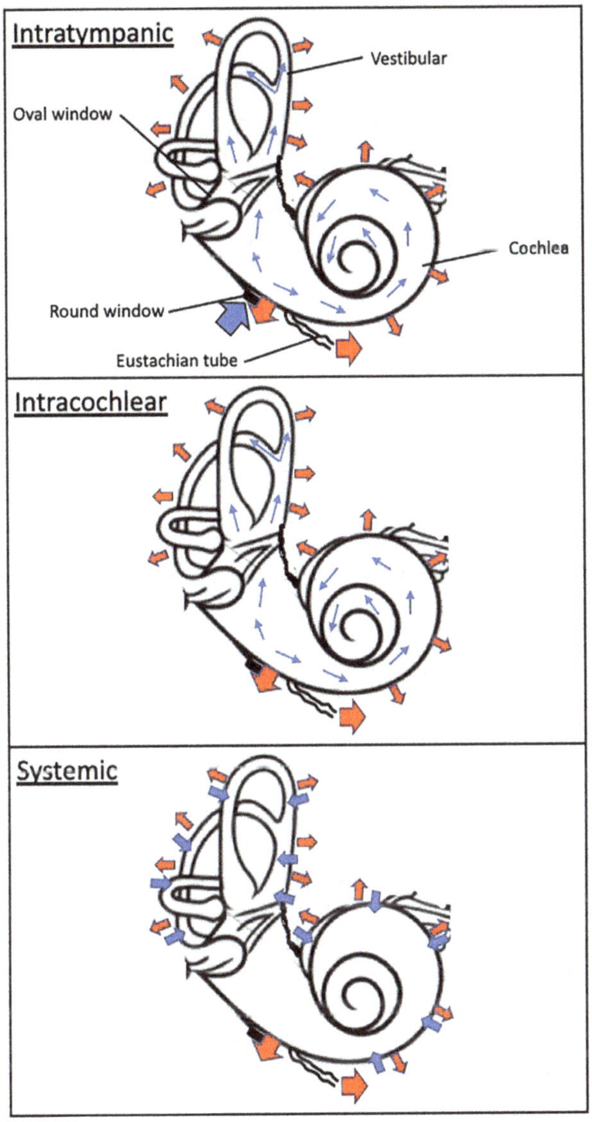

FIGURE 2 | Schematic of drug absorption and elimination following intratympanic, intracochlear, and systemic administration. The wide blue arrows indicate drug absorption to the inner ear compartment, including the cochlea and vestibular. The thin blue arrows denote distribution within the inner drug compartment. The wide red arrows depicts elimination from the otic compartment through (1) the inner ear blood circulatory system which interfaces throughout the cochlea and vestibular apparatus, (2) loss to the cochlear aqueduct and (3) loss to the middle ear. The black disk symbolizes the round window.

spiral ligament. This structure is surrounded by a network of endothelial cells connected via tight junctions, protecting the cochlea from the systemic circulation, and known as the blood-labyrinth barrier (BLB) (Juhn et al., 2001). Experimental studies have demonstrated that the BLB is an effective structure in limiting diffusion from the bloodstream into the cochlea, with rates of entry on average 4–6% of the total plasma concentration (Inamura and Salt, 1992). The BLB exhibits some functional attributes comparable to the blood-brain barrier (BBB), but also some differences. The BLB largely prevents the passage of substances from the blood into the inner ear, is seemingly less permeable to several ions (sodium, calcium, and calcium) than the BBB and differentially modulates the passage of larger substances as a function of the molecular weight compared to the BBB (Juhn et al., 2001). These differences in functionality are ascribed in part to the tight junction composition, permeability enhancers and receptors mediating endocytosis or transcytosis making up the BLB (Nyberg et al., 2019). Hence, the physicochemical properties of systemically administered drug will drive their diffusion across the BLB. As a result, drug exposure to the inner ear following systemic administration is limited and highly variable. For instance, Bird and colleagues noted a large inter-variability spanning three orders of magnitude in perilymph concentrations between human patients after systemic administration of a methylprednisolone aqueous solution (Bird et al., 2007) or a dexamethasone solution (Bird et al., 2011).

In contrast, following intratympanic administration, local absorption from the middle ear takes place via the round window, the oval window and the bony otic capsule. The RWM is considered a primary passage of intratympanic drugs but also a physical barrier to inner ear delivery. The oval window may be a promising delivery route to target the vestibular system and associated disorders. These structures provide access primarily to the cochlea, and through a diffusion process to the vestibular apparatus (Goycoolea, 2001; Imamura and Adams, 2003; Banerjee and Parnes, 2004). The round window membrane (RWM) is the most accessible of these structures; absorption of drugs through the RWM is dependent upon permeability properties and the contact duration of the applied drug substances. For instance, RWM permeability is markedly affected by the presence of additives such as membrane permeation enhancers (Li et al., 2018) and preservatives (Mikulec et al., 2008), certain attributes of the pharmacological agent such as molecular weight (Chelikh et al., 2003) and chemical properties (Salt et al., 2018; Salt and Plontke, 2018). Animal studies as well as computer simulations have demonstrated that prolonging the drug contact duration of aqueous solutions with the round window membrane results in increased drug levels in the inner ear (Plontke and Salt, 2006; Plontke et al., 2007a). Transport across the RWM relies on additional processes such as passive diffusion and active transport. While it has been suggested that the oval window offers an alternate route of absorption to the inner ear, its contribution and impact remain to be ascertained (Tanaka and Motomura, 1981; Takumida and Anniko, 2004). It has been proposed that drug substances could passively diffuse through the thin bone structure of the stapes and the walls of the oval window niche. Drug diffusion to the apex of the cochlea has been demonstrated to be possible in rodents through the bony otic capsule (Mikulec et al., 2008). However, the anatomical differences between rodents and humans, in particular the fact that the human cochlea is largely embedded in the temporal bone, suggest that this route of entry may be is significantly more challenging in humans.

Distribution of drugs in the inner ear is mostly governed by passive diffusion (**Figure 2**). Unlike the circulatory system, the perilymphatic and endolymphatic fluids of the inner ear display extremely slow rates of volume flow (Salt et al., 1986; Ohyama et al., 1988; Salt and Ma, 2001). Because passive diffusion is a non-linear process over distance, gradients along the length of the cochlea are observed when drugs are deposited at the base of the cochlea (round window niche) (Salt et al., 1986; Plontke et al., 2007a). Additionally, drugs passively diffuse into tissues and fluid spaces (Salt et al., 1991a,b). This interscalar distribution contributes to a net loss of drug to the cochlear blood flow the magnitude of which is believed to be significant (Salt and Plontke, 2005). Since the inner ear distribution of substances is primarily driven by concentration gradients, any changes in these gradients will affect drug availability to the local compartment in a process coined "redistribution." Finally, studies of the perilymph suggest that protein binding of acidic and lipophilic drugs could alter drug distribution in the perilymph by trapping pharmacological agents (Swan et al., 2009).

The elimination or clearance of drugs in the inner ear fluids is primarily driven by metabolism, which is dependent upon the nature of the drugs themselves. Building on the initial study by Thalmann et al. (1994), it was recently demonstrated that the perilymphatic compartment contains proteins such as albumin, alpha-1 acid protein, lipoproteins as well as enzymes (Swan et al., 2009). Protein binding to drug substances would protect them from being metabolized rapidly, while serving as drug reservoirs and carriers. To date, only a few studies have investigated the enzymatic processes taking place in inner fluids. Examples illustrate that the prodrug dexamethasone-phosphate is converted into its active moiety dexamethasone (Mikulec et al., 2008), and the activity of purines is modulated by ectonucleosidases (Chelikh et al., 2003). Other clearance mechanisms have been described, including loss to the fluid spaces in the cochlea, uptake into intercellular spaces, loss to the cerebrospinal fluid via the cochlear aqueduct, and to the middle ear via the round window and oval window membranes (Salt and Plontke, 2009).

INNER EAR DRUG DELIVERY

Systemic delivery may seem to be the preferred approach for therapeutic treatment of inner ear disorders because of its convenience. However, systemic routes of administration (such as oral and intravenous) may result in limited therapeutic access to inner ear target structures, with drug levels being several orders of magnitude lower than following local intratympanic administration (Bird et al., 2007, 2011). The protection imparted by blood-labyrinth barrier against the diffusion of substances from the circulatory system into the inner ear, the different metabolic pathways and various routes of excretion, all contribute to a variable fate of the drug in the inner ear, hence possibly resulting in variable clinical outcome (Paulson et al., 2008). Consequently, dosing regimens have aimed at delivering high drug levels systemically in the hope of achieving adequate inner ear therapeutic efficacy, creating potential systemic side effect liabilities.

Because of the limitations of systemic delivery, alternative means to efficiently deliver medications to the inner ear have been explored. Since the initial work by Ersner et al. (1951) and decades later by others (Sakata et al., 1986; Shea and Ge, 1996) demonstrating the clinical potential of locally administered drugs in the ear, there has been a trend in clinical practice to recognize and implement local delivery procedures as a more effective approach (Hu and Parnes, 2009; MCcall et al., 2010).

Comparison of different approaches for drug delivery to the inner ear compartment is summarized in **Table 2**.

Intracochlear Delivery

Intracochlear delivery devices are currently being developed to deliver drugs directly to the inner ear. These are largely modifications of existing technologies such as cochlear implants, osmotic pumps and microperfusion systems surgically implanted into the inner ear. By modifying cochlear implant electrodes and coupling them to an external pump system, Paasche et al. (2006)

TABLE 2 | Comparison of different routes of administration to the inner ear.

	Benefits	Limitations
Systemic	- Non-invasive - Ease of administration	- Limited inner ear exposure due to poor drug absorption across BLB - Large systemic exposure with potential for dose limitation, and associated risks of adverse effects
Intracochlear	- Direct exposure to the inner ear - Prolonged and controlled cochlear drug delivery via perfusion/devices - Limited systemic exposure	- Invasive (surgical procedure required) - Risks of infection of the inner ear - Device performance restrictions
Intratympanic Extracochlear implants	- Significant exposure to the inner ear - Prolonged and controlled drug delivery via perfusion/devices - Limited systemic exposure	- Required drug diffusion across the RWM into inner ear - Moderately invasive (incision of the ear drum) - Risks of persistent ear drum perforation, ear infection - Risks of hearing degradation
Intratympanic Natural polymers Synthetic polymers Nanoparticulates	- Minimally invasive - Significant exposure to the inner ear - Limited systemic exposure	- Required drug diffusion across the RWM into inner ear - Depending on polymer, may require several injections due to limited duration of exposure - Depending on polymer, risks of middle ear inflammation/fibrosis
Intratympanic Poloxamer	- Minimally invasive - Significant and prolonged exposure to the inner ear (weeks to months) following a single administration - Limited systemic exposure	- Required drug diffusion across the RWM into inner ear

demonstrated the possibility of delivering a bioactive molecule directly to the inner ear. The coating of cochlear electrodes with a biopolymer loaded with a bioactive agent has also been investigated and demonstrates encouraging preliminary findings (Hendricks et al., 2008; Richardson et al., 2009).

Controlled delivery devices can offer the benefit of managing the rate and duration of drug release. Advance of these technologies is dependent upon the miniaturization and integration of multiple functions in a single implant. To date, some osmotic pumps have been approved for non-otic medical use, but are of limited benefit because of non-adjustable dosing regimen, limited duration of drug delivery, and no on/off control of the pump's actions (MCcall et al., 2010). Microfluidic systems, on the other hand, incorporate flexibility of programming drug infusion rates. Advances have been made recently in this area leading to the development of a self-contained, programmable device (Chen et al., 2005; Fiering et al., 2009; Sewell et al., 2009; Peppi et al., 2018). Cochlear infusion of a glutamate receptor antagonist in guinea pigs was achieved for 30 days using a microfluidic system (Fiering et al., 2009). More recently, an open label study was conducted in tinnitus patients under a compassionate treatment protocol. The NMDA receptor antagonist gacyclidine was administered intracochlearly via a DurectRWmuCath^{TM} into the round window niche for a period of 3–4 days (Wenzel et al., 2010). Four of the six treated patients demonstrated a transient improvement in their tinnitus perception. Another human study explored the safety of dexamethasone-eluting cochlear implant electrodes, and demonstrated lower impedances in these subjects (Plontke et al., 2016). In general, the most obvious drawback to these technologies is the requirement for surgical implantation and potential for device performance issues once implanted.

Intratympanic Delivery

The interconnections between the cochlea and the vestibular structures enable any pharmacological agent administered intratympanically to potentially reach, via the round window, all of the inner ear substructures. Thus, tractable delivery is possible via intratympanic administration, especially in humans where the inner ear is embedded into the skull near the brainstem, resulting in extreme inaccessibility except via an intratympanic approach.

Implantable Extracochlear Catheters

One of the first attempts at developing a sustained release system for delivery onto the RWM was the MicroWick (Silverstein, 1999). This device consists of a polyvinyl acetate wick (1 mm in diameter by 9 mm in length) applied to the round window niche through a ventilation tube placed in the tympanic membrane (myringotomy). Patients would then self-administer the medication into the external canal. A typical dosing regimen requires multiple daily applications for several weeks. Since its inception, a few studies have been published demonstrating the effectiveness of the Microwick in the treatment of Meniere's disease using gentamicin (Hill et al., 2006; Suryanarayanan et al., 2009), SSNHL using steroids (Herr and Marzo, 2005; Van Wijck et al., 2007) and AIED using a TNFα blocker (Van Wijk et al., 2006). In the Meniere's disease studies, long term vertigo control with gentamicin was observed in the majority of patients at the 24-month follow-up. In the SSNHL studies, significant improvement in hearing (~25 dB) as measured by pure tone average was observed in 8 out of 12 patients. The AIED study reported that the delivery of the TNFα blocker once weekly for 4 weeks resulted in hearing improvement and reduction in disease relapse. However, complications from the Microwick were observed in small fraction of patients (~25%) and consisted of a persistent perforation of the tympanum, ear infection, the development of fibrosis in the middle ear, and hearing degradation (Herr and Marzo, 2005; Suryanarayanan et al., 2009).

Round window microcatheters, such as μ-Cath and e-Cath, consist of several lumens: a first one for drug administration, a second one for middle ear fluid drainage, and sometimes a third one incorporating an electrode to monitor ear signals (MCcall et al., 2010). Implantable catheters are anchored in the round window bony niche and protrude through the tympanic membrane into the external ear canal. Drug is usually administered using a microperfusion pump device, which ensures continuous drug delivery at a constant flow rate over a period of several weeks. Several clinical studies using microcatheters in the treatment of Meniere's disease (Schoendorf et al., 2001; Plontke et al., 2009) and SSNHL (Kopke et al., 2001; Lefebvre and Staecker, 2002; Herr and Marzo, 2005; Plontke et al., 2005, 2006) have been published, almost exclusively with steroids. Two non-randomized pilot studies delivered steroids to SSNHL patients who failed oral steroids; improvements in hearing and speech discrimination were observed in a majority of patients. A randomized placebo control study of similar design demonstrated a tendency toward better hearing in the treatment group, but did not reach statistical significance. Overall, success in clinical outcome has been variable but noted improvements in clinical endpoints were seen for the majority of the patients. Similarly to the Microwick, implantable catheters can be associated with catheter dislocation and/or obstruction, persistent tympanic perforation and ear infection (Plontke et al., 2005).

Intratympanic Injection

Current intratympanic injection approaches focus on the off-label use of approved drug formulations that were initially formulated and developed for intravenous administration. An empirical approach has been employed to define the dose selection and dosing schedule in the off-label clinical use of these drugs for inner ear therapy. For instance, corticosteroids have been widely used in the treatment of Meniere's disease (Silverstein et al., 1998, 2009; Araujo et al., 2005; Garduno-Anaya et al., 2005; Kitahara et al., 2008a) and SSNHL (Chandrasekhar, 2001; Kopke et al., 2001; Xenellis et al., 2006; Battaglia et al., 2008; Plontke et al., 2009) Dosing schedules and regimen vary considerably between clinicians, with the total dose received differing by more than two orders of magnitude and with intratympanic injections given as often as once daily for 10 consecutive days (Peng et al., 2008) or as rarely as a single injection (Haynes et al., 2007). Furthermore, patients are asked to remain in a supine position for up to an hour and counseled not to swallow, as these behaviors can lead to rapid elimination of solution out of the middle ear via the Eustachian tube. The confluence of these variables is an important factor in the reported variability in clinical outcomes observed among patients in these studies. Bird and colleagues noted a large inter-variability in perilymph concentrations between patients after intratympanic administration of a methylprednisolone (Bird et al., 2007) or a dexamethasone (Bird et al., 2011) solution, providing a rationale for the reported variable clinical successes. Several factors can positively influence the clinical outcome. More than the absolute dose given at each administration or the total cumulative dose, the number of injections and the interval between them emerge as better predictors of a positive clinical outcome. These findings appear to be valid across drug classes (dexamethasone, methylprednisolone) and disease modalities (MD, SSNHL). Therefore, a more effective approach resides in developing delivery systems that prolong the drug exposure in the inner ear compartment. In addition, such systems might minimize the risks associated with multiple intratympanic injections over a short period of time, including perforation of the tympanic membrane, ear infection and otorrhea.

NOVEL FORMULATIONS FOR INNER EAR DELIVERY

The intratympanic delivery strategies discussed above underscores the need for developing more effective delivery systems that prolong the drug exposure in the inner ear compartment following a single administration, primarily by overcoming delivery barriers and improving drug retention. Such systems typically rely on the use of various classes of polymers to temporally modulate drug release. In addition, these approaches might minimize the risks associated with multiple intratympanic injections over a short period of time, including perforation of the tympanic membrane, ear infection and otorrhea. A summary of novel formulations for inner ear delivery that have entered clinical development is presented in **Table 3**.

Natural and Synthetic Polymers

Polymers are macromolecular networks that can serve as controlled release drug delivery vehicles. These systems have been developed for a number of therapeutic applications, and recently their potential for local delivery to the inner ear has been investigated [reviewed in Wise and Gillespie (2012), Liu et al. (2013), El Kechai et al. (2015)].

The mechanism of drug absorption and release can vary substantially between the different classes of polymers (Van Tomme et al., 2008). Gelatin, a natural polymer, can be modified to present a negatively or positively charged profile, therefore allowing the binding of drugs through polyion complexation. Hyaluronic acid, another natural polymer of anionic charge, can also serve as a drug carrier. Drug release from these classes of polymers occurs via enzymatic hydrolysis of the polymer (Nakagawa and Ito, 2007). In contrast, with other biopolymers such as alginate and chitosan, drugs are released through diffusion out of the matrix. The use of synthetic polymers can confer additional benefits, especially in-situ gelling properties. A biological trigger, such as temperature or pH, would ensure the self-assembly of the matrix, that is the transition from a solution to a gel form. In some instances, this process can be reversible such as with triblock copolymers including poloxamer 407 (Dumortier et al., 2006). Other polymers such as poly(lactic-co-glycolic acid) or PLGA are organized as nanoparticles, that release drug into intracellular compartments following an endocytic absorption process (Xu et al., 2009).

Gelatin, in the form of Gelfoam, has been administered to the middle ear of both laboratory animals (Endo et al., 2005; Iwai et al., 2006; Lee et al., 2007; Inaoka et al., 2009) and humans (Arriaga and Goldman, 1998; Kitahara et al., 2008b; Nakagawa et al., 2014). Because the isoelectric point of gelatin can be engineered to create a positively or negatively charged polymer, it is a potentially useful carrier for proteins and nucleic acids. Growth factors such as BDNF, IGF-1 and HGF delivered to the inner ear in gelatin hydrogels showed detectable levels in the perilymph for up to 1 week and were effective in improving hearing in an animal model of NIHL (Iwai et al., 2006; Inaoka et al., 2009). Open-label clinical studies of Gelfoam dexamethasone in patients with Meniere's disease showed inconsistent results with one study finding limited benefits (Arriaga and Goldman, 1998) and a second reporting long-term hearing improvement as measured by pure tone average and speech discrimination (Kitahara et al., 2008b). Histological assessments in animals have noted the significant

TABLE 3 | Novel formulations for intratympanic delivery that have entered clinical development.

Drug	Active pharmaceutical ingredient	Therapeutic class	Indication	Drug delivery system	Clinical status
OTIPRIO	Ciprofloxacin	Antibacterial	Otitis media with effusion undergoing tympanostomy tube placement Acute otitis externa	Poloxamer	FDA approved
OTIVIDEX	Dexamethasone	Steroid	Vertigo associated with Meniere's disease	Poloxamer	Phase III
AM-101	S-Ketamine	NMDA antagonist	Tinnitus	Hyaluronic acid	Phase III
AM-111	D-JNKI-1	JNK inhibitor	Hearing loss	Hyaluronic acid	Phase III
FX-322	Progenitor Cell Activation	Several	Hearing loss	Poloxamer	Phase I/II
OTO-311	Gacyclidine	NMDA antagonist	Tinnitus	Poloxamer	Phase I

ototoxic liability of gelatin hydrogels, especially the presence of a severe acute inflammatory response and the development of fibrosis in the middle ear, but the toxic findings did not extend to the cochlear and vestibular structures (Sheppard et al., 2004; Kitahara et al., 2008b).

Several classes of drugs have been loaded into hyaluronate polymers, including dexamethasone, S-ketamine, gentamicin, and kinase inhibitors which have been investigated in animal models of hearing loss and tinnitus (Yildirim et al., 2005; Barkdull et al., 2007; Coleman et al., 2007; James et al., 2008). Unlike Gelfoam, hyaluronate polymers appear safe to use and are not associated with persistent middle ear inflammation nor fibrosis but only provide a few days of exposure (Kelly et al., 1999).

Hyaluronic acid (Healon) delivery of dexamethasone has been evaluated in several small, open-label clinical studies of Meniere's disease (Shea and Ge, 1996; Shea, 1997; Silverstein et al., 1998; Selivanova et al., 2005) and SSNHL (Gouveris et al., 2005; Stenner et al., 2006) patients with positive benefits reported. A randomized placebo-controlled Phase II clinical study reported on the safety and efficacy of AM-101 (S-Ketamine in hyaluronic acid) in acute tinnitus patients (van de Heyning et al., 2014). AM-101 was administered as three intratympanic injections over the course of 3 days and resulted in improvement in some tinnitus measures (loudness, annoyance) in a subset of tinnitus patients; however, these results were not replicated in Phase III studies[1]. The dosing regimen used in these clinical study highlights the limited prolonged exposure benefit of such a delivery approach. AM-111 (D-JNK inhibitor peptide in hyaluronic acid) is being developed for the treatment of SSNHL. Preclinical studies have demonstrated the activity of AM-111 in various models of otoprotection (Eshraghi et al., 2018). The current clinical experience demonstrated in a randomized placebo-controlled Phase II study improvements in hearing and speech in a subpopulation of patients with severe to profound acute SSNHL, but not in the overall study population (mild to profound acute SNHL) (Suckfuell et al., 2014).

There are only a few published pre-clinical studies and no clinical studies evaluating alginate and chitosan matrices in otologic conditions. Both polymers appear to only yield a few days of drug exposure in the inner ear, typically less than a week. Alginate can be tailored to deliver a variety of substances from small molecules to proteins to cells (Tonnesen and Karlsen, 2002). Noushi et al. (2005) reported administration of alginate beads to the middle ear of guinea pigs does not produce signification tissue inflammation or fibrosis. Chitosan polymers can also accommodate various biological materials, because of the positively charged nature of the matrix. Its drug sustained release properties can be tailored primarily by altering the sensitivity to lysozyme degradation. The only animal study describing the drug release profile of chitosan polymers indicated a short period of drug exposure in the inner ear of mice, of 3 to 5 days (Paulson et al., 2008). Chitosan polymers were not found to be associated with toxicity in the inner ear of guinea pigs (Saber et al., 2009).

[1]https://ir.aurismedical.com/news-releases/news-release-details/auris-medical-provides-business-update, press release March 13, 2018.

Nanoparticulate Systems

Nanoparticulate systems ranging from silica-based materials to liposomes and nanogels (Pyykko et al., 2016) represent an additional approach to otic formulation of drugs. PLGA nanoparticles can encapsulate bioactive molecules of various physicochemical properties (Bala et al., 2004; Nakagawa and Ito, 2007). Drug delivery to the cochlea using PLGA has been investigated in guinea pigs (Tamura et al., 2005), where deposition in the middle ear allowed delivery of rhodamine to the cochlea within 10 min of administration and present for the duration of the study (2 h). Similar findings were made in chinchillas following application of PLGA encapsulated iron oxide nanoparticles (40 min post-application) (Ge et al., 2007). Lidocaine loaded PLGA particles provided sustained release into the inner ear of guinea pigs for a short period of approximately 3 days (Horie et al., 2010) with no significant inflammation of the middle ear mucosa. The use of nanoparticle systems for delivery of growth factors has recently been explored – Nerve Growth Factor conjugated to lipid-based crystalline nanoparticles (Bu et al., 2015) applied to the RWM of guinea pigs resulted in exposure to the inner ear, but lasting only several hours. To date, no nanoparticulate systems have been evaluated clinically for otic delivery.

Poloxamer-Based Polymers

Poloxamers, a group of triblock copolymers, are a particularly versatile class of polymer for inner ear delivery. They differ largely from other classes of polymers due to their amphiphilic nature, unique self-assembly properties, thermoreversible attributes and versatility of composition which make poloxamers amenable to broad applications (Bodratti and Alexandridis, 2018). Poloxamers consist of ethylene oxide and propylene oxide blocks arranged in a tripartite PEO-PPO-PEO configuration (Van Tomme et al., 2008). These copolymers display amphiphilic properties which are highly dependent upon the number of PEO and PPO units. The size, lipophilicity and hydrophilicity properties of poloxamers can be widely tailored.

Poloxamers exhibit thermoreversible and mucoadhesive properties, which make them particularly suitable for intratympanic inner ear drug delivery. Above the critical gelation concentration, PEO-PPO-PEO polymers exhibit a temperature dependent transition from a solution to a gel state in water. The transition temperature is determined by the copolymer composition, especially the ratio of PPO to PEO and the molecular weight of the polymer and thus can be set at body temperature. Further, poloxamers share bioadhesive characteristics that can be enhanced by the addition of various solvents and ionic agents. The bioadhesiveness typically increases as a function of gel strength and is associated with increased residence time.

Poloxamers are effective drug delivery vehicles for bioactive substances in the inner ear, ranging from small molecules to large proteins. In preclinical studies, dexamethasone levels in the inner ear are sustained for several weeks following a single intratympanic administration of OTIVIDEX (OTO-104, a micronized dexamethasone loaded P407 hydrogel formulation)

(Wang et al., 2009; Piu et al., 2011). Similarly, a poloxamer formulation of the steroid triamcinolone acetonide yielded inner ear drug levels for at least 10 days (Honeder et al., 2014). Lee et al. (2004) reported that intratympanic administration of a poloxamer-based formulation of the antibiotic vancomycin successfully addressed MRSA infection in chronic otitis media. The pharmacokinetic profile can be altered by changing the nature and composition of the formulation, especially when non-aqueous soluble forms of a drug substance are used: insoluble forms of both dexamethasone and methylprednisolone, when formulated in a P407 hydrogel, yield significantly longer exposure in the inner ear than aqueous soluble forms (Wang et al., 2011). In all, an intricate interrelation exists between the pharmaceutical agent and the poloxamer copolymer. By modifying various parameters specific to the poloxamer hydrogel and bioactive molecule, a tailored drug release profile from a few days to several months can be developed, with a more homogenous basal-apical concentration gradient (Plontke et al., 2007b), relative to aqueous solutions. The addition of poloxamer to a PLGA-PEG-PLGA copolymer increased the inner ear exposure to the antiviral agent cidofovir while maintaining the absence of ototoxicity (Feng et al., 2014). Finally, poloxamers are listed on the FDA's Generally Regarded As Safe (GRAS) list, and their administration is deemed safe in humans (Singh-Joy and McLain, 2008). While poloxamers are not biodegradable, their administration in the middle ear results in their rapid disappearance from that compartment within a couple of weeks, the elimination being a function of the poloxamer concentration (Engmer Berglin et al., 2015). In conditions where the middle ear was filled, intratympanic administration of poloxamer, but also other polymers, was associated with transient conductive hearing loss, consistent with the high viscosity of the polymers (Engmer Berglin et al., 2015). However, no evidence of toxicity was noted in the middle ear, cochlear and vestibular structures in preclinical studies when the dosing volume covered only the round window niche (Wang et al., 2011).

Poloxamer-based delivery systems have been evaluated in several neurotology clinical trials. OTIVIDEX (OTO-104, a micronized dexamethasone loaded P407 hydrogel formulation) is currently being developed for the treatment of Meniere's disease. Findings from Phase 2 and 3 clinical studies reported that OTIVIDEX was well tolerated with no safety concerns identified (Lambert et al., 2012, 2016). A Phase 1 study conducted in healthy volunteers reported that OTO-311, a P407 based formulation of the non-competitive N-methyl-D-aspartate (NMDA) receptor antagonist gacyclidine being developed for the treatment of tinnitus, was well tolerated with no safety concerns identified (Anderson et al., 2019). Another poloxamer-based hydrogel formulation FX-322, a combinational therapy dubbed PCA (Progenitor Cell Activation), was evaluated in a Phase 1 clinical trial in adult patients with stable sensorineural loss scheduled for cochlear implantation[2]. The investigators reported that FX-322 was well tolerated with no drug related adverse events[3]. More recently a Phase 1/2 study of FX-322 in the same patient population completed enrollment[4], but to date no results have been reported. Finally, only a single poloxamer-based delivery system has been approved for otic delivery: OTIPRIO® (an otic suspension of the fluoroquinolone antibacterial ciprofloxacin in poloxamer 407) is approved for two indications: (1) treatment of pediatric patients with bilateral otitis media with effusion undergoing tympanostomy tube placement and (2) acute otitis externa (Mair et al., 2015, 2016; Park et al., 2016; Dohar et al., 2018).

CONCLUSION

Means to efficiently and reliably deliver therapeutic drugs to the inner ear compartment are being developed, with local delivery approaches now largely favored. In particular, a procedure that has been gaining acceptance in the physician's practice is intratympanic injection. Combining intratympanic administration with the use of otic-specific formulations provides an effective approach to deliver reliable and sustained therapeutic levels to the inner ear. This approach has been tested in a number of neurotology clinical trials and several drugs employing this method are under development for the treatment of neurotology disorders.

AUTHOR CONTRIBUTIONS

Both authors contributed to the conception and designed the manuscript, revised the manuscript, read and approved the submitted version of the manuscript. FP wrote the first draft of the manuscript.

REFERENCES

Anderson, J., Hou, J., Wang, X., Fernandez, R., Tsikovskaia, N., and Piu, F. (2019). "Clinical development of intratympanic sustained exposure formulation of the NMDA receptor antagonist gacyclidine for the treatment of tinnitus," in *Proceedings of the 42nd Annual MidWinter Meeting - Association for Research in Otolaryngology*, Baltimore, MD.

Araujo, M. F., Oliveira, C. A., and Bahmad, F. M. (2005). Intratympanic dexamethasone injections as a treatment for severe, disabling tinnitus: Does it work? *Arch. Otolaryngol. Head Neck Surg.* 131, 113–117.

Arriaga, M. A., and Goldman, S. (1998). Hearing results of intratympanic steroid treatment of endolymphatic hydrops. *Laryngoscope* 108, 1682–1685.

Bala, I., Hariharan, S., and Kumar, M. N. (2004). PLGA nanoparticles in drug delivery: the state of the art. *Crit. Rev. Ther. Drug Carrier Syst.* 21, 387–422.

Banerjee, A., and Parnes, L. S. (2004). The biology of intratympanic drug administration and pharmacodynamics of round window drug absorption. *Otolaryngol. Clin. North Am.* 37, 1035–1051.

Barkdull, G. C., Hondarrague, Y., Meyer, T., Harris, J. P., and Keithley, E. M. (2007). AM-111 reduces hearing loss in a guinea pig model of acute labyrinthitis. *Laryngoscope* 117, 2174–2182. doi: 10.1097/MLG.0b013e3181461f92

Barritt, L. (2008). Meniere's disease. *XPharm* 3, 1–6.

Battaglia, A., Burchette, R., and Cueva, R. (2008). Combination therapy (intratympanic dexamethasone + high-dose prednisone taper) for the treatment of idiopathic sudden sensorineural hearing loss. *Otol. Neurotol.* 29, 453–460. doi: 10.1097/MAO.0b013e318168da7a

Bird, P. A., Begg, E. J., Zhang, M., Keast, A. T., Murray, D. P., and Balkany, T. J. (2007). Intratympanic versus intravenous delivery of methylprednisolone to cochlear perilymph. *Otol. Neurotol.* 28, 1124–1130.

Bird, P. A., Murray, D. P., Zhang, M., and Begg, E. J. (2011). Intratympanic versus intravenous delivery of dexamethasone and dexamethasone sodium phosphate to cochlear perilymph. *Otol. Neurotol.* 32, 933–936. doi: 10.1097/MAO.0b013e3182255933

Bodratti, A. M., and Alexandridis, P. (2018). Formulation of poloxamers for drug delivery. *J. Funct. Biomater.* 9:E11. doi: 10.3390/jfb9010011

Bu, M., Tang, J., Wei, Y., Sun, Y., Wang, X., Wu, L., et al. (2015). Enhanced bioavailability of nerve growth factor with phytantriol lipid-based crystalline nanoparticles in cochlea. *Int. J. Nanomedicine* 10, 6879–6889. doi: 10.2147/IJN.S82944

Chan, Y. (2009). Tinnitus: ediology, classification, characteristics, and treatment. *Discov. Med.* 8, 133–136.

Chandrasekhar, S. S. (2001). Intratympanic dexamethasone for sudden sensorineural hearing loss: clinical and laboratory evaluation. *Otol. Neurotol.* 22, 18–23.

Chelikh, L., Teixeira, M., Martin, C., Sterkers, O., Ferrary, E., and Couloigner, V. (2003). High variability of perilymphatic entry of neutral molecules through the round window. *Acta Otolaryngol.* 123, 199–202.

Chen, Z., Kujawa, S. G., Mckenna, M. J., Fiering, J. O., Mescher, M. J., Borenstein, J. T., et al. (2005). Inner ear drug delivery via a reciprocating perfusion system in the guinea pig. *J. Control Release* 110, 1–19.

Coleman, J. K., Littlesunday, C., Jackson, R., and Meyer, T. (2007). AM-111 protects against permanent hearing loss from impulse noise trauma. *Hear. Res.* 226, 70–78.

D'aldin, C., Cherny, L., Devriere, F., and Dancer, A. (1999). Treatment of acoustic trauma. *Ann. N. Y. Acad. Sci.* 884, 328–344.

Dohar, J. E., Don, D., Koempel, J., Lu, C. H., Hakanson, D., and Chan, K. H. (2018). Safety and efficacy of intratympanic ciprofloxacin otic suspension post-tubes in a real-world pediatric population. *Am. J. Otolaryngol.* 39, 101–106. doi: 10.1016/j.amjoto.2017.12.016

Dumortier, G., Grossiord, J. L., Agnely, F., and Chaumeil, J. C. (2006). A review of poloxamer 407 pharmaceutical and pharmacological characteristics. *Pharm. Res.* 23, 2709–2728.

El Kechai, N., Agnely, F., Mamelle, E., Nguyen, Y., Ferrary, E., and Bochot, A. (2015). Recent advances in local drug delivery to the inner ear. *Int. J. Pharm.* 494, 83–101. doi: 10.1016/j.ijpharm.2015.08.015

Endo, T., Nakagawa, T., Kita, T., Iguchi, F., Kim, T. S., Tamura, T., et al. (2005). Novel strategy for treatment of inner ears using a biodegradable gel. *Laryngoscope* 115, 2016–2020.

Engmer Berglin, C., Videhult Pierre, P., Ekborn, A., Bramer, T., Edsman, K., Hultcrantz, M., et al. (2015). Local treatment of the inner ear: a study of three different polymers aimed for middle ear administration. *Acta Otolaryngol.* 135, 985–994. doi: 10.3109/00016489.2015.1058534

Ersner, M. S., Spiegel, E. A., and Alexander, M. H. (1951). Transtympanic injection of anesthetics for the treatment of Meniere's syndrome. *AMA Arch. Otolaryngol.* 54, 43–52.

Eshraghi, A. A., Aranke, M., Salvi, R., Ding, D., Coleman, J. K. M., Ocak, E., et al. (2018). Preclinical and clinical otoprotective applications of cell-penetrating peptide D-JNKI-1 (AM-111). *Hear. Res.* 368, 86–91. doi: 10.1016/j.heares.2018.03.003

Feng, L., Ward, J. A., Li, S. K., Tolia, G., Hao, J., and Choo, D. I. (2014). Assessment of PLGA-PEG-PLGA copolymer hydrogel for sustained drug delivery in the ear. *Curr. Drug Deliv.* 11, 279–286.

Fiering, J., Mescher, M. J., Leary Swan, E. E., Holmboe, M. E., Murphy, B. A., Chen, Z., et al. (2009). Local drug delivery with a self-contained, programmable, microfluidic system. *Biomed. Microdevices* 11, 571–578. doi: 10.1007/s10544-008-9265-5

Garduno-Anaya, M. A., Couthino De Toledo, H., Hinojosa-Gonzalez, R., Pane-Pianese, C., and Rios-Castaneda, L. C. (2005). Dexamethasone inner ear perfusion by intratympanic injection in unilateral Meniere's disease: a two-year prospective, placebo-controlled, double-blind, randomized trial. *Otolaryngol. Head Neck Surg.* 133, 285–294.

Ge, X., Jackson, R. L., Liu, J., Harper, E. A., Hoffer, M. E., Wassel, R. A., et al. (2007). Distribution of PLGA nanoparticles in chinchilla cochleae. *Otolaryngol. Head Neck Surg.* 137, 619–623.

Gouveris, H., Selivanova, O., and Mann, W. (2005). Intratympanic dexamethasone with hyaluronic acid in the treatment of idiopathic sudden sensorineural hearing loss after failure of intravenous steroid and vasoactive therapy. *Eur. Arch. Otorhinolaryngol.* 262, 131–134.

Goycoolea, M. V. (1992). The round window membrane under normal and pathological conditions. *Acta Otolaryngol. Suppl.* 493, 43–55.

Goycoolea, M. V. (2001). Clinical aspects of round window membrane permeability under normal and pathological conditions. *Acta Otolaryngol.* 121, 437–447.

Gupta, R., and Sataloff, R. T. (2003). Noise-induced autoimmune sensorineural hearing loss. *Ann. Otol. Rhinol. Laryngol.* 112, 569–573.

Harris, J. P., and Salt, A. N. (2007). "Meniere's disease," in *Handbook of the Senses*, ed. P. Dallos (Cambridge, MA: Academic Press).

Haynes, D. S., O'malley, M., Cohen, S., Watford, K., and Labadie, R. F. (2007). Intratympanic dexamethasone for sudden sensorineural hearing loss after failure of systemic therapy. *Laryngoscope* 117, 3–15.

Hendricks, J. L., Chikar, J. A., Crumling, M. A., Raphael, Y., and Martin, D. C. (2008). Localized cell and drug delivery for auditory prostheses. *Hear. Res.* 242, 117–131. doi: 10.1016/j.heares.2008.06.003

Herr, B. D., and Marzo, S. J. (2005). Intratympanic steroid perfusion for refractory sudden sensorineural hearing loss. *Otolaryngol. Head Neck Surg.* 132, 527–531.

Hill, S. L. III, Digges, E. N., and Silverstein, H. (2006). Long-term follow-up after gentamicin application via the Silverstein MicroWick in the treatment of Meniere's disease. *Ear Nose Throat J.* 85:494.

Honeder, C., Engleder, E., Schopper, H., Gabor, F., Reznicek, G., Wagenblast, J., et al. (2014). Sustained Release of Triamcinolone Acetonide from an Intratympanically Applied Hydrogel Designed for the Delivery of High Glucocorticoid Doses. *Audiol. Neurootol.* 19, 193–202. doi: 10.1159/000358165

Horie, R. T., Sakamoto, T., Nakagawa, T., Tabata, Y., Okamura, N., Tomiyama, N., et al. (2010). Sustained delivery of lidocaine into the cochlea using poly lactic/glycolic acid microparticles. *Laryngoscope* 120, 377–383. doi: 10.1002/lary.20713

Hu, A., and Parnes, L. S. (2009). Intratympanic Steroids for Inner Ear Disorders: A Review. *Audiol. Neurootol.* 14, 373–382. doi: 10.1159/000241894

Imamura, S., and Adams, J. C. (2003). Distribution of gentamicin in the guinea pig inner ear after local or systemic application. *J. Assoc. Res. Otolaryngol.* 4, 176–195.

Inamura, N., and Salt, A. N. (1992). Permeability changes of the blood-labyrinth barrier measured in vivo during experimental treatments. *Hear. Res.* 61, 12–18.

Inaoka, T., Nakagawa, T., Kikkawa, Y. S., Tabata, Y., Ono, K., Yoshida, M., et al. (2009). Local application of hepatocyte growth factor using gelatin hydrogels attenuates noise-induced hearing loss in guinea pigs. *Acta Otolaryngol.* 129, 453–457. doi: 10.1080/00016480902725197

Iwai, K., Nakagawa, T., Endo, T., Matsuoka, Y., Kita, T., Kim, T. S., et al. (2006). Cochlear protection by local insulin-like growth factor-1 application using biodegradable hydrogel. *Laryngoscope* 116, 529–533.

James, D. P., Eastwood, H., Richardson, R. T., and O'leary, S. J. (2008). Effects of round window dexamethasone on residual hearing in a Guinea pig model of cochlear implantation. *Audiol. Neurootol.* 13, 86–96.

Juhn, S. K., Hunter, B. A., and Odland, R. M. (2001). Blood-labyrinth barrier and fluid dynamics of the inner ear. *Int. Tinnitus J.* 7, 72–83.

Kelly, R. M., Meyer, J. D., Matsuura, J. E., Shefter, E., Hart, M. J., Malone, D. J., et al. (1999). In vitro release kinetics of gentamycin from a sodium hyaluronate gel delivery system suitable for the treatment of peripheral vestibular disease. *Drug Dev. Ind. Pharm.* 25, 15–20.

Kitahara, T., Doi, K., Maekawa, C., Kizawa, K., Horii, A., Kubo, T., et al. (2008a). Meniere's attacks occur in the inner ear with excessive vasopressin type-2 receptors. *J. Neuroendocrinol.* 20, 1295–1300. doi: 10.1111/j.1365-2826.2008.01792.x

Kitahara, T., Kubo, T., Okumura, S., and Kitahara, M. (2008b). Effects of endolymphatic sac drainage with steroids for intractable Meniere's disease: a long-term follow-up and randomized controlled study. *Laryngoscope* 118, 854–861. doi: 10.1097/MLG.0b013e3181651c4a

Kopke, R. D., Hoffer, M. E., Wester, D., O'leary, M. J., and Jackson, R. L. (2001). Targeted topical steroid therapy in sudden sensorineural hearing loss. *Otol. Neurotol.* 22, 475–479.

Lambert, P. R., Carey, J., Mikulec, A. A., Lebel, C., and Otonomy Meniere's Study Group (2016). Intratympanic sustained-exposure dexamethasone thermosensitive gel for symptoms of Meniere's disease: randomized phase 2b safety and efficacy trial. *Otol. Neurotol.* 37, 1669–1676.

Lambert, P. R., Nguyen, S., Maxwell, K. S., Tucci, D. L., Lustig, L. R., Fletcher, M., et al. (2012). A randomized, double-blind, placebo-controlled clinical study to assess safety and clinical activity of OTO-104 given as a single intratympanic injection in patients with unilateral Meniere's disease. *Otol. Neurotol.* 33, 1257–1265. doi: 10.1097/MAO.0b013e318263d35d

Lee, K. Y., Nakagawa, T., Okano, T., Hori, R., Ono, K., Tabata, Y., et al. (2007). Novel therapy for hearing loss: delivery of insulin-like growth factor 1 to the cochlea using gelatin hydrogel. *Otol. Neurotol.* 28, 976–981.

Lee, S. H., Lee, J. E., Baek, W. Y., and Lim, J. O. (2004). Regional delivery of vancomycin using pluronic F-127 to inhibit methicillin resistant Staphylococcus aureus (MRSA) growth in chronic otitis media in vitro and in vivo. *J. Control Release* 96, 1–7.

Lefebvre, P. P., and Staecker, H. (2002). Steroid perfusion of the inner ear for sudden sensorineural hearing loss after failure of conventional therapy: a pilot study. *Acta Otolaryngol.* 122, 698–702.

Li, W., Hartsock, J. J., Dai, C., and Salt, A. N. (2018). Permeation enhancers for intratympanically-applied drugs studied using fluorescent dexamethasone as a marker. *Otol. Neurotol.* 39, 639–647. doi: 10.1097/MAO.0000000000001786

Liu, H., Hao, J., and Li, K. S. (2013). Current strategies for drug delivery to the inner ear. *Acta Pharm. Sin. B* 3, 86–96.

Liu, X. Z., and Yan, D. (2007). Ageing and hearing loss. *J. Pathol.* 211, 188–197.

Mair, E. A., Moss, J. R., Dohar, J. E., Antonelli, P. J., Bear, M., and Lebel, C. (2015). Randomized clinical trial of a sustained-exposure ciprofloxacin for intratympanic injection during tympanostomy tube surgery. *Ann. Otol. Rhinol. Laryngol.* 125, 105–114. doi: 10.1177/0003489415599001

Mair, E. A., Park, A. H., Don, D., Koempel, J., Bear, M., and Lebel, C. (2016). Safety and efficacy of intratympanic ciprofloxacin otic suspension in children with middle ear effusion undergoing tympanostomy tube placement: two randomized clinical trials. *JAMA Otolaryngol. Head Neck Surg.* 142, 444–451. doi: 10.1001/jamaoto.2016.0001

McCall, A. A., Swan, E. E., Borenstein, J. T., Sewell, W. F., Kujawa, S. G., and Mckenna, M. J. (2009). Drug delivery for treatment of inner ear disease: current state of knowledge. *Ear Hear.* 31, 156–165.

MCcall, A. A., Swan, E. E., Borenstein, J. T., Sewell, W. F., Kujawa, S. G., and Mckenna, M. J. (2010). Drug delivery for treatment of inner ear disease: current state of knowledge. *Ear Hear.* 31, 156–165. doi: 10.1097/AUD.0b013e3181c351f2

Mikulec, A. A., Hartsock, J. J., and Salt, A. N. (2008). Permeability of the round window membrane is influenced by the composition of applied drug solutions and by common surgical procedures. *Otol. Neurotol.* 29, 1020–1026. doi: 10.1097/MAO.0b013e31818658ea

Nakagawa, T., and Ito, J. (2007). Drug delivery systems for the treatment of sensorineural hearing loss. *Acta Otolaryngol. Suppl.* 127, 30–35.

Nakagawa, T., Kumakawa, K., Usami, S., Hato, N., Tabuchi, K., Takahashi, M., et al. (2014). A randomized controlled clinical trial of topical insulin-like growth factor-1 therapy for sudden deafness refractory to systemic corticosteroid treatment. *BMC Med.* 12:219. doi: 10.1186/s12916-014-0219-x

National Institute of Health (2000). *Sudden Deafness*. Bethesda, MD: National Institutes of Health.

Neitzel, R. L., Swinburn, T. K., Hammer, M. S., and Eisenberg, D. (2017). Economic impact of hearing loss and reduction of noise-induced hearing loss in the United States. *J. Speech Lang. Hear. Res.* 60, 182–189. doi: 10.1044/2016_JSLHR-H-15-0365

Noushi, F., Richardson, R. T., Hardman, J., Clark, G., and O'leary, S. (2005). Delivery of neurotrophin-3 to the cochlea using alginate beads. *Otol. Neurotol.* 26, 528–533.

Nyberg, S., Abbott, N. J., Shi, X., Steyger, P. S., and Dabdoub, A. (2019). Delivery of therapeutics to the inner ear: the challenge of the blood-labyrinth barrier. *Sci. Transl. Med.* 11:eaao0935. doi: 10.1126/scitranslmed.aao0935

Ohyama, K., Salt, A. N., and Thalmann, R. (1988). Volume flow rate of perilymph in the guinea-pig cochlea. *Hear Res.* 35, 119–129.

Paasche, G., Bogel, L., Leinung, M., Lenarz, T., and Stover, T. (2006). Substance distribution in a cochlea model using different pump rates for cochlear implant drug delivery electrode prototypes. *Hear Res.* 212, 74–82.

Panda, N. K., Verma, R. K., and Saravanan, K. (2008). Sudden sensorineural hearing loss: have we got a cure? *J. Otolaryngol. Head Neck Surg.* 37, 807–812.

Park, A. H., White, D. R., Moss, J. R., Bear, M., and Lebel, C. (2016). Phase 3 trials of thermosensitive ciprofloxacin gel for middle ear effusion in children with tubes. *Otolaryngol. Head Neck Surg.* 155, 324–331. doi: 10.1177/0194599816645526

Paulson, D. P., Abuzeid, W., Jiang, H., Oe, T., O'malley, B. W., and Li, D. (2008). A novel controlled local drug delivery system for inner ear disease. *Laryngoscope* 118, 706–711. doi: 10.1097/MLG.0b013e31815f8e41

Peng, Y., Xiong, S., Cheng, Y., Qi, Y. F., and Yang, Y. (2008). [Clinical investigation of different routes of administration of dexamethasone on sudden deafness]. *Lin Chung Er Bi Yan Hou Tou Jing Wai Ke Za Zhi* 22, 442–445.

Peppi, M., Marie, A., Belline, C., and Borenstein, J. T. (2018). Intracochlear drug delivery systems: a novel approach whose time has come. *Expert Opin. Drug Deliv.* 15, 319–324.

Piu, F., Wang, X., Fernandez, R., Dellamary, L., Harrop, A., Ye, Q., et al. (2011). OTO-104: a sustained-release dexamethasone hydrogel for the treatment of otic disorders. *Otol. Neurotol.* 32, 171–179. doi: 10.1097/MAO.0b013e3182009d29

Plontke, S., Lowenheim, H., Preyer, S., Leins, P., Dietz, K., Koitschev, A., et al. (2005). Outcomes research analysis of continuous intratympanic glucocorticoid delivery in patients with acute severe to profound hearing loss: basis for planning randomized controlled trials. *Acta Otolaryngol.* 125, 830–839.

Plontke, S., and Zenner, H. P. (2002). Pharmacokinetic considerations in intratympanic drug delivery to the inner ear. *Acta Otorhinolaryngol. Belg.* 56, 369–370.

Plontke, S. K., Gotze, G., Rahne, T., and Liebau, A. (2016). Intracochlear drug delivery in combination with cochlear implants: current aspects. *HNO* 65(Suppl. 1), 19–28.

Plontke, S. K., Lowenheim, H., Mertens, J., Engel, C., Meisner, C., Weidner, A., et al. (2009). Randomized, double blind, placebo controlled trial on the safety and efficacy of continuous intratympanic dexamethasone delivered via a round window catheter for severe to profound sudden idiopathic sensorineural hearing loss after failure of systemic therapy. *Laryngoscope* 119, 359–369.

Plontke, S. K., Mynatt, R., Gill, R. M., Borgmann, S., and Salt, A. N. (2007a). Concentration gradient along the scala tympani after local application of gentamicin to the round window membrane. *Laryngoscope* 117, 1191–1198.

Plontke, S. K., and Salt, A. N. (2006). Simulation of application strategies for local drug delivery to the inner ear. *ORL J. Otorhinolaryngol. Relat. Spec.* 68, 386–392.

Plontke, S. K., Siedow, N., Wegener, R., Zenner, H. P., and Salt, A. N. (2007b). Cochlear pharmacokinetics with local inner ear drug delivery using a three-dimensional finite-element computer model. *Audiol. Neurootol.* 12, 37–48.

Plontke, S. K., Zimmermann, R., Zenner, H. P., and Lowenheim, H. (2006). Technical note on microcatheter implantation for local inner ear drug delivery: surgical technique and safety aspects. *Otol. Neurotol.* 27, 912–917.

Pyykko, I., Zou, J., Schrott-Fischer, A., Glueckert, R., and Kinnunen, P. (2016). An overview of nanoparticle based delivery for treatment of inner ear disorders. *Methods Mol. Biol.* 1427, 363–415. doi: 10.1007/978-1-4939-3615-1_21

Richardson, R. T., Wise, A. K., Thompson, B. C., Flynn, B. O., Atkinson, P. J., Fretwell, N. J., et al. (2009). Polypyrrole-coated electrodes for the delivery of charge and neurotrophins to cochlear neurons. *Biomaterials* 30, 2614–2624. doi: 10.1016/j.biomaterials.2009.01.015

Saber, A., Strand, S. P., and Ulfendahl, M. (2009). Use of the biodegradable polymer chitosan as a vehicle for applying drugs to the inner ear. *Eur. J. Pharm. Sci.* 39, 110–115. doi: 10.1016/j.ejps.2009.11.003

Sakata, E., Kitago, Y., Murata, Y., and Teramoto, K. (1986). [Treatment of Meniere's disease. Middle ear infusion with lidocaine and steroid solution]. *Auris Nasus Larynx* 13, 79–89.

Salt, A. N. (2006). Pharmacokinetics of drug entry into cochlear fluids. *Volta Rev.* 105, 277–298.

Salt, A. N., Hartsock, J. J., Piu, F., and Hou, J. (2018). Dexamethasone and dexamethasone phosphate entry into perilymph compared for middle ear applications in guinea pigs. *Audiol. Neurootol.* 23, 245–257. doi: 10.1159/000493846

Salt, A. N., and Ma, Y. (2001). Quantification of solute entry into cochlear perilymph through the round window membrane. *Hear Res.* 154, 88–97.

Salt, A. N., Ohyama, K., and Thalmann, R. (1991a). Radial communication between the perilymphatic scalae of the cochlea, I: estimation by tracer perfusion. *Hear Res.* 56, 29–36.

Salt, A. N., Ohyama, K., and Thalmann, R. (1991b). Radial communication between the perilymphatic scalae of the cochlea, II: estimation by bolus injection of tracer into the sealed cochlea. *Hear Res.* 56, 37–43.

Salt, A. N., and Plontke, S. K. (2005). Local inner-ear drug delivery and pharmacokinetics. *Drug Discov. Today* 10, 1299–1306.

Salt, A. N., and Plontke, S. K. (2009). Principles of local drug delivery to the inner ear. *Audiol. Neurootol.* 14, 350–360. doi: 10.1159/000241892

Salt, A. N., and Plontke, S. K. (2018). Pharmacokinetic principles in the inner ear: influence of drug properties on intratympanic applications. *Hear Res.* 368, 28–40. doi: 10.1016/j.heares.2018.03.002

Salt, A. N., Thalmann, R., Marcus, D. C., and Bohne, B. A. (1986). Direct measurement of longitudinal endolymph flow rate in the guinea pig cochlea. *Hear Res.* 23, 141–151.

Schoendorf, J., Neugebauer, P., and Michel, O. (2001). Continuous intratympanic infusion of gentamicin via a microcatheter in Meniere's disease. *Otolaryngol. Head Neck Surg.* 124, 203–207.

Selivanova, O. A., Gouveris, H., Victor, A., Amedee, R. G., and Mann, W. (2005). Intratympanic dexamethasone and hyaluronic acid in patients with low-frequency and Meniere's-associated sudden sensorineural hearing loss. *Otol. Neurotol.* 26, 890–895.

Sewell, W. F., Borenstein, J. T., Chen, Z., Fiering, J., Handzel, O., Holmboe, M., et al. (2009). Development of a microfluidics-based intracochlear drug delivery device. *Audiol. Neurootol.* 14, 411–422. doi: 10.1159/000241898

Shea, J. J. (1997). The role of dexamethasone or streptomycin perfusion in the treatment of Meniere's disease. *Otolaryngol. Clin. North Am.* 30, 1051–1059.

Shea, J. J., and Ge, X. (1996). Dexamethasone perfusion of the labyrinth plus intravenous dexamethasone for Meniere's disease. *Otolaryngol. Clin. North Am.* 29, 353–358.

Sheppard, W. M., Wanamaker, H. H., Pack, A., Yamamoto, S., and Slepecky, N. (2004). Direct round window application of gentamicin with varying delivery vehicles: a comparison of ototoxicity. *Otolaryngol. Head Neck Surg.* 131, 890–896.

Silverstein, H. (1999). Use of a new device, the MicroWick, to deliver medication to the inner ear. *Ear Nose Throat J.* 78, 595–598, 600.

Silverstein, H., Farrugia, M., and Van Ess, M. (2009). Dexamethasone inner ear perfusion for subclinical endolymphatic hydrops. *Ear Nose Throat J.* 88, 778–785.

Silverstein, H., Isaacson, J. E., Olds, M. J., Rowan, P. T., and Rosenberg, S. (1998). Dexamethasone inner ear perfusion for the treatment of Meniere's disease: a prospective, randomized, double-blind, crossover trial. *Am. J. Otol.* 19, 196–201.

Singh-Joy, S. D., and McLain, V. C. (2008). Safety assessment of poloxamers 101, 105, 108, 122, 123, 124, 181, 182, 183, 184, 185, 188, 212, 215, 217, 231, 234, 235, 237, 238, 282, 284, 288, 331, 333, 334, 335, 338, 401, 402, 403, and 407, poloxamer 105 benzoate, and poloxamer 182 dibenzoate as used in cosmetics. *Int. J. Toxicol.* 27(Suppl. 2), 93–128. doi: 10.1080/10915810802244595

Stenner, M., Jecker, P., Gouveris, H., and Mann, W. (2006). [Treatment of sensorineural hearing loss in acute viral otitis media with intratympanic dexamethasone and hyaluronic acid in comparison with intravenous therapy]. *Laryngorhinootologie* 85, 32–37.

Suckfuell, M., Lisowska, G., Domka, W., Kabacinska, A., Morawski, K., Bodlaj, R., et al. (2014). Efficacy and safety of AM-111 in the treatment of acute sensorineural hearing loss: a double-blind, randomized, placebo-controlled phase II study. *Otol. Neurotol.* 35, 1317–1326. doi: 10.1097/MAO.0000000000000466

Suryanarayanan, R., Srinivasan, V. R., and O'sullivan, G. (2009). Transtympanic gentamicin treatment using Silverstein MicroWick in Meniere's disease patients: long term outcome. *J. Laryngol. Otol.* 123, 45–49. doi: 10.1017/S0022215108002776

Swan, E. E., Mescher, M. J., Sewell, W. F., Tao, S. L., and Borenstein, J. T. (2008). Inner ear drug delivery for auditory applications. *Adv. Drug Deliv. Rev.* 60, 1583–1599. doi: 10.1016/j.addr.2008.08.001

Swan, E. E., Peppi, M., Chen, Z., Green, K. M., Evans, J. E., Mckenna, M. J., et al. (2009). Proteomics analysis of perilymph and cerebrospinal fluid in mouse. *Laryngoscope* 119, 953–958. doi: 10.1002/lary.20209

Swartz, R., and Longwell, P. (2005). Treatment of vertigo. *Am. Fam. Phys.* 71, 1115–1122.

Takumida, M., and Anniko, M. (2004). Localization of endotoxin in the inner ear following inoculation into the middle ear. *Acta Otolaryngol.* 124, 772–777.

Tamura, T., Kita, T., Nakagawa, T., Endo, T., Kim, T. S., Ishihara, T., et al. (2005). Drug delivery to the cochlea using PLGA nanoparticles. *Laryngoscope* 115, 2000–2005.

Tanaka, K., and Motomura, S. (1981). Permeability of the labyrinthine windows in guinea pigs. *Arch. Otorhinolaryngol.* 233, 67–73.

Thalmann, I., Kohut, R. I., Ryu, J., Comegys, T. H., Senarita, M., and Thalmann, R. (1994). Protein profile of human perilymph: in search of markers for the diagnosis of perilymph fistula and other inner ear disease. *Otolaryngol. Head Neck Surg.* 111, 273–280.

Tonnesen, H. H., and Karlsen, J. (2002). Alginate in drug delivery systems. *Drug Dev. Ind. Pharm.* 28, 621–630.

van de Heyning, P., Muehlmeier, G., Cox, T., Lisowska, G., Maier, H., Morawski, K., et al. (2014). Efficacy and Safety of AM-101 in the treatment of acute inner ear tinnitus-A double-blind, randomized, placebo-controlled phase II study. *Otol. Neurotol.* 35, 589–597. doi: 10.1097/MAO.0000000000000268

Van Tomme, S. R., Storm, G., and Hennink, W. E. (2008). In situ gelling hydrogels for pharmaceutical and biomedical applications. *Int. J. Pharm.* 355, 1–18. doi: 10.1016/j.ijpharm.2008.01.057

Van Wijck, F., Staecker, H., and Lefebvre, P. P. (2007). Topical steroid therapy using the Silverstein Microwick in sudden sensorineural hearing loss after failure of conventional treatment. *Acta Otolaryngol.* 127, 1012–1017.

Van Wijk, F., Staecker, H., Keithley, E., and Lefebvre, P. P. (2006). Local perfusion of the tumor necrosis factor alpha blocker infliximab to the inner ear improves autoimmune neurosensory hearing loss. *Audiol. Neurootol.* 11, 357–365.

Wang, X., Dellamary, L., Fernandez, R., Harrop, A., Keithley, E. M., Harris, J. P., et al. (2009). Dose-dependent sustained release of dexamethasone in inner ear cochlear fluids using a novel local delivery approach. *Audiol. Neurootol.* 14, 393–401. doi: 10.1159/000241896

Wang, X., Dellamary, L., Fernandez, R., Ye, Q., Lebel, C., and Piu, F. (2011). Principles of inner ear sustained release following intratympanic administration. *Laryngoscope* 121, 385–391. doi: 10.1002/lary.21370

Wenzel, G. I., Warnecke, A., Stover, T., and Lenarz, T. (2010). Effects of extracochlear gacyclidine perfusion on tinnitus in humans: a case series. *Eur. Arch. Otorhinolaryngol.* 267, 691–699. doi: 10.1007/s00405-009-1126-1

Wise, A. K., and Gillespie, L. N. (2012). Drug delivery to the inner ear. *J. Neural Eng.* 9:065002. doi: 10.1088/1741-2560/9/6/065002

Xenellis, J., Papadimitriou, N., Nikolopoulos, T., Maragoudakis, P., Segas, J., Tzagaroulakis, A., et al. (2006). Intratympanic steroid treatment in idiopathic sudden sensorineural hearing loss: a control study. *Otolaryngol. Head Neck Surg.* 134, 940–945.

Xu, P., Gullotti, E., Tong, L., Highley, C. B., Errabelli, D. R., Hasan, T., et al. (2009). Intracellular drug delivery by poly(lactic-co-glycolic acid) nanoparticles, revisited. *Mol. Pharm.* 6, 190–201. doi: 10.1021/mp800137z

Yildirim, A., Coban, L., Satar, B., Yetiser, S., and Kunt, T. (2005). Effect of intratympanic dexamethasone on noise-induced temporary threshold shift. *Laryngoscope* 115, 1219–1222.

11

Otoprotection to Implanted Cochlea Exposed to Noise Trauma with Dexamethasone Eluting Electrode

Adrien A. Eshraghi[1,2,3], Amit Wolfovitz[1], Rasim Yilmazer[1], Carolyn Garnham[4], Ayca Baskadem Yilmazer[1], Esperanza Bas[1], Peter Ashman[1], Jonathan Roell[1], Jorge Bohorquez[3], Rahul Mittal[1], Roland Hessler[4], Daniel Sieber[4] and Jeenu Mittal[1]*

[1]Department of Otolaryngology, University of Miami Hearing Research Laboratory, Miller School of Medicine, Miami, FL, United States, [2]Department of Neurological Surgery, Miller School of Medicine, Miami, FL, United States, [3]Department of Biomedical Engineering, University of Miami, Miami, Coral Gables, FL, United States, [4]MED-EL Hearing Implants, Innsbruck, Austria

***Correspondence:**
Adrien A. Eshraghi
aeshraghi@med.miami.edu

Cochlear implantation (CI) is now widely used to provide auditory rehabilitation to individuals having severe to profound sensorineural hearing loss (SNHL). However, CI can lead to electrode insertion trauma (EIT) that can cause damage to sensory cells in the inner ear resulting in loss of residual hearing. Even with soft surgical techniques where there is minimal macroscopic damage, we can still observe the generation of molecular events that may initiate programmed cell death *via* various mechanisms such as oxidative stress, the release of pro-inflammatory cytokines, and activation of the caspase pathway. In addition, individuals with CI may be exposed to noise trauma (NT) due to occupation and leisure activities that may affect their hearing ability. Recently, there has been an increased interest in the auditory community to determine the efficacy of drug-eluting electrodes for the protection of residual hearing. The objective of this study is to determine the effect of NT on implanted cochlea as well as the otoprotective efficacy of dexamethasone eluting electrode to implanted cochlea exposed to NT in a guinea pig model of CI. Animals were divided into five groups: EIT with dexamethasone eluting electrode exposed to NT; EIT exposed to NT; NT only; EIT only and naïve animals (control group). The hearing thresholds were determined by auditory brainstem recordings (ABRs). The cochlea was harvested and analyzed for transcript levels of inflammation, apoptosis and fibrosis genes. We observed that threshold shifts were significantly higher in EIT, NT or EIT + NT groups compared to naïve animals at all the tested frequencies. The dexamethasone eluting electrode led to a significant decrease in hearing threshold shifts in implanted animals exposed to NT. Proapoptotic tumor necrosis factor-α [TNF-α, TNF-α receptor 1a (TNFαR1a)] and pro-fibrotic transforming growth factor β1 (TGFβ) genes were more than two-fold up-regulated following EIT and EIT + NT compared to the control group. The use of dexamethasone releasing electrode significantly decreased the transcript levels of pro-apoptotic and pro-fibrotic genes. The dexamethasone releasing electrode has shown promising results for hearing protection in implanted animals exposed to NT. The results of this study suggest that dexamethasone releasing electrode holds great potential in developing effective treatment modalities for NT in the implanted cochlea.

Keywords: drug-eluting electrodes, otoprotection, noise trauma, hearing loss, local drug delivery, dexamethasone, cochlear implantation

INTRODUCTION

Cochlear implantation (CI) is long known as the modality of choice for hearing rehabilitation in individuals with severe to profound sensorineural hearing loss (SNHL; Eshraghi et al., 2012; Lenarz et al., 2013; Macherey and Carlyon, 2014; Akçakaya et al., 2019). In recent years, CI indications have expanded to include candidates with substantial residual hearing and consequently, measures to preserve this residual hearing have become an important area of interest (Raveh et al., 2015; Eshraghi et al., 2017). The strategies for hearing preservation focus both on electrode design (softer, less traumatic and possibly drug-eluting) and on new surgical techniques that will enable minimal traumatic implantation (Eshraghi et al., 2011; Miranda et al., 2014; Khater and El-Anwar, 2017). The mechanisms involved in the loss of residual hearing following CI have been studied and demonstrate early and delayed loss of this hearing (Eshraghi et al., 2005; Dedhia et al., 2016; Quesnel et al., 2016). Early loss of residual hearing starts soon after the introduction of the electrode into cochlea that may lead to direct structural damage and consequent necrosis of cochlear sensory cells (Jia et al., 2013). This process is followed by the initiation of extrinsic and intrinsic molecular pathways of cochlear damage (Eshraghi and Van de Water, 2006). These pathways are triggered by oxidative stress and the expression of pro-inflammatory cytokines (Dinh et al., 2015). These cytokines, and oxidative damage, in turn, lead to activation of pro-apoptotic pathways, mitogen-activated protein kinases/c-Jun-N-terminal kinases (MAPK/JNK), that lead to programmed cell death in the affected cells within the first 24 h following electrode insertion trauma (EIT; Eshraghi et al., 2010, 2015). These pathways may continue with expression of pro-fibrogenic cytokines that produce fibrogenesis and angiogenesis beginning around 96 h post-implantation. The activation of these inflammatory and apoptotic pathways may further be accelerated by exposure of implanted individuals to noise trauma (NT). This NT may include both acoustic NT and electric overstimulation. There is a growing number of people with CI for whom the effect of NT is unclear, compared to the non-implanted population. NIHL has been reported as the etiology of deafness in implanted individuals, with a prevalence ranging from 2% (CI) to 20% (CI with electroacoustic stimulation; Simpson et al., 1993; Lazard et al., 2012). Currently, we can only speculate on the extent to which the SNHL in these implanted individuals can be attributed to noise exposure or due to a combination of other underlying predisposing factors. For example, implanted individuals may be exposed to high levels of noise due to occupation and leisure activities such as attending musical concerts. However, the effect of this NT on the hearing ability of implanted individuals is still not known. Therefore, the objective of the present study is to assess the effect of NT on the hearing in an implanted cochlea with and without dexamethasone eluting electrodes.

MATERIALS AND METHODS

Experimental Groups

Both male and female pigmented guinea pigs (Cady Hill Farms, MA) weighing approximately 350 g were used in this study. Animals were divided into five groups: EIT with dexamethasone eluting electrode (10%) exposed to NT (n = 13); EIT exposed to NT (n = 13); NT only (n = 13); EIT only (n = 13) and naïve animals separate for EIT or NT group and EIT/NT or EIT/NT/Dex group (control group; n = 13 each separately for these two different groups). The separate group of control animals was used for EIT or NT group and EIT/NT or EIT/NT/Dex group to avoid unnecessary exposure of animals to auditory brainstem recording (ABR) recordings. In the EIT or NT group, ABRs were done on days 1, 3, 7, 14 and 30 after implantation or exposing to high noise whereas in EIT/NT or EIT/NT/Dex group, the animals were first implanted, subjected to NT 7 days post-implantation and then ABRs were performed. A separate cohort of animals was used for gene expression (RT-PCR) studies (N = 6 for each above mentioned five groups). The production and physical characteristics of dexamethasone eluting electrodes have been described in detail in our previous studies (Bas et al., 2016). The electrode was made up of a sterile silicone rod with one recording contact at 1 mm from the tip (**Figure 1A**). It was designed for the guinea pig basal turn with a diameter of 0.3 mm at the tip, increasing gradually in size to be 0.5 mm in diameter at a distance of 4 mm from the tip. After implantation, dexamethasone from the drug-eluting electrode is released into the surrounding perilymph in the cochlea. The dexamethasone release rate from 10% eluting electrode has been demonstrated to be higher during the initial period of 5 days (166 ng/day) that goes down to 49 ng/day by 91 day determined by high performance liquid chromatography-mass spectrometry (HPLC-MS) in an *in vitro* study (Wilk et al., 2016). Another *in vitro* study also confirmed the comparable levels and similar patterns of dexamethasone release from drug-eluting electrode using a similar approach (Bas et al., 2016). For NT, awake animals were exposed to the sound level of 120 dB, 6–10 kHz centered at 8 kHz for 2 h. A number of studies have exposed awake animals to high NT without any undue pain and distress to the animals (Housley et al., 2013; Yang et al., 2015; Tuerdi et al., 2017; Vlajkovic et al., 2017; Chen et al., 2019). For noise exposure, animals were kept in individual cages and placed in an electrically shielded, double-walled sound-attenuating chamber.

The sound was generated by a waveform generator, amplified by an audio amplifier (Pioneer Electronics, Long Beach, CA, USA), and presented in an open field through speakers (Pioneer Electronics, Long Beach, CA, USA) placed 10 cm in front of the animal's cage. The noise level was determined using sound meter (Extech, Waltham, MA, USA) that measures sound from 35 to 130 dB. Animals were subjected to NT for 7 days post-CI surgery. Hearing thresholds of animals were determined at various time-periods before and after the surgery or NT. The experimental timeline of this study has been shown in **Figure 1B**.

All animal procedures used in this study were approved by the University of Miami Institutional Animal Care and Use Committee and followed NIH guidelines for the use and care of animals in biomedical research.

Surgical Procedures

The guinea pigs were anesthetized with intraperitoneal ketamine (40 mg/kg) and xylazine (5 mg/kg). Local anesthesia was administered with a 1% lidocaine subcutaneous injection. The operated ear was randomly assigned for implantation. Using sterile techniques and a binocular operating microscope, a retro-auricular incision was made to expose the bulla of the experimental ear. The bulla was opened with a scalpel, the round window membrane (RWM) and promontory were identified, and a cochleostomy was performed in the basal turn of the cochlea using a diamond drill of 0.8 mm. An electrode (dexamethasone eluting or non-eluting) was slowly inserted *via* the cochleostomy for a length of 4 mm into the scala tympani as described in our previous studies (Eshraghi et al., 2013, 2015; Bas et al., 2016). The electrode was then secured in place with a fascia graft at the cochleostomy site. Once the stability of the électrode array was established, the defect in the temporal bone bulla was closed with carboxylate dental cement. A burr hole was made in the skull at 1 mm anterior to the lambda suture and a stainless steel screw was implanted superficial to the dura ("epidural") to record auditory brainstem responses. The post-auricular incision was closed using several interrupted sutures. Intraperitoneal buprenorphine (0.05 mg/kg) was given for analgesia at the time of surgery and twice a day for two more days post-surgery.

Auditory Brainstem Recording (ABR)

The hearing of both ears of all guinea pigs was measured by ABR responses to pure-tone stimuli (1, 4, 8, and 16 kHz). The ABR frequencies were selected based on previous studies (Eshraghi et al., 2013; Bas et al., 2016). The ABRs were obtained using recording electrodes placed in the superior postauricular area (−) and in the vertex (+) of the guinea pig's scalp. The ground electrode was inserted in a deep muscle of the left leg. Intelligent Hearing Systems (IHS Smart EP, Miami, FL, USA) hardware and software were used to record ABR responses. Stimuli were delivered at a rate of 29 Hz to the cochlea tested by using an Etymotic Research ER2 insert earphone (Etymotic Research, Elk Grove Village, IL, USA) with a custom-made silicone ear tip that fits the guinea pig's ear canal diameter. The responses were amplified using an Opti-Amp bio amplifier from IHS that was connected to the Smart EP system. The intensity of stimulation was decreased by 10-dB decrements until no ABR response was identifiable by software developed by IHS to establish threshold values. These threshold values were confirmed by visual inspection of the responses by two of the investigators blinded to the study groups.

Quantitative RT-PCR Analyses

Total RNA was extracted from whole cochlear tissues with TRIzol reagent (Invitrogen, Carlsbad, CA, USA) following the manufacturer's protocol. RNA purity and concentration were determined by the absorbance at 260 and 280 nm using NanoDrop ND-1000 (Thermo Fisher Scientific, Waltham, MA, USA; Bas et al., 2019). cDNA was synthesized using an iScript kit (Bio-Rad, Hercules, CA, USA). Quantitative real-time PCR was performed in duplicate by using iQ SYBR Green Supermix (Bio-Rad, Hercules, CA, USA) on an iCycler Real-Time CFX96 detection system (Bio-Rad, Hercules, CA, USA). The mRNA level was normalized by using the housekeeping gene GAPDH. The primers were designed based on the cDNA sequences obtained from Ensemble Genome Browser[1] and NCBI nucleotide database[2] as described in previous studies (Bas et al., 2012). Melting curves were also performed to ensure primer specificity and to evaluate for any contamination. Relative changes in mRNA levels of genes were assessed using the 2(-ΔΔ CT) method (Livak and Schmittgen, 2001) and normalized to the house-keeping gene GAPDH. They were then normalized to the expression levels obtained from the control. Six whole cochlear tissue explants per group were used for each time point and three independent replicates were done. The average fold change compared to control group was calculated.

Statistical Analysis

Two-way ANOVA with Bonferroni *post hoc* testing was used for ABR threshold comparisons between groups at different time points. For gene expression studies, student's *t*-test was used. $P < 0.05$ was considered statistically significant.

RESULTS

Effect of Dexamethasone Eluting Electrodes on Hearing Thresholds in a Guinea Pig Model

To determine the effect of EIT and NT on hearing, guinea pigs were subjected to ABRs. Unimplanted naïve animals served as the control group. In agreement with our previous studies, hearing threshold shifts were significantly higher in implanted animals compared to the control group at 1, 4, 8 and 16 kHz at all post-implanted time periods ($P < 0.001$; **Figures 2A–D**). The threshold shifts were significantly higher in the noise-exposed unimplanted animals compared to the group with an implanted cochlea (EIT) at all tested frequencies ($P < 0.05$).

Next, we determined the hearing thresholds of animals implanted with non-eluting or dexamethasone eluting electrodes. We observed higher threshold shifts in animals that were exposed

[1] http://www.ensembl.org

[2] http://www.ncbi.nlm.nih.gov/nuccore

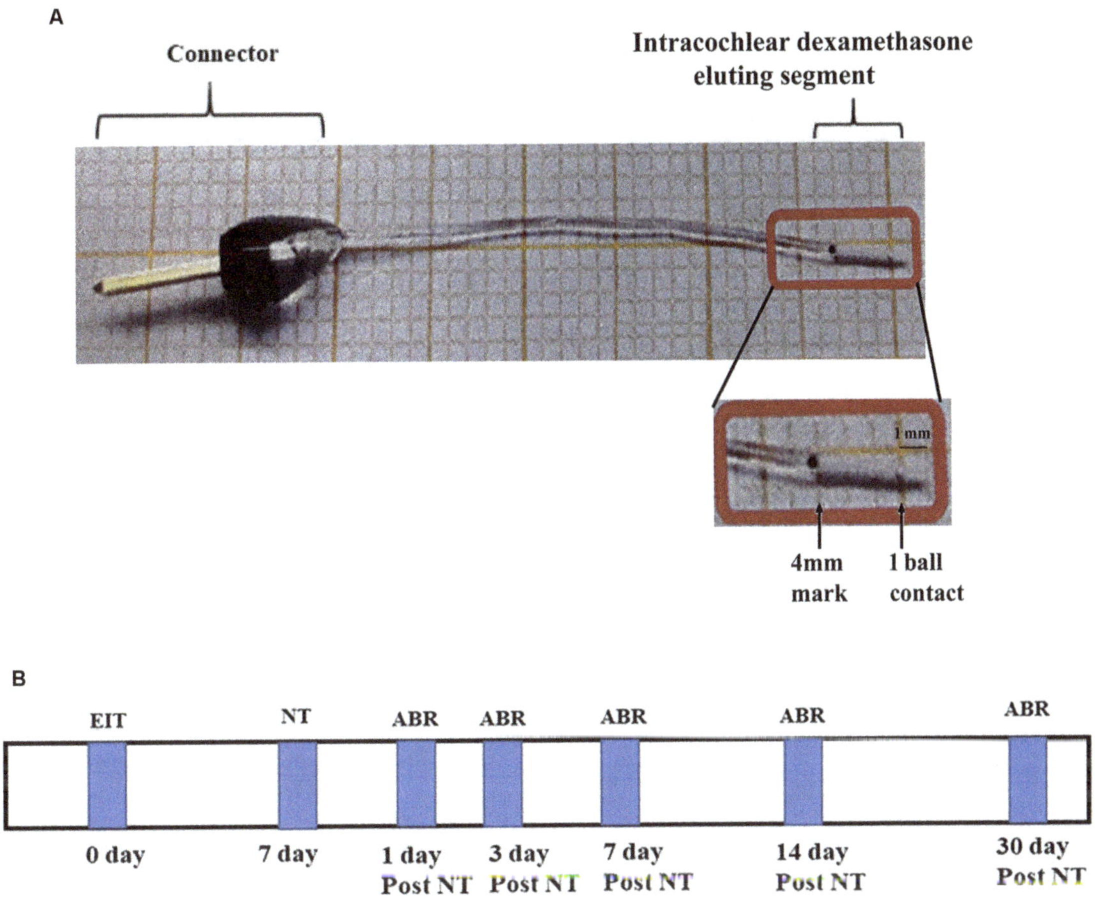

FIGURE 1 | Drug-eluting electrode and timeline. **(A)** Dexamethasone eluting electrode showing a connector and intracochlear segment with one electrical ball contact at the distal end. **(B)** Experimental timeline.

to NT with non-eluting electrodes at all tested frequencies compared to the control group (**Figures 3A–D**; $P < 0.001$). Threshold shifts in the animals implanted with dexamethasone eluting electrodes and subjected to NT (7 days after post-CI surgery) were consistently smaller compared to the threshold shift that was observed in guinea pigs with the non-eluting electrodes exposed to NT starting from day 3 up to day 30 (**Figures 3A–D**; $P < 0.01$). These results suggest that dexamethasone provides otoprotection against NT and EIT.

Changes in Transcript Levels of Cytokine and Receptors in Cochleae of Guinea Pigs Exposed to NT

Previous studies have demonstrated that cytokines, namely tumor necrosis factor-α (TNF-α) and transforming growth factor β1 (TGF β1), play a significant role in the initiation of apoptotic pathways and fibrosis leading to sensory cell damage following cochlear insults (Dinh et al., 2015; Bas et al., 2019). The binding of TNF-α to its receptors, TNF-α receptor 1a (TNFαR1a) and TNF-α receptor 1b (TNFαR1b), can initiate downstream host signaling cascade leading to apoptosis of auditory hair cells (Morrill and He, 2017). Therefore we determined the transcript levels of TNFα and TGF β1 as well as TNFαR1a and TNFαR1b in the cochlear tissues of guinea pigs exposed to NT using real-time PCR at different time periods post-NT. There was a significant upregulation in transcript levels of TNFα at 2 and 12 h post-NT, followed by a slight decrease in levels at 24 h and 8 days post-NT (**Figure 4A**). Increased transcript levels of TNFαR1a were observable with an increase in the post-NT time period from 2 h to 8 days (**Figure 4B**). TNFαR1b was initially significantly up-regulated in the first 2 h post NT followed by decreased levels in the later time intervals (**Figure 4C**). TGF β1 showed the highest transcript levels at 8-day post-NT. These results suggest that NT induces significant upregulation of inflammatory and fibrotic gene expression in the cochlea exposed to NT (**Figure 4D**).

Expression of Cytokine and Receptors in Cochleae From Implanted Animals

To determine the effect of EIT on cytokine and receptors, the transcript levels of TNF-α, TNFαR1a, TNFαR1b and TGF β1 were determined in the cochlear tissues of implanted animals

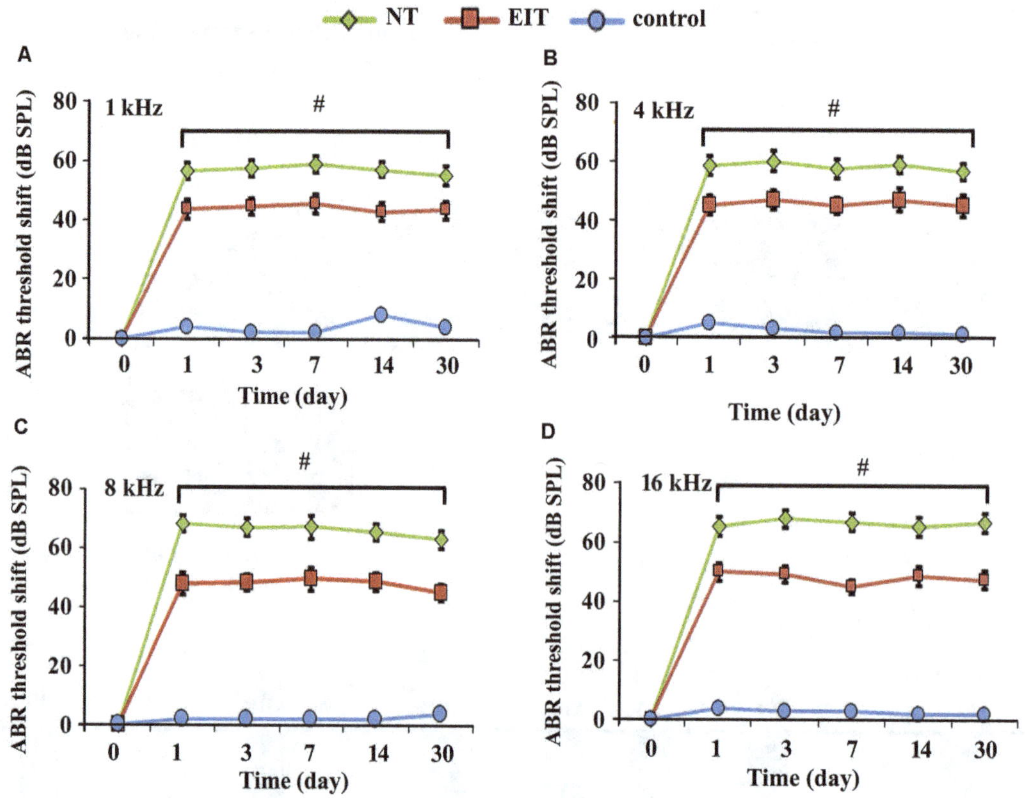

FIGURE 2 | Auditory brainstem recording (ABR) threshold shifts. Hearing threshold shifts in control, electrode insertion trauma (EIT) group, and animals exposed to noise trauma (NT) at 1 kHz **(A)**, 4 kHz **(B)**, 8 kHz **(C)** and 16 kHz **(D)** at different time-periods. ABR threshold shifts were significantly higher in NT groups compared to implanted animals. $^{\#}P < 0.05$ compared to the EIT group. Data represent mean ± standard deviation.

at 24 h and 7-day post-EIT. High transcript levels of TNF-α were observable at 24 h post-EIT showing significantly elevated expression at 7-day post-EIT (**Figure 5A**). A similar pattern of expression of TNFαR1a was observed showing high production at 7-day post-EIT (**Figure 5B**). On the other hand, elevated levels of TNFαR1b were observed only at 24 h post-EIT, followed by decreased expression at 7-day post-EIT (**Figure 5C**). High levels of TGF β1 were observable at 7-day post-EIT that are consistent with its role in fibrosis and scar formation following electrode insertion (**Figure 5D**).

DEX Eluting Electrode Significantly Decreases the Transcript Levels of Cytokine and Receptors

We compared the transcript levels of TNF-α, TNFαR1a, TNFαR1b and TGF β1 in the cochlear tissues of animals implanted with dexamethasone eluting and non-eluting electrodes exposed to NT. The cochlear tissues harvested from animals implanted with non-eluting electrodes and exposed to NT showed high transcript levels of TNF-α, TNFαR1a and TGF β1 (**Figures 6A,B,D**). However, a significant downregulation of TNF-α, TNFαR1a, and TGF β1 was observed in the cochlear tissues of guinea pigs implanted with dexamethasone eluting electrodes and subjected to NT (**Figures 6A,B,D**; $P < 0.001$). An insignificant increase in elevation of TNFαR1b was observed in the inner ear tissues from animals implanted with dexamethasone eluting electrode ($P > 0.05$; **Figure 6C**).

DISCUSSION

Macroscopic damage to the cochlea occurring right after implantation results in the activation of intrinsic and extrinsic molecular pathways in the cochlea leading to sensory cell damage (Eshraghi and Van de Water, 2006; Dinh et al., 2015). By 24 h, oxidative stress induced by mechanical trauma, pro-inflammatory cytokines (mainly TNFα), and enzymes are released (Eshraghi et al., 2015). The caspase pathway is then activated leading to a pro-apoptotic signal cascade and programmed cell death. The expression of pro-apoptotic molecules (such as c-Jun, p-Jun, and caspase 3) was observed in immunohistochemistry studies to be expressed in hair cells and supporting cells as early as 6 h post-EIT (Eshraghi et al., 2015). By 96 h, pro-inflammatory cytokines and enzymes return to baseline level and fibrogenesis is initiated by growth factors such as TGF β1. The activation of inflammatory and apoptotic pathways may further be exacerbated following exposure to acoustic

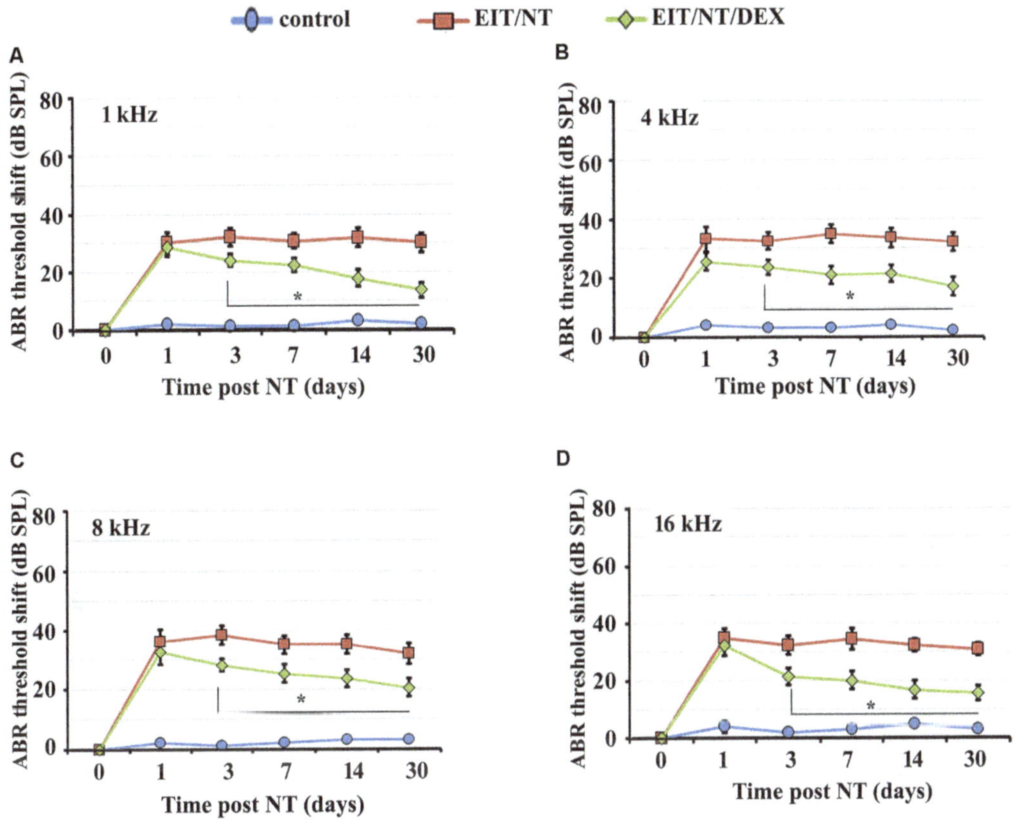

FIGURE 3 | Dexamethasone eluting electrodes provides otoprotection. Guinea pigs were implanted with dexamethasone eluting or non eluting electrode and subjected to NT. ABR thresholds were significantly lower in animals implanted with dexamethasone eluting electrodes compared to guinea pigs receiving non-eluting electrodes at 1 kHz **(A)**, 4 kHz **(B)**, 8 kHz **(C)** and 16 kHz **(D)** at all time-periods. Time period zero indicates baseline ABRs before EIT and NT. $^{*}P < 0.01$ compared to EIT/NT group. Data represent mean ± standard deviation.

NT or electric overstimulation. Since there is an ever-growing population of implanted individuals exposed to the unchecked noise levels of daily living, it is still unknown what would be the influence of these unchecked noise levels on those individuals with impaired inner ear anatomy and cochlear sound wave conduction. This influence of NT on implanted ears has not been assessed to the best of our knowledge.

Recently, there has been an increased interest in the auditory community for the delivery of otoprotective agents into the cochlea through drug-eluting electrodes. Mostly silicone polymer is used for the delivery of otoprotective agents that are embedded into the electrode array (Farahmand-Ghavi et al., 2010). The utility of a drug-eluting electrode was initially demonstrated by an *in vitro* study (Paasche et al., 2003). Using a modified electrode attached to a pump, it was shown that it is possible to deliver the drugs in temporal bones, which was used as a surrogate model of the human cochlea. Another study showed improvement in hearing thresholds as evident by ABR and distortion product otoacoustic emission (DPOAE) values in guinea pigs implanted with 2% dexamethasone eluting rods compared to animals having non-eluting control rods (Liu et al., 2015). The cochleae of animals that received dexamethasone eluting rods also showed less fibrosis and lower levels of TNFα compared to the control group. Pharmacokinetic studies demonstrated peak dexamethasone concentration at 30 min postoperatively. It was observed that dexamethasone eluting rods can deliver the drug up to 1-week post-implantation in *in vivo* studies. In agreement with these findings, another investigation using a guinea pig model showed that dexamethasone eluting electrode provided otoprotection to the cochlea against elevation in hearing thresholds, loss of hair cells, damage to neural elements, increases in impedance and fibrosis that result from EIT-initiated damage in a dose-dependent manner up to 90 days (Bas et al., 2016). It has also been shown that dexamethasone eluting electrode (1 and 10%) promotes short-term preservation of residual hearing 4–6 weeks post-implantation in a gerbil model (Douchement et al., 2015). However, in this study, the long-term preservation of residual hearing (after 1-year post-EIT) was observed only at higher frequencies (16,000 Hz) and not at lower frequencies (500 and 1,000 Hz). All these studies demonstrate the efficacy of dexamethasone eluting electrode in providing otoprotection and promoting the preservation of residual hearing following EIT. In our study, we observed that the dexamethasone eluting electrode not only provides

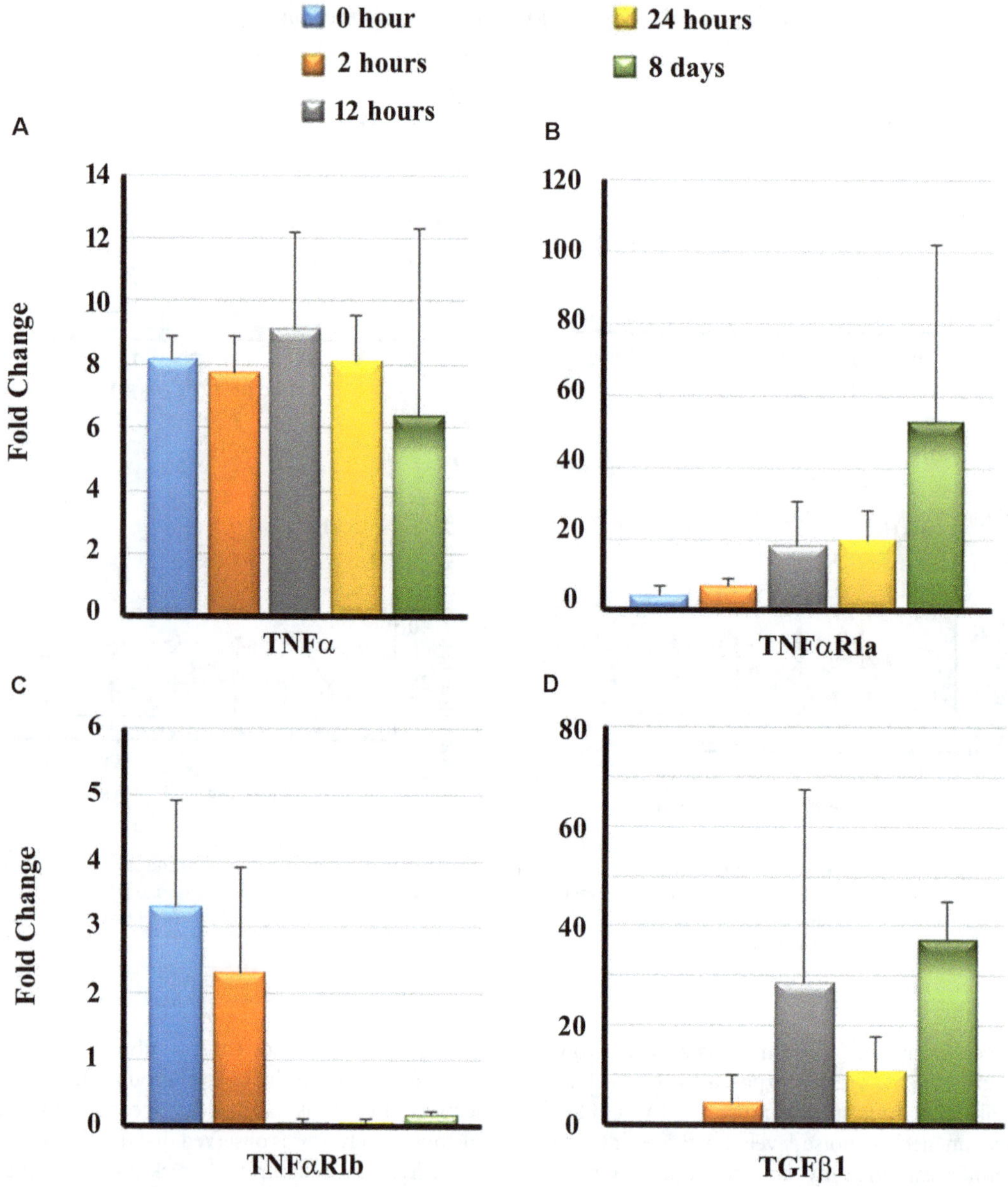

FIGURE 4 | Transcripts levels of pro-inflammatory and pro-fibrogenic genes in the cochleae. Guinea pigs were subjected to NT and cochleae were harvested at different post-NT time periods. The expression of tumor necrosis factor-α (TNF-α; **A**), TNF-α receptor 1a (TNFαR1a; **B**), TNFαR1b **(C)** and transforming growth factor β1 (TGF β1; **D**) was determined by real-time PCR. Time zero represents cochleae harvested immediately after NT. Data are expressed as fold change compared to the control group and represents mean ± standard deviation.

otoprotection against EIT but also for NT in our guinea pig model.

It is also interesting to note that in the present study, we observed that ABR thresholds were lower in implanted animals subjected to NT compared to implanted animals or those exposed to NT alone Although the precise reasons for this effect are still not known, it is possible that implanted animals actually receive less sound due to the electrode in the cochlea compared to non-implanted animals. In addition, there is a release of growth factors as well as heat shock proteins (HSP) in the inner ear following CI (Warnecke et al., 2019). Higher insulin-like growth factor binding protein 1 (IGFBP-1) levels have been observed in the perilymph of implanted individuals (Warnecke et al., 2019). IGFBP1 regulates the action of IGF-1 that plays a crucial role in the embryonic and postnatal development of the cochlea (Camarero et al., 2001; Digicaylioglu et al., 2004; Bach, 2015). Studies have shown that IGF-1 can act as a potent otoprotective agent and provide protection against auditory hair cell damage (Hayashi et al., 2013, 2014; Yamamoto et al., 2014; Yamahara et al., 2015, 2019). The local administration of

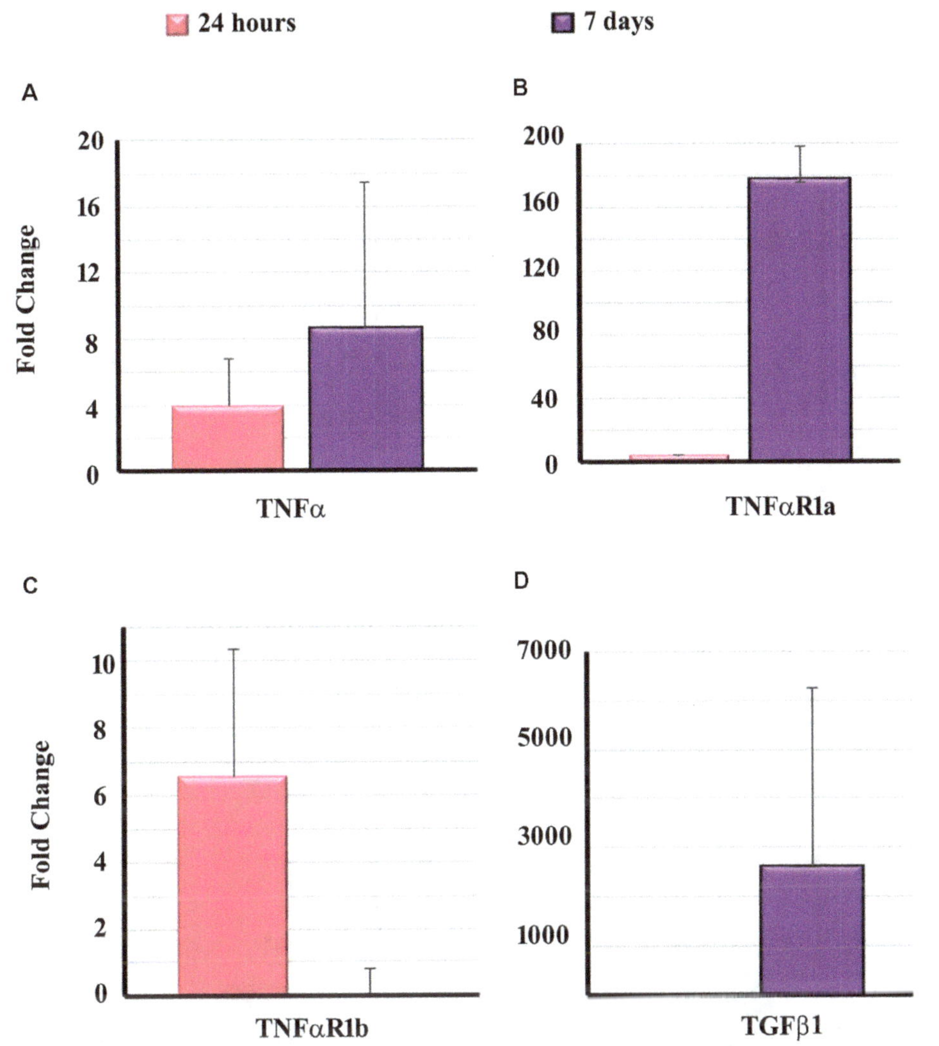

FIGURE 5 | Expression of pro-inflammatory and pro-fibrogenic genes in the cochleae of implanted animals. Cochleae from guinea pigs implanted with non-drug eluting electrodes were harvested at the different post-EIT time period and subjected to real-time PCR to determine the levels of TNF-α **(A)**, TNFαR1a **(B)**, TNFαR1b **(C)** and TGF β1 **(D)**. Data are expressed as fold change compared to the control group and represents mean ± standard deviation.

IGF-1 in a hydrogel provides protection against acoustic NT in both guinea pig and rat animal models (Iwai et al., 2006; Lee et al., 2007). The elevated levels of HSPs such as HSP70 have also been observed in the perilymph of implanted individuals (Schmitt et al., 2018). Geldanamycin-induced HSP70 has been demonstrated to provide otoprotection against gentamicin-mediated ototoxicity (Yu et al., 2009). This pre-availability of these growth factors and HSPs may account for the otoprotection observed in implanted animals exposed to NT. Further studies are warranted to understand the precise molecular mechanisms that provide otoprotection to implanted animals exposed to NT.

Cochlear insults such as EIT and NT induce the generation of proinflammatory cytokines such as TNFα (Fujioka et al., 2006). The binding of TNFα to its receptor, TNFαR1a, and TNFαR1b initiates downstream signaling cascades that can play a crucial role in sensory cell damage in the cochlea (Dinh et al., 2015). In this study, we observed that NT induced a significant up-regulation of TNFα and its receptor, TNFαR1a, within the first 24 h. TNFα levels remained relatively constant initially but gradually decreased 8 days post-implantation. On the other hand, TNFαR1a continued to be exponentially up-regulated even 8 days post-implantation, thus promoting pro-apoptotic pathways even at that time. TNFαR1b was significantly up-regulated within the first 2 h. It was then significantly down-regulated within 12 h post-NT. TNFα receptors are known to promote nuclear entry of the transcription factor NF-κB that can induce transcription of pro-inflammatory genes as well as activation of the apoptosis pathway (Aggarwal, 2003; Hayden and Ghosh, 2014). TGF β1, a strong mediator of fibrogenesis, inflammatory, and immune response in the cochlea (Bas et al., 2019), was significantly up-regulated within 2 h post-NT leading to a decrease in the pro-apoptotic pathways

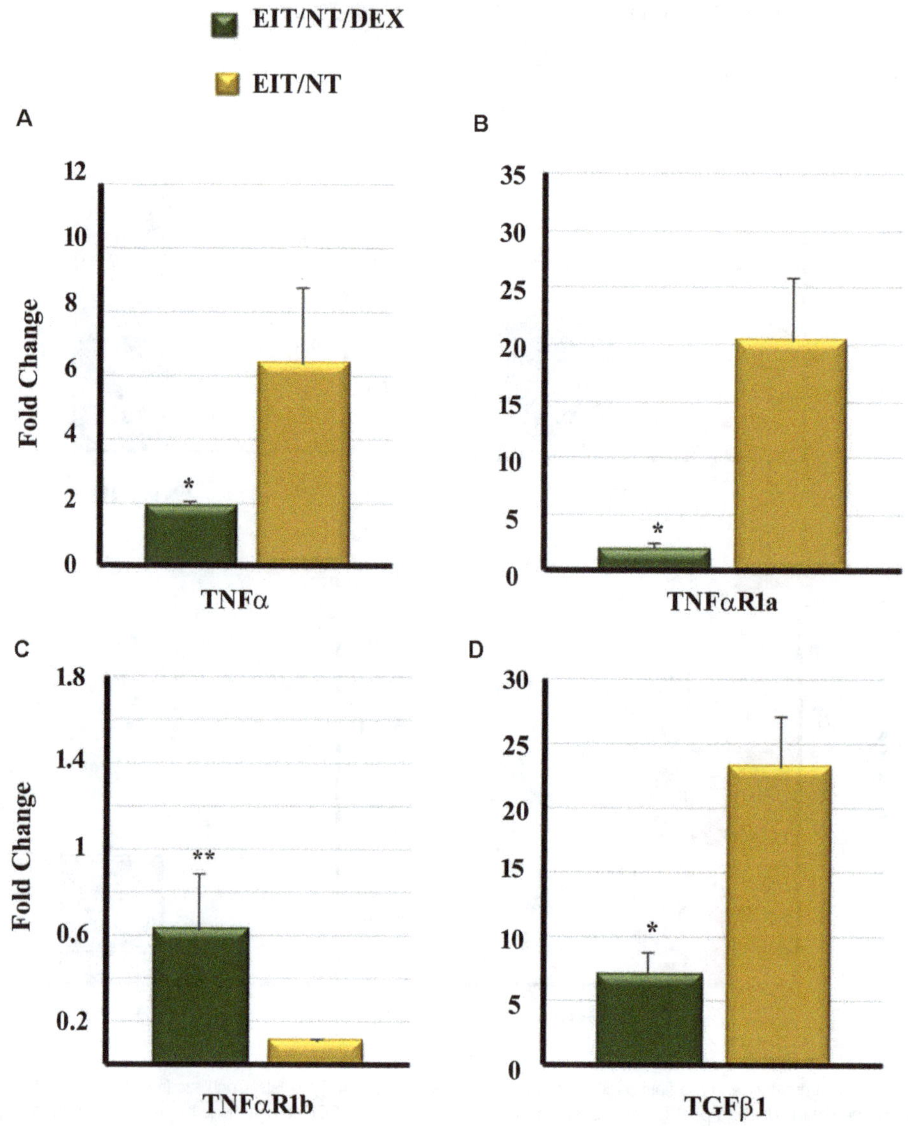

FIGURE 6 | Dexamethasone significantly decreases the expression of pro-inflammatory and pro-fibrogenic genes in the cochleae. Guinea pigs were implanted with dexamethasone or non-drug-eluting electrodes and subjected to NT. Cochleae were harvested at different time periods. The expression of TNF-α **(A)**, TNFαR1a **(B)**, TNFαR1b **(C)** and TGF β1 **(D)** was determined by real-time PCR. $^*P < 0.01$ or $^{**}P > 0.05$ compared to EIT/NT group. Data are expressed as fold change compared to control group and represents the mean ± standard deviation.

on the one hand but an increase in fibrosis on the other. EIT led to a significant up-regulation of inflammatory and fibrotic gene expression (TNFα, TNFαR1a, and TGF β1) in 24 h and even more significantly after 7 days. The inflammatory and fibrotic gene expression was significantly decreased with the dexamethasone eluting electrode. Our results are in agreement with a previous study that showed a significant reduction in recruitment of inflammatory cells such as fibrocyte, lymphocyte macrophage, and giant cells in the cochlea of animals implanted with a dexamethasone-loaded silicone elastomer shaped like a CI electrode when compared to animals receiving non-eluting electrode (Farhadi et al., 2013).

In summary, the present study demonstrated that both the ABR threshold shift and the expression of pro-apoptotic and pro-fibrogenic genes were significantly decreased in dexamethasone implanted animals exposed to NT compared to animals implanted with non-drug eluting electrodes or subjected to either NT or EIT alone. One of the limitations of the present study is that the NT used in this investigation is artificial and NT in CI patients may be of a different origin, leading to different pathological changes in the ear, which needs to be deciphered in future studies. However, our study is very close to the situations where implanted individuals are exposed to acoustic trauma such as while attending musical concerts. Another limitation of our study that we tested the hearing thresholds in our guinea pig model only at lower frequencies. The higher frequencies can provide information on direct trauma impact and therapeutic results of dexamethasone releasing electrode. This is relevant in view of the electrode position and dexamethasone release in the basal region of the cochlea. Further studies will help in determining the effect of NT on hearing thresholds at higher frequencies in the implanted cochlea. Despite these limitations, our study and published literature strongly suggest the potential of dexamethasone eluting electrodes in providing otoprotection and preservation of residual hearing post-CI. However, dexamethasone downregulates immune responses in the cochlea, which may increase predisposition to infections. Due to the proximity of the ear to the brain and the presence of cochlear as well as vestibular aqueduct, cochlear infections are a potential risk factor for developing meningitis. Therefore, long-term safety studies are warranted to determine the optimum doses of dexamethasone. In addition, there is a need to discover novel otoprotective agents that can be delivered through drug-eluting electrodes which can promote the preservation of residual hearing post-CI. Drug-eluting electrodes hold great translational potential for the delivery of therapeutics to the inner ear. Due to the complex anatomy of the inner ear, cochlear drug delivery is associated with significant challenges. It is expected that drug-eluting electrodes will revolutionize the field of drug delivery into the inner ear leading to the efficient administration of therapeutics into the cochlea. Based on the results of this study, it can be concluded that dexamethasone eluting rods can protect the cochlea from EIT and NT alone and also from a combination of EIT and NT in a guinea pig model. Further studies using a larger cohort of animals will help in confirming the results of the present study and will open up avenues for potential translation of drug-eluting electrodes from bench to bedside.

ETHICS STATEMENT

All animal procedures used in this study were approved by the University of Miami Institutional Animal Care and Use Committee and followed NIH guidelines for the use and care of animals in biomedical research.

AUTHOR CONTRIBUTIONS

All authors listed have made a substantial, direct and intellectual contribution to the work, and approved it for publication.

REFERENCES

Aggarwal, B. B. (2003). Signalling pathways of the TNF superfamily: a double-edged sword. *Nat. Rev. Immunol.* 3, 745–756. doi: 10.1038/nri1184

Akçakaya, H., Doğan, M., Gürkan, S., Koçak, Ö., and Yücel, E. (2019). Early cochlear implantation: verbal working memory, vocabulary, speech intelligibility and participant variables. *Cochlear Implants Int.* 20, 62–73. doi: 10.1080/14670100.2019.1565077

Bach, L. A. (2015). Insulin-like growth factor binding proteins—an update. *Pediatr. Endocrinol. Rev.* 13, 521–530.

Bas, E., Anwar, M. R., and Van De Water, T. R. (2019). TGF β-1 and WNT signaling pathways collaboration associated with cochlear implantation trauma-induced fibrosis. *Anat. Rec.* doi: 10.1002/ar.24064 [Epub ahead of print].

Bas, E., Bohorquez, J., Goncalves, S., Perez, E., Dinh, C. T., Garnham, C., et al (2016). Electrode array-eluted dexamethasone protects against electrode insertion trauma induced hearing and hair cell losses, damage to neural elements, increases in impedance and fibrosis: a dose response study. *Hear. Res.* 337, 12–24. doi: 10.1016/j.heares.2016.02.003

Bas, E., Gupta, C., and Van De Water, T. R. (2012). A novel organ of corti explant model for the study of cochlear implantation trauma. *Anat. Rec. (Hoboken)* 295, 1944–1956. doi: 10.1002/ar.22585

Camarero, G., Avendano, C., Fernandez-Moreno, C., Villar, A., Contreras, J., de Pablo, F., et al. (2001). Delayed inner ear maturation and neuronal loss in postnatal Igf-1-deficient mice. *J. Neurosci.* 21, 7630–7641. doi: 10.1523/JNEUROSCI.21-19-07630.2001

Chen, H., Xing, Y., Zhang, Z., Tao, S., Wang, H., Aiken, S., et al. (2019). Coding-in-noise deficits are not seen in responses to amplitude modulation in subjects with cochlear synaptopathy induced by a single noise exposure. *Neuroscience* 400, 62–71. doi: 10.1016/j.neuroscience.2018.12.048

Dedhia, K., Worman, T., Meredith, M. A., and Rubinstein, J. T. (2016). Patterns of long-term hearing loss in hearing preservation cochlear implant surgery. *Otol. Neurotol.* 37, 478–486. doi: 10.1097/mao.0000000000001011

Digicaylioglu, M., Garden, G., Timberlake, S., Fletcher, L., and Lipton, S. A. (2004). Acute neuroprotective synergy of erythropoietin and insulin-like growth factor I. *Proc. Natl. Acad. Sci. U S A* 101, 9855–9860. doi: 10.1073/pnas.0403172101

Dinh, C. T., Goncalves, S., Bas, E., Van De Water, T. R., and Zine, A. (2015). Molecular regulation of auditory hair cell death and approaches to protect sensory receptor cells and/or stimulate repair following acoustic trauma. *Front. Cell. Neurosci.* 9:96. doi: 10.3389/fncel.2015.00096

Douchement, D., Terranti, A., Lamblin, J., Salleron, J., Siepmann, F., Siepmann, J., et al. (2015). Dexamethasone eluting electrodes for cochlear implantation: effect on residual hearing. *Cochlear Implants Int.* 16, 195–200. doi: 10.1179/1754762813Y.0000000053

Eshraghi, A. A., Ahmed, J., Krysiak, E., Ila, K., Ashman, P., Telischi, F. F., et al. (2017). Clinical, surgical and electrical factors impacting residual hearing in cochlear implant surgery. *Acta Otolaryngol.* 137, 384–388. doi: 10.1080/00016489.2016.1256499

Eshraghi, A. A., Dinh, C. T., Bohorquez, J., Angeli, S., Abi-Hachem, R., and Van De Water, T. R. (2011). Local drug delivery to conserve hearing: mechanisms of action of eluted dexamethasone within the cochlea. *Cochlear Implants Int.* 12, S51–S53. doi: 10.1179/146701011x13001035753254

Eshraghi, A. A., Gupta, C., Van De Water, T. R., Bohorquez, J. E., Garnham, C., Bas, E., et al. (2013). Molecular mechanisms involved in cochlear implantation trauma and the protection of hearing and auditory sensory cells by inhibition of c-Jun-N-terminal kinase signaling. *Laryngoscope* 123, S1–S14. doi: 10.1002/lary.23902

Eshraghi, A. A., Hoosien, G., Ramsay, S., Dinh, C. T., Bas, E., Balkany, T. J., et al. (2010). Inhibition of the JNK signal cascade conserves hearing against electrode insertion trauma-induced loss. *Cochlear Implants Int.* 11, 104–109. doi: 10.1179/146701010x12671177544104

Eshraghi, A. A., Lang, D. M., Roell, J., Van De Water, T. R., Garnham, C., Rodrigues, H., et al. (2015). Mechanisms of programmed cell death signaling in hair cells and support cells post-electrode insertion trauma. *Acta Otolaryngol.* 135, 328–334. doi: 10.3109/00016489.2015.1012276

Eshraghi, A. A., Nazarian, R., Telischi, F. F., Rajguru, S. M., Truy, E., and Gupta, C. (2012). The cochlear implant: historical aspects and future prospects. *Anat. Rec.* 295, 1967–1980. doi: 10.1002/ar.22580

Eshraghi, A. A., Polak, M., He, J., Telischi, F. F., Balkany, T. J., and Van De Water, T. R. (2005). Pattern of hearing loss in a rat model of cochlear implantation trauma. *Otol. Neurotol.* 26, 442–447. doi: 10.1097/01.mao.0000169791.53201.e1

Eshraghi, A. A., and Van de Water, T. R. (2006). Cochlear implantation trauma and noise-induced hearing loss: apoptosis and therapeutic strategies. *Anat. Rec. A Discov. Mol. Cell. Evol. Biol.* 288, 473–481. doi: 10.1002/ar.a.20305

Farahmand-Ghavi, F., Mirzadeh, H., Imani, M., Jolly, C., and Farhadi, M. (2010). Corticosteroid- releasing cochlear implant: a novel hybrid of biomaterial and drug delivery system. *J. Biomed. Mater. Res. Part B Appl. Biomater.* 94, 388–398. doi: 10.1002/jbm.b.31666

Farhadi, M., Jalessi, M., Salehian, P., Ghavi, F. F., Emamjomeh, H., Mirzadeh, H., et al. (2013). Dexamethasone eluting cochlear implant: histological study in animal model. *Cochlear Implants Int.* 14, 45–50. doi: 10.1179/1754762811y.0000000024

Fujioka, M., Kanzaki, S., Okano, H. J., Masuda, M., Ogawa, K., and Okano, H. (2006). Proinflammatory cytokines expression in noise-induced damaged cochlea. *J. Neurosci. Res.* 83, 575–583. doi: 10.1002/jnr.20764

Hayashi, Y., Yamamoto, N., Nakagawa, T., and Ito, J. (2013). Insulin-like growth factor 1 inhibits hair cell apoptosis and promotes the cell cycle of supporting cells by activating different downstream cascades after pharmacological hair cell injury in neonatal mice. *Mol. Cell. Neurosci.* 56, 29–38. doi: 10.1016/j.mcn.2013.03.003

Hayashi, Y., Yamamoto, N., Nakagawa, T., and Ito, J. (2014). Insulin-like growth factor 1 induces the transcription of Gap43 and Ntn1 during hair cell protection in the neonatal murine cochlea. *Neurosci. Lett.* 560, 7–11. doi: 10.1016/j.neulet.2013.11.062

Hayden, M. S., and Ghosh, S. (2014). Regulation of NF-κB by TNF family cytokines. *Semin. Immunol.* 26, 253–266. doi: 10.1016/j.smim.2014.05.004

Housley, G. D., Morton-Jones, R., Vlajkovic, S. M., Telang, R. S., Paramananthasivam, V., Tadros, S. F., et al. (2013). ATP-gated ion channels mediate adaptation to elevated sound levels. *Proc. Natl. Acad. Sci. U S A* 110, 7494–7499. doi: 10.1073/pnas.1222295110

Iwai, K., Nakagawa, T., Endo, T., Matsuoka, Y., Kita, T., Kim, T. S., et al. (2006). Cochlear protection by local insulin-like growth factor-1 application using biodegradable hydrogel. *Laryngoscope* 116, 529–533. doi: 10.1097/01.mlg.0000200791.77819.eb

Jia, H., Wang, J., François, F., Uziel, A., Puel, J. L., and Venail, F. (2013). Molecular and cellular mechanisms of loss of residual hearing after cochlear implantation. *Ann. Otol. Rhinol. Laryngol.* 122, 33–39. doi: 10.1177/000348941312200107

Khater, A., and El-Anwar, M. W. (2017). Methods of hearing preservation during cochlear implantation. *Int. Arch. Otorhinolaryngol.* 21, 297–301. doi: 10.1055/s-0036-1585094

Lazard, D. S., Vincent, C., Venail, F., Van de Heyning, P., Truy, E., Sterkers, O., et al. (2012). Pre-, per- and postoperative factors affecting performance of postlinguistically deaf adults using cochlear implants: a new conceptual model over time. *PLoS One* 7:e48739. doi: 10.1371/journal.pone.0048739

Lee, K. Y., Nakagawa, T., Okano, T., Hori, R., Ono, K., Tabata, Y., et al. (2007). Novel therapy for hearing loss: delivery of insulin-like growth factor 1 to the cochlea using gelatin hydrogel. *Otol. Neurotol.* 28, 976–981. doi: 10.1097/mao.0b013e31811f40db

Lenarz, T., Pau, H. W., and Paasche, G. (2013). Cochlear implants. *Curr. Pharm. Biotechnol.* 14, 112–123. doi: 10.2174/1389201011314010014

Liu, Y., Jolly, C., Braun, S., Janssen, T., Scherer, E., Steinhoff, J., et al. (2015). Effects of a dexamethasone-releasing implant on cochleae: a functional, morphological and pharmacokinetic study. *Hear Res.* 327, 89–101. doi: 10.1016/j.heares.2015.04.019

Livak, K. J., and Schmittgen, T. D. (2001). Analysis of relative gene expression data using real-time quantitative PCR and the $2^{-\Delta\Delta CT}$ method. *Methods* 200125, 402–408. doi: 10.1006/meth.2001.1262

Macherey, O., and Carlyon, R. P. (2014). Cochlear implants. *Curr. Biol.* 24, R878–R884. doi: 10.1016/j.cub.2014.06.053

Miranda, P. C., Sampaio, A. L., Lopes, R. A., Ramos Venosa, A., and de Oliveira, C. A. (2014). Hearing preservation in cochlear implant surgery. *Int. J. Otolaryngol.* 2014:468515. doi: 10.1155/2014/468515

Morrill, S., and He, D. Z. Z. (2017). Apoptosis in inner ear sensory hair cells. *J. Otol.* 12, 151–164. doi: 10.1016/j.joto.2017.08.001

Paasche, G., Gibson, P., Averbeck, T., Becker, H., Lenarz, T., and Stöver, T. (2003). Technical report: modification of a cochlear implant electrode for drug delivery to the inner ear. *Otol. Neurotol.* 24, 222–227. doi: 10.1097/00129492-200303000-00016

Quesnel, A. M., Nakajima, H. H., Rosowski, J. J., Hansen, M. R., Gantz, B. J., and Nadol, J. B. Jr. (2016). Delayed loss of hearing after hearing preservation cochlear implantation: human temporal bone pathology and implications for etiology. *Hear. Res.* 333, 225–234. doi: 10.1016/j.heares.2015.08.018

Raveh, E., Attias, J., Nageris, B., Kornreich, L., and Ulanovski, D. (2015). Pattern of hearing loss following cochlear implantation. *Eur. Arch. Otorhinolaryngol.* 272, 2261–2266. doi: 10.1007/s00405-014-3184-2

Schmitt, H., Roemer, A., Zeilinger, C., Salcher, R., Durisin, M., Staecker, H., et al. (2018). Heat shock proteins in human perilymph: implications for cochlear implantation. *Otol. Neurotol.* 39, 37–44. doi: 10.1097/mao.0000000000001625

Simpson, T. H., McDonald, D., and Stewart, M. (1993). Factors affecting laterality of standard threshold shift in occupational hearing conservation programs. *Ear Hear.* 14, 322–331. doi: 10.1097/00003446-199310000-00003

Tuerdi, A., Kinoshita, M., Kamogashira, T., Fujimoto, C., Iwasaki, S., Shimizu, T., et al. (2017). Manganese superoxide dismutase influences the extent of noise-induced hearing loss in mice. *Neurosci. Lett.* 642, 123–128. doi: 10.1016/j.neulet.2017.02.003

Vlajkovic, S. M., Ambepitiya, K., Barclay, M., Boison, D., Housley, G. D., and Thorne, P. R. (2017). Adenosine receptors regulate susceptibility to noise-induced neural injury in the mouse cochlea and hearing loss. *Hear. Res.* 345, 43–51. doi: 10.1016/j.heares.2016.12.015

Warnecke, A., Prenzler, N. K., Schmitt, H., Daemen, K., Keil, J., Dursin, M., et al. (2019). Defining the inflammatory microenvironment in the human cochlea by perilymph analysis: toward liquid biopsy of the cochlea. *Front. Neurol.* 10:665. doi: 10.3389/fneur.2019.00665

Wilk, M., Hessler, R., Mugridge, K., Jolly, C., Fehr, M., Lenarz, T., et al. (2016). Impedance changes and fibrous tissue growth after cochlear implantation are correlated and can be reduced using a dexamethasone eluting electrode. *PLoS One* 11:e0147552. doi: 10.1371/journal.pone.0147552

Yamahara, K., Asaka, N., Kita, T., Kishimoto, I., Matsunaga, M., Yamamoto, N., et al. (2019). Insulin-like growth factor 1 promotes cochlear synapse regeneration after excitotoxic trauma *in vitro*. *Hear. Res.* 374, 5–12. doi: 10.1016/j.heares.2019.01.008

Yamahara, K., Yamamoto, N., Nakagawa, T., and Ito, J. (2015). Insulin-like growth factor 1: a novel treatment for the protection or regeneration of cochlear hair cells. *Anat. Rec.* 330, 2–9. doi: 10.1016/j.heares.2015.04.009

Yamamoto, N., Nakagawa, T., and Ito, J. (2014). Application of insulin-like growth factor-1 in the treatment of inner ear disorders. *Front. Pharmacol.* 5:208. doi: 10.3389/fphar.2014.00208

Yang, D., Zhou, H., Zhang, J., and Liu, L. (2015). Increased endothelial progenitor cell circulation and VEGF production in a rat model of noise-induced hearing loss. *Acta Otolaryngol.* 135, 622–628. doi: 10.3109/00016489.2014.1003092

Yu, Y., Szczepek, A. J., Haupt, H., and Mazurek, B. (2009). Geldanamycin induces production of heat shock protein 70 and partially attenuates ototoxicity caused by gentamicin in the organ of Corti explants. *J. Biomed. Sci.* 16:79. doi: 10.1186/1423-0127-16-79

12

Advances and Challenges in Pharmaceutical Therapies to Prevent and Repair Cochlear Injuries from Noise

Eric C. Bielefeld[1]* *and Megan J. Kobel*[1,2]

[1] *Department of Speech and Hearing Science, The Ohio State University, Columbus, OH, United States,*

[2] *Department of Otolaryngology-Head & Neck Surgery, The Ohio State University Wexner Medical Center, Columbus, OH, United States*

Correspondence:
Eric C. Bielefeld
bielefeld.6@osu.edu

Noise induces a broad spectrum of pathological injuries to the cochlea, reflecting both mechanical damage to the delicate architecture of the structures of the organ of Corti and metabolic damage within the organ of Corti and lateral wall tissues. Unlike ototoxic medications, the blood-labyrinth barrier does not offer protection against noise injury. The blood-labyrinth barrier is a target of noise injury, and can be weakened as part of the metabolic pathologies in the cochlea. However, it also offers a potential for therapeutic intervention with oto-protective compounds. Because the blood-labyrinth barrier is weakened by noise, penetration of blood-borne oto-protective compounds could be higher. However, systemic dosing for cochlear protection from noise offers other significant challenges. An alternative option to systemic dosing is local administration to the cochlea through the round window membrane using a variety of drug delivery techniques. The review will discuss noise-induced cochlear pathology, including alterations to the blood-labyrinth barrier, and then transition into discussing approaches for delivery of oto-protective compounds to reduce cochlear injury from noise.

Keywords: noise, cochlea, blood-labyrinth barrier, pharmaceutical, otoprotection, rescue

INTRODUCTION

Noise-induced hearing loss is a highly prevalent condition due to the combination of high-level noise in the workplace and in different non-occupational settings. Many countries have imposed occupational noise standards to minimize the number of workers sustaining NIHL. However, these standards are predicated upon a significant period of recovery during non-work hours. As recreational or simply non-occupational noise sources increase, the recovery interval for those exposed to noise decreases. Thus, NIHL continues to be a significant health hazard for many societies. In many of those societies, acoustic protection devices are widely available, but the expense, diminished auditory input, and discomfort associated with wearing them reduces their

---

Abbreviations: BLB, blood-labyrinth barrier; CSF, cerebrospinal fluid; IHC, inner hair cell; i.p., intra-peritoneal; IT, intratympanic; IV, intravenous; JNK, c-jun-N-terminal protein kinase; MP, methylprednisolone; NAC, n-acetyl, l-cysteine; NIHL, noise-induced hearing loss; OHC, outer hair cell; PTS, permanent threshold shift; RWM, round window membrane; s.c., sub-cutaneous; SGN, spiral ganglion neuron; TAAC, triamcinolone acetonide; TTS, temporary threshold shift.

use in several vulnerable populations. In addition, for the devices to be effective, they must be used properly, which can be challenging for some who are without access to specific training. Further, they are impractical in a number of settings where communication is needed, environmental noise perception is critical for safety, or where the noise exposures cannot be anticipated. Therefore, there has been an ongoing need to develop pharmaceutical approaches to reduce susceptibility to cochlear injury from noise.

Pharmaceutical protection from hearing loss has been explored against a number of the causes of acquired sensorineural hearing loss, including noise (see below), ototoxic medications (Campbell et al., 1996; Chen et al., 2007; Bielefeld et al., 2013), auto-immune disorders (Trune et al., 1999; Van Wijk et al., 2006), and aging (Bielefeld et al., 2008; Vlajkovic et al., 2011). These conditions have several common sites of pathology in the cochlea and share many of the same underlying mechanisms. All of the pharmaceutical approaches to preventing cochlear injury share the same challenges of the barriers of tissue uptake into the cochlea, and cellular uptake into the populations most vulnerable to injury. Despite the commonalities across these different cochlear insults, there are also many differences, and each carries its own set of challenges. For example, pharmaceutical protection from ototoxic drug-induced hearing loss has the advantage of a well-defined window for when cochlear injury might take place because the schedule of ototoxic drug delivered is clearly defined for the clinical patient. However, pharmaceutical protection is complicated because it must occur without comprising the health benefits the ototoxic drug offers. For auto-immune disorders, the onset is often sudden and without any warning. For that reason, pharmaceutical treatment is limited to rescue approaches. In rescue approaches, the treatment compound is given after the insult to minimize the amount of permanent injury. For age-related hearing loss, the challenge lies with the fact the hearing loss occurs gradually over a long period of time without a clearly identifiable underlying pathology that is consistent from patient to patient.

Noise presents a unique insult to the cochlea. However, addressing a pharmaceutical protection strategy for noise requires consideration of many of the challenges associated with other cochlear insults. Noise can induce simultaneous metabolic and mechanical changes that can injure the organ of Corti in both overlapping and separate ways (Henderson et al., 2006). The relative contribution of metabolic and mechanical damage to the cochlea is dictated by the sound pressure level, the duration, the frequency content, and the kurtosis factor of the noise exposure. Kurtosis factor estimates the deviation of a sample from the Gaussian distribution (Qiu et al., 2006) and can be used as a measure of the randomness of a noise exposure over time, with sensitivity to the peaks present in the exposure (Hamernik et al., 2003). Noise also offers challenges to pharmaceutical protection from the timing and dosing perspectives. Hazardous noise exposures can occur repeatedly over a period of months, years, or decades. In those cases, pharmaceutical protection from noise requires a compound with high efficacy that can be delivered to the cochlea without the systemic side effects associated with repeated dosing. Noise exposures can also occur suddenly without any opportunity to prepare. In those instances, there is a therapeutic window for rescue after the noise exposure in which the damage can be potentially mitigated pharmaceutically. This rescue approach carries an urgent need for the compound to reach the injured cells as quickly as possible in potentially high doses.

Further complicating the issue of drug delivery into the noise-exposed cochlea is the potential for noise exposure to alter blood flow to the cochlea, and to alter the BLB (discussed in more detail below). These alterations to the BLB may have the effect of increasing the penetration of rescue compounds into cochlear tissue, but also may change the distribution of the compounds within the different compartments and cells of the cochlea.

The current review will describe the myriad of strategies that have been tested with the goal of achieving pharmaceutical protection from noise injury, with a focus on the different approaches that have been taken to optimize drug delivery into the noise-exposed cochlea. Particular emphasis will be placed on the drug delivery challenges that are unique to noise protection. The review will begin with a description of the pathophysiologic changes that occur in the cochlea during and after exposure to hazardous noise. The impact of noise on the BLB will be discussed, along with implications that those changes may have on drug delivery. Finally, a review of different approaches that have been taken to treat the ear pharmaceutically through local drug delivery to the cochlea or systemic delivery in protection (drug delivery before noise exposure) and rescue (drug delivery after noise exposure) paradigms will be presented in order to critically evaluate the approaches that offer the most promise for clinical application in the noise-exposed patient population.

NOISE-INDUCED INJURY TO THE COCHLEA AND BLOOD-LABYRINTH BARRIER

Noise exposure causes a broad set of physical changes in cochlear structures, including the organ of Corti, neuronal terminals, spiral ligament, and stria vascularis (Wang Y. et al., 2002; Henderson et al., 2006; Ohlemiller, 2008). Mechanical injuries in the organ of Corti can result in holes in the reticular lamina (Ahmad et al., 2003), damaged stereocilia (Slepecky et al., 1981), and disconnection of the hair cells from supporting cells (Henderson et al., 2006). Metabolic stress includes proliferation of reactive oxygen species in the cochlea (Yamane et al., 1995; Ohlemiller et al., 1999; Yamashita et al., 2004). OHC loss has frequently been linked to PTS, and OHCs are known to be vulnerable to acoustic-related injury (Bohne and Harding, 2000; Wang Y. et al., 2002; Chen and Fechter, 2003). However, there is a poor correlation between OHC loss and degree of PTS in many mammalian species (Ohlemiller et al., 2000; Chen, 2002; Chen and Fechter, 2003), and in those cases, IHC loss can be better correlated with PTS (Nordmann et al., 2000; Harding et al., 2002). IHC loss after noise exposure is considerably smaller than OHC loss and generally occurs after OHC loss (Nordmann et al., 2000; Harding et al., 2002).

In addition to hair cell damage and loss, noise exposure can also lead to damage to Type I afferent neurons and their peripheral processes, which may underlie TTS (Robertson, 1983; Puel et al., 1998; Pujol and Puel, 1999). Swelling and vacuolization of afferent terminals after noise exposure may be due to glutamate excitotoxicity (Puel et al., 1998). After hair cell loss due to noise exposure, SGNs can undergo secondary degeneration, especially in regions with destroyed IHCs (Stankovic et al., 2004; Sugawara et al., 2005). Long-term survival of neurons is enhanced by the presence of intact supporting cells (Stankovic et al., 2004; Sugawara et al., 2005). Supporting cells sit in close proximity to the unmyelinated portion of the SGNs near the hair cell synapses and express many markers similar to the glial cells in the central nervous system that provide necessary trophic support (Rio et al., 2002; Stankovic et al., 2004). In cochlear regions with IHC loss, degeneration of peripheral axons has been detected at 1 week after noise exposure, and degeneration of cell bodies at 8 weeks after noise exposure (Wang Y. et al., 2002).

Since hair cell loss occurs directly after noise exposure and SGN degeneration follows a much longer time course, this degeneration was believed to occur secondarily to hair cell loss (Stankovic et al., 2004; Kujawa and Liberman, 2009). However, evidence suggests that primary SGN loss can occur in the absence of hair cell loss over a period of several months to years after noise exposure (Kujawa and Liberman, 2006, 2009; Lin et al., 2011).

Protection of the cochlea and vestibular end organs from invasion by external pathogens comes in part from the BLB. The cochlea is characterized by the presence of three distinct fluid compartments, two of which are filled with perilymph and one with endolymph. Perilymph is characterized by its 0 mV electrical charge and ionic composition consistent with blood plasma or CSF. Scala media also contains cortilymph in the space underneath the reticular lamina, but above the basilar membrane. This fluid is ionically the same as perilymph, and bathes the cells of the organ of Corti below their apical surfaces. See **Figure 1A** for a representative cross section of the cochlea showing the three chambers. The exact origins of perilymph and cortilymph from within the body are unknown, as it may be filtered from plasma or be CSF that has entered the labyrinth through the cochlear aqueduct (Kaupp and Giebel, 1980) or via the internal auditory meatus (Glueckert et al., 2018). Endolymph is the fluid of scala media above the reticular lamina that drives the depolarization of the hair cells through its positive endocochlear electrical potential and its high K+ concentration. The endocochlear potential is generated by the active mechanism in the marginal cells of stria vascularis. Therefore, in order to restrict access to cells of the organ of Corti, the BLB must restrict access from the bloodstream into both the endolymph, via stria vascularis, and the perilymph/cortilymph. The intra-strial barrier is characterized by many of the same mechanisms that define the blood-brain barrier. Materials must cross from the bloodstream, through the capillaries within stria vascularis, and those capillary walls represent a major site of the BLB. See **Figure 1B** for a schematic of a cross section of the stria vascularis and the capillaries that run through it (Jin et al., 2009). The endothelial cells on the walls of the strial capillaries are connected by tight junctions (Juhn, 1988). Those endothelial cells are supported by a basement membrane and population of pericyte cells (Shi, 2009), the latter of which may have a regulatory role in cochlear blood flow (Dai et al., 2009). Further, the BLB at the level of the strial capillaries is formed in part by processes from perivascular resident macrophage type-melanocyte cells to further seal the capillary walls (Shi, 2010; Zhang et al., 2012). See Shi (2016) for a detailed review of the structure of the strial capillary BLB. The pericytes and perivascular resident macrophage type-melanocytes help to control the expression of the tight junctions between the endothelial cells (Neng et al., 2013). The blood-perilymph barrier is more difficult to characterize, due to the multiple possible origin points for the perilymph. If perilymph is derived from CSF through the cochlear aqueduct, then the blood-CSF barrier at the level of choroid plexi is separating the perilymph from the blood. In the choroid plexi, the blood-CSF barrier is formed by tight junctions between epithelial cells (Dando et al., 2014). Tight junctions of the epithelial cells of the arachnoid mater aid the blood-CSF barrier (Dando et al., 2014), as do tight junction of endothelial cells in the venous system within the sub-arachnoid space (Abbott, 2013). Locally at the level of the cochlea itself, tight junctions have been detected between the endothelial cells of capillaries in the modiolus ("M" on **Figure 1A**) and the mesothelial cells of the capillaries of spiral limbus ("SpLim" on **Figure 1A**; Jahnke, 1980), indicating a direct blood-perilymph barrier in the cochlea. Overall, due to the many possible points of entry from the blood to the perilymph, it is difficult to assess the blood-perilymph barrier anatomically. However, there has been research on noise effects on the transport of mannitol from the blood into the perilymph, and the finding was that impulse noise exposure does not alter the blood-perilymph barrier (Laurell et al., 2008). In contrast, there is evidence that noise exposure can damage the BLB at the level of stria vascularis. In stria vascularis, the pericyte cells' connections to the capillary endothelial cells are weakened by high-level noise exposure (Shi, 2009). Horseradish peroxidase was found to leak from chinchillas' strial blood vessels into the intra-strial spaces when the horseradish peroxidase was injected 25–30 min after a 22-min noise exposure at 122 dB SPL (Hukee and Duvall, 1985). Further, polyethyleneimine transport from strial blood vessels into cochlear tissues, specifically Reissner's membrane, was increased in the ears of guinea pigs that had been exposed to a 105-dB SPL noise for 30 min (Suzuki et al., 2002). Such increases were not detected in spiral ligament, spiral limbus, or the basilar membrane. Increased permeability for lanthanum nitrate particles from cochlear blood vessels into strial tissue after 115 dB SPL noise for 4 or 6 h/day for 2 days was detected in albino guinea pigs (Wu et al., 2014). The noise-induced increase in permeability of the BLB has been attributed to noise-induced depletion of ATP causing a reduction in activity of the Na^+-K^+-ATPase pump, which in turn, increases permeability of the tight junctions that characterize the functionality of the BLB (Yang et al., 2011).

Overall, the literature indicates that noise can cause a breakdown of the BLB at the level of the strial vasculature (Hukee and Duvall, 1985; Suzuki et al., 2002; Wu et al., 2014). The exact timing of those changes and recovery of the BLB after noise exposure are not explicitly clear, nor are the different

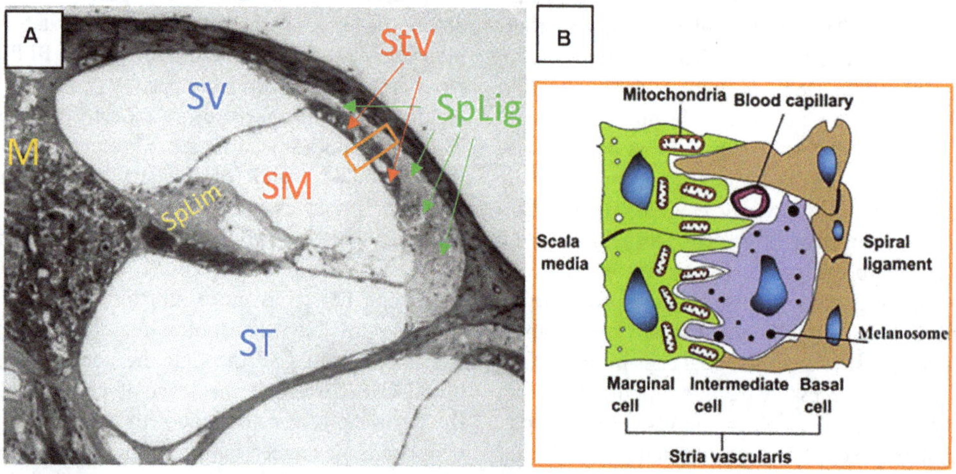

FIGURE 1 | (A) Cross section of the cochlea. SV, scala vestibuli; SM, scala media; ST, scala tympani; StV, stria vascularis; SpLig, spiral ligament; M, modiolus; SpLim, spiral limbus. Note how spiral ligament surrounds stria vascularis, as it represents a connection point between substances in the perilymph of scala vestibuli and scala tympani, with the endolymph of scala media through the stria vascularis. The orange rectangle is a cross section of stria vascularis and spiral ligament that is schematized in panel **(B)**. **(B)** The schematic structure of the stria vascularis. Please note the capillary running through the middle of the stria vascularis between the basal and marginal cells and above the intermediate cell. Tight junctions, the basement membrane, pericytes, and perivascular resident macrophage type-melanocytes create the BLB separating the blood from the intra-strial space. Panel **(A)** is an image kindly supplied by Dr. Jianxin Bao of Northeast Ohio Medical University.

dynamics of changes to the BLB with different noise parameters (level, duration, frequency content, and kurtosis). The reduction in the BLB seen after noise exposures indicates that, at least for a window of time after noise exposure, the cochlea may be maximally accessible for drug delivery. In the cases of oto-protective compounds, this could offer a window for optimal delivery of compounds in rescue paradigms.

RESCUE APPROACHES USING SYSTEMIC DRUG DELIVERY

Systemic drug delivery methods are those delivered to the entire body, with the goal of getting a portion of the compound into the tissue that is in need. Systemic approaches offer the advantages of ease of drug delivery and the potential for repeated dosing to enhance therapeutic benefit. The disadvantages include exposure of other tissue systems in the body to compounds that could affect them negatively (side effects), potentially lower drug penetration into tissues that are sequestered from the blood, such as the brain or labyrinth, and uncertainty about pharmacokinetics of the compounds when delivered through different approaches. Because of the compromised BLB seen after noise exposure, drug access to cochlear fluids may be higher during a window of time after the noise has ended. That window of cochlear access may contribute to the effectiveness of rescue approaches to reduce NIHL. In pharmaceutical rescue from noise, i.p. and s.c. injections, have been tested extensively. A rescue approach to noise oto-protection is defined as one in which the pharmaceutical is delivered exclusively after the completion of the noise, and can be contrasted with a protection paradigm in which the oto-protective compound is delivered before the noise. Many protection paradigms also include dosing after the noise has finished, but the key distinction between protection and rescue is when the first dose of the oto-protective compound is delivered. For protection, that first dose is before the noise, and for rescue, the first dose (and all subsequent doses) is delivered after the noise. It should be noted that a very large number of additional pharmaceuticals have demonstrated oto-protective capabilities in protection paradigms, but the focus here is on rescue experiments in which the compounds are first delivered after the noise has ended. Therefore, we are excluding protection experiments that used systemic dosing that began before the noise exposure, even if the dosing continued after the noise exposure finished. For the following experiments reviewed, the experimental conditions are broadly summarized in **Table 1** for comparisons.

Riluzole, a wide-spectrum neuroprotective agent that can inhibit apoptosis and necrosis, was found to promote recovery from compound action potential threshold shift when given by i.p. injection daily for 5 days after a 30-min noise exposure (Wang J. et al., 2002). Injections beginning at 30 min and 1 h after the noise promoted recovery that was equivalent to when the drug was injected 30 min before the noise. When the first injection was at 3 h, the effectiveness diminished, and diminished further when the injections started at six or 12 h. By 24 h, the rescue effect was gone. This indicated a maximum window for the onset of therapeutic intervention between 12 and 24 h post-noise.

Glucocorticoids have been used in several different paradigms as an oto-protectant against NIHL (see below for local delivery approaches). Systemic rescue with MP was achieved, with partial, but statistically significant, reduction in PTS when MP was

TABLE 1 | The experiments and noise exposure, drug, and animal model variables listed for each systemic rescue experiment discussed in Section "Rescue Approaches Using Systemic Drug Delivery."

Experiment	Compound	Animal	Route	Noise duration and dB SPL	Time of first injection after noise	Subsequent injections	Efficacy of rescue
Wang Y. et al., 2002	Riluzole	Guinea pig	i.p.	30 min – 120 dB SPL	30 min, 1, 3, 6, 12, or 24 h	Once per day for 5 days	Partial
Tabuchi et al., 2006	MP	ddY mouse	unknown	4 h – 128 dB SPL	Immediate or 3 h	None	Partial
Bao et al., 2013	MP	C57BL/6J mouse	i.p.	30 min–110 dB SPL	24 h	None	Partial
Han et al., 2015	Dexamethasone	C57BL/6J mouse	i.p.	1 h – 110 dB SPL	1 day	Once on day 4	Nearly complete
Zhou et al., 2009	MP	Guinea pig	i.m.	60 impulses – 165 dB pSPL	1 h	3 injections within 48 h	Partial
Campbell et al., 2007	D-methionine	Chinchilla	i.p.	6 h – 105 dB SPL	1 h	5 injections, one every 12 h	Nearly complete
Campbell et al., 2011	D-methionine	Chinchilla	i.p.	6 h – 105 dB SPL	3, 5, or 7 h	5 injections, one every 12 h	Nearly complete
Lo et al., 2013	D-methionine	Albino guinea pig	i.p.	6 h – 105 dB SPL	1 h	5 injections, one every 12 h	Partial
Coleman et al., 2007a	NAC or acetyl carnitine	Chinchilla	i.p.	6 h – 105 dB SPL	1, 4, or 12 h	5 injections, one every 12 h	Partial
Coleman et al., 2007b	AM-111	Chinchilla	i.p.	150 impulses – 155 dB pSPL	1 or 4 h	None	Partial
Bielefeld et al., 2011	KX1-004 or KX1-004+NAC	Chinchilla	s.c.	1 h – 112 dB SPL	1 and 24 h	None	Partial
Park et al., 2014	Renexin	C57BL/6 mice	Intra-gastric	1 h – 110 dB SPL	24 h	Once per day for 7 days	Nearly complete
Yamashita et al., 2005	Salicylate and trolox	Guinea pig	s.c. and i.p	5 h – 120 dB SPL	1 h, 1, 3, or 5 days	Twice daily until day 14	Partial
Vlajkovic et al., 2014	Adenosine amine congener	Wistar rat	i.p.	2 h – 110 dB SPL	12 h, 1, 2, or 3 days	Once every 24 h for 5 days	Partial

delivered immediately after noise to ddY mice. When given 3 h after the noise, there was no rescue effect on PTS. It should be noted that method of systemic delivery was not reported (Tabuchi et al., 2006). In contrast to the evidence that the window of rescue with MP is closed within 3 h of the noise, MP delivered to C57BL/6J mice via i.p. injection was able to reduce PTS when given at 24 h post-noise (Bao et al., 2013). Similarly, dexamethasone delivered by i.p.in C57BL/6J mice was able to provide nearly complete protection, measured 7 days after noise, when the dexamethasone was delivered one and 4 days after noise (Han et al., 2015). MP has also been used to induce rescue from impulse noise injury. Guinea pigs exposed to 165 dB pSPL impulses showed lower threshold shifts at 4 weeks when rescue treated with intra-muscular MP beginning at 1 h after the noise (Zhou et al., 2009).

D-methionine has been used to reduce oxidative stress-mediated cochlear injury from noise (Kopke et al., 2002) and ototoxic compounds (Campbell et al., 2007). As a rescue agent, it was delivered to chinchillas via i.p. injection starting 1 h after a 6-h noise exposure, with another four injections, one every 12 h, thereafter. The D-methionine injections reduced PTS across frequencies compared to controls injected with saline vehicle (Campbell et al., 2007). The rescue effect was also detected, without significant weakening, when the injections started at 3, 5, or 7 h after the same noise exposure (Campbell et al., 2011). A dose-dependent effect was also produced in the albino guinea pig, exposed to a 6-h noise and given i.p. injections D-methionine starting 1 h post-noise, and repeated every 12 h (Lo et al., 2013). The same experimental noise paradigm used by Campbell et al. (2007, 2011), injection pattern (every 12 h after initial dose), and animal model was also used to test the rescue effect of NAC and acetyl carnitine. Significant PTS reduction was found when the injections began 1 or 4 h after the noise concluded, but the effect was weaker when the injections began at 4 h compared to one. When the injections began at 12 h, no protection was found (Coleman et al., 2007a). AM-111, a proprietary compound containing D-JNK-1, a JNK inhibitor targeted to prevent noise-induced apoptosis, was also tested in chinchillas via i.p. injection 1 or 4 h after a noise exposure of repeated 155 dB pSPL impulses. Both injection times yielded significantly reduced PTS, with a slightly weaker effect from the 4-h injections (Coleman et al., 2007b). KX1-004, a Src-protein tyrosine kinase inhibitor, was also able to reduce PTS in chinchillas when given by s.c. injection one and 24 h after a 1-h noise exposure, either alone or in combination with NAC given i.p. (Bielefeld et al., 2011). Unpublished data from the authors of Bielefeld et al. (2011) using a rescue approach also indicated that additional injections after 24 h were not effective in creating a stronger rescue effect. These sets of findings corroborated the general notion that rescue intervention within a 12-h window after noise could significantly reduce PTS.

Despite the finding with riluzole that the critical window closes between 12 and 24 h after exposure, several studies have found rescue effects for interventions that commenced after 12 h post-noise. Renexin, a proprietary compound whose effects in the cochlea are believed to include increased blood flow and suppression of superoxide, improved recovery of thresholds by ~5–10 dB in mice when given after a 1-h noise exposure (Park et al., 2014). The dosing was delivered intragastrically, beginning at 24 h post-exposure. Salicylate acts as a free radical scavenger, and has been shown to reduce gentamicin ototoxicity (Chen et al., 2007). Salicylate was also given s.c. in combination with i.p. trolox, an analog of vitamin E, as rescue agents against NIHL. The series of injections began at different times, 1 h, 1, 3, or 5 days after the 5-h noise exposure concluded. The injections were delivered twice daily until an endpoint of 14 days post-noise. Each of the injection series significantly attenuated PTS, OHC loss, and oxidative stress from the noise. However, the protective effect got progressively weaker with each delay in the onset of the injections, with the strongest protection from the injections starting at 1 h, and the weakest protection when the injections started at 5 days (Yamashita et al., 2005). Rescue after a 2-h noise exposure in rats with an adenosine amine congener, delivered i.p., reduced PTS when injections commenced 12 or 24 h after the noise, and the effect was equally strong with either starting time. There was a small protective effect when the injections began at 48 h, but no effect when started at 72 h (Vlajkovic et al., 2014).

Collectively, the experiments on rescue after noise exposure indicate that the optimal intervention time is essentially as soon as possible after the noise, and that the effect is weaker when the intervention begins after 24 h. However, they also indicate that intervention at or after 24 h can produce some rescue effect in some models. What remains uncertain is how much of a role the type of compound used, the animal model, the route of administration, the dose levels, the number and type of subsequent injections, and the acoustic parameters of the noise exposure have on the rescue effect. Finally, though the BLB is compromised after noise exposure, it is unknown whether increased permeability of the BLB affected any of the rescue efficacy of the compounds described. Drug penetration into the cells vulnerable to injury from noise is inferred by the efficacy of the compounds in conferring rescue. Pharmacokinetics studies after systemic dosing are needed to further understand how/when the drugs are reaching the cochlear cells, to assess the effects of noise-induced changes to the BLB, and to determine how to optimize drug penetration to the cells in need.

LOCAL DELIVERY OF OTO-PROTECTIVE COMPOUNDS TO THE COCHLEA

For protection or rescue from noise injury, a prime target has been local delivery of compounds directly into the cochlea. This approach avoids major concerns about systemic side effects. Access to the cochlea through diffuse through the RWM and/or the oval window membrane provide direct access to the perilymph of scala tympani and scala vestibule directly, as does a cochleostomy [see **Figure 2** from Zou et al. (2016) for schematic representation of access to the perilymph through the oval window and RWM]. This would provide access to the cells of the organ of Corti via diffusion from the cortilymph (see blue arrow on the inset cross section diagram of **Figure 2**). Scala media and the endolymph are much harder to access, and therefore local delivery does not necessarily circumvent the BLB at the level of stria vascularis (**Figure 1**). Thus, compounds that are dependent upon crossing from the endolymph through the transduction channels of the stereocilia in order to penetrate the hair cells may not be effective in local delivery. Further, there are challenges with sustaining the compound within the cochlear tissues and optimizing drug delivery in the least invasive manner possible. Drug delivery to the cochlea through local delivery via the RWM has received significant attention due to increases in perilymph concentration (Salt and Plontke, 2009; Plontke and Salt, 2018) and reduction in plasma serum levels (Parnes et al., 1999; Chandrasekhar et al., 2000; Chen et al., 2003a; Bird et al., 2007; Salt and Plontke, 2009). However, applicability of RWM application clinically is restricted to agents that are efficacious when administered after trauma, as patients are unlikely to elect to undergo an invasive procedure prior to known exposure. The RWM acts as a semi-permeable membrane and application can be accomplished via IT injection into the middle ear space or, for more precise and sustained deliveries, using hydrogel formulations (Paulson et al., 2008; Borden et al., 2011) or osmotic mini-pump perfusion (Salt and Plontke, 2005). The assumed route of drug delivery is diffusion across the RMW with secondary diffusion through the oval window (Bachmann

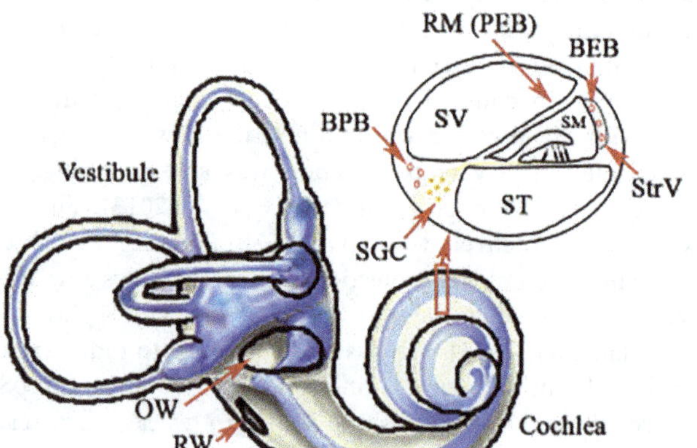

FIGURE 2 | Illustration of the inner ear, with highlights of the oval (OW) and round windows (RW). The inset displays a cross section of the cochlear chambers. Scala vestibuli (SV) and scala tympani (ST) are filled with perilymph and are accessible through local delivery of compounds into the middle ear space or through a cochleostomy. Scala media (SM) is filled with endolymph and separated from the blood by the blood-strial barrier in stria vascularis (StrV).

et al., 2001; Salt et al., 2012a; Salt and Hirose, 2018) and possible entrance via the otic capsule in some animal models (Mikulec et al., 2009). The bony otic capsule in the apical turns is very thin in some species, such as guinea pigs and chinchillas. Drugs applied filling the entire bulla rather than irrigating against the RWM, showed significantly higher apical concentrations suggesting permeability of the bony otic capsule (Mikulec et al., 2009). Drugs applied via IT injections can be lost in the middle ear via the Eustachian tube, middle ear vasculature and lymphatics (Salt and Plontke, 2018), and the use of gel formulations has been shown to stabilize retention in the middle ear (Wang et al., 2009, 2011). Protective effects from noise exposure are achieved through actions on multiple pathways underlying NIHL, including anti-inflammatory (Chi et al., 2011), anti-apoptotic (Wang et al., 2007) and antioxidant and free radical scavenging (Alagic et al., 2011). Overall protective effects for local application are typically greater than systemic delivery methods (Wang J. et al., 2002; Han et al., 2015) due to the presumed higher level of detectable concentrations in the cochlea. Similarly, prolonged applications rather than single applications have been seen to be more efficacious (Harrop-Jones et al., 2016) due to the presumed increase in duration of delivery.

Perilymphatic fluid is the primary medium for local pharmacotherapeutic administration. Inner ear fluids do not show appreciable movement or "stirring" and locally applied drugs are dependent on passive diffusion rates (Salt and Ma, 2001; Salt, 2002; Salt and Plontke, 2005). Dependent on perilymph sampling methods, local administration results in substantial base-to-apex gradients in agent concentration (Laurell et al., 2002; Mynatt et al., 2006; Bird et al., 2007; Plontke et al., 2007; Salt, 2008; Creber et al., 2018), as reflected in cochlear tissue labeling (Laurell et al., 2002; Grewal et al., 2013; Creber et al., 2018). These gradients are lower for hydrogel applications (Salt et al., 2011) or intracochlear injections in comparison to IT solution injections into the middle ear space (Hahn et al., 2012). Additionally, a significant variability in perilymph concentrations is seen between individual humans or animal species for RWM local delivery (Bird et al., 2007) which is diminished for hydrogel (Borden et al., 2011; Salt et al., 2011) and intra-cochlear delivery (Hahn et al., 2012).

Glucocorticoids, including MP and dexamethasone, have received significant research in inner ear pharmacokinetics and tissue uptake, more so than for other agents, as local administration is used clinically for treatment of several inner ear disorders including NIHL (Bird et al., 2007; Swan et al., 2008; Zhou et al., 2009; Stachler et al., 2012; Trune and Canlon, 2012). Glucocorticoids are effective for protection from hazardous impact of noise through suppression of cochlear responses to oxidative stress, ischemia, and inflammation. Glucocorticoids have been shown to modulate the inflammatory response through inhibition of tumor necrosis factor α–induced cytokine secretion from cochlear spiral ligament fibrocytes *in vitro*, increasing cochlear blood flow *in vivo*, and enhancing glutathione biosynthesis in the cochlear spiral ganglion (Shirwany et al., 1998; Maeda et al., 2005; Nagashima and Ogita, 2006). While several have investigated the impact of RWM drug administration on noise exposure and many studies have examined the pharmacokinetics of glucocorticoids in the inner ear, there have been relatively few studies examining both in the same population.

In general, local administration of MP or dexamethasone leads to greater perilymph concentration than systemic application (Bird et al., 2007; Yang et al., 2008; Grewal et al., 2013; Creber et al., 2018; Lee et al., 2018). For example, in humans, local IT administration of 40 mg of MP led to a 126-fold greater perilymph concentration after a single 1 mg/kg IV injection and 33-fold increase after 10 mg/kg IV infusion (Bird et al., 2007). After RWM application of 20% dexamethasone in guinea pigs, a higher tissue uptake and greater perilymph concentration of approximately two orders of magnitude than that after systemic IV delivery of 2 mg/kg (Creber et al., 2018). Additionally, higher and more prolonged intracochlear uptake was seen after administration of 3 IT injections of 20 μL of 10 mg/mL of fluorescein isothiocyanate-labeled dexamethasone in comparison to 3 i.p. injections of 60 μG/100 g (Lee et al., 2018). Tissue labeling after local administration mirrors glucocorticoid receptor distribution with the highest labeling in the SGNs, organ of Corti, and lateral walls (Lee et al., 2018) corresponding to the highest concentration of receptors in cochlear structures (Zuo et al., 1995). Dexamethasone perilymph elimination half-life has been calculated to be 111 min (Salt et al., 2012b) with peak glucocorticoid receptor activation, dexamethasone tissue labeling, and perilymph concentration 60 min after local application (Hargunani et al., 2006; Yang et al., 2008; Grewal et al., 2013). After this, perilymph concentrations after IT injection show elimination from perilymph by around 6 h (Parnes et al., 1999; Bird et al., 2007; Yang et al., 2008). Dexamethasone labeling in cochlear tissue is present up to 7 days after administration (Lee et al., 2018), but significant decreases in uptake and labeling are seen by 12 h (Wang et al., 2011; Grewal et al., 2013). Greater dexamethasone uptake and immunofluorescent labeling has been reported in IHCs compared to OHCs in mice (Grewal et al., 2013), but this selective uptake has not been seen across species (Creber et al., 2018). Cochlear tissue penetration exhibited a base-to-apex gradient, similar to perilymph concentrations, suggesting that tissue penetration is proportionally related to perilymph concentrations (Grewal et al., 2013; Creber et al., 2018). However, this gradient was not seen in receptor activation in SGNs in guinea pigs (Creber et al., 2018), which indicates a dissociation between end organ target receptor activation and perilymph concentrations.

Local glucocorticoid administration prior to noise exposure has been shown to protect against compound threshold shifts measured 7 days after exposure (Takemura et al., 2004; Harrop-Jones et al., 2016). For the following experiments reviewed, the broad experimental parameters and protective effects are provided in **Table 2** to allow comparison. Efficacy of pre-exposure IT injections are time-dependent with reduced protection seen by 24 h prior suggesting that early administration is limited due to clearance from the perilymph at the time of injury (Yildirim et al., 2005; Harrop-Jones et al., 2016). Sustained release using thermoreversible hydrogels as a drug carrier has been shown to increase dexamethasone concentrations and provide lasting exposure in guinea pigs and sheep for days to weeks (Wang

TABLE 2 | The experiments and noise exposure, drug, and animal model variables listed for each systemic rescue experiment discussed in Section "Local delivery of Oto-Protective Compounds to the Cochlea."

Experiment	Compound	Animal	Compound delivery	Noise duration and dB SPL	Time of first injection	Subsequent Injections	Efficacy
Zhu et al., 2018	Dexamethasone or TAAC	Guinea pig	Hydrogel	3 h – 120 dB SPL	Immediately post-noise	None	None (TAAC), Partial (DEX)
Mamelle et al., 2018	Dexamethasone	Guinea pig	Hydrogel	1 h – 100 dB SPL	48 h post-noise	None	None
Harrop-Jones et al., 2016	OTO-104 or Dexamethasone	Guinea pig	Hydrogel (OTO-104), solution (DEX)	2 h – 105 or 110 dB SPL	1 day prior, 2, 3, or 4 days post-noise	None	Partial (OTO-104), None (DEX)
Chi et al., 2011	Dexamethasone	Albino guinea pig	Gelfoam	80 impulses – 167 dB pSPL	1 day post-noise	None	Partial
Sendowski et al., 2006	MP	Guinea pig	Intracochlear osmotic pump	3 impulses – 170 dB pSPL	Immediately post-noise	Continuously for 7 days	Partial
Zhou et al., 2009	MP	Guinea pig	Solution	60 impulses – 165 dB pSPL	1 h	4 injections, one every 48 h	Partial
Han et al., 2015	Dexamethasone	C57BL.6J mice	Solution	1 h – 110 dB SPL	1 day post-noise	4 days after noise	Nearly complete
Alagic et al., 2011	D-methionine	Guinea pig	Solution	45 min – 100 dB	90 min prior	None	Partial
Zou et al., 2003	NAC	Guinea pig	Gelfoam	15 min vibration – 108 dB	24, 48, or 72 h or 7 days prior	None	None
Bielefeld et al., 2013	4-[2-amino-ethyl]benzenesulfonyl fluoride	Chinchilla	Solution	6 h – 106 dB SPL or 75 impulses – 155 dB pSPL	Immediately prior	None	Partial (impulse), none (continuous noise)
Wang et al., 2007	D-JNK-1	Guinea pig	Osmotic pump onto RWM or hydrogel	15 min – 130 dB SPL	30 min before, 1, 4, 6, 12 or 24 h post	Continuously for 7 days (osmotic pump), None (hydrogel)	Nearly complete if within 12 h
Wang et al., 2003	D-JNK-1	Guinea pig	Intracochlear osmotic pump	30 min – 120 dB SPL	2 days prior	Continuously for 7 days	Nearly complete
Coleman et al., 2007b	AM-111	Chinchilla	Hyrdogel or osmotic pump	150 impulses – 155 dB pSPL	1 or 4 h	None	Partial
Wang J. et al., 2002	Riluzole	Guinea pig	Intracochlear osmotic pump	30 min – 120 dB SPL	2 days prior	Continuously for 7 days	Partial
Chen et al., 2003b	Caroverine	Guinea pig	Gelfoam	1 h – 110 dB SPL	1 or 24 h post	None	Partial if 1 h, None if 24 h
Chen et al., 2004	Caroverine	Guinea pig	Gelfoam	1 h – 110 dB SPL	10 min prior	None	Partial

et al., 2009, 2011; Borden et al., 2011). However, protective effects have been limited (Yildirim et al., 2005; Harrop-Jones et al., 2016; Mamelle et al., 2018; Zhu et al., 2018). Zhu et al. (2018) utilized hydrogels containing 6% dexamethasone or 30% TAAC prior to a 3-h 120 dB SPL noise exposure in guinea pigs. No PTS protection was achieved 28 days after exposure, but a small protective effect was noted at 7 days. As well, there was significantly higher preserved SGN density in the first turn in the dexamethasone group, suggesting possible protection against supra-threshold ABR amplitude loss (hidden hearing loss). No protection in thresholds or cochlear structures was noted for TAAC (Zhu et al., 2018). A similar lack of threshold protection was seen with 1% dexamethasone hydrogel application 48 h after a 1-h 100 dB SPL noise exposure in guinea pigs (Mamelle et al., 2018). However, use of 2 or 6% OTO-104, a poloxamer hydrogel containing dexamethasone, 1 day prior and up to 3 days after a 2-h 105 dB SPL noise exposure yielded significant functional protection, as assessed through ABR thresholds 7 days after exposure. No protective effect was noted at any time point utilizing IT injections of dexamethasone sodium phosphate solution (Harrop-Jones et al., 2016). The differing results between these studied utilizing hydrogels may be secondary to differences in drug formulation and noise exposure parameters which induced a larger threshold shift in the Zhu et al. (2018) study. Both Zhu et al. (2018) and Harrop-Jones et al. (2016) noted some protective effect at 7 days after exposure. However, the final time point in Zhu et al. (2018) was 28 days and animals were not followed to this time point by Harrop-Jones et al. (2016). Additionally, while a significant rescue effect was noted by Harrop-Jones et al. (2016) this was not seen by Mamelle et al. (2018) which may be attributed to differences in drug formulation or dosages (1% vs. 2% or 6%).

Rescue paradigms with delivery through an osmotic pump, or gelatin sponge, or IT injections has mixed effects on PTS protection despite reduction in HC loss (Sendowski et al., 2006; Zhou et al., 2009; Chi et al., 2011; Han et al., 2015). Chi et al. (2011) applied dexamethasone to the round window niche in guinea pigs using gelfoam 1 day after exposure to repeated 167 dB pSPL impulses. After application, perilymph sampling revealed a peak concentration at 15 min (over 5000 ug/ml) with a 17-fold decrease in concentration by 6 h (~300 ug/ml). Significant reductions in threshold shifts and HC loss were noted 3 weeks post-exposure without accompanying protection of SGN morphology (Chi et al., 2011). In contrast, intracochlear MP for 7 days initiated immediately after exposure to 170 dB pSPL impulses in guinea pigs showed functional protection of threshold shifts at 48 h but not 14 days. However, IHC and OHC loss 14 days post-exposure was reduced from 30 to 46%, respectively, to 8 and 16% (Sendowski et al., 2006). Single rescue IT injections after exposure have been shown to provide functional protection of ABR thresholds and DPOAE amplitudes with accompanying HC protection when initiated within 24 h after the noise (Zhou et al., 2009; Han et al., 2015). In a patient population presenting for treatment 3 days to 2 weeks after noise exposure, IT MP injections given in conjunction with standard systemic therapy showed a larger improvement in thresholds than systemic therapy alone (Zhou et al., 2013).

Antioxidants and ROS scavengers have undergone significant investigation through multiple administration routes; however, RWM application has received less attention in part due to limited functional protection. Laurell et al. (2002) studied kinetics and distribution of radioactive D-methionine and thiourea, small sulfur-containing molecules, in rats. Both D-methionine and thiourea showed peak concentrations at the earliest sample time of 17 min with a terminal half-life of 0.57 and 0.77 h after microinfusion to the RW niche for 1 h. Tracer expression was highest in the basal stria vascularis and organ of Corti, which was attributed to the diffusion gradient, as sampling did not allow direct measurement of perilymph concentration gradients (Laurell et al., 2002). Local D-methionine solution administered to the RW niche 90 min prior to noise exposure showed a reduction in TTS at 24 h post-noise exposure. D-methionine was still present in perilymph at 24 h post-application, which was the latest time point measured (Alagic et al., 2011).

While NAC has been seen to provide significant functional and morphologic protection to noise trauma when used through other routes of administration (Kopke et al., 2007), local application has been shown to cause a temporary increase in thresholds in the basal turn (Zou et al., 2003; Eastwood et al., 2010). As such, NAC failed to provide functional or morphologic protection in guinea pigs against a vibration-induced hearing loss model (Zou et al., 2003). Bielefeld (2013) delivered an NADPH oxidase inhibitor across the RWM in chinchillas immediately prior to octave band or impulse noise. A reduction in PTS after exposure to the impulse noise was seen in treated animals; however, a significant effect was not seen for exposure to the octave band noise or in OHC counts for either exposure.

Substantial research supports that the JNK pathway underlies sensory cell death and cochlear inflammation (Eshraghi et al., 2013). D-JNK-1, a chemically synthesized cell permeable JNK ligand, has demonstrated protective effects via RWM local application when administered prior to noise exposure (Wang et al., 2003, 2007; Eshraghi et al., 2018). There is decreasing efficiency in rescue therapy in a time-dependent manner, with some efficacy of treatment seen as late as 6 h post-insult (Wang et al., 2007). While Eshraghi et al. (2018) report a "relatively flat" perilymph gradient on D-JNK-1 within hours after RWM application in the chinchilla, Wang et al. (2007) demonstrated a significant base-to-apex gradient in fluorescent labeling after one 30-min perfusion of FITC-conjugated D-JNK-1 peptides onto the RWM. In contrast to other small molecules, clearance of D-JNK-1 is relatively slow. Fluorescent staining was seen in hair cells and neurons throughout the scala tympani, with the exception of the stria vascularis, and extended into the scala vestibuli. Labeling was stable until 7 days after application, with decline starting at 14 days and limited detection at 21 days (Wang et al., 2007). However, whether strength of fluorescent staining correlates with pharmacologic activity has yet to be determined. Additionally, there is a relatively short time window for intervention blocking apoptotic processes using local application of D-JNK-1 after injury (Wang et al., 2007). Thus, extended cochlear presence may not provide additional therapeutic benefit. Prolonged exposure through intracochlear perfusion of D-JNK-1 initiated 2 days prior to exposure and continuing for 5 days after almost completely prevented permanent hearing loss and cochlear hair cell death (Wang et al., 2003). A similar effect was seen with application onto the intact RWM using either an osmotic pump or hydrogel formulation in a dose- and time-dependent manner (Wang et al., 2003; Coleman et al., 2007b). Single dose IT injections of AM-111, administered to 11 patients presenting within 24 h after firecracker injury, showed a possible therapeutic effect for some patients. However, due to the small number of patients and lack of control group, a potential effect was limited (Doz et al., 2007).

Riluzole, discussed above in systemic delivery, was also delivered intracochlearly for 2 days prior and 5 days after a 30-min noise exposure. The intracochlear riluzole treatment reduced compound action potential threshold shift and HC loss in guinea pigs. Reductions in mitochondrial damage, translocation of cytochrome c, and DNA fragmentation were also seen (Wang J. et al., 2002).

Caroverine, an AMPA and NMDA antagonist and antioxidant, has been shown to provide significant dose-dependent protection against noise in albino guinea pigs with local administration either immediately prior or up to 1 h post-exposure through blocking excitotoxic pathways (Chen et al., 2003b, 2004). However, the therapeutic window is relatively narrow, and application at 24 h failed to provide functional protection (Chen et al., 2004). Pharmacokinetics in the guinea pig after local gelfoam application of 15 μL of 1.6 or 12.8 mg/ml of caroverine showed peak perilymph concentrations 30 min post-administration, and they were 20 and 80 times higher than systemic administration of 4 mg/kg. Elimination from the perilymph was seen by 3 h for the lower dose and 6 h for the higher dose. Additionally, caroverine has been shown to cause a temporary increase in ABR thresholds and delay in ABR wave I latency up to 24 h after application, more so in the basal region with the highest assumed concentrations and at time points with highest detected perilymph concentrations, presumably through blocking glutamatergic activity (Chen et al., 2003a).

While RWM application has significant benefits due to the reduction in systemic side effects, generalizability of studies between species is limited by anatomic variation in the cochlea.

Dimensions of fluid spaces vary within species (Erixon et al., 2009; Avci et al., 2014) and considerably across species (Thorne et al., 1999). Additionally, the fluid space and scala tympani is significantly longer in larger mammals, including humans, which may further limit local application of an agent to more limited regions than seen in small animal models (Wang et al., 2011; Glueckert et al., 2018). Dexamethasone perilymph concentrations at the basal turn of the cochlea were 17- to 27- fold higher in guinea pigs than sheep after 2% dexamethasone application of 50 or 600 μL, respectively, to the round window niche (Wang et al., 2011). Additionally, there is substantial inter-individual variability in response to treatment, which may be related to the high variability in perilymph concentrations measured (Bird et al., 2007).

CONCLUSION

Noise exerts a complex and highly variable set of effects on the cochlea. Among those effects are those that impair the cochlea's sensitivity to acoustic stimuli (hair cell injury, reduction of the endocochlear potential, de-afferentation of the IHCs) and those that affect the homeostasis of the organ as a whole (blood flow changes, increased permeability of the BLB). Changes in permeability of the BLB can have injurious effects, such as increasing the penetration of ototoxic compounds into scala media. However, BLB permeability changes can also have beneficial effects, such as creating a window in which drugs delivered systemically can more easily access the organ of Corti. Indeed a window for rescue interventions, in which drugs are delivered after noise to promote recovery and decrease permanent injury, are clearly effective through 12–24 h after noise. This indicates that, clinically, unanticipated noise exposures can potentially be treated to minimize hearing loss. Further, local administration of drugs can increase cochlear access to compounds that are restricted by the BLB with the goal of rendering the ear less susceptible to permanent NIHL.

AUTHOR CONTRIBUTIONS

All authors listed have made a substantial, direct and intellectual contribution to the work, and approved it for publication.

ACKNOWLEDGMENTS

We thank Ryan Harrison and Riley DeBacker for their assistance in the preparation of this manuscript.

REFERENCES

Abbott, N. J. (2013). Blood-brain barrier structure and function and the challenges for CNS drug delivery. *J. Inherit. Metab. Dis.* 36, 437–449. doi: 10.1007/s10545-013-9608-0

Ahmad, M., Bohne, B. A., and Harding, G. W. (2003). An in vivo tracer strategy of noise-induced damage to the reticular lamina. *Hear. Res.* 185, 82–100. doi: 10.1016/s0378-5955(02)00713-x

Alagic, Z., Goiny, M., and Canlon, B. (2011). Protection against acoustic trauma by direct application of D-methionine to the inner ear. *Acta Otolaryngol.* 131, 802–808. doi: 10.3109/00016489.2011.564652

Avci, E., Nauwelaers, T., Lenarz, T., Hamacher, V., and Kral, A. (2014). Variations in microanatomy of the human cochlea. *J. Comp. Neurol.* 522, 3245–3261. doi: 10.1002/cne.23594

Bachmann, G., Su, J., Zumegen, C., Wittekindt, C., and Michel, O. (2001). [Permeability of the round window membrane for prednisolone-21-hydrogen succinate. Prednisolone content of the perilymph after local administration vs. systemic injection]. *HNO* 49, 538–542.

Bao, J., Hugerford, M., Luxmore, R., Ding, D., Qui, Z., Lei, D., et al. (2013). Prophylactic and therapeutic functions of drug combinations against noise-induced hearing loss. *Hear. Res.* 304, 33–40. doi: 10.1016/j.heares.2013.06.004

Bielefeld, E. C. (2013). Reduction in impulse noise-induced permanent threshold shift with intracochlear application of an NADPH oxidase inhibitor. *J. Am. Acad. Audiol.* 24, 461–473. doi: 10.3766/jaaa.24.6.3

Bielefeld, E. C., Coling, D., Chen, G. D., and Henderson, D. (2008). Multiple dosing strategies with acetyl L-carnitine (ALCAR) fail to alter age-related hearing loss in the Fischer 344/NHsd rat. *J. Negat. Results Biomed.* 7:4. doi: 10.1186/1477-5751-7-4

Bielefeld, E. C., Tanaka, C., Chen, G. D., Coling, D., Li, M., Henderson, D., et al. (2013). An Src-protein tyrosine kinase inhibitor to reduce cisplatin ototoxicity while preserving its antitumor effect. *Anticancer Drugs* 24, 43–51. doi: 10.1097/CAD.0b013e32835739fd

Bielefeld, E. C., Wantuck, R., and Henderson, D. (2011). Postexposure treatment with a Src-PTK inhibitor in combination with N-l-acetyl cysteine to reduce noise-induced hearing loss. *Noise Health* 13, 292–298. doi: 10.4103/1463-1741.82962

Bird, P. A., Begg, E. J., Zhang, M., Keast, A. T., Murray, D. P., and Balkany, T. J. (2007). Intratympanic versus intravenous delivery of methylprednisolone to cochlear perilymph. *Otol. Neurotol.* 28, 1124–1130. doi: 10.1097/MAO.0b013e31815aee21

Bohne, B. A., and Harding, G. W. (2000). Degeneration in the cochlear after noise damage: primary versus secondary events. *Am. J. Otol.* 21, 505–509.

Borden, R. C., Saunders, J. E., Berryhill, W. E., Krempl, G. A., Thompson, D. M., and Queimado, L. (2011). Hyaluronic acid hydrogel sustains the delivery of dexamethasone across the round window membrane. *Audiol. Neurootol.* 16, 1–11. doi: 10.1159/000313506

Campbell, K., Claussen, A., Meech, R., Verhulst, S., Fox, D., and Hughes, L. (2011). D-methionine (D-met) significantly rescues noise-induced hearing loss: timing studies. *Hear. Res.* 282, 138–144. doi: 10.1016/j.heares.2011.08.003

Campbell, K. C., Meech, R. P., Klemens, J. J., Gerberi, M. T., Dyrstad, S. S., Larsen, D. L., et al. (2007). Prevention of noise- and drug-induced hearing loss with D-methionine. *Hear. Res.* 226, 92–103. doi: 10.1016/j.heares.2006.11.012

Campbell, K. C., Rybak, L. P., Meech, R. P., and Hughes, L. (1996). D-methionine provides excellent protection from cisplatin ototoxicity in the rat. *Hear. Res.* 102, 90–98. doi: 10.1016/s0378-5955(96)00152-9

Chandrasekhar, S. S., Rubinstein, R. Y., Kwartler, J. A., Gatz, M., Connelly, P. E., Huang, E., et al. (2000). Dexamethasone pharmacokinetics in the inner ear: comparison of route of administration and use of facilitating agents. *Otolaryngol. Head Neck Surg.* 122, 521–528. doi: 10.1067/mhn.2000.102578

Chen, G., and Fechter, L. D. (2003). The relationship between noise-induced hearing loss and hair cell loss in rats. *Hear. Res.* 177, 81–90. doi: 10.1016/s0378-5955(02)00802-x

Chen, G. D. (2002). Effect of hypoxia on noise-induced auditory impairment. *Hear. Res.* 172, 186–195. doi: 10.1016/s0378-5955(02)00582-8

Chen, Y., Huang, W. G., Zha, D. J., Qiu, J. H., Wang, J. L., Sha, S. H., et al. (2007). Aspirin attenuates gentamicin ototoxicity: from the laboratory to the clinic. *Hear. Res.* 226, 178–182. doi: 10.1016/j.heares.2006.05.008

Chen, Z., Duan, M., Lee, H., Ruan, R., and Ulfendahl, M. (2003a). Pharmacokinetics of caroverine in the inner ear and its effects on cochlear function after systemic and local administrations in guinea pigs. *Audiol. Neurootol.* 8, 49–56. doi: 10.1159/000067893

Chen, Z., Ulfendahl, M., Ruan, R., Tan, L., and Duan, M. (2003b). Acute treatment of noise trauma with local caroverine application in the guinea pig. *Acta Otolaryngol.* 123, 905–909. doi: 10.1080/00016480310000638

Chen, Z., Ulfendahl, M., Ruan, R., Tan, L., and Duan, M. (2004). Protection of auditory function against noise trauma with local caroverine administration in guinea pigs. *Hear. Res.* 197, 131–136. doi: 10.1016/J.HEARES.2004.03.021

Chi, F.-L., Yang, M.-Q., Zhou, Y.-D., and Wang, B. (2011). Therapeutic efficacy of topical application of dexamethasone to the round window niche after acoustic trauma caused by intensive impulse noise in guinea pigs. *J. Laryngol. Otol.* 125, 673–685. doi: 10.1017/S0022215111000028

Coleman, J. K., Kopke, R. D., Liu, J., Ge, X., Harper, E. A., and Jones, G. E. (2007a). Pharmacological rescue of noise induced hearing loss using N-acetylcysteine and acetyl-L-carnitine. *Hear. Res.* 226, 104–113. doi: 10.1016/j.heares.2006.08.008

Coleman, J. K., Littlesunday, C., Jackson, R., and Meyer, T. (2007b). AM-111 protects against permanent hearing loss from impulse noise trauma. *Hear. Res.* 226, 70–78. doi: 10.1016/J.HEARES.2006.05.006

Creber, N. J., Eastwood, H. T., Hampson, A. J., Tan, J., and O'Leary, S. J. (2018). A comparison of cochlear distribution and glucocorticoid receptor activation in local and systemic dexamethasone drug delivery regimes. *Hear. Res.* 368, 75–85. doi: 10.1016/J.HEARES.2018.03.018

Dai, M., Nuttall, A., Yang, Y., and Shi, X. (2009). Visualization and contractile activity of cochlear pericytes in the capillaries of the spiral ligament. *Hear. Res.* 254, 100–107. doi: 10.1016/j.heares.2009.04.018

Dando, S. J., Mackay-Sim, A., Norton, R., Currie, B. J., St John, J. A., Ekberg, J. A., et al. (2014). Pathogens penetrating the central nervous system: infection pathways and the cellular and molecular mechanisms of invasion. *Clin. Microbiol. Rev.* 27, 691–726. doi: 10.1128/CMR.00118-13

Doz, P., Suckfuell, M., Canis, M., Strieth, S., Scherer, H., and Haisch, A. (2007). Intratympanic treatment of acute acoustic trauma with a cell-permeable JNK ligand: a prospective randomized phase I/II study Intratympanic treatment of acute acoustic trauma with a cell-permeable JNK ligand: a prospective randomized phase I/II study. *Acta Otolaryngol.* 127, 938–942. doi: 10.1080/00016480601110212

Eastwood, H., Pinder, D., James, D., Chang, A., Galloway, S., Richardson, R., et al. (2010). Permanent and transient effects of locally delivered n-acetyl cysteine in a guinea pig model of cochlear implantation. *Hear. Res.* 259, 24–30. doi: 10.1016/J.HEARES.2009.08.010

Erixon, E., Högstorp, H., Wadin, K., and Rask-Andersen, H. (2009). Variational anatomy of the human cochlea. *Otol. Neurotol.* 30, 14–22. doi: 10.1097/MAO.0b013e31818a08e8

Eshraghi, A. A., Aranke, M., Salvi, R., Ding, D., Coleman, J. K. M., Ocak, E., et al. (2018). Preclinical and clinical otoprotective applications of cell-penetrating peptide D-JNKI-1 (AM-111). *Hear. Res.* 368, 86–91. doi: 10.1016/j.heares.2018.03.003

Eshraghi, A. A., Gupta, C., Van De Water, T. R., Bohorquez, J. E., Garnham, C., Bas, E., et al. (2013). Molecular mechanisms involved in cochlear implantation trauma and the protection of hearing and auditory sensory cells by inhibition of c-jun-N-terminal kinase signaling. *Laryngoscope* 123, S1–S14. doi: 10.1002/lary.23902

Glueckert, R., Johnson Chacko, L., Rask-Andersen, H., Liu, W., Handschuh, S., and Schrott-Fischer, A. (2018). Anatomical basis of drug delivery to the inner ear. *Hear. Res.* 368, 10–27. doi: 10.1016/J.HEARES.2018.06.017

Grewal, A. S., Nedzelski, J. M., Chen, J. M., and Lin, V. Y. (2013). Dexamethasone uptake in the murine organ of Corti with transtympanic versus systemic administration. *J. Otolaryngol. Head Neck Surg.* 42:19. doi: 10.1186/1916-0216-42-19

Hahn, H., Salt, A. N., Biegner, T., Kammerer, B., Delabar, U., Hartsock, J. J., et al. (2012). Dexamethasone levels and base-to-apex concentration gradients in the scala tympani perilymph after intracochlear delivery in the guinea pig. *Otol. Neurotol.* 33, 660–665. doi: 10.1097/MAO.0b013e318254501b

Hamernik, R. P., Qiu, W., and Davis, B. (2003). The effects of the amplitude distribution of equal energy exposures on noise-induced hearing loss: the kurtosis metric. *J. Acoust. Soc. Am.* 114, 386–395. doi: 10.1121/1.1582446

Han, M. A., Back, S. A., Kim, H. L., Park, S. Y., Yeo, S. W., and Park, S. N. (2015). Therapeutic effect of dexamethasone for noise-induced hearing loss. *Otol. Neurotol.* 36, 755–762. doi: 10.1097/MAO.0000000000000759

Harding, G. W., Bohne, B. A., and Ahmad, M. (2002). DPOAE level shifts and ABR threshold shifts compared to detailed analysis of histopathological damage from noise. *Hear. Res.* 174, 158–171. doi: 10.1016/s0378-5955(02)00653-6

Hargunani, C. A., Kempton, J. B., DeGagne, J. M., and Trune, D. R. (2006). Intratympanic injection of dexamethasone. *Otol. Neurotol.* 27, 564–569. doi: 10.1097/01.mao.0000194814.07674.4f

Harrop-Jones, A., Wang, X., Fernandez, R., Dellamary, L., Ryan, A. F., LeBel, C., et al. (2016). The sustained-exposure dexamethasone formulation OTO-104 offers effective protection against noise-induced hearing loss. *Audiol. Neurootol.* 21, 12–21. doi: 10.1159/000441814

Henderson, D., Bielefeld, E. C., Harris, K. C., and Hu, B. H. (2006). Role of oxidative stress in noise-induced hearing loss. *Ear Hear.* 27, 1–19. doi: 10.1097/01.aud.0000191942.36672.f3

Hukee, M. J., and Duvall, A. J. III (1985). Cochlear vessel permeability to horseradish peroxidase in the normal and acoustically traumatized chinchilla: a reevaluation. *Ann. Otol. Rhinol. Laryngol.* 94, 297–303.

Jahnke, K. (1980). The blood-perilymph barrier. *Arch. Otorhinolaryngol.* 228, 29–34. doi: 10.1007/bf00455891

Jin, Z., Uhlen, I., Wei-Jia, K., and Mao-li, D. (2009). Cochlear homeostasis and its role in genetic deafness. *J. Otol.* 4, 15–22. doi: 10.1016/s1672-2930(09)50003-7

Juhn, S. K. (1988). Barrier systems in the inner ear. *Acta Otolaryngol. Suppl.* 458, 79–83. doi: 10.3109/00016488809125107

Kaupp, H., and Giebel, W. (1980). Distribution of marked perilymph to the subarachnoidal space. *Arch. Otorhinolaryngol.* 229, 245–253. doi: 10.1007/bf02565527

Kopke, R. D., Coleman, J. K., Liu, J., Campbell, K. C., and Riffenburgh, R. H. (2002). Candidate's thesis: enhancing intrinsic cochlear stress defenses to reduce noise-induced hearing loss. *Laryngoscope* 112, 1515–1532. doi: 10.1097/00005537-200209000-00001

Kopke, R. D., Jackson, R. L., Coleman, J. K. M., Liu, J., Bielefeld, E. C., and Balough, B. J. (2007). NAC for noise: from the bench top to the clinic. *Hear. Res.* 226, 114–125. doi: 10.1016/j.heares.2006.10.008

Kujawa, S. G., and Liberman, M. C. (2006). Acceleration of age-related hearing loss by early noise exposure: evidence of a misspent youth. *J. Neurosci.* 26, 2115–2123. doi: 10.1523/jneurosci.4985-05.2006

Kujawa, S. G., and Liberman, M. C. (2009). Adding insult to injury: cochlear nerve degeneration after "Temporary" noise-induced hearing loss. *J. Neurosci.* 29, 14077–14085. doi: 10.1523/JNEUROSCI.2845-09.2009

Laurell, G., Teixeira, M., Sterkers, O., Bagger-Sjöbäck, D., Eksborg, S., Lidman, O., et al. (2002). Local administration of antioxidants to the inner ear. Kinetics and distribution(1). *Hear. Res.* 173, 198–209. doi: 10.1016/s0378-5955(02)00613-5

Laurell, G. F., Teixeira, M., Duan, M., Sterkers, O., and Ferrary, E. (2008). Intact blood-perilymph barrier in the rat after impulse noise trauma. *Acta Otolaryngol.* 128, 608–612. doi: 10.1080/00016480701644102

Lee, J. J., Jang, J. H., Choo, O.-S., Lim, H. J., and Choung, Y.-H. (2018). Steroid intracochlear distribution differs by administration method: systemic versus intratympanic injection. *Laryngoscope* 128, 189–194. doi: 10.1002/lary.26562

Lin, H. W., Furman, A. C., Kujawa, S., and Liberman, M. C. (2011). Primary neural degenerations in the guinea pig cochlea after reversible noise-induced threshold shift. *J. Assoc. Res. Otolaryngol.* 12, 605–616. doi: 10.1007/s10162-011-0277-0

Lo, W. C., Liao, L. J., Wang, C. T., Young, Y. H., Chang, Y. L., and Cheng, P. W. (2013). Dose-dependent effects of D-methionine for rescuing noise-induced permanent threshold shift in guinea-pigs. *Neuroscience* 254, 222–229. doi: 10.1016/j.neuroscience.2013.09.027

Maeda, K., Yoshida, K., Ichimiya, I., and Suzuki, M. (2005). Dexamethasone inhibits tumor necrosis factor-(-induced cytokine secretion from spiral ligament fibrocytes. *Hear. Res.* 202, 154–160. doi: 10.1016/J.HEARES.2004.08.022

Mamelle, E., El Kechai, N., Adenis, V., Nguyen, Y., Sterkers, O., Agnely, F., et al. (2018). Assessment of the efficacy of a local steroid rescue treatment administered 2 days after a moderate noise-induced trauma in guinea pig. *Acta Otolaryngol.* 138, 610–616. doi: 10.1080/00016489.2018.1438659

Mikulec, A. A., Plontke, S. K., Hartsock, J. J., Salt, A. N. (2009). Entry of substances into perilymph through the bone of the otic capsule after intratympanic applications in guinea pigs: implications for local drug delivery in humans. *Otol. Neurotol.* 30, 131–138. doi: 10.1097/MAO.0b013e318191bff8

Mynatt, R., Hale, S. A., Gill, R. M., Plontke, S. K., and Salt, A. N. (2006). Demonstration of a longitudinal concentration gradient along scala tympani by sequential sampling of perilymph from the cochlear apex. *J. Assoc. Res. Otolaryngol.* 7, 182–193. doi: 10.1007/s10162-006-0034-y

Nagashima, R., and Ogita, K. (2006). Enhanced biosynthesis of glutathione in the spiral ganglion of the cochlea after in vivo treatment with dexamethasone in mice. *Brain Res.* 1117, 101–108. doi: 10.1016/J.BRAINRES.2006.07.113

Neng, L., Zhang, F., Kachelmeier, A., and Shi, X. (2013). Endothelial cell, pericyte, and perivascular resident macrophage-type melanocyte interactions regulate cochlear intrastrial fluid-blood barrier permeability. *J. Assoc. Res. Otolaryngol.* 14, 175–185. doi: 10.1007/s10162-012-0365-9

Nordmann, A. S., Bohne, B. S., and Harding, G. W. (2000). Histopathological differences between temporary and permanent threshold shift. *Hear. Res.* 139, 13–30. doi: 10.1016/s0378-5955(99)00163-x

Ohlemiller, K. K. (2008). Recent findings and emerging questions in cochlear noise injury. *Hear. Res.* 245, 5–17. doi: 10.1016/j.heares.2008.08.007

Ohlemiller, K. K., McFadden, S. L., Ding, D. L., Lear, P. M., and Ho, Y. S. (2000). Targeted mutation of the gene for cellular glutathione peroxidase (Gpx1) increases noise-induced hearing loss in mice. *J. Assoc. Res. Otolaryngol.* 1, 243–254. doi: 10.1007/s101620010043

Ohlemiller, K. K., Wright, J. S., and Dugan, L. L. (1999). Early elevation of cochlear reactive oxygen species following noise exposure. *Audiol. Neurootol.* 4, 229–236. doi: 10.1159/000013846

Park, S. Y., Back, S. A., Kim, H. L., Kim, D. K., Yeo, S. W., and Park, S. N. (2014). Renexin as a rescue regimen for noise-induced hearing loss. *Noise Health* 16, 257–264. doi: 10.4103/1463-1741.140497

Parnes, L. S., Sun, A.-H., and Freeman, D. J. (1999). Corticosteroid pharmacokinetics in the inner ear fluids: an animal study followed by clinical application. *Laryngoscope* 109, 1–17. doi: 10.1097/00005537-199907001-00001

Paulson, D. P., Abuzeid, W., Jiang, H., Oe, T., O'Malley, B. W., and Li, D. (2008). A novel controlled local drug delivery system for inner ear disease. *Laryngoscope* 118, 706–711. doi: 10.1097/MLG.0b013e31815f8e41

Plontke, S. K., Mynatt, R., Gill, R. M., Borgmann, S., and Salt, A. N. (2007). Concentration gradient along the scala tympani after local application of gentamicin to the round window membrane. *Laryngoscope* 117, 1191–1198. doi: 10.1097/MLG.0b013e318058a06b

Plontke, S. K., and Salt, A. N. (2018). Local drug delivery to the inner ear: principles, practice, and future challenges. *Hear. Res.* 368, 1–2. doi: 10.1016/J.HEARES.2018.06.018

Puel, J. L., Ruel, K., d'Aldin, C. G., and Pujol, R. (1998). Excitotoxicity and repair of cochlear synapses after noise-trauma induced hearing loss. *Neuroreport* 9, 2109–2114. doi: 10.1097/00001756-199806220-00037

Pujol, R., and Puel, J. L. (1999). Excitotoxicity, synaptic repair, and functional recovery in the mammalian cochlea: a review of recent findings. *Ann. N. Y. Acad. Sci.* 884, 249–254. doi: 10.1111/j.1749-6632.1999.tb08646.x

Qiu, W., Hamernik, R. P., and Davis, B. (2006). The kurtosis metric as an adjunct to energy in the prediction of trauma from continuous, nonGaussian noise exposures. *J. Acoust. Soc. Am.* 120, 3901–3906. doi: 10.1121/1.2372455

Rio, C., Dikker, P., Liberman, M. C., and Corfas, G. (2002). Glial fibrillary acidic protein expression and promoter activity in the inner ear of developing and adult mice. *J. Comp. Neurol.* 442, 156–162. doi: 10.1002/cne.10085

Robertson, D. (1983). Functional significance of dendritic swelling after loud sounds in the guinea-pig cochlea. *Hear. Res.* 9, 263–278. doi: 10.1016/0378-5955(83)90031-x

Salt, A. N. (2002). Simulation of methods for drug delivery to the cochlear fluids. *Adv. Otorhinolaryngol.* 59, 140–148. doi: 10.1159/000059251

Salt, A. N. (2008). Dexamethasone concentration gradients along scala tympani after application to the round window membrane. *Otol. Neurotol.* 29, 401–406. doi: 10.1097/MAO.0b013e318161aaae

Salt, A. N., Hartsock, J., Plontke, S., LeBel, C., and Piu, F. (2011). Distribution of dexamethasone and preservation of inner ear function following intratympanic delivery of a gel-based formulation. *Audiol. Neurootol.* 16, 323–335. doi: 10.1159/000322504

Salt, A. N., Hartsock, J. J., Gill, R. M., Piu, F., and Plontke, S. K. (2012a). Perilymph pharmacokinetics of markers and dexamethasone applied and sampled at the lateral semi-circular canal. *J. Assoc. Res. Otolaryngol.* 13, 771–783. doi: 10.1007/s10162-012-0347-y

Salt, A. N., and Hirose, K. (2018). Communication pathways to and from the inner ear and their contributions to drug delivery. *Hear. Res.* 362, 25–37. doi: 10.1016/j.heares.2017.12.010

Salt, A. N., King, E. B., Hartsock, J. J., Gill, R. M., and O'Leary, S. J. (2012b). Marker entry into vestibular perilymph via the stapes following applications to the round window niche of guinea pigs. *Hear. Res.* 283, 14–23. doi: 10.1016/J.HEARES.2011.11.012

Salt, A. N., and Ma, Y. (2001). Quantification of solute entry into cochlear perilymph through the round window membrane. *Hear. Res.* 154, 88–97. doi: 10.1016/s0378-5955(01)00223-4

Salt, A. N., and Plontke, S. K. (2009). Principles of local drug delivery to the inner ear. *Audiol. Neurootol.* 14, 350–360. doi: 10.1159/000241892

Salt, A. N., and Plontke, S. K. (2018). Pharmacokinetic principles in the inner ear: influence of drug properties on intratympanic applications. *Hear. Res.* 368, 28–40. doi: 10.1016/j.heares.2018.03.002

Salt, A. N., and Plontke, S. K. R. (2005). Local inner-ear drug delivery and pharmacokinetics. *Drug Discov. Today* 10, 1299–1306. doi: 10.1016/S1359-6446(05)03574-9

Sendowski, I., Abaamrane, L., Raffin, F., Cros, A., and Clarençon, D. (2006). Therapeutic efficacy of intra-cochlear administration of methylprednisolone after acoustic trauma caused by gunshot noise in guinea pigs. *Hear. Res.* 221, 119–127. doi: 10.1016/J.HEARES.2006.08.010

Shi, X. (2009). Cochlear pericyte responses to acoustic trauma and the involvement of hypoxia-inducible factor-1alpha and vascular endothelial growth factor. *Am. J. Pathol.* 174, 1692–1704. doi: 10.2353/ajpath.2009.080739

Shi, X. (2010). Resident macrophages in the cochlear blood-labyrinth barrier and their renewal via migration of bone-marrow-derived cells. *Cell Tissue Res.* 342, 21–30. doi: 10.1007/s00441-010-1040-2

Shi, X. (2016). Pathophysiology of the cochlear intrastrial fluid-blood barrier (review). *Hear. Res.* 338, 52–63. doi: 10.1016/j.heares.2016.01.010

Shirwany, N. A., Seidman, M. D., and Tang, W. (1998). Effect of transtympanic injection of steroids on cochlear blood flow, auditory sensitivity, and histology in the guinea pig. *Am. J. Otol.* 19, 230–235.

Slepecky, N., Hamernik, R., Henderson, D., and Coling, D. (1981). Ultrastructural changes to the cochlea resulting from impulse noise. *Arch. Otorhinolaryngol.* 230, 273–278. doi: 10.1007/bf00456329

Stachler, R. J., Chandrasekhar, S. S., Archer, S. M., Rosenfeld, R. M., Schwartz, S. R., Barrs, D. M., et al. (2012). Clinical practice guideline. *Otolaryngol. Head Neck Surg.* 146, S1–S35. doi: 10.1177/0194599812436449

Stankovic, K., Rio, C., Xia, A., Sugawara, M., Adams, J. C., Liberman, M. C., et al. (2004). Survival of adult spiral ganglion neurons requires erbB receptor signaling in the inner ear. *J. Neurosci.* 24, 8651–8661. doi: 10.1523/jneurosci.0733-04.2004

Sugawara, M., Corfas, G., and Liberman, M. C. (2005). Influence of supporting cells on neuronal degeneration after hair cell loss. *J. Assoc. Res. Otolaryngol.* 6, 136–147. doi: 10.1007/s10162-004-5050-1

Suzuki, M., Yamasoba, T., Ishibashi, T., Miller, J. M., and Kaga, K. (2002). Effect of noise exposure on blood-labyrinth barrier in guinea pigs. *Hear. Res.* 164, 12–18. doi: 10.1016/s0378-5955(01)00397-5

Swan, E. E. L., Mescher, M. J., Sewell, W. F., Tao, S. L., and Borenstein, J. T. (2008). Inner ear drug delivery for auditory applications. *Adv. Drug Deliv. Rev.* 60, 1583–1599. doi: 10.1016/J.ADDR.2008.08.001

Tabuchi, K., Murashita, H., Sakai, S., Hoshino, T., Uemaetomari, I., and Hara, A. (2006). Therapeutic time window of methylprednisolone in acoustic injury. *Otol. Neurotol.* 27, 1176–1179. doi: 10.1097/01.mao.0000226313.82069.3f

Takemura, K., Komeda, M., Yagi, M., Himeno, C., Izumikawa, M., Doi, T., et al. (2004). Direct inner ear infusion of dexamethasone attenuates noise-induced trauma in guinea pig. *Hear. Res.* 196, 58–68. doi: 10.1016/j.heares.2004.06.003

Thorne, M., Salt, A. N., DeMott, J. E., Henson, M. M., Henson, O. W., and Gewalt, S. L. (1999). Cochlear fluid space dimensions for six species derived from reconstructions of three-dimensional magnetic resonance images. *Laryngoscope* 109, 1661–1668. doi: 10.1097/00005537-199910000-00021

Trune, D. R., and Canlon, B. (2012). Corticosteroid therapy for hearing and balance disorders. *Anat. Rec.* 295, 1928–1943. doi: 10.1002/ar.22576

Trune, D. R., Wobig, R. J., Kempton, J. B., and Hefeneider, S. H. (1999). Steroid treatment in young MRL.MpJ-Fas(lpr) autoimmune mice prevents cochlear dysfunction. *Hear. Res.* 137, 167–173. doi: 10.1016/s0378-5955(99)00148-3

Van Wijk, F., Staecker, H., Keithley, E., and Lefebvre, P. P. (2006). Local perfusion of the tumor necrosis factor alpha blocker infliximab to the inner ear improves autoimmune neurosensory hearing loss. *Audiol. Neurootol.* 11, 357–365. doi: 10.1159/000095897

Vlajkovic, S. M., Chang, H., Paek, S. Y., Chi, H. H., Sreebhavan, S., Telang, R. S., et al. (2014). Adenosine amine congener as a cochlear rescue agent. *Biomed Res. Int.* 2014:841489. doi: 10.1155/2014/841489

Vlajkovic, S. M., Guo, C. X., Telang, R., Wong, A. C., Paramananthasivam, V., Boison, D., et al. (2011). Adenosine kinase inhibition in the cochlea delays the onset of age-related hearing loss. *Exp. Gerontol.* 46, 905–914. doi: 10.1016/j.exger.2011.08.001

Wang, J., Dib, M., Lenoir, M., Vago, P., Eybalin, M., Hameg, A., et al. (2002). Riluzole rescues cochlear sensory cells from acoustic trauma in the guinea-pig. *Neuroscience* 111, 635–648. doi: 10.1016/s0306-4522(02)00004-0

Wang, J., Ruel, J., Ladrech, S., Bonny, C., van de Water, T. R., and Puel, J.-L. (2007). Inhibition of the c-Jun N-terminal kinase-mediated mitochondrial cell death pathway restores auditory function in sound-exposed animals. *Mol. Pharmacol.* 71, 654–666. doi: 10.1124/mol.106.028936

Wang, J., Van De Water, T. R., Bonny, C., de Ribaupierre, F., Puel, J. L., and Zine, A. (2003). A peptide inhibitor of c-Jun N-terminal kinase protects against both aminoglycoside and acoustic trauma-induced auditory hair cell death and hearing loss. *J. Neurosci.* 23, 8596–8607. doi: 10.1523/JNEUROSCI.23-24-08596.2003

Wang, X., Dellamary, L., Fernandez, R., Harrop, A., Keithley, E. M., Harris, J. P., et al. (2009). Dose-dependent sustained release of dexamethasone in inner ear cochlear fluids using a novel local delivery approach. *Audiol. Neurootol.* 14, 393–401. doi: 10.1159/000241896

Wang, X., Fernandez, R., Dellamary, L., Harrop, A., Ye, Q., Lichter, J., et al. (2011). Pharmacokinetics of dexamethasone solution following intratympanic injection in guinea pig and sheep. *Audiol. Neurootol.* 16, 233–241. doi: 10.1159/000320611

Wang, Y., Hirose, K., and Liberman, M. C. (2002). Dynamics of noise-induced cellular injury and repair in the mouse cochlea. *J. Assoc. Res. Otolayrngol.* 3, 248–268. doi: 10.1007/s101620020028

Wu, Y. X., Zhu, G. X., Liu, X. Q., Sun, F., Zhou, K., Wang, S., et al. (2014). Noise alters guinea pig's blood-labyrinth barrier ultrastructure and permeability along with a decrease of cochlear claudin-5 and occludin. *BMC Neurosci.* 15:136. doi: 10.1186/s12868-014-0136-0

Yamane, H., Nakai, Y., Takayama, M., Konishi, K., Iguchi, H., Nakagawa, T., et al. (1995). The emergence of free radicals after acoustic trauma and strial blood flow. *Acta Otolaryngol. Suppl.* 51, 87–92. doi: 10.3109/00016489509121877

Yamashita, D., Jiang, H. Y., Le Prell, C. G., Schacht, J., and Miller, J. M. (2005). Post-exposure treatment attenuates noise-induced hearing loss. *Neuroscience* 134, 633–642. doi: 10.1016/j.neuroscience.2005.04.015

Yamashita, D., Jiang, H. Y., Schacht, J., and Miller, J. M. (2004). Delayed production of free radicals following noise exposure. *Brain Res.* 1019, 201–209. doi: 10.1016/j.brainres.2004.05.104

Yang, J., Wu, H., Zhang, P., Hou, D.-M., Chen, J., and Zhang, S.-G. (2008). The pharmacokinetic profiles of dexamethasone and methylprednisolone concentration in perilymph and plasma following systemic and local administration. *Acta Otolaryngol.* 128, 496–504. doi: 10.1080/00016480701558906

Yang, Y., Dai, M., Wilson, T. M., Omelchenko, I., Klimek, J. E., and Wilmarth, P. A. (2011). Na(/K(-ATPase (1 identified as an abundant protein in the blood-labyrinth barrier that plays an essential role in the barrier integrity. *PLoS One* 6:e16547. doi: 10.1371/journal.pone.0016547

Yildirim, A., Coban, L., Satar, B., Yetiser, S., and Kunt, T. (2005). Effect of intratympanic dexamethasone on noise-induced temporary threshold shift. *Laryngoscope* 115, 1219–1222. doi: 10.1097/01.MLG.0000163748.55350.89

Zhang, W., Dai, M., Fridberger, A., Hassan, A., Degagne, J., Neng, L., et al. (2012). Perivascular-resident macrophage-like melanocytes in the inner ear are essential for the integrity of the intrastrial fluid-blood barrier. *Proc. Natl. Acad. Sci. U.S.A.* 109, 10388–10393. doi: 10.1073/pnas.1205210109

Zhou, Y., Zheng, G., Zheng, H., Zhou, R., Zhu, X., and Zhang, Q. (2013). Primary observation of early transtympanic steroid injection in patients with delayed treatment of noise-induced hearing loss. *Audiol. Neurootol.* 18, 89–94. doi: 10.1159/000345208

Zhou, Y., Zheng, H., Shen, X., Zhang, Q., and Yang, M. (2009). Intratympanic administration of methylprednisolone reduces impact of experimental intensive impulse noise trauma on hearing. *Acta Otolaryngol.* 129, 602–607. doi: 10.1080/00016480802342424

Zhu, C., Gausterer, J. C., Schöpper, H., Nieratschker, M., Saidov, N., Ahmadi, N., et al. (2018). Evaluation of sustained-release steroid hydrogels in a guinea pig model for noise-induced hearing loss. *Audiol. Neurootol.* 23, 73–81. doi: 10.1159/000487662

Zou, J., Bretlau, P., Pyykkö, I., Toppila, E., Olovius, N. P., Stephanson, N., et al. (2003). Comparison of the protective efficacy of neurotrophins and antioxidants for vibration-induced trauma. *ORL J. Otorhinolaryngol. Relat. Spec.* 65, 155–161. doi: 10.1159/000072253

Zou, J., Pyykkö, I., Hyttinen, J. (2016). Inner ear barriers to nanomedicine-augmented drug delivery and imaging. *J. Otol.* 11, 165–177. doi: 10.1016/j.joto.2016.11.002

Zuo, J., Curtis, L. M., Yao, X., ten Cate, W. J. F., Bagger-Sjöbäck, D., Hultcrantz, M., et al. (1995). Glucocorticoid receptor expression in the postnatal rat cochlea. *Hear. Res.* 87, 220–227. doi: 10.1016/0378-5955(95)00092-I

13

Drug Diffusion Along an Intact Mammalian Cochlea

Ildar I. Sadreev[1], George W. S. Burwood[2†], Samuel M. Flaherty[2], Jongrae Kim[3], Ian J. Russell[2], Timur I. Abdullin[4] and Andrei N. Lukashkin[2,5]**

[1] Department of Medicine, Faculty of Medicine, Imperial College, London, United Kingdom, [2] Sensory Neuroscience Research Group, School of Pharmacy and Biomolecular Sciences, University of Brighton, Brighton, United Kingdom, [3] School of Mechanical Engineering, Institute of Design, Robotics and Optimisation, Aerospace Systems Engineering, University of Leeds, Leeds, United Kingdom, [4] Department of Biochemistry, Biotechnology and Pharmacology, Institute of Fundamental Medicine and Biology, Kazan Federal University, Kazan, Russia, [5] Centre for Regenerative Medicine and Devices, University of Brighton, Brighton, United Kingdom

***Correspondence:**
Ildar I. Sadreev
i.sadreev@imperial.ac.uk
Andrei N. Lukashkin
a.lukashkin@brighton.ac.uk

†Present Address:
George W. S. Burwood,
Oregon Hearing Research Center
(OHSU), Portland, OR, United States

Intratympanic drug administration depends on the ability of drugs to pass through the round window membrane (RW) at the base of the cochlea and diffuse from this location to the apex. While the RW permeability for many different drugs can be promoted, passive diffusion along the narrowing spiral of the cochlea is limited. Earlier measurements of the distribution of marker ions, corticosteroids, and antibiotics demonstrated that the concentration of substances applied to the RW was two to three orders of magnitude higher in the base compared to the apex. The measurements, however, involved perforating the cochlear bony wall and, in some cases, sampling perilymph. These manipulations can change the flow rate of perilymph and lead to intake of perilymph through the cochlear aqueduct, thereby disguising concentration gradients of the delivered substances. In this study, the suppressive effect of salicylate on cochlear amplification via block of the outer hair cell (OHC) somatic motility was utilized to assess salicylate diffusion along an intact guinea pig cochlea *in vivo*. Salicylate solution was applied to the RW and threshold elevation of auditory nerve responses was measured at different times and frequencies after application. Resultant concentrations of salicylate along the cochlea were calculated by fitting the experimental data using a mathematical model of the diffusion and clearing of salicylate in a tube of variable diameter combined with a model describing salicylate action on cochlear amplification. Concentrations reach a steady-state at different times for different cochlear locations and it takes longer to reach the steady-state at more apical locations. Even at the steady-state, the predicted concentration at the apex is negligible. Model predictions for the geometry of the longer human cochlea show even higher differences in the steady-state concentrations of the drugs between cochlear base and apex. Our findings confirm conclusions that achieving therapeutic drug concentrations throughout the entire cochlear duct is hardly possible when the drugs are applied to the RW and are distributed via passive diffusion. Assisted methods of drug delivery are needed to reach a more uniform distribution of drugs along the cochlea.

Keywords: cochlea, drug delivery, salicylate, cochlear amplifier, cochlear round window

INTRODUCTION

The mammalian cochlea is one of the least accessible organs for drug delivery (Salt and Plontke, 2009; Rivera et al., 2012; El Kechai et al., 2015; Hao and Li, 2019). Systemic administration of many drugs, notably the most frequently used corticosteroids, and aminoglycoside antibiotics, is severely limited by the blood-labyrinth barrier (Salt and Hirose, 2018). Local intratympanic administration (Schuknecht, 1956; Bowe and Jacob, 2010) would be a preferable option for these drugs and local delivery is the only option for many old and newly emerging classes of drugs and therapies including local anesthetics, antioxidants, apoptosis inhibitors, neurotransmitters and their antagonists, monoclonal antibodies, growth factors, signaling pathway regulators, and genetic material (see Devare et al., 2018; Hao and Li, 2019 for the latest reviews). Intratympanic administration of drugs relies on their remaining in contact with the round window membrane (RW) (a membranous opening in the bony wall of the cochlea into the middle ear) long enough to allow their diffusion into the perilymph of the scala tympani (ST). The ability of drugs to pass through the RW does not, however, guarantee their sufficient distribution along the cochlear spiral. Drug distribution in the ST is limited by the low flow rate of perilymph within the cochlea and by cochlear geometry. The longitudinal flow of perilymph in the cochlea has been shown to be relatively slow, if present at all (Ohyama et al., 1988), and drug distribution in the perilymph is dominated by passive diffusion. Passive diffusion along the ST is, however, constrained because the cochlea is a relatively long and narrow tube with a cochlear cross-section that decreases gradually from the RW at the base to the apex. It is in the cochlear apex where human speech processing is initiated (e.g., Nuttall et al., 2018) and where drug delivery to the cochlea has greatest potential therapeutic and socioeconomic impact.

However, direct measurements of the distribution of marker ions and contrasting agents (Salt and Ma, 2001; Haghpanahi et al., 2013), corticosteroids (Plontke et al., 2008; Creber et al., 2018) and antibiotics (Mynatt et al., 2006; Plontke et al., 2007a) or measurements of the physiological effects of drugs (Chen et al., 2005; Borkholder et al., 2010) demonstrated that the concentration of substances applied to the RW was much higher in the cochlear base than in the apex. These measurements, however, involved perforating the cochlear bony wall and, in some cases, sampling perilymph. These manipulations can change the flow rate of perilymph (Ohyama et al., 1988; Salt and Ma, 2001) and lead to the intake of cerebrospinal fluid through the cochlear aqueduct (Salt et al., 2003), thereby disguising concentration gradients of the delivered substances.

A few studies investigated the distribution of substances applied to the RW in the intact cochlea without breaking cochlear boundaries. This was done mainly in morphological studies investigating the distribution of dexamethasone and other substances along the cochlea after their intratympanic administration (Saijo and Kimura, 1984; Imamura and Adams, 2003; Hargunani et al., 2006; Grewal et al., 2013). While these studies confirmed the existence of base-to-apex gradients, the actual concentrations of substances along the cochlea were not measured. Borkholder et al. (2014) measured the threshold elevation of distortion product otoacoustic emissions (DPOAE) produced by primary tones of different frequencies after intratympanic application of salicylate. Salicylate affects cochlear amplification in a concentration-dependent manner but the DPOAE is a non-linear phenomenon and the dependence of DPOAE thresholds on the primary tone level and cochlear amplification is complex (Lukashkin et al., 2002). As a result, salicylate concentrations along the cochlear spiral cannot be easily derived from the DPOAE threshold elevations.

The purpose of the current study is to quantify drug diffusion from the RW along an intact guinea pig cochlea, to identify the factors that limit passive drug diffusion along the cochlea, and to analyse possible solutions to overcome these limitations. Salicylate was used as a model drug with well-characterized physiological effects. A mathematical model, which includes a diffusion component and a biophysical component describing the action of salicylate on the cochlear amplifier was validated using experimental data and used to assess the distribution of substances along the human cochlea.

MATERIALS AND METHODS

Animals

Pigmented guinea pigs of similar weight (350–360 g) were anesthetized with the neurolept anesthetic technique (0.06 mg/kg body weight atropine sulfate s.c., 30 mg/kg pentobarbitone i.p., 500 μl/kg Hypnorm i.m.). Additional injections of Hypnorm were given every 40 min. Additional doses of pentobarbitone were administered as needed to maintain a non-reflexive state. The heart rate was monitored with a pair of skin electrodes placed on both sides of the thorax. The animals were tracheotomized and artificially respired, and their core temperature was maintained at 38°C with a heating blanket and a heated head holder. All procedures involving animals were performed in accordance with UK Home Office regulations with approval from the local ethics committee.

Signal Generation and Recording

The middle ear cavity of the ear used for the measurements was opened to reveal the RW. Compound action potentials (CAPs) of the auditory nerve were measured from the cochlear bony ridge in the proximity of the RW membrane using Teflon-coated silver wire coupled to laboratory designed and built extracellular amplifier (James Hartley). Thresholds of the N1 peak of the CAP were estimated visually using 10 ms tone stimuli at a repetition rate of 10 Hz.

For acoustic stimulation, sound was delivered to the tympanic membrane by a closed acoustic system comprising two Bruel and Kjaer 4134 ½″ microphones for delivering tones and a single Bruel and Kjaer 4133 ½″ microphone for monitoring sound pressure at the tympanum. The microphones were coupled to the ear canal via 1 cm long, 4 mm diameter tubes to a conical speculum, the 1 mm diameter opening of which was placed about 1 mm from the tympanum. The closed sound system was calibrated *in situ* for frequencies between 1 and 50 kHz. Known sound pressure levels were expressed in dB SPL re 2×10^{-5} Pa.

All acoustic stimuli in this work were shaped with raised cosines of 0.5 ms duration at the beginning and at the end of stimulation. White noise for acoustical calibration and tone sequences for auditory stimulation were synthesized by a Data Translation 3010 board at 250 kHz and delivered to the microphones through low-pass filters (100 kHz cut-off frequency). Signals from the acoustic measuring amplifier (James Hartley) were digitized at 250 kHz using the same board and averaged in the time domain. Experimental control, data acquisition, and data analysis were performed using a PC with programmes written in MATLAB (The MathWorks. Inc. 2018a).

Five microliters of sodium salicylate solution (either 100 mM in experiments on salicylate diffusion in the ST or 1M in experiments with complete block of the cochlear amplifier) in Hanks' Balanced Salt Solution were placed on the RW using pipettes. The solution was removed from the RW using paper wicks to observe the wash out effect.

Model Overview

Diffusion and Clearing Equation

For the purpose of modeling, the ST is approximated by a tube with a decreasing diameter similar to that described in previous models, for example by Plontke et al. (2007b) (**Figure 1A**). The radii of the tube, $r(0)$ and $r(l)$, are equal to a and b at $x = 0$ and $x = l$, respectively, where l is the ST length. All the dimensions are known (Thorne et al., 1999) and symmetry along y and z axes is assumed. Zero longitudinal perilymph flow in the compartment is assumed (Ohyama et al., 1988) and only the passive diffusion of a drug (salicylate) with diffusion coefficient k_d is considered. In addition to diffusion, there is also clearing of the drug characterized by the clearing coefficient k_c. This clearing can be represented simply as a leak through the scala boundary (e.g., loss to the vasculature and tissues, and to other cochlear compartments). The diffusion and clearing processes are assumed to be completely independent. Because the tube radius is much smaller than its length, i.e., $r(x) \ll l$ for all x in $[0, l]$, only diffusion along x axis is considered and the concentration $c(x, t)$ within each cross-section for a fixed instance t is assumed to be constant, i.e., it does not change along the y axis. If the area of the cross-section is $S(x)$ then the diffusion can be described by the following partial differential equation (see **Appendix** for detailed derivation):

$$\frac{dc(x,t)}{dt} = \frac{1}{S(x)} \cdot \frac{d}{dx}\left(S(x) \cdot k_d \cdot \frac{dc(x,t)}{dx}\right) - c(x,t) \cdot \frac{2k_c}{r(x)}, \quad (1)$$

with the boundary conditions

$$c(0,t) = c_{rw}, \quad (2)$$

$$k_d \frac{dc(l,t)}{dx} = 0 \quad (3)$$

and initial conditions

$$c(0,0) = c_{rw}; x = 0, \quad (4)$$

$$c(x,0) = 0; x > 0. \quad (5)$$

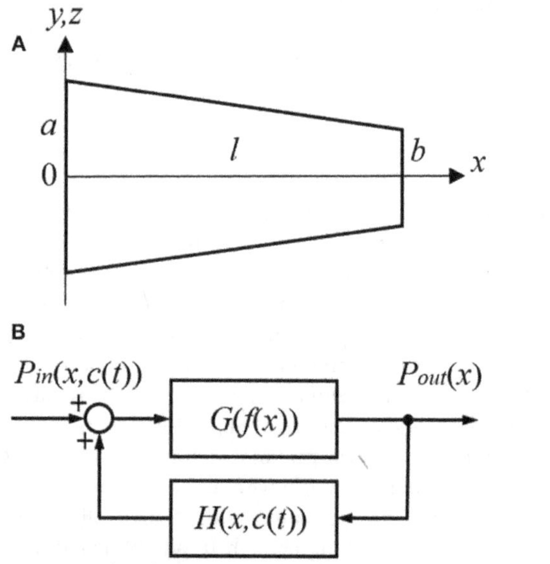

FIGURE 1 | Schematic presentation of **(A)** the scala tympani (ST) approximated by a tube of decreasing diameter and **(B)** the cochlear amplifier modeled as a system with positive feedback provided by the outer hair cells (OHCs).

The diffusion coefficient k_d is known (Lide, 2002) but the clearing coefficient k_c is unknown. The ratio of the diffusion and clearing coefficients can, however, be found via fitting the experimental data. The physical meaning of k_d/k_c can be described as the ratio between the amount of substance that diffuses through a unit surface normal to the direction of diffusion for a unit concentration gradient and the amount of drug that is cleared through a unit surface normal to the direction of substance exit for a unit substance concentration, both for unit time duration. The diffusion/clearing equation was validated using experimental data on the physiological effect of salicylate on the CAP thresholds. Because the salicylate concentrations could not be directly inferred from the physiological effect of salicylate, a biophysical element of the model was developed allowing calculations of the salicylate concentrations along the cochlea.

Link Between Position and Frequency

The dependence between frequency of stimulation f and frequency position along the length x of the basilar membrane for the guinea pig cochlea is defined by the Greenwood equation (Greenwood, 1990)

$$f(\tilde{x}) = A \cdot \left(10^{\alpha\tilde{x}} - \beta\right), \quad (6)$$

where $A = 0.35$, $\alpha = 2.1/18.5$, $\beta = 0.85$ and $\tilde{x} = l - x$ meaning that the starting point for $\tilde{x}$ in Greenwood (1990) is at the apex and not the base of the cochlea, as in this study.

Cochlear Amplifier

The cochlear amplifier is represented by a positive feedback system (**Figure 1B**) with feedback gain $H(x, c(t))$ due to force generation by the OHCs (Mountain et al., 1983; Yates, 1990;

Lukashkin and Russell, 1999). The following assumptions are made for a small signal, linear regime:

1. The CAP threshold is observed for different sound pressure $P_{in}(x, c(t))$ at the tympanum but for the same BM displacements, i.e., for the same constant pressure $P_{out}(x)$ at the BM for any given frequency/place x during manipulations with the cochlear amplifier. The assumption is based on good correspondence between neural and BM thresholds at the CF (Ruggero et al., 2000; Temchin et al., 2008).
2. Feedback gain $H(x, c(t))$ is proportional to the outer hair cell (OHC) force $F(x, c(t))$ for any given frequency/place in the cochlea

$$H(x, c(t)) = \alpha \cdot F(x, c(t)), \tag{7}$$

   where α is the gain constant. The initial feedback gain $H(x, 0)$ for any frequency/place before application of salicylate can be found empirically (see below).
3. Salicylate changes only feedback gain $H(x, c(t))$ through changes in $F(x, c(t))$.
4. In line with other modeling studies (e.g., Meaud and Grosh, 2014; Ni et al., 2016), it is assumed that pressure/displacement at the BM is a linear combination of the passive BM response due to acoustic stimulation and active response due to the OHC forces.

The link between local salicylate concentration $c(x, t)$ and reduction in force $FR(x, c(t))$ generated by the OHCs can be described by the Hill function (Hallworth, 1997)

$$FR(x, c(t)) = V_{\max} \cdot \frac{c(x, t)^n}{k^n + c(x, t)^n}, \tag{8}$$

where $V_{\max} = 0.71629$, $k = 0.101$, and $n = 0.983$.

The reduction in force is linked to the force before $F(x, 0)$ and after $F(x, c(t))$ salicylate application as

$$FR(x, c(t)) = \frac{F(x, 0) - F(x, c(t))}{F(x, 0)} = 1 - \frac{F(x, c(t))}{F(x, 0)} \tag{9}$$

or,

$$F(x, c(t)) = F(x, 0) \cdot \left(1 - FR(x, c(t))\right). \tag{10}$$

It can be written for any given frequency/place before salicylate application at $t = 0$ (**Figure 1B**)

$$\frac{P_{out}(x)}{P_{in}(x, 0)} = \frac{G}{1 - G \cdot H(x, 0)}, \tag{11}$$

where G is the open loop gain. Similarly, at time t after salicylate application

$$\frac{P_{out}(x)}{P_{in}(x, c(t))} = \frac{G}{1 - G \cdot H(x, c(t))}. \tag{12}$$

Dividing (11) by (12) and taking into account (7), it could be written

$$\frac{P_{in}(x, c(t))}{P_{in}(x, 0)} = \frac{1 - G \cdot \alpha \cdot F(x, c(t))}{1 - G \cdot \alpha \cdot F(x, 0)}. \tag{13}$$

Substituting $F(x, c(t))$ from (10) into (13) and using (7), one can obtain

$$\frac{P_{in}(x, c(t))}{P_{in}(x, 0)} = \frac{1 - G \cdot H(x, 0) \cdot (1 - FR(x, c(t)))}{1 - G \cdot H(x, 0)}. \tag{14}$$

The left part of (14) is measured in the experiment. $FR(x, c(t))$ is calculated using the Hill function (8) with $c(x, t)$ in this equation being calculated using the diffusion/clearing equation (1).

An analytical form of empirical dependence $H(x, 0)$, i.e., feedback gain before salicylate application for different frequencies/locations, can be obtained as follows. Feedback from the OHCs can be completely blocked in experiments using a high concentration of salicylate. In this case $H(x, c(t)) = 0$ in (12) and the transfer function of the feedback system (**Figure 1B**) is equal to the open loop gain G. Then similar to (11) and (12)

$$\frac{P_{out}(x)}{P_{inBlock}(x)} = G, \tag{15}$$

where $P_{inBlock}(x)$ is the sound pressure required to produce a response from the auditory nerve in preparations where the cochlear amplifier is completely blocked, and it does not depend on time. Dividing (11) by (15) and rearranging gives the following equation

$$H(x, 0) = \frac{1}{G} \cdot \left(1 - \frac{P_{in}(x, 0)}{P_{inBlock}(x)}\right), \tag{16}$$

where $P_{inBlock}(x)/P_{in}(x, 0)$ is measured in separate experiments.

G has frequently been assumed to be constant along the cochlea (e.g., Mountain et al., 1983; Yates, 1990; Lukashkin and Russell, 1999). In spite of the special design of the cochlea, which minimized energy losses when the BM traveling wave moves from the base to apex (Jones et al., 2013), some energy dissipation is still expected during wave propagation in a viscous environment. To account for energy losses, we assumed a simple linear dependence of the open loop gain $G(f(x))$ on frequency

$$G(f(x)) = s \cdot f(x) + i, \tag{17}$$

where s is the slope and i is the intercept defined as $i = 1 - s \cdot f_l$, with $f_l = 49.9165$ kHz specifying the upper frequency limit of linear dependence for $G(f(x))$. Hence, $G(f(x))$ effectively depends only on a single parameter s, which could be found by fitting the experimental data.

Initial Model Parameters

Ratio $P_{inBlock}(x)/P_{in}(x, 0)$ was measured as a function of frequency f. Equation (6) shows how this frequency can be converted to a coordinate. An arbitrary Hill type function

$$\frac{P_{inBlock}}{P_{in}}(f) = m_1 \frac{f^{m_2}}{m_3^{m_2} + f^{m_2}} + m_4 \tag{18}$$

was fitted to the experimental data with $20\log_{10}$ transformation for dB using the Genetic Algorithm (GA) tool in MATLAB (The MathWorks. Inc. 2018a) (initial local fit). The obtained m_1, m_2,

m_3, and m_4 (**Table 1**) were then used for the later optimization procedures described below (final global fit). The feedback gain before application of salicylate $H(x, 0) = H(f(x), 0)$ was obtained according to (16) and (18) as

$$H(f, 0) = \frac{1}{G} \cdot \left(1 - 1/\left(m_1 \frac{f^{m_2}}{m_3^{m_2} + f^{m_2}} + m_4\right)\right). \quad (19)$$

Initial values for the all parameters used in the model before the optimization procedure are shown in **Table 1**.

Optimized Model Parameters

Equation (14) with $20\log_{10}$ transformation for dB was solved in MATLAB (The MathWorks. Inc. 2018a) using pdepe solver for partial differential equations and fitted to the entire set of experimental data for all frequencies and salicylate concentrations using Genetic Algorithm (GA) tool in MATLAB (The MathWorks. Inc. 2018a). The sum of squared errors

$$SE = \sum_{i=1}^{n} (M_i - E_i)^2$$

was used as a cost function for minimization, where M are the model predictions and E are the experimental data for points $i = 1...n$. It is worth noting that only three model parameters were fitted during the global fit/optimization. These parameters are the cochlear length l, k_d/k_c ratio and slope s of the open loop gain $G(f(x))$.

TABLE 1 | Model parameter values.

Parameter	Unit	Initial value	Optimized value	Source of the initial value
a	mm	0.56	Fixed	Thorne et al., 1999
b	mm	0.18	Fixed	Thorne et al., 1999
l	mm	18–19	19	Thorne et al., 1999
k_d	mm^2/s	0.959e-3	Fixed	Lide, 2002
$ratio = k_d/k_c$	mm	1–10	1.6968	Initial guess
c_{rw}	mM	100	Fixed	Experiment
A	kHz	0.35	Fixed	Greenwood, 1990
α	1/mm	2.1/18.5	Fixed	Greenwood, 1990
β	–	0.85	Fixed	Greenwood, 1990
k	mM	0.101	Fixed	Hallworth, 1997
n	–	0.983	Fixed	Hallworth, 1997
$V_{\max}$	–	0.71629	Fixed	Hallworth, 1997
m_1	–	1011.2	Fixed	Experiment
m_2	–	8.1406	Fixed	Experiment
m_3	kHz	3.4816	Fixed	Experiment
m_4	–	31.686	Fixed	Experiment
s	1/kHz	0–0.0261	0.00014742	Initial guess

RESULTS

Cochlear Amplifier Gain

Gain of the cochlear amplifier and corresponding feedback gain of the model, $H(x, 0) = H(f(x), 0)$ [equation (16)] was determined empirically from elevation of the CAP thresholds after application of 1M salicylate solution to the RW which caused a consistent and steady increase in threshold over the entire frequency range (**Figure 2**, black circles). Values for m_1, m_2, m_3, and m_4 (**Table 1**) were determined through fit of the experimental data points by equation (18) (**Figure 2**, red curve) using the Genetic Algorithm (GA) tool in MATLAB (The MathWorks. Inc. 2018a). These values were used for the general optimization procedure performed at later stages.

Distribution of Salicylate Along the Guinea Pig Cochlea

One hundred mM solution of salicylate applied to the RW caused a rapid increase followed by saturation of CAP thresholds for high frequency tones (**Figure 3A**). CAP threshold increase for tones of lower frequencies was observed after an initial delay and did not reach saturation during the time of observation. Any changes in CAP threshold due to application of salicylate were below the noise floor of measurements for tone frequencies lower than 5 kHz, which corresponds to approximately the apical 55% of cochlear length [(Greenwood, 1990); equation (6)]. A partial recovery of the CAP threshold was observed after salicylate solution was washed out from the RW confirming that threshold elevation during application of salicylate was due to specific action of salicylate and not because of general deterioration of preparations.

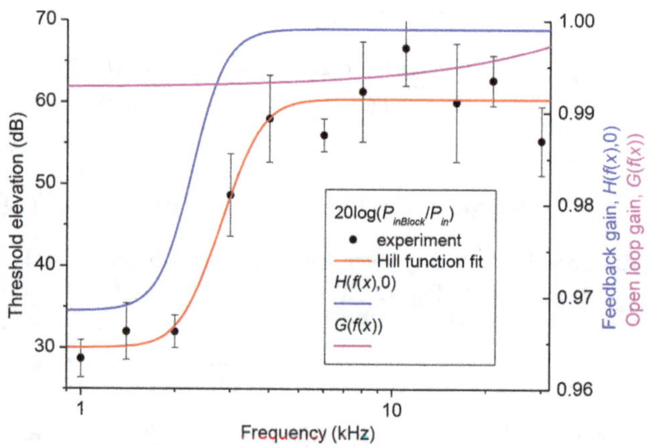

FIGURE 2 | Elevation of CAP thresholds after complete block of the cochlear amplifier (left Y-axis) and corresponding value of the open loop and feedback gain (right Y-axis). Black circles show the experimental values of threshold elevation (mean ± SD, $n = 3$). Red curve indicates fit of the experimental data points by Equation (18). Related values of the parameters m_1, m_2, m_3 and m_4 are given in **Table 1**. Value of the open loop (magenta curve) and feedback (blue curve) gains after the final global optimization procedure were calculated using Equations (17) and (19), respectively, with the optimized value of parameter s (**Table 1**).

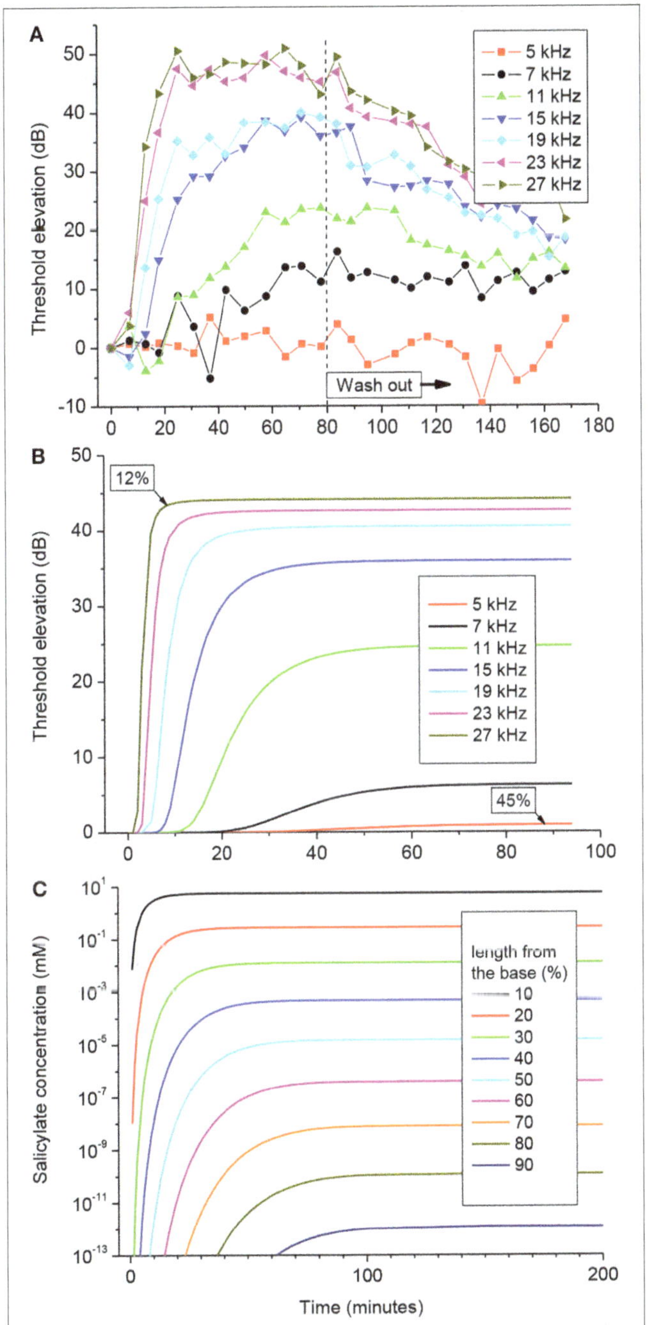

FIGURE 3 | CAP threshold elevation **(A,B)** and salicylate distribution **(C)** in the guinea pig cochlea after application of 100 mM of salicylate solution to the RW at time = 0. **(A)** Representative example of the CAP threshold elevation in a single preparation. Salicylate was washed out after 80 min of application. **(B)** Combined best fit of the entire set of experimental data on CAP threshold elevation for five preparations (**Figure S1**) using the parameter optimization procedure. Labels indicate percentage of the total cochlear length from the base. **(C)** Salicylate concentration along the cochlear length calculated using the optimized values of the model parameters (**Table 1**).

Pooled data from five animals were used to find an optimized set of the model parameters via fitting the entire set of experimental data using the Genetic Algorithm (GA) tool in MATLAB (The MathWorks. Inc. 2018a) (see Materials and Methods). The combined best fit to the entire set of experimental data for the optimized set of parameters is illustrated in **Figure 3B**. **Figure S1** shows the same plots for each of the frequencies along the corresponding experimental data. It is worth noting, that the optimization procedure was performed over the entire experimental set in order to fit the data for all the experimental frequencies simultaneously (**Figure S1**). The optimized set of model parameters (**Table 1**) found due to the general optimization procedure was used to predict cochlear responses and concentrations of salicylate (**Figure 3C**) along the entire cochlear length and over arbitrary time duration.

The absence of CAP threshold changes at frequencies below 5 kHz was due to poor diffusion of salicylate from the RW into the cochlear apex. It required increasingly longer times for the salicylate concentration to reach steady-state in the more apical regions of the cochlea, but at 90% of cochlear length (10% from the apex), salicylate concentration was about 12 orders of magnitude smaller than at the base even at steady-state (**Figure 3C**). The model suggests that this steep concentration gradient is due mainly to the fast clearing of salicylate from the ST which is reflected in the small k_d/k_c ratio found in the optimization (**Table 1**). Because the flux J is proportional to the concentration gradient [equation (A1)], changes in salicylate concentration at the RW will not lead to changes in the concentration gradient between the cochlear base and apex. In this case all steady-state curves for different concentrations of salicylate at the RW are scaled versions of each other (data not shown). Hence, for a specific substance (i.e., for specific diffusion (k_d) and clearing (k_c) coefficients) and for a given cochlear geometry, the ratio of steady-state concentrations at the base, and apex of the cochlea is a constant and does not depend on substance concentration at the RW. This was further assessed for the human cochlea.

Diffusion of an Arbitrary Substance in the Human Cochlea

Hence, the validity of the diffusion/clearing equation has been confirmed using the experimental data on salicylate block of the cochlear amplifier, the equation can be used to make conclusions about the distribution of arbitrary substances along the human cochlea (**Figure 4**). Decrease in the relative contribution of clearing into the distribution of a substance along the ST, i.e.,. increase of k_d/k_c ratio, leads to a dramatic reduction in the steady-state, base-to-apex gradient of the substance concentration (**Figure 4A**) calculated using the non-dimensional form of the diffusion equation (A14). This result is expected because a larger amount of the substance is available for diffusion into the cochlear apex in this case. For salicylate, however, the difference between the basal and apical concentrations is even larger in the human cochlea (red cross in **Figure 4A**) compared to guinea pigs and reaches 16 orders of magnitude because of the increased length of the human cochlea.

Figure 4A provides theoretical estimates of the minimal gradients which can be reached along the ST due to passive diffusion, when substances are in contact with the RW long enough to establish a concentration equilibrium distribution. Reduction in the base-to-apex gradient for substances with

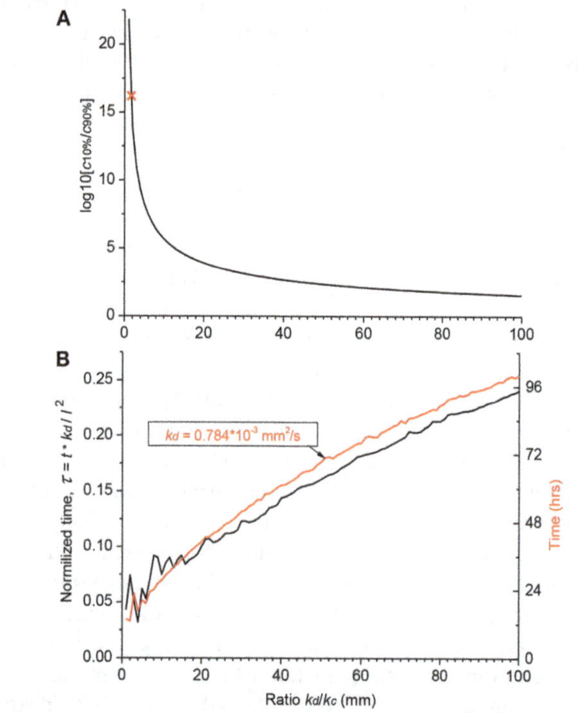

FIGURE 4 | Theoretical distribution of an arbitrary substance in the human cochlea. **(A)** Dependence of the ratio of basal (c10%) and apical (c90%) steady-state concentrations on the ratio of diffusion (k_d) and clearing (k_c) coefficients. Red cross indicates the point for salicylate ($k_d/k_c = 1.7$). **(B)** Normalized time (black curve, left ordinate) required to reach steady-state concentration at the cochlear apex for substances with different ratio of the diffusion (k_d) and clearing (k_c) coefficients. Red curve shows a specific example of the absolute time (right ordinate) for a substance with the diffusion coefficient (k_d) similar to that of dexamethasone. The steady-state was defined as the normalized difference between consecutive numerical values of concentration $<10^{-4}$. Jitter in the curves for small k_d/k_c ratios is due to very low apical concentrations. The following geometrical parameters for human cochlea were used for calculations using the non-dimensional form of the diffusion equation (A14) $a = 0.7981$, $b = 0.3990$, and $l = 28.46$ mm (Thorne et al., 1999).

higher k_d/k_c ratios, which are better retained in the ST, comes at the expense of the much longer substance exposure times required to reach steady-state concentration gradients (**Figure 4B**). For example, for a drug with the diffusion coefficient k_d similar to dexamethasone, for which the clearing coefficient is unknown, it takes days of retention at the RW when realistic k_d/k_c ratios are assumed (red curve in **Figure 4B**). The problem is that, while it is theoretically possible to achieve smaller base-to apex concentration gradients for a drug with high k_d/k_c ratios, in practice, if the drug is active, it will be cleared from the ST into the cochlear tissue, hence k_c cannot be arbitrarily small. In this case, the minimal theoretical difference in the base-to-apex concentrations of the drug is still a few orders of magnitude.

DISCUSSION

The existence of a base-to-apex drug concentration gradient, when drugs are applied to the RW, has been well-established. From this point of view, this study quantifies these gradients for the intact cochlea when the flow of perilymph in the ST is very small (Ohyama et al., 1988). This study does not investigate the problem of the RW permeability which is a separate challenge and requires specific considerations for particular drugs and formulations (Salt and Plontke, 2018). Instead, sodium salicylate which easily passes through the RW was used to ensure high concentrations at the cochlear base. Though, passive proton-mediated diffusion of salicylate across biomembranes is observed at micromolar concentrations (Takagi et al., 1998), the RW diffusional barrier could, presumably, be overcome by the drug at the much higher, submolar concentrations used in this study. While the RW membrane is highly permeable to salicylate and the CAP threshold elevation at high frequencies started within seconds after salicylate application, the model assumption that salicylate concentrations on both RW sides were the same might introduce some error in the calculated absolute concentrations. We would like to emphasize, however, that an error in calculation of the absolute concentrations (note that the absolute concentrations were calculated using Hallworth's (1997) empirical dependence between salicylate concentration and the OHC force reduction) does not lead to an error in calculation of the concentration gradient which is the basis for the conclusions in this study. This is true because the flux J is proportional to the concentration gradient [equation (A1)] and gradient curves calculated for different salicylate concentrations at the RW are scaled versions of each other with the same gradients. It is worth noting that, from discoveries we made in our preliminary experiments, salicylate concentrations higher than 100 mM used to study diffusion in this work caused elevation of CAP thresholds throughout the entire frequency range. This flooding of the whole cochlea with salicylate was due apparently to overloading of the cochlear clearing and other possible mechanisms involved. In this case, the dynamic equilibrium between diffusion and clearing and steady-state salicylate concentrations cannot be reached and our model cannot be applied. From an experimental standpoint, the use of higher concentrations of salicylate also made time-dependent estimates of diffusion impossible for high frequencies because the clearing mechanism in the basal turn became almost immediately saturated following salicylate application. As a result of the clearing overload and other unidentified processes, salicylate is accumulated throughout the cochlea affecting all the frequencies as it was observed in our experiments where we applied 1M salicylate to the RW. Of course, therapeutic use of concentrated drug formulations in order to overcome the issues raised by this study could be problematic due to likely side effects and/or restricted aqueous solubility and thus is not a practical solution.

While the steady-state distribution of concentrations, which is the basis for conclusions in this study, is fitted well by the simple diffusion model, the responses for the lower frequencies became gradually slower compared to the model predictions (**Figure S1**). This may happen because salicylate action on the cochlear amplifier is not limited by its block of the OHC motility (e.g., Russell and Schauz, 1995; Wu et al., 2010) as it is assumed in the model. A compensatory effect from a hypothetical mechanism maintaining cochlear homeostasis and

OHC sensitivity and responsible for the "bounce" phenomenon after exposure to loud sounds (Kirk et al., 1997; Drexl et al., 2014) may also explain delayed threshold elevation at subtle salicylate concentrations in the low-frequency cochlear region. Finally, salicylate concentration at the cochlear base may be diluted by the cerebrospinal fluid coming through the cochlear aqueduct into the perilymph which becomes hyperosmotic due to relatively high salicylate concentration at the base. None of these mechanisms should, however, affect our conclusion about the magnitude of the steady-state concentration gradients along the ST.

For a cochlea of given geometry, the concentration gradient along the ST depends only on the relationship between diffusion and clearing and is drug specific. In terms of the current study, it is the value of k_d/k_c, which defines the ratio between the amount of drug entering through a unit surface of the ST normal to the direction of diffusion and leaving it through a unit area of the side walls within the same time period. Salicylate, which is readily cleared from the ST ($k_d/k_c = 1.6968$), does not in practice diffuse into the cochlear apex and the resultant theoretical base-to-apex concentration gradient is extremely high (red cross in **Figure 4A**). Drugs which are better retained in the ST (i.e., have higher k_d/k_c ratio) form smaller concentration gradients, but this is traded for the considerably longer time it takes for these drugs to reach steady-state concentrations in the cochlear apex (**Figure 4B**). Hence, this approach may not be practical when there is only a short time window for the treatment of a specific cochlear disorder. Also, using a drug form which is better retained in the ST will lead to larger concentration differences between the ST and surrounding tissue. This may be a problem for drugs with narrow therapeutic windows unless an inactive form of the drug is used for even distribution along the ST through diffusion and it is activated only when the drug is cleared into the surrounding tissue.

Because the retention of a drug at the RW does not lead to a leveling of its concentration along the cochlear spiral (see also Plontke et al., 2007b), different strategies for drug delivery to the cochlear apex should be employed. Stable drug loaded nanocarriers (Zou et al., 2014; Li et al., 2017; Kamalov et al., 2018) which can stay in the ST long enough without being cleared into the surrounding tissue may be a feasible option. When the concentration of nanocarriers along the ST reaches a constant level, the encapsulated drug could be released from the carriers through thermal or light activation (Karimi et al., 2016, 2017; Yuan et al., 2017) to obtain sufficient drug concentrations along the entire cochlear spiral. A potential problem with this approach is the substantial increase in time required to reach the equilibrium base-to-apex gradient of nanocarrier concentrations, due to the substantially smaller diffusion coefficients of even the smallest liposomes and micelles, compared to lone drug molecules (**Figure 4B**) (del Amo et al., 2017).

Drug loaded nanoparticles, however, could be used to take advantage of anatomical and cellular features of the cochlea which enable drug uptake through routes and pathways other than the ST route (Glueckert et al., 2018). Disulfiram loaded nanoparticles, for example, were observed in the apical part of the spiral ganglion just 1 day after their application to the RW and elevation of auditory brainstem response thresholds, due to disulfiram induced apoptosis of the ganglion neurons, was detected for frequencies corresponding to the cochlear apex within 2 days after application (Buckiová et al., 2012). Nanoparticles can also be effectively driven and distributed along the entire cochlea. Assisted diffusion of magnetically driven, prednisolone-loaded magnetic nanoparticle along the cochlea resulted in a significant increase in the protective effect of the drug against cisplatin-induced ototoxicity compared to intratympanic injections of prednisolone (Ramaswamy et al., 2017).

This study investigates passive drug diffusion along the intact cochlea when the drug is applied to the RW and highlights intrinsic problems with this method of local drug administration into the inner ear. Retaining drugs at the RW for an arbitrarily long time does not decrease its base-to-apex concentration gradient, which, at steady state, depends solely upon the relationship between drug diffusion along and clearing from the ST. Usage of drug-loaded nanocarriers which utilize the anatomical and cellular properties of the cochlea, and which can be actively distributed along the entire length of the cochlea seems to be a more promising approach.

ETHICS STATEMENT

All procedures involving animals were performed in accordance with UK Home Office regulations with approval from the University of Brighton Animal Welfare and Ethical Review Body.

AUTHOR CONTRIBUTIONS

AL, IR, and TA conceived and designed the study. GB, SF, and AL performed the experiments and analyzed experimental results. IS, JK, and AL developed the model. IS performed numerical simulations and fitting to the experimental data. All authors contributed to analysis and discussion of the results. IS and AL wrote the manuscript with contribution from all authors.

ACKNOWLEDGMENTS

The authors thank Vadim Biktashev for his helpful advice and comments on the diffusion part of the model.

REFERENCES

Borkholder, D. A., Zhu, X., and Frisina, R. D. (2014). Round window membrane intracochlear drug delivery enhanced by induced advection. *J. Control. Release* 174, 171–176. doi: 10.1016/j.jconrel.2013.11.021

Borkholder, D. A., Zhu, X., Hyatt, B. T., Archilla, A. S., Livingston, I. I. I., W. J. III, and Frisina, R. D. (2010). Murine intracochlear drug delivery: reducing concentration gradients within the cochlea. *Hear. Res.* 268, 2–11. doi: 10.1016/j.heares.2010.04.014

Bowe, S. N., and Jacob, A. (2010). Round window perfusion dynamics: implications for intracochlear therapy. *Curr. Opin. Otolaryngol. Head Neck Surg.* 18, 377–385. doi: 10.1097/MOO.0b013e32833d30f0

Buckiová, D., Ranjan, S., Newman, T. A., Johnston, A. H., Sood, R., Kinnunen, P. K., et al. (2012). Minimally invasive drug delivery to the cochlea through application of nanoparticles to the round window membrane. *Nanomedicine* 7, pp., 1339–1354. doi: 10.2217/nnm.12.5

Chen, Z., Kujawa, S. G., McKenna, M. J., Fiering, J. O., Mescher, M. J., Borenstein, J. T., et al. (2005). Inner ear drug delivery via a reciprocating perfusion system in the guinea pig. *J. Control. Release* 110, pp., 1–19. doi: 10.1016/j.jconrel.2005.09.003

Creber, N. J., Eastwood, H. T., Hampson, A. J., Tan, J., and O'Leary, S. J. (2018). A comparison of cochlear distribution and glucocorticoid receptor activation in local and systemic dexamethasone drug delivery regimes. *Hear. Res.* 368, 75–85. doi: 10.1016/j.heares.2018.03.018

del Amo, E. M., Rimpelä, A. K., Heikkinen, E., Kari, O. K., Ramsay, E., Lajunen, T., et al. (2017). Pharmacokinetic aspects of retinal drug delivery. *Prog. Retin. Eye Res.* 57, 134–185. doi: 10.1016/j.preteyeres.2016.12.001

Devare, J., Gubbels, S., and Raphael, Y. (2018). Outlook and future of inner ear therapy. *Hear. Res.* 368, 127–135. doi: 10.1016/j.heares.2018.05.009

Drexl, M., Überfuhr, M., Weddell, T. D., Lukashkin, A. N., Wiegrebe, L., Krause, E., et al. (2014). Multiple indices of the 'bounce' phenomenon obtained from the same human ears. *J. Assoc. Res. Otolaryngol.* 15, 57–72. doi: 10.1007/s10162-013-0424-x

El Kechai, N., Agnely, F., Mamelle, E., Nguyen, Y., Ferrary, E., and Bochot, A. (2015). Recent advances in local drug delivery to the inner ear. *Int. J. Pharm.* 494, 83–101. doi: 10.1016/j.ijpharm.2015.08.015

Glueckert, R., Chacko, L. J., Rask-Andersen, H., Wei, L., Handschuh, S., and Schrott-Fischer, A. (2018). Anatomical basis of drug delivery to the inner ear. *Hear. Res.* 368, 10–27. doi: 10.1016/j.heares.2018.06.017

Greenwood, D. D. (1990). A cochlear frequency-position function for several species—29 years later. *J. Acoust. Soc. Am.* 87, 2592–2605. doi: 10.1121/1.399052

Grewal, A. S., Nedzelski, J. M., Chen, J. M., and Lin, V. Y. (2013). Dexamethasone uptake in the murine organ of Corti with transtympanic versus systemic administration. *J. Otolaryngol.-Head N.* 42, :19. doi: 10.1186/1916-0216-42-19

Haghpanahi, M., Gladstone, M. B., Zhu, X., Frisina, R. D., and Borkholder, D. A. (2013). Noninvasive technique for monitoring drug transport through the murine cochlea using micro-computed tomography. *Ann. Biomed. Eng.* 41, 2130–2142. doi: 10.1007/s10439-013-0816-4

Hallworth, R. (1997). Modulation of outer hair cell compliance and force by agents that affect hearing. *Hear. Res.* 114, 204–212. doi: 10.1016/S0378-5955(97)00167-6

Hao, J., and Li, S. K. (2019). Inner ear drug delivery: recent advances, challenges, and perspective. *Eur. J. Pharm. Sci.* 126, 82–92. doi: 10.1016/j.ejps.2018.05.020

Hargunani, C. A., Kempton, J. B., DeGagne, J. M., and Trune, D. R. (2006). Intratympanic injection of dexamethasone: time course of inner ear distribution and conversion to its active form. *Otol. Neurotol.* 27, 564–569. doi: 10.1097/01.mao.0000194814.07674.4f

Imamura, S. I., and Adams, J. C. (2003). Distribution of gentamicin in the guinea pig inner ear after local or systemic application. *J. Assoc. Res. Otolaryngol.* 4, 176–195. doi: 10.1007/s10162-002-2036-8

Jones, G. P., Lukashkina, V. A., Russell, I. J., Elliott, S. J., and Lukashkin, A. N. (2013). Frequency-dependent properties of the tectorial membrane facilitate energy transmission and amplification in the cochlea. *Biophys. J.* 104, 1357–1366. doi: 10.1016/j.bpj.2013.02.002

Kamalov, M. I., Dǎng, T., Petrova, N. V., Laikov, A. V., Luong, D., Akhmadishina, R. A., et al. (2018). Self-assembled nanoformulation of methylprednisolone succinate with carboxylated block copolymer for local glucocorticoid therapy. *Colloids Surf. B Biointerfaces* 164, pp. 78–88. doi: 10.1016/j.colsurfb.2018.01.014

Karimi, M., Sahandi Zangabad, P., Baghaee-Ravari, S., Ghazadeh, M., Mirshekari, H., and Hamblin, M. R. (2017). Smart nanostructures for cargo delivery: uncaging and activating by light. *J. Am. Chem. Soc.* 139, 4584–4610. doi: 10.1021/jacs.6b08313.

Karimi, M., Sahandi Zangabad, P., Ghasemi, A., Amiri, M., Bahrami, M., Malekzad, H., et al. (2016). Temperature-responsive smart nanocarriers for delivery of therapeutic agents: applications and recent advances. *ACS Appl. Mater. Interfaces* 8, 21107–21133. doi: 10.1021/acsami.6b00371

Kirk, D. L., Moleirinho, A., and Patuzzi, R. B. (1997). Microphonic and DPOAE measurements suggest a micromechanical mechanism for the 'bounce' phenomenon following low-frequency tones. *Hear. Res.* 112, 69–86. doi: 10.1016/S0378-5955(97)00104-4

Li, L., Chao, T., Brant, J., O'Malley Jr, B., Tsourkas, A., and Li, D. (2017). Advances in nano-based inner ear delivery systems for the treatment of sensorineural hearing loss. *Adv. Drug Deliv. Rev.* 108, 2–12. doi: 10.1016/j.addr.2016.01.004

Lide, D. R. (2002). *CRC Handbook of Chemistry and Physics, 83rd Edn.* Boca Raton, FL: CRC Press.

Lukashkin, A. N., Lukashkina, V. A., and Russell, I. J. (2002). One source for distortion product otoacoustic emissions generated by low- and high-level primaries. *J. Acoust. Soc. Am.* 111, 2740–2748. doi: 10.1121/1.1479151

Lukashkin, A. N., and Russell, I. J. (1999). Analysis of the f2- f1 and 2f1- f2 distortion components generated by the hair cell mechanoelectrical transducer: Dependence on the amplitudes of the primaries and feedback gain. *J. Acoust. Soc. Am.* 106, 2661–2668. doi: 10.1121/1.428096

Meaud, J., and Grosh, K. (2014). Effect of the attachment of the tectorial membrane on cochlear micromechanics and two-tone suppression. *Biophys. J.* 106, 1398–1405. doi: 10.1016/j.bpj.2014.01.034

Mountain, D. C., Hubbard, A. E., and McMullen, T. A. (1983). "Electromechanical processes in the cochlea," in *Mechanics of Hearing*, eds. E. de Boer and M. A. Viergever (Dordrecht: Springer), 119–126.

Mynatt, R., Hale, S. A., Gill, R. M., Plontke, S. K., and Salt, A. N. (2006). Demonstration of a longitudinal concentration gradient along scala tympani by sequential sampling of perilymph from the cochlear apex. *J. Assoc. Res. Otolaryngol.* 7, 182–193. doi: 10.1007/s10162-006-0034-y

Ni, G., Elliott, S. J., and Baumgart, J. (2016). Finite-element model of the active organ of Corti. *J. R. Soc. Interface* 13, :20150913. doi: 10.1098/rsif.2015.0913

Nuttall, A. L., Ricci, A. J., Burwood, G., Harte, J. M., Stenfelt, S., Cayé-Thomasen, P., et al. (2018). A mechanoelectrical mechanism for detection of sound envelopes in the hearing organ. *Nat. Commun.* 9, :4175. doi: 10.1038/s41467-018-06725-w

Ohyama, K., Salt, A. N., and Thalmann, R. (1988). Volume flow rate of perilymph in the guinea-pig cochlea. *Hear. Res.* 35, 119–129. doi: 10.1016/0378-5955(88)90111-6

Plontke, S. K., Biegner, T., Kammerer, B., Delabar, U., and Salt, A. N. (2008). Dexamethasone concentration gradients along scala tympani after application to the round window membrane. *Otol. Neurotol.* 29, 401–406. doi: 10.1097/MAO.0b013e318161aaae

Plontke, S. K., Mynatt, R., Gill, R. M., Borgmann, S., and Salt, A. N. (2007a). Concentration gradient along the scala tympani after local application of gentamicin to the round window membrane. *Laryngoscope*, 117, 1191–1198. doi: 10.1097/MLG.0b013e318058a06b

Plontke, S. K., Siedow, N., Wegener, R., Zenner, H. P., and Salt, A. N. (2007b). Cochlear pharmacokinetics with local inner ear drug delivery using a three-dimensional finite-element computer model. *Audiol. Neurotol.* 12, 37–48. doi: 10.1159/000097246

Ramaswamy, B., Roy, S., Apolo, A. B., Shapiro, B., and Depireux, D. A. (2017). Magnetic nanoparticle mediated steroid delivery mitigates cisplatin induced hearing loss. *Front. Cell. Neurosci.* 11, :268. doi: 10.3389/fncel.2017.00268

Rivera, T., Sanz, L., Camarero, G., and Varela-Nieto, I. (2012). Drug delivery to the inner ear: strategies and their therapeutic implications for sensorineural hearing loss. *Curr. Drug Deliv.* 9, 231–242. doi: 10.2174/156720112800389098

Ruggero, M. A., Narayan, S. S., Temchin, A. N., and Recio, A. (2000). Mechanical bases of frequency tuning and neural excitation at the base of the cochlea: comparison of basilar-membrane vibrations and auditory-nerve-fiber responses in chinchilla. *Proc. Natl. Acad. Sci. U.S.A.* 97, 11744–11750. doi: 10.1073/pnas.97.22.11744

Russell, I. J., and Schauz, C. (1995). Salicylate ototoxicity: effects on stiffness and electromotility of outer hair cells isolated from the guinea pig cochlea. *Auditory Neurosci.* 1, 309–319.

Saijo, S., and Kimura, R. S. (1984). Distribution of HRP in the inner ear after injection into the middle ear cavity. *Acta Otolaryngol.* 97, 593–610. doi: 10.3109/00016488409132937

Salt, A. N., and Hirose, K. (2018). Communication pathways to and from the inner ear and their contributions to drug delivery. *Hear. Res.* 362, 25–37. doi: 10.1016/j.heares.2017.12.010

Salt, A. N., Kellner, C., and Hale, S. (2003). Contamination of perilymph sampled from the basal cochlear turn with cerebrospinal fluid. *Hear. Res.* 182, 24–33. doi: 10.1016/S0378-5955(03)00137-0

Salt, A. N., and Ma, Y. (2001). Quantification of solute entry into cochlear perilymph through the round window membrane. *Hear. Res.* 154, 88–97. doi: 10.1016/S0378-5955(01)00223-4

Salt, A. N., and Plontke, S. K. (2009). Principles of local drug delivery to the inner ear. *Audiol. Neurotol.* 14, 350–360. doi: 10.1159/000241892

Salt, A. N., and Plontke, S. K. (2018). Pharmacokinetic principles in the inner ear: influence of drug properties on intratympanic applications. *Hear. Res.* 368, 28–40. doi: 10.1016/j.heares.2018.03.002

Schuknecht, H. F. (1956). Ablation therapy for the relief of Meniere's disease. *Laryngoscope* 66, 859–859. doi: 10.1288/00005537-195607000-00005

Takagi, M., Taki, Y., Sakane, T., Nadai, T., Sezaki, H., Oku, N., et al. (1998). A new interpretation of salicylic acid transport across the lipid bilayer: implications of pH-dependent but not carrier-mediated absorption from the gastrointestinal tract. *J. Pharmacol. Exp. Ther.* 285, 1175–1180.

Temchin, A. N., Rich, N. C., and Ruggero, M. A. (2008). Threshold tuning curves of chinchilla auditory-nerve fibers. I. Dependence on characteristic frequency and relation to the magnitudes of cochlear vibrations. *J. Neurophysiol.* 100, 2889–2898. doi: 10.1152/jn.90637.2008

Thorne, M., Salt, A. N., DeMott, J. E., Henson, M. M., Henson, O. W. Jr., and Gewalt, S. L. (1999). Cochlear fluid space dimensions for six species derived from reconstructions of three-dimensional magnetic resonance images. *Laryngoscope* 109, 1661–1668. doi: 10.1097/00005537-199910000-00021

Wu, T., Lv, P., Kim, H. J., Yamoah, E. N., and Nuttall, A. L. (2010). Effect of salicylate on KCNQ4 of the guinea pig outer hair cell. *J. Neurophysiol.* 103, 1969–1977. doi: 10.1152/jn.01057.2009

Yates, G. K. (1990). Basilar membrane nonlinearity and its influence on auditory nerve rate-intensity functions. *Hear. Res.* 50, 145–162. doi: 10.1016/0378-5955(90)90041-M

Yuan, A., Huan, W., Liu, X., Zhang, Z., Zhang, Y., Wu, J., et al. (2017). NIR light-activated drug release for synergetic chemo-photothermal therapy. *Mol. Pharm.* 14, 242–251. doi: 10.1021/acs.molpharmaceut.6b00820

Zou, J., Sood, R., Zhang, Y., Kinnunen, P. K., and Pyykkö, I. (2014). Pathway and morphological transformation of liposome nanocarriers after release from a novel sustained inner-ear delivery system. *Nanomedicine* 9, 2143–2155. doi: 10.2217/nnm.13.181

14

Developments in Bio-Inspired Nanomaterials for Therapeutic Delivery to Treat Hearing Loss

Christopher Rathnam[1], Sy-Tsong Dean Chueng[1], Yu-Lan Mary Ying[2], Ki-Bum Lee[1,3] and Kelvin Kwan[3,4]**

[1] Department of Chemistry and Chemical Biology, Rutgers, The State University of New Jersey, Piscataway, NJ, United States, [2] Department of Otolaryngology Head and Neck Surgery, Rutgers New Jersey Medical School, Newark, NJ, United States, [3] Stem Cell Research Center and Keck Center for Collaborative Neuroscience, Rutgers, The State University of New Jersey, Piscataway, NJ, United States, [4] Department of Cell Biology and Neuroscience, Rutgers, The State University of New Jersey, Piscataway, NJ, United States

***Correspondence:**
Ki-Bum Lee
kblee@rutgers.edu
Kelvin Kwan
kwan@dls.rutgers.edu

Sensorineural hearing loss affects millions of people worldwide and is a growing concern in the aging population. Treatment using aminoglycoside antibiotics for infection and exposure to loud sounds contribute to the degeneration of cochlear hair cells and spiral ganglion neurons. Cell loss impacts cochlear function and causes hearing loss in ~ 15% of adult Americans (~36 million). The number of individuals with hearing loss will likely grow with increasing lifespans. Current prosthesis such as hearing aids and cochlear implants can ameliorate hearing loss. However, hearing aids are ineffective if hair cells or spiral ganglion neurons are severely damaged, and cochlear implants are ineffective without properly functioning spiral ganglion neurons. As such, strategies that alleviate hearing loss by preventing degeneration or promoting cell replacement are urgently needed. Despite showing great promise from *in vitro* studies, the complexity and delicate nature of the inner ear poses a huge challenge for delivering therapeutics. To mitigate risks and complications associated with surgery, new technologies and methodologies have emerged for efficient delivery of therapeutics. We will focus on biomaterials that allow controlled and local drug delivery into the inner ear. The rapid development of microsurgical techniques in conjunction with novel bio- and nanomaterials for sustained drug delivery appears bright for hearing loss treatment.

Keywords: inner ear, nanoparticle, hydrogel, drug delivery, hearing loss

INTRODUCTION

Drugs for Treating Inner Ear Disease

Sudden sensorineural hearing loss (SSHL), Meniere's disease (MD), and autoimmune inner ear disease are prevalent inner ear disorders seen in the clinic. Sudden sensorineural hearing loss affects 1–6 people per 5,000 every year (National Institute on Deafness and Other Communication Disorders) and is characterized as an idiopathic hearing loss that occurs suddenly or rapidly over a few days. Often, SSHL is associated with tinnitus, a ringing, or other auditory perception in the absence of an external stimulus (Schreiber et al., 2010). Meniere's disease is a disorder of the inner ear with unknown etiology. The symptoms of MD include episodes of spontaneous, recurrent vertigo accompanied by fluctuating hearing loss, intermittent tinnitus and characterized by endolymphatic hydrops (Havia et al., 2002; Nakashima et al., 2016). Autoimmune ear diseases (AIED) are characterized by the bilateral progressive sensorineural hearing loss that occurs over the course of weeks to months, with patients responding to the administration of immunosuppressants. Primary AIED has restricted pathology to the ear but may involve secondary autoimmunity. Although the etiology of the disorder is likely immune-mediated, there is no direct evidence that autoimmunity is the underlying cause of the disease. Autoimmune inner ear diseases include Cogan syndrome, Wegener granulomatosis, systemic lupus erythematosus, and various vasculitis (Ruckenstein, 2004).

In the clinic, patients diagnosed with SSHL or MD are treated with steroids, aminoglycosides, antioxidants (L-N-acetylcysteine), apoptosis inhibitors, or *N*-methyl-D-aspartate (NMDA) inhibitors. For AIED, cytotoxic agent cyclophosphamide is used. To date, only steroids and aminoglycoside are clinically available therapies for intratympanic administration to the inner ear. Intratympanic steroid injection is the most prevalent clinical application to restore acute hearing loss in all inner ear diseases. While the specific action of the steroids in the hearing apparatus is uncertain, steroid treatment likely improves hearing by reducing inflammation and swelling in the hearing organs. Use of intratympanic dexamethasone injections to treat sudden hearing loss may also attenuate symptoms of tinnitus (Garduno-Anaya et al., 2005). A number of clinical studies have been published on intratympanic injection of steroids for the treatment of acute hearing loss and vertigo exacerbation in MD, in addition to systemic therapy (Schoo et al., 2017). Furthermore, intratympanic administration of aminoglycosides (i.e., gentamicin) to chemically ablate vestibular hair cells is now an alternative and less invasive procedure for achieving chemical labyrinthectomy for uncontrolled vertigo spells in MD while preserving auditory function (Hill et al., 2006).

CURRENT STRATEGIES FOR INNER EAR DRUG DELIVERY

The current treatment standard for inner ear disorders is the intratympanic injection of liquid formulations of drugs. While intratympanic injection is the most common method for delivery of drugs to the inner ear, other methods such as intracochlear delivery are also available for extreme cases. In either case, several barriers need to be overcome for efficient drug delivery.

Intratympanic Drug Delivery

The tympanic membrane (TM) is a thin, cone-shaped membrane that separates the external ear from the middle ear. The TM has low permeability to most substances and is considered an impenetrable barrier for drug delivery to the inner ear. For intratympanic drug delivery, the integrity of TM is compromised before drugs are injected into the middle ear cavity where diffusion into the inner ear occurs. The shape of the external canal and differences in cone angle and depth of TM in humans hinder direct and precise administration of drugs (Volandri et al., 2011). Successful employment of steroids by intratympanic delivery for inner ear disease treatment was first reported about three decades ago (Itoh and Sakata, 1991). Since then, intratympanic injections are the preferred delivery method for treatment of SSHL, MD or vertigo because local delivery avoids the many side effects associated with systemic drug delivery (Chandrasekhar, 2001; Doyle et al., 2004). To date, delivery of either steroids or aminoglycosides is done by intratympanic injection to avoid the bony structure of the otic capsule and the TM. Delivery of small molecules or biologics in the inner ear by intratympanic injections still need to overcome several physical and cellular barriers (Chandrasekhar, 2001; Doyle et al., 2004). Physical barriers such as the RWM and other membranous partitions prevent drugs from diffusing from the middle ear cavity where the therapeutics reside.

The majority of small molecules delivered intratympanically likely enter through the RWM by passive diffusion into the inner ear. Diffusion of small molecules after intratympanic delivery results in large gradients along the length of the cochlea (Salt and Plontke, 2009). Extraneous obstructions due to anatomic variations in the round window niche contribute to the wide variability in delivery and dosage of drugs thus limiting reproducible clinical efficacy (Alzamil and Linthicum, 2000). Intratympanic injections are performed either without assisted visualization or with a micro-endoscope to assist in removing potential round window niche obstructions (Plontke et al., 2002). Once injected, the liquids in the middle ear cavity will eventually drain into the Eustachian tube that connects the middle ear cavity into the nasopharynx. The TM heals after the surgical procedure while the efficacy of treatment is monitored. The inconsistent nature of intratympanic injections due to anatomical variations, variability in treatment protocols and the different biological effects of various inner ear cell types influence treatment efficacy.

Drug Entry Through the Round and Oval Windows

For intratympanic administration, drugs in the middle ear cavity can diffuse into the basal cochlear turn through the RWM, and possibly through the oval window. The RWM is a semi-permeable membrane separating the middle ear from the inner ear. It is composed of three layers: an outer epithelial layer, a middle connective layer, and an inner cellular layer facing the scala tympani perilymph of the cochlea. RWM permeability is affected by many factors in normal and pathological conditions (Goycoolea, 2001). The varied shapes of the ear canal in humans often introduce difficulty in visualizing RWM during intratympanic administration and the obstruction of RWM by plugs of connective or fibrosis tissue can lead to interpatient variability in intratympanic administration (Salt and Plontke, 2005).

The oval window allows access to the scala vestibule of the inner ear from the middle ear cavity. The oval window is covered by the footplate of the stapes and is attached by the annular ligament. Experimental results suggest that the oval window is more permeable to compounds than RWM, likely due to the cellular composition of the structure. Delivery through the oval window may be useful in treating vestibular dysfunction and provides a promising route of drug delivery to the vestibular system, which houses the saccule, utricle, and semi-circular canals (**Figure 1**; King et al., 2011, 2013, 2017).

Intracochlear Drug Administration

To overcome drug loss from the middle ear space, intracochlear administration allows direct drug entry into the cochlea. To this end, several methods have been developed to provide direct access to the cochlea, including canalostomy followed by direct injection, osmotic pumps, or cochlear implant mediated delivery (Ayoob and Borenstein, 2015). Achieving even distribution of therapeutics throughout the cochlear turns may be difficult. This is due to the varying diameters of the coiled cochlea, slow diffusion rate from base to apex of the cochlea, poor control of targeted delivery to the cells in different cochlear turns and delayed intracochlear fibrosis that develops over time. Direct access to the cochlea is generally avoided because it requires surgical and destructive techniques that can lead to co-morbidities and exacerbate inner ear damages (Borenstein, 2011). Clinicians typically employ intracochlear delivery only as the last option or if they are already performing surgery for other ailments.

BARRIERS TO INNER EAR DRUG DELIVERY

The bony otic capsule housing the cochlea and vestibular organs is the major anatomic and physiological barrier to inner ear drug delivery. It is both the densest bone and most inaccessible location in the human body for surgical procedures. To avoid the otic capsule, systemic drug delivery allows drugs to enter the inner ear intravascularly through the blood vessels. The intravascular route is an attractive, non-invasive strategy to avoid the inaccessible anatomy. The drugs likely travel through the labyrinthine artery, which branches into the spiral modiolar artery, vestibulocochlear artery, and the anterior vestibular artery. The spiral modiolar artery supplies blood into the stria vascularis and organ of Corti and allows drugs to enter into these regions. The permeability of drug through the blood-labyrinth barrier (BLB) at the luminal surface of inner ear capillaries restricts the entry of many blood-borne compounds into inner ear tissues. Similar to the blood-brain-barrier, the BLB is characterized by endothelial cells that seal the luminal surface of the inner ear capillaries using tight and adherent junctions. The BLB preferentially excludes high molecular weight compounds and decreases their entry into the inner ear. Local administration avoids BLB restricted systemic delivery into the inner ear.

Drug Clearance From the Middle Ear Cavity

In the middle ear cavity, the round and oval window membranes are potential physical barriers that prevent drug permeation and accumulation in the cochlea. In intratympanic delivery, while drugs reside in the middle ear cavity, the liquid drains from the Eustachian tube, a canal that connects the middle ear cavity to the throat and the back of the nasal cavity. Drainage is facilitated by mucociliary flow, causing drug loss and short drug residence time in the middle ear space. Increasing drug residence in the middle ear cavity allows for sustained drug delivery and limits drug clearance by drainage through the Eustachian canal or excretion out of the inner ear BLB (Salt, 2005; Salt and Plontke, 2005). Effective drug clearance in the middle ear causes short drug residence time and decreases drug concentrations after administration resulting in less effective treatment.

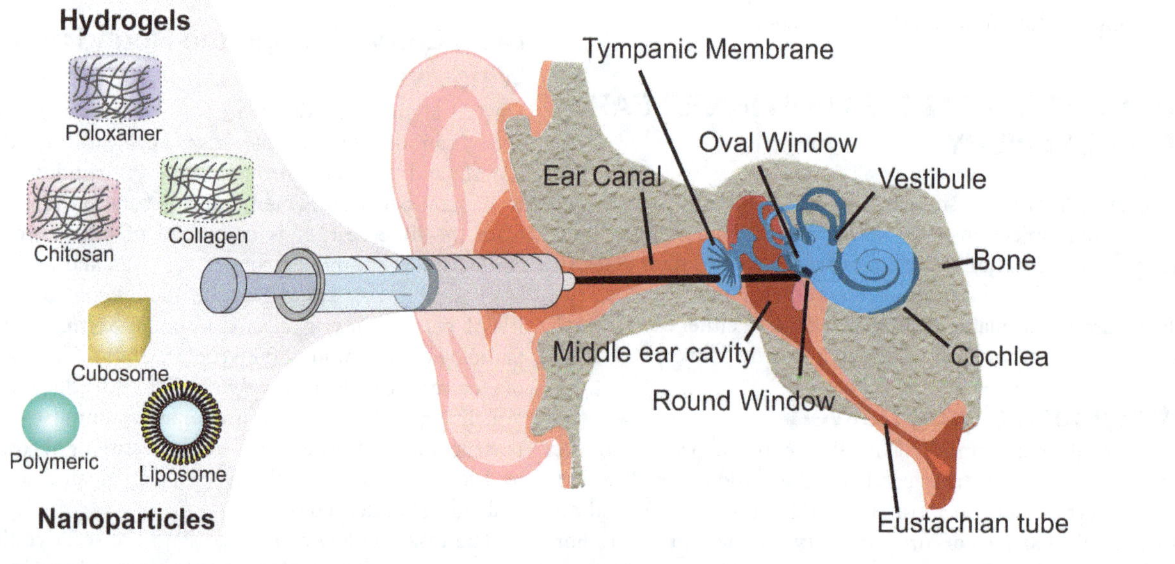

FIGURE 1 | Scheme of intratympanic injection of biomaterials to the round window for inner ear therapy.

Drug Clearance From the Cochlea

Once cochlear delivery is achieved, the residence of therapeutics in the cochlea affects the efficacy of treatment. A cross-section of the cochlea reveals three separate compartments: the scala vestibuli, scala media, and scala tympani. Tight cellular barriers separate the Na^+ rich perilymph in the scala media and scala vestibule from the K^+ rich endolymph in the scala media. These barriers vary in the degree of permeability, which complicates the assessment of pharmacokinetic spread and elimination of drugs. Fluid exchange and maintenance of salt concentrations in the cochlea alter residence time and drug concentrations in the cochlea duct (Salt and Plontke, 2005). Unlike other bodily fluids, cochlear fluid composition, cochlear fluid homeostasis, and generation and regulation of the endocochlear potential by K^+ secretion contributes to the distribution of drugs throughout the cochlea (Wangemann, 2006) and results in highly variable or unpredictable pharmacokinetics.

A potential route that decreases the residence time of therapeutics in the inner ear is drainage through the cochlear aqueduct, which connects the perilymphatic space of the cochlear basal turn to the subarachnoid space of the posterior cranial fossa. The cochlear aqueduct maintains fluid and pressure balance between the inner ear perilymph and cerebral spinal fluid (CSF) (Gopen et al., 1997). Perilymph sampling from the basal turn of scala tympani for pharmacokinetic studies of inner ear drug delivery systems is contaminated by CSF (Salt and Hirose, 2018). CSF dilutes and hinders effective concentration of drugs after intratympanic or intracochlear administration at the cochlear base. Understanding the microanatomy, fluid flow, and characteristics of the different cell types in the inner ear are important to achieve a uniform and sustained delivery of drugs or therapeutics in the cochlea.

BIOMATERIALS FOR LOCAL DRUG DELIVERY

The fragile nature of the inner ear, the numerous membranous structures and the complex biological barriers designed to protect the inner ear from harmful exogenous materials make delivery to the inner ear extremely challenging. Developing non-ototoxic biomaterials that can bypass the tissue-specific biological barriers are required for efficient delivery. Systemically administered drug or biologic must cross the blood labyrinth barrier to reach the inner ear (Juhn et al., 1982). Usually, only a small amount of the therapeutic reaches the inner ear. Therefore, high doses of therapeutics are required to achieve effective concentrations for efficacious treatments. Systemic administration of high drug concentrations, particularly steroids, has numerous side effects. To avoid such side effects, intratympanic injection of therapeutics to the middle ear cavity allows local organ targeted delivery.

Even though intratympanic injection allows for local drug delivery, it results in variable drug kinetics and lack of cellular specificity. Newer approaches for drug delivery into inner ear have considered these limitations and employed novel biomaterials to sustain prolonged drug exposure to targeted cells with minimal systemic side effects. Such delivery methods will allow for a single local administration without repeated dosing in an office-based procedure. Development of biomaterials that overcome cellular toxicity, control degradation kinetics and modulate drug distribution after delivery need to be addressed.

To sustain delivery, limit degradation and allow even distribution in the inner ear, two major classes of biomaterials have been developed: hydrogels and nanoparticles. Soluble drugs can be loaded into hydrogels placed at the RWM for controlled and sustained drug diffusion from the middle ear space. Coupling drugs to nanoparticles impede drug degradation and can be tuned for fast diffusion and cell-specific targeting in the inner ear. When designing such biomaterials, additional considerations include efficacy, toxicity, and long-term degradation. Delivery of biomaterials is well studied in a variety of organs such as the eye, bones, heart. Requirements for each targeted organ entails a unique design and modifications to safely and effectively function as therapeutic carriers (Langer and Peppas, 1981; Panyam and Labhasetwar, 2003; Couvreur, 2013; Li and Mooney, 2016). To this end, recent advances in material science and nanochemistry have led to the rapid development of biomaterial systems for inner ear drug delivery (**Table 1**).

Hydrogels for Drug Retention and Controlled Release of Therapeutics

A major hurdle of intratympanic or intracochlear delivery is controlling residence time and sustained release to achieve therapeutic drug concentrations in the inner ear. Hydrogels helps retain drugs for sustained release. Hydrogels are hydrophilic polymeric networks that retain water and swell with a very large water fraction. Hydrogels are of particular interest for drug delivery because of their chemical functionality, biocompatibility, tunable physical properties, drug loading capability, and degradation capability (Peppas and Sahlin, 1996; Hoare and Kohane, 2008). Hydrogel-based drug delivery systems into the inner ear involve introducing a liquid that gels in the middle ear cavity near the RWM. Retaining the drug in the solidified hydrogel allows the drug to persist in a local region, prolong diffusion across the RWM and release of drugs at therapeutically meaningful concentrations (El Kechai et al., 2015). Viscosity of hydrogels increases the retention time of drugs, improves drug kinetics by increasing residence time and allows equilibrium to be reached for even distribution. Hydrogels vary in their molecular interactions, ionic charge, physical appearance, and chemical composition such as the source of the monomer (**Figure 2**; Li and Mooney, 2016), but can be classified into natural and synthetic products. Natural products are some of the best-studied hydrogels due to biocompatibility as observed by the lack of cellular toxicity and negligible immune response after introducing the biomaterial into the human body. Synthetic hydrogels are becoming more prevalent due to increased control over chemical functionality, mechanical properties, drug loading, and degradation kinetics (Ahmed, 2015).

Synthetic Poloxamer Hydrogels

Poloxamers are synthetic polymers made of a central block of poly (propylene oxide) (PPO) and two flanking blocks of poly

TABLE 1 | Common biomaterial used for drug delivery to the inner ear.

Material	Structure	Key advantage	Method of drug loading	References
Poloxamers	Hydrogel/Nanoparticles	Thermogelation, tunable drug release, biodegradable, chemically defined, porosity	Encapsulation, chemical linking	Dumortier et al., 2006; Wang et al., 2009, 2011; Salt et al., 2011; Engleder et al., 2014; Honeder et al., 2014;
Chitosan	Hydrogel/Nanoparticles	Cationic, mucoadhesive, biocompatible, biodegradable, porosity	Electrostatic, encapsulation, chemical linking	Dai et al., 2018; Kayyali et al., 2018
Collagen/Gelatin	Hydrogel/Nanoparticles	Naturally found in humans, biocompatible, biodegradable gelatin-low immunogenicity	Encapsulation, chemical linking	Endo et al., 2005; Iwai et al., 2006; Lee et al., 2007; Inaoka et al., 2009; Kikkawa et al., 2009; Van Vlierberghe et al., 2011; Lambert et al., 2016
PLGA	Hydrogel/Nanoparticles	Biodegradable, tunable size, tunable degradation, chemically defined, FDA approved, porosity	Encapsulation, tethering	Tamura et al., 2005; Zou et al., 2010b; Cai et al., 2014, 2017; Dai et al., 2018
SPION	Nanoparticles	T2 MRI contrast agent, magnetofection, FDA approved for imaging	Adsorption, Tethering	Thaler et al., 2011; Ramaswamy et al., 2017; Zou et al., 2017
Polymersomes	Nanoparticles	Ease of functionalization, biocompatible, versatile drug loading, chemically synthesized	Encapsulation, tethering	Meng et al., 2009; Roy et al., 2010; Zhang et al., 2011a, 2012; Surovtseva et al., 2012
BSA	Nanoparticles	Biocompatible, biodegradable	Encapsulation	Yu et al., 2014
Lipid nanocapsules	Nanoparticles	Small size, physical stability, ease of manufacture, high hydrophobic drug loading, chemically and structurally defined	Encapsulation	Zou et al., 2008; Zhang et al., 2011b
Liposomes	Nanoparticles	Biocompatible, FDA approved, hydrophobic and hydrophilic drugs	Encapsulation, tethering	Fröhlich, 2012; Kayyali et al., 2018; Yang et al., 2018
Cubosomes	Nanoparticles	Biodegradable, loads all drug types, high drug loading, physical stability, chemically and structurally defined	Encapsulation	Azmi et al., 2015; Bu et al., 2015
Silver nanoparticles	Nanoparticles	Anti-fungal, Anti-bacterial, ease of synthesis, chemically and structurally defined	Tethering, adsorption	Zou et al., 2015
Silica	Nanoparticles	Biodegradable, ease of surface tuning/modification, porosity, chemically and structurally defined	Adsorption, tethering	Praetorius et al., 2007; Wise et al., 2016; Xu et al., 2018

(ethylene glycol) (PEG). Poloxamers are extensively developed for drug delivery because their gel transition temperature can be adjusted by varying the concentration of poloxamer. The poloxamer can form a thermo-responsive gel that is a liquid at room temperature for handling ease, resuspension, and injection of a drug, while triggered to gel at body temperature *in situ* when applied to the RWM. Of the many poloxamers studied, poloxamer 407, where the 40 represents the PPO molecular mass (4,000 g/mol), and the 7 represents the PEG content (70%), is the main synthetic hydrogel used for inner ear delivery. This poloxamer has been used to deliver a variety of different drug types into the inner ear (Dumortier et al., 2006). Compared to intratympanic injection of dexamethasone, poloxamer 407 loaded with micronized dexamethasone (mDex) delivered to the guinea pig round window provided sustained release of the drug, increased the overall concentration in the perilymph by ~1.6-fold and increased the residence time of the drug by ~24 fold. Injected dexamethasone solutions show an initial spike in concentration before clearing from the perilymph within 12 h, while the mDex hydrogel formulations result in 10 days of sustained release. Use of poloxamer 407 highlights its suitability for long term drug delivery (Wang et al., 2009). Prolonged-release of dexamethasone would be more beneficial for the treatment of inner ear disease rather than a single bolus dose that is rapidly cleared. The study also demonstrates that mDex delivery using poloxamer 407 led to more homogenous distribution of dexamethasone along the length of the cochlea (Salt et al., 2011).

Another advantage of using poloxamers is the ability to deliver low solubility therapeutics. Formation of micelles in the hydrogel facilitates loading of hydrophobic drugs and gel formation (Engleder et al., 2014). Low solubility drugs such as dexamethasone and methylprednisolone are more easily incorporated in the poloxamer hydrogel compared to aqueous solution (Wang et al., 2011). Triamcinolone Acetonide (TAAc), a glucocorticoid for treatment of inner ear disease, was loaded into poloxamer 407 hydrogels. Intratympanic injection of the TAAc loaded hydrogels near the round window allowed for 10 days of sustained drug release at high levels. Levels of TAAc were significantly higher (up to 600 fold) in the perilymph than in the plasma, suggesting local release of drug through the RWM with minimal release into the circulatory system. Hydrogel treatment, however, showed temporary ABR threshold shifts which returned

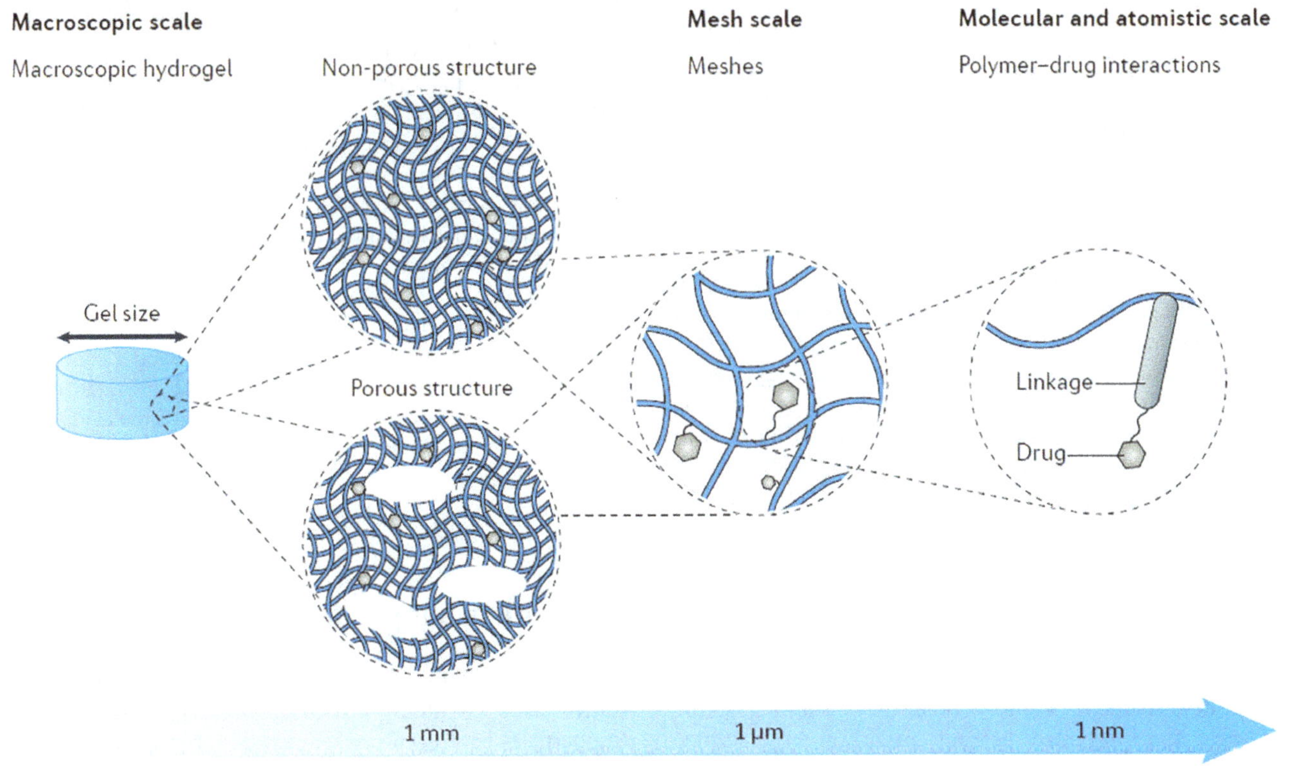

FIGURE 2 | Schematic showing the multi-scale tunability of hydrogels for drug delivery applications, showcasing the versatility of drug delivery properties based on material characteristics. By modulating material properties such as composition, porosity, and intramolecular bonding the degradation and drug release kinetics can be tuned as well as other properties such as gelation temperature and shear thinning mechanics.

back to normal 10 days without histological damage or reduction in hair cell numbers. Intratympanic injection of the hydrogel into the middle ear likely prevents movement of the middle ear bones and perturbs sound transmission to the inner ear. Degradation of the hydrogel reverses the temporary ABR threshold shift (Honeder et al., 2014). These examples demonstrate sustained drug delivery through the RWM using poloxamers.

Natural Chitosan Hydrogels

Natural polymer hydrogels are based on collagen, hyaluronic acid, and chitosan. The main advantage of using these polymers are biocompatibility, making them excellent non-toxic drug delivery systems. Chitosan has been developed for many years due to its biocompatibility and biodegradability. Chitosan is found in the outer skeleton of shellfish and has cationic characteristics that confer mucoadhesive property which allows it to adhere to the outer epithelium of the RWM by electrostatic interactions (Sogias et al., 2008). The selective attachment of chitosan allows for specific placement at the RWM. Chitosan glycerophosphate (CGP) has also been used to make hydrogels due to its favorable thermoresponsive properties to gel at body temperature, its mucoadhesive properties, and its ability to harbor a variety of payloads. Delivery of dexamethasone into the murine inner ear using CGP hydrogels demonstrate they adhere to the round window niche and shows release of a high percentage (92%) of the dexamethasone in the perilymph after 5 days (Paulson et al., 2008).

In addition to corticosteroids, CGP hydrogels have been used to treat MD by delivering the ototoxic drug gentamicin to chemically ablate vestibular hair cells. By intratympanic injection, gentamicin enters both the vestibule and the cochlea but selectively accumulates in vestibular hair cells allowing for preferential vestibular hair cell ablation (Lyford-Pike et al., 2007). CGP hydrogel delivery allowed sustained gentamicin release over 7 days compared to an injection of liquid gentamicin which declined after 1 day (Xu et al., 2010). Despite sustained release, a gentamicin concentration gradient developed in the cochlea from the base-to-apex, exposing gentamicin to the basal portion of the cochlea at higher doses and for a longer period (Luo and Xu, 2012). The side effect of increased gentamicin at the base of the cochlea may lead to high-frequency hearing loss.

To gain more control over the timed-release of drugs, the addition of chitosanase, an enzyme that degrades chitosan hydrogel can be used to "turn off" drug delivery. Treatment with chitosanase quickly degrades the CGP-hydrogel, which is then cleared through the Eustachian tube. This results in burst release and accumulation of low drug concentrations in the perilymph. The "turn off" system for CGP-based hydrogel drug delivery can be employed to quickly terminate drug delivery and avoid unwanted side-effects from sustained or prolonged drug exposure (Lajud et al., 2013). Chitosan gels can be used to deliver many different drugs, but the intended use and effects of the drugs for inner ear treatment can be tuned for slow sustained delivery or controlled burst release. These studies demonstrate the flexibility for chitosan-based hydrogels as a controllable local drug delivery system to the inner ear (Lajud et al., 2015).

Natural Collagen or Gelatin Hydrogels

Another natural polymer commonly used for inner ear delivery is collagen or its denatured form gelatin. Both are found in the human body and are biocompatible. When combined with various types of cross-linkers, collagen and gelatin can form hydrogels for controlled drug release (Van Vlierberghe et al., 2011). Delivery of biologics, such as growth factors that promote inner ear cell survival, are limited by the short half-life of these proteins. Use of the biocompatible natural hydrogels ensure that the proteins retain biological activity, reduce degradation and allow for prolonged release.

Gelatin hydrogel delivery of insulin-like growth factor 1 (IGF1) to the inner ear after noise-induced hearing loss in guinea pigs increased outer hair cell survival. The positively charged recombinant human IGF1 protein electrostatically interacts with negatively charged gelatin hydrogel. IGF1 release over 7 days reduced auditory brainstem recording (ABR) thresholds and prevented hearing loss (Iwai et al., 2006; Lee et al., 2007). Exogenous hepatocyte growth factor (HGF) has been shown to be otoprotective and promote hair cell survival after toxic insults (Kikkawa et al., 2009). HGF soaked gelatin hydrogel administered to the round window of a noise-damaged guinea pig prevented ABR threshold increase and outer hair cell loss in the basal region of the cochlea (Inaoka et al., 2009). Brain-derived neurotrophic factor (BDNF), a factor that increases spiral ganglion neuron survival after ototoxic damage, was delivered to the RWM by gelatin hydrogel. Sustained delivery by encapsulating BDNF in the gelatin hydrogel increased BDNF concentration in the perilymph over 100 fold, which was detected even after 7 days. Sustained exposure to BDNF prevented elevated ABR thresholds and preserved spiral ganglion neurons from ototoxic insult (Endo et al., 2005).

Use of hydrogels for slow release of drugs and biologics into the inner ear can be important for long-term application. Hydrogels are the lowest hanging fruit in terms of biomaterials for delivery to the inner ear because of their non-toxic and biologically safe nature of the material; however, safety and efficacy for the treatment of inner ear disorders in longitudinal studies still need to be validated. In fact, several companies are performing clinical trials for gel-based formulations for the treatment of inner ear disorders (Lambert et al., 2016). While hydrogels have the distinct advantage of increasing retention time and providing sustained drug release at the round window, they do not address the challenges of slowing drug degradation and ensuring cell-specific delivery. Preventing drug degradation allows prolonged residence of effective concentration drugs at the delivery site, while cell-specific delivery increases therapeutic efficacy and limits deleterious side effects.

Nanoparticles for Improved Diffusion and Clearance Prevention

The design of nanoparticles is applicable for delivering a wide variety of therapeutics in different diseases. Coupling therapeutics to nanoparticles can alter drug degradation and diffusion kinetics through tissue barriers. Nanoparticles prevent drug degradation by providing a protective barrier around the molecule. Diffusion kinetics of drugs can be altered by modifying nanoparticle surface properties, such as charge and hydrophobicity to increase drug circulation time, tissue penetration and cellular uptake. Nanotechnology allows tuning of designer nanoparticles properties to increase drug accumulation and stability, as well as provide cell-specific delivery of therapeutics to the tissue of interest (**Figure 3**; Chou et al., 2011). In addition, nanoparticle platforms allow multiple drugs to be loaded in order to increase drug delivery efficiency and efficacy. Nanoparticle-based drug delivery into the inner ear remains relatively unexplored.

Polymeric Nanoparticles

Polymeric nanoparticles are advantageous for drug delivery due to their biocompatibility, small size, degradation tunability, and relatively simple synthesis procedure. Because of this, polymeric nanoparticles have been used in a wide range of drug delivery applications including cancer therapies, diagnostics, molecular imaging, and a myriad of other applications (De Jong and Borm, 2008; Janib et al., 2010). PLGA is one of the most well studied polymeric nanoparticles due to its biocompatibility, ease of surface modification, biodegradability, and ability to encapsulate drugs. Early studies utilizing a rhodamine-conjugated poly (lactic-co-glycolic acid) (PLGA) nanoparticles were detected by fluorescence microscopy. Systematic delivery of rhodamine-conjugated PLGA nanoparticles accumulated in the liver, kidney, and cochlea of guinea pigs. Long-term residence of the nanoparticles was observed only in the liver but not in the cochlea or kidney. Limited accumulation was likely due to tissue-specific barriers, increased clearance or rapid degradation of particles. To enhance local concentrations in the cochlea, PLGA nanoparticles were suspended in gelfoam, a substance similar to hydrogel, and placed at the RWM for local delivery. Local administration significantly increased the number of particles in the cochlea but formed a gradient of unevenly distributed nanoparticles with more nanoparticles residing in the cochlear basal turn. These studies established the feasibility of localized nanoparticle delivery across the round window (Tamura et al., 2005).

To increase the accumulation of nanoparticles in the inner ear, key modifications to the size, surface properties, and conjugated ligands can be made to affect diffusion kinetics and residence time of nanoparticles in the inner ear. Changing the size of PLGA nanoparticles to 150 and 300 nm enhanced entry into the inner ear. Functionalizing the surface of the nanoparticles with the non-ionic detergent pluronic acid 127 increased accumulation of particles in the inner ear after intracochlear delivery. Pluronic 127 increases the hydrophilicity of the nanoparticles to increase circulation time, reduce clearance, and enhance bioavailability (Zou et al., 2010b). Modifying particles with chitosan created a

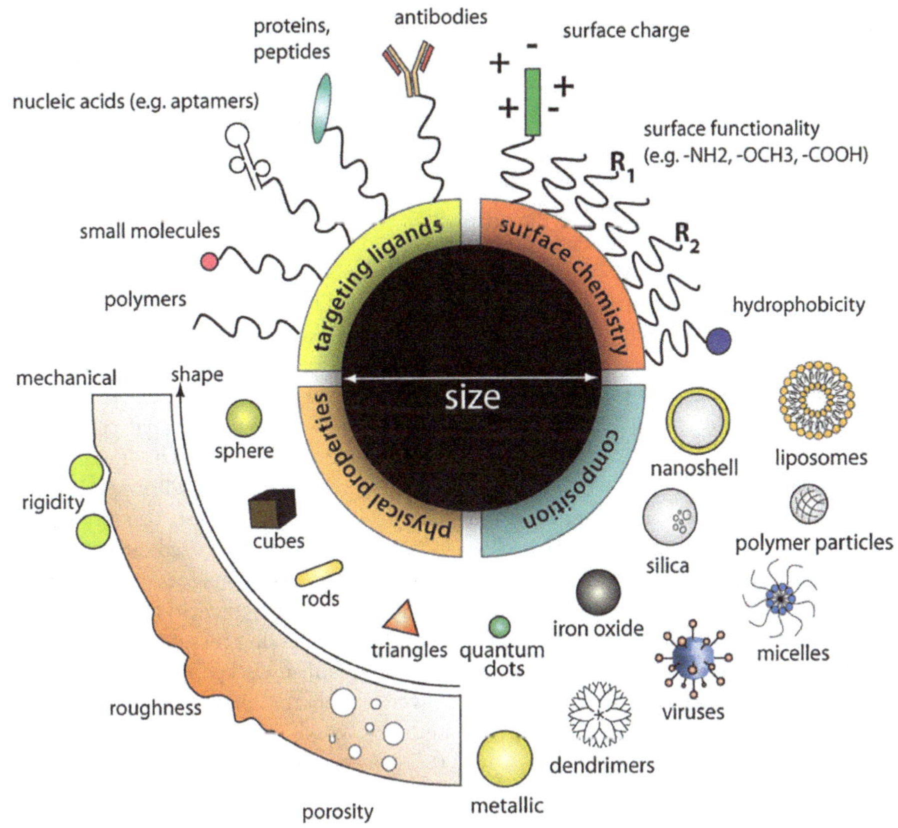

FIGURE 3 | Material composition, surface properties, and functional groups can all be tuned to modulate the functional properties of nanoparticles such as drug loading and release kinetics, fluorescence, cell targeting, diffusion, cellular uptake, and many more. The modular nature of nanoparticles makes them ideal for optimizing the delivery of molecules for specific bioapplications.

positively charged surface that increases the kinetics at which these particles enter the inner ear. Modifying nanoparticles with a hydrophilic surface using poloxamer 407 resulted in greater penetration and increased accumulation of particles in the perilymph. Lastly, tethering cell-penetrating peptide ligands to the surface, such as TAT peptides, could increase the transport of the nanoparticles into the inner ear through the round window. These studies demonstrate that facile surface functionalization can enhance nanoparticle delivery to the inner ear (Cai et al., 2017).

While PLGA nanoparticles can encapsulate drugs and allow delivery of a single drug, it can also be used to deliver multiple therapeutics for synergistic drug actions. To this end, the ability of PLGA nanoparticles to deliver a combination of three drugs, notoginsenoside R1, ginsenoside Rg1, and ginsenoside Rb1 to protect spiral ganglion neurons from cochlear ischemia was done. The total amount of R1, Rg1, and Rb1 in the perilymph increased 4. 0-, 3. 1-, and 7.1-fold, respectively, compared to the delivery of free drug solution. This demonstrated the ability of PLGA nanoparticles to simultaneously deliver multiple drugs to the inner ear for a potentially greater therapeutic effect (Cai et al., 2014).

For controlled delivery after injection, nanoparticles such as polymersomes can easily be modified, making them controllable by pH, magnetic fields and other factors (Meng et al., 2009). Polymersomes consisting of polyethylene glycol-polycaprolactone (PEG-PCL) diblock polymers encapsulate hydrophobic drugs into the center of the nanoparticles. Dye-labeled polymersomes delivered transtympanically or by cochleostomy showed a significant number of nanoparticles in the spiral ligament, the organ of Corti, and the spiral ganglion cells (Zhang et al., 2011a; Buckiová et al., 2012).

Amino acid and protein-based nanoparticles are biocompatible and increase drug retention time during delivery. Bovine serum albumin (BSA) proteins are biodegradable and can be used as a nanoparticle delivery system. Distribution of rhodamine-labeled BSA nanoparticles after intratympanic delivery increases the retention time of drugs in the middle ear. While BSA does not easily pass through the round window, it is thought to serve a similar purpose as hydrogels by increasing retention time at the round window and slowing degradation of drugs (Yu et al., 2014). Poly-amino acid-based nanoparticles such as poly (2-hydroxyethyl aspartamide) (PHEA) have been used for inner ear delivery. Dye encapsulated PHEA showed significant uptake in the organ of Corti, with dye accumulating in inner hair cells. PHEA nanoparticles may be advantageous for the delivery of therapeutics to the inner hair cells (Kim et al., 2015). While there is no known ligand on PHEA nanoparticles to target inner hair cells, preferential accumulation in inner hair cells may be attributed to their physical and chemical properties such as the surface charge and hydrophilicity of the particles and how they bind to the surface of inner hair cells before endocytosis of the nanoparticles.

Although size, surface properties, and surface functionalization can clearly affect polymeric nanoparticle retention time, degradation rate and uptake into cells, the mechanism by which each of these occurs will depend on nanoparticle design and the unique properties of different cell types. Structural, compositional, and functional interactions between nanoparticle and cells *in vivo* will likely constrain the efficiency of delivery and further studies are needed to fully elucidate the functional relationships between nanoparticles properties and their pharmacokinetic effects.

Non-polymeric Nanoparticles

While polymeric nanoparticles are well studied for inner ear drug delivery, lipid-based, silica-based, and metallic nanoparticles have not been as well explored. Many of these non-polymeric nanoparticles are unique because of their magnetic, anti-microbial, tunable properties. Despite some of the useful qualities of non-polymeric nanoparticles, many are expensive, difficult to manufacture and only allow limited changes in surface properties.

Lipid-based nanoparticles can be used to deliver a range of therapeutics such as gadolinium to serve as an imaging contrasting agent (Zou et al., 2010a, 2012), doxorubicin for cancer treatment (Doxil) (Barenholz, 2012) and a transgene for gene therapy (Wareing et al., 1999). Lipid-based nanoparticles allow loading of large amounts of hydrophobic drugs, however, control over degradation and surface properties of the nanoparticle is limited. Fluorescently labeled lipid nanocapsules (LNCs) saturated in gelfoam and placed at the RWM can reach the spiral ganglion neuron cell bodies, nerve fibers, and spiral ligament fibrocytes within 30 min (Zou et al., 2008). LNCs did not cause hearing loss, cell death, or morphological changes in the inner ear, for up to 28 days suggesting low cytotoxicity (Zhang et al., 2011b).

Surface charge and hydrophilicity in lipid-based nanoparticles can change uptake and targeting. Addition of cationic and cationic-PEG (with a hydrophilic PEG chain) to phospholipid-based nanoparticle enhances entry into the RWM but showed a high level of cytotoxicity (Fröhlich, 2012). Using cationic-PEG particles to deliver dexamethasone to the mouse RWM provided a protective anti-inflammatory effect from kanamycin and furosemide treatment (Yang et al., 2018). Addition of cationic charge and increase of hydrophilicity at of phospholipid based nanoparticle can potentially be used for inner ear delivery if cytotoxicity is limited.

Lipid-based crystalline nanoparticles, called cubosomes formed from phytantriol lipids are of specific interest because they have a high drug loading capacity due to their large surface area. They are biodegradable and can incorporate hydrophobic, hydrophilic, and amphiphilic drugs into their matrix (Azmi et al., 2015). When nerve growth factor (NGF) was loaded into the phytantriol lipid-crystal nanoparticles (PHY-NGF) and delivered to the RWM, there was a significant 3.28 fold enhanced drug transport across the round window and a 4.8 fold increased maximum drug concentration compared to unloaded NGF treatment (Bu et al., 2015).

Metallic nanoparticles made of noble metals or iron oxide are used because of their bio-inert features, properties as MRI contrast imaging or ability for magnetofection. Fe_3O_4 nanoparticles oxidized by ceric ammonium nitrate (CAN) forms a CAN-Fe_2O_3 nanoparticle system that can cross both the round and oval window after delivery to the rat middle ear. The CAN-Fe_2O_3 accumulated in Reissner's membrane, basilar membrane, and cochlear lateral wall. In the lateral wall, nanoparticles were found in the mesothelial cells of the scala tympani, the spiral ligament, and the stria vascularis. After 14 days all the nanoparticles were cleared from the inner ear (Zou et al., 2017). To improve tissue delivery of metallic nanoparticles, a magnetic field was used after intratympanic injection of prednisolone loaded magnetic nanoparticles in cisplatin-treated mice. Using a magnetic field to deliver drugs showed a significant reduction of hearing loss and increased outer hair cell survival from cisplatin-induced ototoxicity (Ramaswamy et al., 2017). Silver nanoparticles also have anti-microbial properties and serve as good contrasting agents for computed tomography (CT) heavy metal detection in the body. Distribution of silver nanoparticles assessed by micro-CT after transtympanic delivery was detected in the middle ear, ossicular chain, RWM, oval window, scala tympani, and Eustachian tube after 4 and 24 h. A distinct concentration gradient was found with fewer particles deeper into the inner ear. It was determined that entry to the inner ear was through the round and oval windows (Zou et al., 2015).

Lastly, silica-based nanoparticles are used because of their biocompatibility, biodegradability, and ease of surface modification and tuning. Distribution of Cy3 labeled silica nanoparticles in the inner ear after placement on the round window showed nanoparticle uptake in the inner hair cells, outer hair cells, spiral ganglion neurons, and supporting cells without any harmful effects on hearing (Praetorius et al., 2007). This demonstrated the safety and feasibility of using silica-based nanoparticles for inner ear drug delivery. Delivery of silica nanoparticle-based BDNF as neuroprotectant to deafened guinea pigs showed a significant improvement in SGN survival after noise-induced hearing loss (Wise et al., 2016). Similarly, hollow mesoporous silica nanoparticles with a zeolitic imidazolate shell can also be used for *in vitro* and *in vivo* delivery into inner ear cells (Xu et al., 2018).

The use of non-polymeric nanoparticles can greatly increase the variety of drugs for encapsulation and allow for a greater variety of physical and surface properties that are beneficial for developing drug delivery systems. While ease of modification and fine control of properties may not be as easy to control for non-polymeric nanoparticles, some of their innate properties such as magnetism, anti-microbial surface, and extremely high drug loading can make them attractive candidates for certain applications.

Modified Nanoparticles for Cell-Specific Delivery

While nanoparticles themselves provide several advantages for increasing drug circulation time and preventing premature degradation of compounds, many drugs or therapeutics would ideally be delivered to a specific inner ear cell type for targeted therapies. Several different ligands have been used to enhance the cell-specific targeting of nanoparticles in the inner ear. Ligand-receptor mediated delivery allows the nanoparticles to bind to the cell surface of a specific cell type and have the nanoparticle endocytosed into the cell. Although the accumulation of nanoparticles into cells has been shown, the mechanism of uptake has not been rigorously tested. The rate and efficiency of uptake would depend on the endocytosis mechanisms in the cell type of interest.

Use of a human Nerve Growth Factor-derived peptide (hNGF_EE) conjugated to the surface of polymersomes drastically increased targeting to spiral ganglion neurons. Binding of the hNFG_EE peptide to the NGF receptor at the cell surface, presumably allows the nanoparticle to home into a cell, adhere to the cell and promote endocytosis of the nanoparticle into neurons. In addition to spiral ganglion neurons, Schwann cells, and nerve fibers can be targeted in organotypic cochlear cultures using the tyrosine kinase receptors and p75 neurotrophin receptors (Roy et al., 2010). Using polymersomes functionalized with a TET1 peptide allowed targeting to the cochlear nerve. The TET1 peptide binds to trisialoganglioside clostridial toxin receptor on nerve fibers to deliver nanoparticles (Zhang et al., 2012).

To target outer hair cells, PRESTIN binding peptides were identified using phage display and coupled to nanoparticles. PRESTIN is a protein expressed specifically in the lateral wall of the outer hair cells body. Two peptides A665 and A666 that bind to PRESTIN were conjugated to PEG-PCL polymersomes. Uptake of the polymersomes was tested in Chinese Hamster Ovary cells expressing PRESTIN and cochlear explants. Strong uptake of particles in the CHO cells and outer hair cells of rat cochleae was observed (Surovtseva et al., 2012). Using the A666 mediated PEG-PLA nanoparticle, dexamethasone was delivered to the round window prior to cisplatin treatment. A666 ligand conjugated particles were taken up by outer hair cells *in vivo* and promoted cell survival after ototoxic damage (Wang et al., 2018).

Cellular targeting using ligands is a relatively understudied field in inner ear drug delivery. The specificity of ligands for cell type-specific delivery is still lacking and display uptake of particles in unintended cell types. Lack of cellular specificity for delivery may limit the current use for some clinical applications such as cellular regeneration. The strong potential of targeting nanoparticles to specific cell types demonstrate the need for in-depth study of nanoparticle, ligand, and receptor interactions with cells found in the inner ear. While degradability, physical properties, and kinetics of nanoparticle systems have been well studied (Li et al., 2017), the target-specific delivery of nanoparticles an area that still needs to be developed to make a large impact in the field of inner ear therapeutics.

Hybrid Hydrogel and Nanoparticle Systems

While nanoparticles and hydrogels each have advantages that significantly improve the efficacy and kinetics of delivery, combining the two materials allows synergistically increased control of drug delivery to the inner ear. Hydrogels provide prolonged exposure and increased residence time of loaded drugs, while nanoparticles decrease degradation and allow cell-specific delivery to the inner ear. One example of combining the two materials is the encapsulation of iron oxide nanoparticles into a Pluronic F127 hydrogel to create a "ferrogel." Magnetic nanoparticles from the ferrogel cross the round window and are taken up by cells in the spiral ligament and Reissner's membrane in human cadavers (Thaler et al., 2011). Application of a magnetic field could further enhance entry into the inner ear.

The combination of chitosan hydrogels and liposomes is another hybrid delivery platform. Chitosan hydrogels allowed sustained delivery, while liposomes improved the transport of nanoparticles through the round window. Tracking of dye-labeled particles after delivery showed the presence of nanoparticles in the perilymph and murine inner ear cells. Use of chitosan and liposome together increased the number of particles in the inner ear compared to nanoparticles alone (Lajud et al., 2015). This hybrid system was used in conjunction with PRESTIN binding peptides and the c-Jun N-terminal kinase (JNK) inhibitor, D-JNKi-1, to target outer hair cells. PRESTIN binding peptides promoted cell-specific delivery to outer hair cells while of D-JNKi-1 prevents apoptosis. Together targeted delivery of D-JNKi-1 significantly protected hearing loss after noise-induced damage (Kayyali et al., 2018). Another example of a hybrid delivery system is the use of chitosan hydrogel with PLGA nanoparticles. Chitosan loaded with the drug interferon α-2 increased residence time of while PLGA prevented degradation. Use of both chitosan and PLGA increased the total amount of drug delivered to the perilymph (Dai et al., 2018).

The combination of film-forming agents and drug-loaded microspheres for intratympanic delivery to the round window are another example of a hybrid delivery system. While film-forming agents are not the same as hydrogels, they serve a similar purpose in slowing release kinetics of drug-loaded nanoparticles. These results showed that steady drug release can occur up to 30 days, and the particles in the film-forming agent remain localized on the round window for the same amount of time. This would not be possible with injection of a liquid suspension of nanoparticles. In addition, release kinetics could be tuned by modifying both the film-forming agent as well as the microspheres to allow greater control over delivery parameters depending on the desired application (Dormer et al., 2019). The combination of different materials such as hydrogels and nanoparticles can be used to modulate the pharmacokinetics of drug delivery to the inner ear via intratympanic injections.

Conclusion and Future Perspectives

Microsurgical techniques for introducing therapeutics to the inner ear have shown that intratympanic and intracochlear injections are viable delivery methods. Although for most clinical applications, intratympanic delivery is more practical. When administering therapeutics via intratympanic injections, entry into the inner ear through the round or oval window depends on the molecular weight, charge, and other biophysical properties of the drug as it interacts with round or oval window membranes. The desired drug properties will depend on the inner ear disease to be treated. By tuning the properties of nanoparticles it may be possible to direct drugs to either the vestibular or auditory system by their preferential crossing through the round or oval window. Once inside the appropriate sensory organ, the residence time, binding and biological effect of the drug are affected by drainage, cellular fluid exchange and uptake by cells.

To optimize intratympanic therapeutic delivery, different tunable hydrogels allow for sustained release of drugs from the middle ear cavity and promote entry into the RWM before degradation. Nanoparticle platforms allow multiple drugs or therapeutics to be loaded, and prevent rapid degradation, increase residence time, and target appropriate cell types. By combining the tunable properties of hydrogels and nanoparticles, a versatile delivery platform with the desired properties can be engineered for a variety of drugs that cater to a specific clinical disease.

There still remains a large gap between preclinical and clinical research for employing and optimizing inner ear delivery systems. Studies on the safety and efficacy of biomaterials are still required. However, the promising results from preclinical models suggest that hydrogel and nanoparticle-based biomaterials are viable substrates for inner ear drug delivery based on their ability to pass through many of the physical and cellular barriers. As novel biomaterials are generated and a greater understanding of the inner ear physiology is achieved, biomaterial-based drug delivery to the inner ear will become more amenable for translational use.

AUTHOR CONTRIBUTIONS

CR wrote the nanomaterial part of the manuscript. Y-LY contributed to the description of the surgical procedures. S-TC generated the figures and edited the manuscript. K-BL edited the manuscript. KK contributed to the inner ear portion of the manuscript and edited the manuscript.

REFERENCES

Ahmed, E. M. (2015). Hydrogel: preparation, characterization, and applications: a review. *J. Adv. Res.* 6, 105–121. doi: 10.1016/j.jare.2013.07.006

Alzamil, K. S., and Linthicum, F. H. Jr. (2000). Extraneous round window membranes and plugs: possible effect on intratympanic therapy. *Ann. Otol. Rhinol. Laryngol.* 109, 30–32. doi: 10.1177/000348940010900105

Ayoob, A. M., and Borenstein, J. T. (2015). The role of intracochlear drug delivery devices in the management of inner ear disease. *Expert Opin. Drug Deliv.* 12, 465–479. doi: 10.1517/17425247.2015.974548

Azmi, I. D. M., Moghimi, S. M., and Yaghmur, A. (2015). Cubosomes and hexosomes as versatile platforms for drug delivery. *Ther. Deliv.* 6, 1347–1364. doi: 10.4155/tde.15.81

Barenholz, Y. (2012). Doxil® — the first FDA-approved nano-drug: lessons learned. *J. Control. Release* 160, 117–134. doi: 10.1016/j.jconrel.2012.03.020

Borenstein, J. T. (2011). Intracochlear drug delivery systems. *Expert Opin. Drug Deliv.* 8, 1161–1174. doi: 10.1517/17425247.2011.588207

Bu, M., Tang, J., Wei, Y., Sun, Y., Wang, X., Wu, L., et al. (2015). Enhanced bioavailability of nerve growth factor with phytantriol lipid-based crystalline nanoparticles in cochlea. *Int. J. Nanomed.* 10, 6879–6889. doi: 10.2147/IJN.S82944

Buckiová, D., Ranjan, S., Newman, T. A., Johnston, A. H., Sood, R., Kinnunen, P. K. J., et al. (2012). Minimally invasive drug delivery to the cochlea through application of nanoparticles to the round window membrane. *Nanomedicine* 7, 1339–1354. doi: 10.2217/nnm.12.5

Cai, H., Liang, Z., Huang, W., Wen, L., and Chen, G. (2017). Engineering PLGA nano-based systems through understanding the influence of nanoparticle properties and cell-penetrating peptides for cochlear drug delivery. *Int. J. Pharm.* 532, 55–65. doi: 10.1016/j.ijpharm.2017.08.084

Cai, H., Wen, X., Wen, L., Tirelli, N., Zhang, X., Zhang, Y., et al. (2014). Enhanced local bioavailability of single or compound drugs delivery to the inner ear through application of PLGA nanoparticles via round window administration. *Int. J. Nanomed.* 9, 5591–5601. doi: 10.2147/IJN.S72555

Chandrasekhar, S. S. (2001). Intratympanic dexamethasone for sudden sensorineural hearing loss: clinical and laboratory evaluation. *Otol. Neurotol.* 22, 18–23. doi: 10.1097/00129492-200101000-00005

Chou, L. Y. T., Ming, K., and Chan, W. C. W. (2011). Strategies for the intracellular delivery of nanoparticles. *Chem. Soc. Rev.* 40, 233–245. doi: 10.1039/c0cs00003e

Couvreur, P. (2013). Nanoparticles in drug delivery: past, present and future. *Adv. Drug Deliv. Rev.* 65, 21–23. doi: 10.1016/j.addr.2012.04.010

Dai, J., Long, W., Liang, Z., Wen, L., Yang, F., and Chen, G. (2018). A novel vehicle for local protein delivery to the inner ear: injectable and biodegradable thermosensitive hydrogel loaded with PLGA nanoparticles. *Drug Dev. Ind. Pharm.* 44, 89–98. doi: 10.1080/03639045.2017.1373803

De Jong, W. H., and Borm, P. J. A. (2008). Drug delivery and nanoparticles:applications and hazards. *Int. J. Nanomed.* 3, 133–149.

Dormer, N. H., Nelson-Brantley, J., Staecker, H., and Berkland, C. J. (2019). Evaluation of a transtympanic delivery system in Mus musculus for extended release steroids. *Eur. J. Pharm. Sci.* 126, 3–10. doi: 10.1016/j.ejps.2018.01.020

Doyle, K. J., Bauch, C., Battista, R., Beatty, C., Hughes, G. B., Mason, J., et al. (2004). Intratympanic steroid treatment: a review. *Otol. Neurotol.* 25, 1034–1039. doi: 10.1097/00129492-200411000-00031

Dumortier, G., Grossiord, J. L., Agnely, F., and Chaumeil, J. C. (2006). A review of poloxamer 407 pharmaceutical and pharmacological characteristics. *Pharm. Res.* 23, 2709–2728. doi: 10.1007/s11095-006-9104-4

El Kechai, N., Agnely, F., Mamelle, E., Nguyen, Y., Ferrary, E., and Bochot, A. (2015). Recent advances in local drug delivery to the inner ear. *Int. J. Pharm.* 494, 83–101. doi: 10.1016/j.ijpharm.2015.08.015

Endo, T., Nakagawa, T., Kita, T., Iguchi, F., Kim, T.-S., Tamura, T., et al. (2005). Novel strategy for treatment of inner ears using a biodegradable gel. *Laryngoscope* 115, 2016–2020. doi: 10.1097/01.mlg.0000183020.32435.59

Engleder, E., Honeder, C., Klobasa, J., Wirth, M., Arnoldner, C., and Gabor, F. (2014). Preclinical evaluation of thermoreversible triamcinolone acetonide hydrogels for drug delivery to the inner ear. *Int. J. Pharm.* 471, 297–302. doi: 10.1016/j.ijpharm.2014.05.057

Fröhlich, E. (2012). The role of surface charge in cellular uptake and cytotoxicity of medical nanoparticles. *Int. J. Nanomed.* 7, 5577–5591.

Garduno-Anaya, M. A., Couthino De Toledo, H., Hinojosa-Gonzalez, R., Pane-Pianese, C., and Rios-Castaneda, L. C. (2005). Dexamethasone inner ear perfusion by intratympanic injection in unilateral Meniere's disease: a two-year prospective, placebo-controlled, double-blind, randomized trial. *Otolaryngol. Head Neck Surg.* 133, 285–294. doi: 10.1016/j.otohns.2005.05.010

Gopen, Q., Rosowski, J. J., and Merchant, S. N. (1997). Anatomy of the normal human cochlear aqueduct with functional implications. *Hear. Res.* 107, 9–22. doi: 10.1016/s0378-5955(97)00017-8

Goycoolea, M. V. (2001). Clinical aspects of round window membrane permeability under normal and pathological conditions. *Acta Otolaryngol.* 121, 437–447. doi: 10.1080/000164801300366552

Havia, M., Kentala, E., and Pyykkö, I. (2002). Hearing loss and tinnitus in Meniere's disease. *Auris Nasus Larynx* 29, 115–119.

Hill, S. L. III, Digges, E. N., and Silverstein, H. (2006). Long-term follow-up after gentamicin application via the silverstein microwick in the treatment of Meniere's disease. *Ear Nose Throat. J.* 85, 494, 496, 498.

Hoare, T. R., and Kohane, D. S. (2008). Hydrogels in drug delivery: progress and challenges. *Polymer* 49, 1993–2007. doi: 10.1016/j.polymer.2008.01.027

Honeder, C., Engleder, E., Schöpper, H., Gabor, F., Reznicek, G., Wagenblast, J., et al. (2014). Sustained release of triamcinolone acetonide from an intratympanically applied hydrogel designed for the delivery of high glucocorticoid doses. *Audiol. Neurotol.* 19, 193–202. doi: 10.1159/000358165

Inaoka, T., Nakagawa, T., Kikkawa, Y. S., Tabata, Y., Ono, K., Yoshida, M., et al. (2009). Local application of hepatocyte growth factor using gelatin hydrogels attenuates noise-induced hearing loss in guinea pigs. *Acta Otolaryngol.* 129, 453–457. doi: 10.1080/00016480902725197

Itoh, A., and Sakata, E. (1991). Treatment of vestibular disorders. *Acta Otolaryngol. Suppl.* 481, 617–623.

Iwai, K., Nakagawa, T., Endo, T., Matsuoka, Y., Kita, T., Kim, T.-S., et al. (2006). Cochlear protection by local insulin-like growth Factor-1 application using biodegradable hydrogel. *Laryngoscope* 116, 529–533. doi: 10.1097/01.mlg.0000200791.77819.eb

Janib, S. M., Moses, A. S., and MacKay, J. A. (2010). Imaging and drug delivery using theranostic nanoparticles. *Adv. Drug Deliv. Rev.* 62, 1052–1063. doi: 10.1016/j.addr.2010.08.004

Juhn, S. K., Rybak, L. P., and Fowlks, W. L. (1982). Transport characteristics of the blood–perilymph barrier. *Am. J. Otolaryngol.* 3, 392–396. doi: 10.1016/s0196-0709(82)80016-1

Kayyali, M. N., Wooltorton, J. R. A., Ramsey, A. J., Lin, M., Chao, T. N., Tsourkas, A., et al. (2018). A novel nanoparticle delivery system for targeted therapy of noise-induced hearing loss. *J. Control. Release* 279, 243–250. doi: 10.1016/j.jconrel.2018.04.028

Kikkawa, Y. S., Nakagawa, T., Tsubouchi, H., Ido, A., Inaoka, T., Ono, K., et al. (2009). Hepatocyte growth factor protects auditory hair cells from aminoglycosides. *Laryngoscope* 119, 2027–2031. doi: 10.1002/lary.20602

Kim, D.-K., Park, S.-N., Park, K.-H., Park, C. W., Yang, K.-J., Kim, J.-D., et al. (2015). Development of a drug delivery system for the inner ear using poly(amino acid)-based nanoparticles. *Drug Deliv.* 22, 367–374. doi: 10.3109/10717544.2013.879354

King, E. B., Salt, A. N., Eastwood, H. T., and O'Leary, S. J. (2011). Direct entry of gadolinium into the vestibule following intratympanic applications in Guinea pigs and the influence of cochlear implantation. *J. Assoc. Res. Otolaryngol.* 12, 741–751. doi: 10.1007/s10162-011-0280-5

King, E. B., Salt, A. N., Kel, G. E., Eastwood, H. T., and O'Leary, S. J. (2013). Gentamicin administration on the stapes footplate causes greater hearing loss and vestibulotoxicity than round window administration in guinea pigs. *Hear. Res.* 304, 159–166. doi: 10.1016/j.heares.2013.07.013

King, E. B., Shepherd, R. K., Brown, D. J., and Fallon, J. B. (2017). Gentamicin applied to the oval window suppresses vestibular function in guinea pigs. *J. Assoc. Res. Otolaryngol.* 18, 291–299. doi: 10.1007/s10162-016-0609-1

Lajud, S. A., Han, Z., Chi, F.-L., Gu, R., Nagda, D. A., Bezpalko, O., et al. (2013). A regulated delivery system for inner ear drug application. *J. Control. Release* 166, 268–276. doi: 10.1016/j.jconrel.2012.12.031

Lajud, S. A., Nagda, D. A., Qiao, P., Tanaka, N., Civantos, A., Gu, R., et al. (2015). A novel chitosan-hydrogel-based nanoparticle delivery system for local inner ear application. *Otol. Neurotol.* 36, 341–347. doi: 10.1097/MAO.0000000000000445

Lambert, P. R., Carey, J., Mikulec, A. A., LeBel, C., and Otonomy Ménière's Study Group, (2016). Intratympanic sustained-exposure dexamethasone thermosensitive gel for symptoms of ménière's disease: randomized phase 2b safety and efficacy trial. *Otol. Neurotol.* 37, 1669–1676. doi: 10.1097/mao.0000000000001227

Langer, R. S., and Peppas, N. A. (1981). Present and future applications of biomaterials in controlled drug delivery systems. *Biomaterials* 2, 201–214. doi: 10.1016/0142-9612(81)90059-4

Lee, K. Y., Nakagawa, T., Okano, T., Hori, R., Ono, K., Tabata, Y., et al. (2007). Novel therapy for hearing loss: delivery of insulin-like growth factor 1 to the cochlea using gelatin hydrogel. *Otol. Neurotol.* 28, 976–981. doi: 10.1097/mao.0b013e31811f40db

Li, J., and Mooney, D. J. (2016). Designing hydrogels for controlled drug delivery. *Nat. Rev. Mater.* 1:16071. doi: 10.1038/natrevmats.2016.71

Li, L., Chao, T., Brant, J., O'Malley, B., Tsourkas, A., and Li, D. (2017). Advances in nano-based inner ear delivery systems for the treatment of sensorineural hearing loss. *Adv. Drug Deliv. Rev.* 108, 2–12. doi: 10.1016/j.addr.2016.01.004

Luo, J., and Xu, L. (2012). Distribution of gentamicin in inner ear after local administration via a chitosan glycerophosphate hydrogel delivery system. *Ann. Otol. Rhinol. Laryngol.* 121, 208–216. doi: 10.1177/000348941212100311

Lyford-Pike, S., Vogelheim, C., Chu, E., Della Santina, C. C., and Carey, J. P. (2007). Gentamicin is primarily localized in vestibular type I hair cells after intratympanic administration. *J. Assoc. Res. Otolaryngol.* 8, 497–508. doi: 10.1007/s10162-007-0093-8

Meng, F., Zhong, Z., and Feijen, J. (2009). Stimuli-responsive polymersomes for programmed drug delivery. *Biomacromolecules* 10, 197–209. doi: 10.1021/bm801127d

Nakashima, T., Pyykko, I., Arroll, M. A., Casselbrant, M. L., Foster, C. A., Manzoor, N. F., et al. (2016). Meniere's disease. *Nat. Rev. Dis. Primers* 2:16028. doi: 10.1038/nrdp.2016.28

Panyam, J., and Labhasetwar, V. (2003). Biodegradable nanoparticles for drug and gene delivery to cells and tissue. *Adv. Drug Deliv. Rev.* 55, 329–347. doi: 10.1016/s0169-409x(02)00228-4

Paulson, D. P., Abuzeid, W., Jiang, H., Oe, T., O'Malley, B. W., and Li, D. (2008). A novel controlled local drug delivery system for inner ear disease. *Laryngoscope* 118, 706–711. doi: 10.1097/MLG.0b013e31815f8e41

Peppas, N. A., and Sahlin, J. J. (1996). Hydrogels as mucoadhesive and bioadhesive materials: a review. *Biomaterials* 17, 1553–1561. doi: 10.1016/0142-9612(95)00307-x

Plontke, S. K., Plinkert, P. K., Plinkert, B., Koitschev, A., Zenner, H. P., and Lowenheim, H. (2002). Transtympanic endoscopy for drug delivery to the inner ear using a new microendoscope. *Adv. Otorhinolaryngol.* 59, 149–155. doi: 10.1159/000059253

Praetorius, M., Brunner, C., Lehnert, B., Klingmann, C., Schmidt, H., Staecker, H., et al. (2007). Transsynaptic delivery of nanoparticles to the central auditory nervous system. *Acta Otolaryngol.* 127, 486–490. doi: 10.1080/00016480600895102

Ramaswamy, B., Roy, S., Apolo, A. B., Shapiro, B., and Depireux, D. A. (2017). Magnetic nanoparticle mediated steroid delivery mitigates cisplatin induced hearing loss. *Front. Cell. Neurosci.* 11:268. doi: 10.3389/fncel.2017.00268

Roy, S., Johnston, A. H., Newman, T. A., Glueckert, R., Dudas, J., Bitsche, M., et al. (2010). Cell-specific targeting in the mouse inner ear using nanoparticles conjugated with a neurotrophin-derived peptide ligand: potential tool for drug delivery. *Int. J. Pharm.* 390, 214–224. doi: 10.1016/j.ijpharm.2010.02.003

Ruckenstein, M. J. (2004). Autoimmune inner ear disease. *Curr. Opin. Otolaryngol. Head Neck Surg* 12, 426–430.

Salt, A. N. (2005). Pharmacokinetics of drug entry into cochlear fluids. *Volta Rev.* 105, 277–298.

Salt, A. N., Hartsock, J., Plontke, S., LeBel, C., and Piu, F. (2011). Distribution of dexamethasone and preservation of inner ear function following intratympanic delivery of a gel-based formulation. *Audiol. Neurotol.* 16, 323–335. doi: 10.1159/000322504

Salt, A. N., and Hirose, K. (2018). Communication pathways to and from the inner ear and their contributions to drug delivery. *Hear. Res.* 362, 25–37. doi: 10.1016/j.heares.2017.12.010

Salt, A. N., and Plontke, S. K. (2005). Local inner-ear drug delivery and pharmacokinetics. *Drug Discov. Today* 10, 1299–1306. doi: 10.1016/s1359-6446(05)03574-9

Salt, A. N., and Plontke, S. K. (2009). Principles of local drug delivery to the inner ear. *Audiol. Neurootol.* 14, 350–360. doi: 10.1159/000241892

Schoo, D. P., Tan, G. X., Ehrenburg, M. R., Pross, S. E., Ward, B. K., and Carey, J. P. (2017). Intratympanic (IT) Therapies for Meniere's disease: some consensus among the confusion. *Curr. Otorhinolaryngol. Rep.* 5, 132–141. doi: 10.1007/s40136-017-0153-5

Schreiber, B. E., Agrup, C., Haskard, D. O., and Luxon, L. M. (2010). Sudden sensorineural hearing loss. *Lancet* 375, 1203–1211.

Sogias, I. A., Williams, A. C., and Khutoryanskiy, V. V. (2008). Why is chitosan mucoadhesive? *Biomacromolecules* 9, 1837–1842. doi: 10.1021/bm800276d

Surovtseva, E. V., Johnston, A. H., Zhang, W., Zhang, Y., Kim, A., Murakoshi, M., et al. (2012). Prestin binding peptides as ligands for targeted polymersome mediated drug delivery to outer hair cells in the inner ear. *Int. J. Pharm.* 424, 121–127. doi: 10.1016/j.ijpharm.2011.12.042

Tamura, T., Kita, T., Nakagawa, T., Endo, T., Kim, T.-S., Ishihara, T., et al. (2005). Drug delivery to the cochlea using PLGA nanoparticles. *Laryngoscope* 115, 2000–2005. doi: 10.1097/01.mlg.0000180174.81036.5a

Thaler, M., Roy, S., Fornara, A., Bitsche, M., Qin, J., Muhammed, M., et al. (2011). Visualization and analysis of superparamagnetic iron oxide nanoparticles in the inner ear by light microscopy and energy filtered TEM. *Nanomedicine* 7, 360–369. doi: 10.1016/j.nano.2010.11.005

Van Vlierberghe, S., Dubruel, P., and Schacht, E. (2011). Biopolymer-based hydrogels as scaffolds for tissue engineering applications: a review. *Biomacromolecules* 12, 1387–1408. doi: 10.1021/bm200083n

Volandri, G., Di Puccio, F., Forte, P., and Carmignani, C. (2011). Biomechanics of the tympanic membrane. *J. Biomech.* 44, 1219–1236. doi: 10.1016/j.jbiomech.2010.12.023

Wang, X., Chen, Y., Tao, Y., Gao, Y., Yu, D., and Wu, H. (2018). A666-conjugated nanoparticles target prestin of outer hair cells preventing cisplatin-induced hearing loss. *Int. J. Nanomed.* 13, 7517–7531. doi: 10.2147/IJN.S170130

Wang, X., Dellamary, L., Fernandez, R., Harrop, A., Keithley, E. M., Harris, J. P., et al. (2009). Dose-dependent sustained release of dexamethasone in inner ear cochlear fluids using a novel local delivery approach. *Audiol. Neurotol.* 14, 393–401. doi: 10.1159/000241896

Wang, X., Dellamary, L., Fernandez, R., Ye, Q., LeBel, C., and Piu, F. (2011). Principles of inner ear sustained release following intratympanic administration. *Laryngoscope* 121, 385–391. doi: 10.1002/lary.21370

Wangemann, P. (2006). Supporting sensory transduction: cochlear fluid homeostasis and the endocochlear potential. *J. Physiol.* 576, 11–21. doi: 10.1113/jphysiol.2006.112888

Wareing, M., Mhatre, A. N., Pettis, R., Han, J. J., Haut, T., Pfister, M. H. F., et al. (1999). Cationic liposome mediated transgene expression in the guinea pig cochlea. *Hear. Res.* 128, 61–69. doi: 10.1016/s0378-5955(98)00196-8

Wise, A. K., Tan, J., Wang, Y., Caruso, F., and Shepherd, R. K. (2016). Improved auditory nerve survival with nanoengineered supraparticles for neurotrophin delivery into the deafened cochlea. *PLoS One* 11:e0164867. doi: 10.1371/journal.pone.0164867

Xu, L., Heldrich, J., Wang, H., Yamashita, T., Miyamoto, S., Li, A., et al. (2010). A controlled and sustained local gentamicin delivery system for inner ear applications. *Otol. Neurotol.* 31, 1115–1121. doi: 10.1097/MAO.0b013e3181eb32d1

Xu, X., Chen, H., Wu, X., Chen, S., Qi, J., He, Z., et al. (2018). Hollow mesoporous silica@zeolitic imidazolate framework capsules and their applications for gentamicin delivery. *Neural Plast.* 2018, 2160854–2160854. doi: 10.1155/2018/2160854

Yang, K.-J., Son, J., Jung, S. Y., Yi, G., Yoo, J., Kim, D.-K., et al. (2018). Optimized phospholipid-based nanoparticles for inner ear drug delivery and therapy. *Biomaterials* 171, 133–143. doi: 10.1016/j.biomaterials.2018.04.038

Yu, Z., Yu, M., Zhang, Z., Hong, G., and Xiong, Q. (2014). Bovine serum albumin nanoparticles as controlled release carrier for local drug delivery to the inner ear. *Nanoscale Res. Lett.* 9:343. doi: 10.1186/1556-276X-9-343

Zhang, Y., Zhang, W., Johnston, A. H., Newman, T. A., Pyykkö, I., and Zou, J. (2011a). Comparison of the distribution pattern of PEG-b-PCL polymersomes delivered into the rat inner ear via different methods. *Acta Otolaryngol.* 131, 1249–1256. doi: 10.3109/00016489.2011.615066

Zhang, Y., Zhang, W., Löbler, M., Schmitz, K.-P., Saulnier, P., Perrier, T., et al. (2011b). Inner ear biocompatibility of lipid nanocapsules after round window membrane application. *Int. J. Pharm.* 404, 211–219. doi: 10.1016/j.ijpharm.2010.11.006

Zhang, Y., Zhang, W., Johnston, A. H., Newman, T. A., Pyykkö, I., and Zou, J. (2012). Targeted delivery of Tet1 peptide functionalized polymersomes to the rat cochlear nerve. *Int. J. Nanomed.* 7, 1015–1022. doi: 10.2147/IJN.S28185

Zou, J., Hannula, M., Misra, S., Feng, H., Labrador, R. H., Aula, A. S., et al. (2015). Micro CT visualization of silver nanoparticles in the middle and inner ear of rat and transportation pathway after transtympanic injection. *J. Nanobiotechnol.* 13:5. doi: 10.1186/s12951-015-0065-9

Zou, J., Ostrovsky, S., Israel, L. L., Feng, H., Kettunen, M. I., Lellouche, J.-P., et al. (2017). Efficient penetration of ceric ammonium nitrate oxidant-stabilized gamma-maghemite nanoparticles through the oval and round windows into the rat inner ear as demonstrated by MRI. *J. Biomed. Mater. Res. B Appl. Biomater.* 105, 1883–1891. doi: 10.1002/jbm.b.33719

Zou, J., Saulnier, P., Perrier, T., Zhang, Y., Manninen, T., Toppila, E., et al. (2008). Distribution of lipid nanocapsules in different cochlear cell populations after round window membrane permeation. *J. Biomed. Mater. Res. B Appl. Biomater.* 87B, 10–18. doi: 10.1002/jbm.b.31058

Zou, J., Sood, R., Ranjan, S., Poe, D., Ramadan, U. A., Kinnunen, P. K. J., et al. (2010a). Manufacturing and in vivo inner ear visualization of MRI traceable liposome nanoparticles encapsulating gadolinium. *J. Nanobiotechnol.* 8:32. doi: 10.1186/1477-3155-8-32

Zou, J., Zhang, W., Poe, D., Qin, J., Fornara, A., Zhang, Y., et al. (2010b). MRI manifestation of novel superparamagnetic iron oxide nanoparticles in the rat inner ear. *Nanomedicine* 5, 739–754. doi: 10.2217/nnm.10.45

Zou, J., Sood, R., Ranjan, S., Poe, D., Ramadan, U. A., Pyykkö, I., et al. (2012). Size-dependent passage of liposome nanocarriers with preserved posttransport integrity across the middle-inner ear barriers in rats. *Otol. Neurotol.* 33, 666–673. doi: 10.1097/MAO.0b013e318254590e

15

Local Drug Delivery for Prevention of Hearing Loss

Leonard P. Rybak[1,2*], *Asmita Dhukhwa*[2], *Debashree Mukherjea*[1] *and Vickram Ramkumar*[2]

[1] *Department of Otolaryngology, School of Medicine, Southern Illinois University, Springfield, IL, United States,*

[2] *Department of Pharmacology, School of Medicine, Southern Illinois University, Springfield, IL, United States*

***Correspondence:**
Leonard P. Rybak
lrybak@siumed.edu

Systemic delivery of therapeutics for targeting the cochlea to prevent or treat hearing loss is challenging. Systemic drugs have to cross the blood-labyrinth barrier (BLB). BLB can significantly prevent effective penetration of drugs in appropriate concentrations to protect against hearing loss caused by inflammation, ototoxic drugs, or acoustic trauma. This obstacle may be obviated by local administration of protective agents. This route can deliver higher concentration of drug compared to systemic application and preclude systemic side effects. Protective agents have been administered by intra-tympanic injection in numerous preclinical studies. Drugs such as steroids, etanercept, D and L-methionine, pifithrin-alpha, adenosine agonists, melatonin, kenpaullone (a cyclin-dependent kinase 2 (CDK2) inhibitor) have been reported to show efficacy against cisplatin ototoxicity in animal models. Several siRNAs have been shown to ameliorate cisplatin ototoxicity when administered by intra-tympanic injection. The application of corticosteroids and a number of other drugs with adjuvants appears to enhance efficacy. Administration of siRNAs to knock down AMPK kinase, liver kinase B1 (LKB1) or G9a in the cochlea have been found to ameliorate noise induced hearing loss. The local administration of these compounds appears to be effective in protecting the cochlea against damage from cisplatin or noise trauma. Furthermore the intra-tympanic route yields maximum protection in the basal turn of the cochlea which is most vulnerable to cisplatin ototoxicity and noise trauma. There appears to be very little transfer of these agents to the systemic circulation. This would avoid potential side effects including interference with anti-tumor efficacy of cisplatin. Nanotechnology offers strategies to effectively deliver protective agents to the cochlea. This review summarizes the pharmacology of local drug delivery by intra-tympanic injection to prevent hearing loss caused by cisplatin and noise exposure in animals. Future refinements in local protective agents provide exciting prospects for amelioration of hearing loss resulting from cisplatin or noise exposure.

Keywords: intra-tympanic injection, cisplatin, noise, hearing loss, acoustic trauma, ototoxicity

INTRODUCTION

Blood-Labyrinth Barrier

A wide variety of drugs has been used to treat inner ear diseases. However, the efficacy of systemic drug therapy is frequently limited by restricted uptake into the inner ear by a barrier system, the blood labyrinth barrier (BLB). The BLB was a term that was developed from the fact that the inner ear fluids have a composition that is distinct from blood. These features provide a diffusion barrier that excludes many substances from entering the inner ear from the blood. Tracer studies demonstrated that various substances enter the perilymph slowly after systemic injection (Juhn et al., 1981). The rate of penetration into perilymph is generally inversely proportional to the molecular weight of compounds tested. This blood-perilymph barrier appears to be situated in the blood vessels located in the modiolus of the cochlea. Substances traveling in these vessels are transported from blood into perilymph of the scala tympani and scala vestibuli (Zou et al., 2016). The cochlear glomeruli of Schwalbe form vessel loops of capillaries adjacent to both perilymphatic scalae (Franz et al., 1993). This barrier consists of non-fenestrated capillaries with a continuous endothelial lining with tight junctions between endothelial cells.

The perilymph-endolymph barrier consists of tight junctions between cells lining Reissner's membrane (Zou et al., 2016). Substances contained in perilymph may enter endolymph if they are able to penetrate this barrier.

The blood-endolymph barrier consists of endothelial cells of capillaries in the stria vascularis that separate the contents of blood in the capillary lumen from the interstitial fluid of the stria vascularis. These marginal cells have tight junctions between them that can restrict passage of substances from blood to endolymph. Within the stria vascularis, marginal cells and the basal cells comprise the intrastrial compartment which separates fluid in that compartment from endolymph in the scala media. This barrier is called the the intrastrial fluid-blood barrier (Shi, 2016). Additional components of the blood-strial barrier have been recently identified. These include pericytes and perivascular resident macrophage-type melanocytes. These three cell types: endothelial cells, pericytes and perivascular resident macrophages are connected by an extracellular basement membrane. Collectively, these cells together form a "cochlear-vascular unit" in the stria vascularis (Shi, 2016; Nyberg et al., 2019). Substances contained in the blood vessels of the stria vascularis may enter the intra-strial space through the blood-strial barrier and then gain access to the endolymph through the marginal cells lining scala media. The various inner ear barriers are illustrated in **Figure 1**.

Treatments for hearing disorders such as cisplatin ototoxicity and noise-induced hearing loss could be administered systemically. However, this approach poses several difficulties: The potential protective agent may (1) not readily cross the BLB (size of the substance) and thus not reach its intended target cells in the cochlea in effective concentrations, (2) could interfere with the desired therapeutic effect of cisplatin (e.g., sodium thiosulfate), and (3) could cause off-target unwanted side effects, especially if high doses are needed to provide protection against hearing loss. One of these off-target effects could result in exacerbation of hearing loss instead of its amelioration. Local application by intra-tympanic administration is minimally invasive and allows drugs or other therapeutic agents to gain access to the inner ear with few or no systemic side effects and minimal risks of interference with the anti-tumor action of drugs like cisplatin. Intra-tympanic injection involves the instillation of substances through the tympanic membrane (Sheehan et al., 2018), shown schematically as a flowchart in (**Figure 2**) and in detail in (**Figure 3**). Another approach for localized drug delivery is through the bulla into the middle ear cavity or application of drugs directly to the round window membrane (RWM). This paper reviews preclinical strategies for local delivery of drugs by intra-tympanic injection to prevent hearing loss from cisplatin and noise trauma.

Pharmacokinetics of Local Drug Delivery

Salt and Plontke have described the use of a standard pharmacologic acronym to describe the pharmacokinetics of drugs after intra-tympanic delivery to the cochlea (Salt and Plontke, 2009, 2018). This acronym is LADME. This term includes liberation, absorption, distribution, metabolism, and elimination of drugs applied intra-tympanically.

Liberation indicates the release of the agent from the dosage form administered to the tympanic cavity into the inner ear. The use of simple drug solutions may not provide sufficient duration of protection. Therefore, incorporation of the drug into controlled-release vehicles can prolong the presence of the drug in the middle ear cavity for transfer through the round or oval window membrane. A variety of technologies have been developed to allow extended release of drugs injected intra-tympanically. Some examples of these methods to prolong the release of active protective agents to the round or oval window membrane include:

- Implantation of an osmotic or digital mini pump to provide sustained delivery of various antioxidants to the RWM in guinea pigs (Wimmer et al., 2004).
- The development and utilization of OTO-104 which contains micronized dexamethasone 160 in poloxamer gel. Significant levels of dexamethasone were maintained in perilymph for 3 months in guinea pigs and more than 1 month in sheep (Piu et al., 2011).
- The intratympanic injection of a hyaluronic acid liposomal gel for sustained delivery of dexamethasone was tested in the guinea pig. The gel remained for a long time in the middle ear cavity and in the RWM after intra-tympanic injection without any evidence of ototoxicity. This resulted in sustained release of dexamethasone in perilymph for 1 month (El Kechai et al., 2016). This appears to be a promising way to deliver corticosteroids to the inner ear to provide sustained protection against cochlear insults.
- Dormer et al. have developed an innovative system to provide extended release of drugs for intra-tympanic injection (Dormer et al., 2019). It contains a film forming agent (FFA) and microspheres to provide prolonged delivery of betamethasone in a formulation called ORB-202 to the round window and inner ear in mice. This technology has shown that corticosteroids contained in microspheres with FFA were retained on the RWM for up to 5 weeks on necropsy examination. A recent review discusses various approaches to nanotechnology for inner ear applications. Only a few examples will be presented below.
- Li et al. have developed a nanohydrogel delivery system, which combines nanotechnology with a chitosan-glycerophosphate hydrogel delivery system.

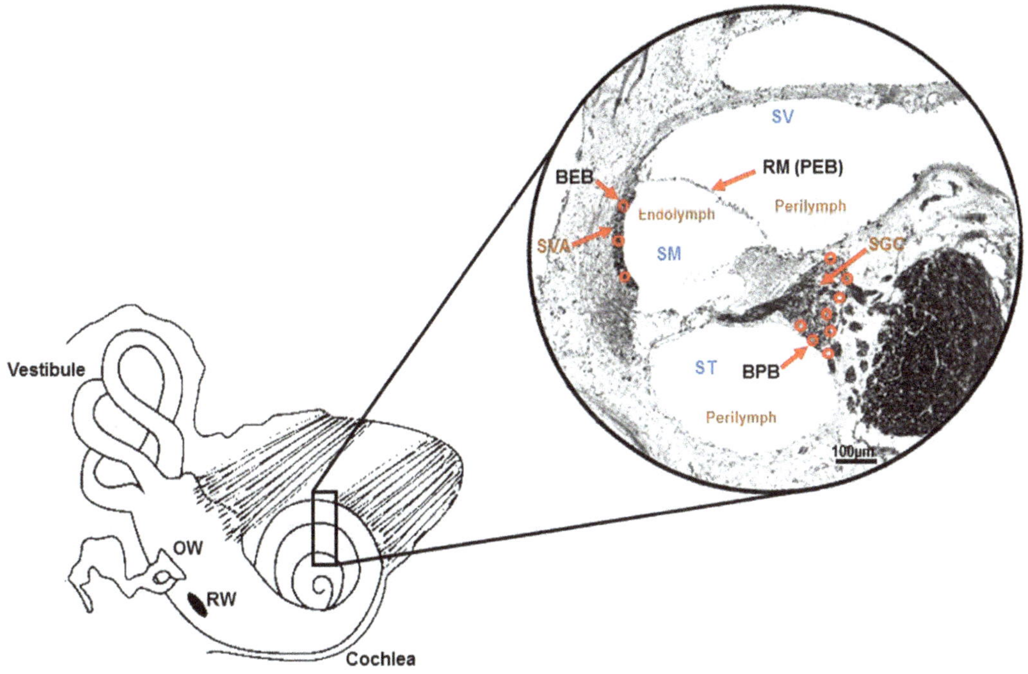

FIGURE 1 | Schematic illustration of barriers within inner ear. Drawing of the cochlea and photomicrograph of a mid-modiolar section of the rat cochlea (stained with Sudan black) demonstrating the various barriers within the inner ear. These include the blood-endolymph barrier (BEB) in the stria vascularis; the blood-perilymph barrier (BPB); and the perilymph-endolymph barrier (PEB) which is formed by Reissner's membrane (RM). Other abbreviations are: SVA (stria vascularis), SGC (spiral ganglion cells), SV (scala vestibuli), ST (scala tympani) and SM (scala media). Perilymph is contained within SV and ST, and endolymph is present in SM. Adapted from Zou et al. (2016).

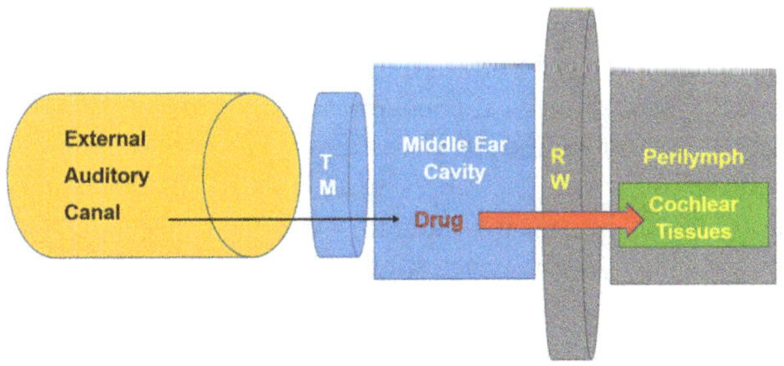

FIGURE 2 | Schematic diagram illustrating method for intra-tympanic injection. The drug is injected through the tympanic membrane (Heinrich et al., 2016) into the middle ear. It then can penetrate the round window membrane (RW) to enter the inner ear fluids (perilymph) and tissues. Modified from the ACS article https://pubs.acs.org/doi/abs/10.1021%2Facs.jmedchem.7b01653 with permission.

These nanoparticles could be delivered across the mouse RWM to reach structures in the scala media (Li et al., 2017).

Liberation can also result from drug generation in the middle ear from gene or cell therapy by which cells are enabled to produce a therapeutic agent (Salt and Plontke, 2018).

A variety of delivery paradigms has been tried to affect liberation. These include rates of injection with pumps, various other devices, and rates of elution among others (Salt and Plontke, 2018).

Absorption describes the passage of the drug from the middle ear cavity to the perilymph through the RWM, oval window or cochlear bone. The RWM in mammals comprises of 3 cellular layers: an epithelial layer that faces the middle ear space; a connective tissue layer in the middle; and a layer that faces the perilymph of the scala tympani (Goycoolea, 1992; Goycoolea and Lundman, 1997). The epithelial layer facing the middle ear cavity has tight junctions between cells (Salt and Plontke, 2009). It appears that the layers of the round window are involved in absorption and secretion of substances to and from the inner ear. Tracer molecules such as cationic ferritin, horseradish peroxidase, and 1 micron latex microspheres instilled into the middle ear pass through RWM, into the inner ear and have been detected in pinocytotic vesicles in the RWM (Goycoolea et al., 1988). Permeability of the RWM depends on molecular weight, solubility in lipids, concentration and charge, as well as the RWM thickness (Goycoolea and Lundman, 1997). Some examples of substances shuttled across RWM are:

- Nanoparticles are translocated across the RWM by endocytosis. This process follows three different mechanisms: macropinocytosis, caveolin-mediated endocytosis, and clathrin-mediated endocytosis (Zhang et al., 2018).

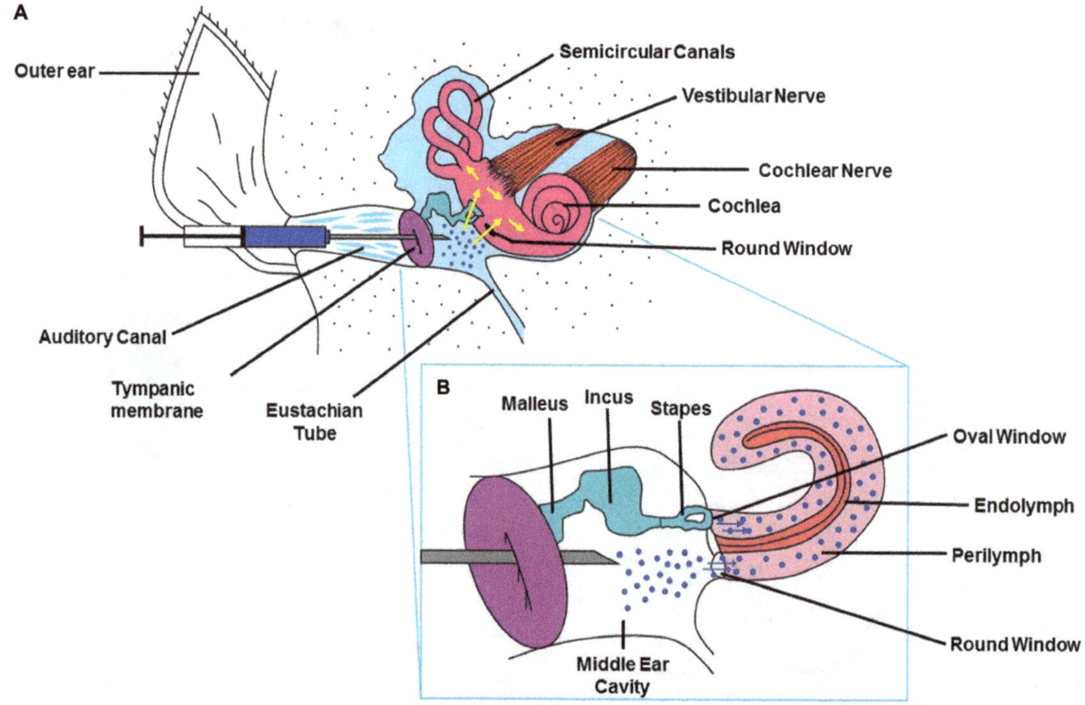

FIGURE 3 | Method for intra-tympanic injection. **(A)** A syringe with an attached 30 gage needle 1/2 to 5/8th of an inch in length is directed through the external ear canal to the tympanic membrane of anesthetized animal with an operating microscope. A single puncture is made in the anterior inferior region. The desired solution is slowly injected into the middle ear and the rat is left undisturbed for 15 min with injected ear facing upward (Sheehan et al., 2018). **(B)** Drawing depicting the injected drug traversing the RWM and entering the cochlea. This figure was modified with permission from the image screenshot at 1:59 of the article https://www.jove.com/video/56564/trans-tympanic-drug-delivery-for-the-treatment-of-ototoxicity.

- A study of RW permeation enhancers was carried out using fluorescein tagged dexamethasone applied to the RW niche in guinea pigs. DMSO, N-methylpyrrolidone and benzyl alcohol provided significantly higher entry than that observed in controls (Li et al., 2018).
- Adjuvants were used to enhance the permeation of dexamethasone through the RWM. Application of dexamethasone on a hyaluronic acid sponge with or without histamine or dexamethasone with histamine provided greater penetration into perilymph in guinea pigs than did dexamethasone alone (Creber et al., 2019).
- A novel method to enhance the delivery of siRNA to the cochlea was developed using a recombination protein, double-stranded RNA-binding domains (TAT-DRBDs). The authors showed efficient siRNA transfection to the cochlea of the chinchilla with this delivery system. They were able to demonstrate successful transfection of Cy3-labeled siRNA into cells of the inner ear through the intact RWM, including the IHCs, OHCs, and vestibular cells in the crista ampullaris, macula utriculi, and macula sacculi (Qi et al., 2014).

The oval window and thin bone of the stapes footplate may provide other routes of entry for drugs applied intra-tympanically. Although the oval window has been shown to be permeable to horseradish peroxidase (Tanaka and Motomura, 1981), it is uncertain how much drug would enter by this route (Salt and Plontke, 2009) unless it were directly applied on the stapes footplate (King et al., 2011) or unless it were applied using nanoparticles. In the latter case, the application of fluorescent chitosan nanoparticles by intra-tympanic injection in guinea pigs was associated with penetration of both RWM and oval window, but with much stronger fluorescence in the vestibule than in the cochlea (Ding et al., 2019). On the other hand King et al. showed with MRI that most of the gadolinium applied through tympanic cavity entered perilymph through stapes (King et al., 2011). The bone of the otic capsule may provide a route of transport from the middle ear to the apical regions of the cochlea in guinea pigs (Salt and Plontke, 2009; Salt and Hirose, 2018).

Distribution includes the mechanism by which the drug is spread within and between perilymph and endolymph and how it passes from inner ear fluids into tissues of the cochlea. The distribution of drugs within the cochlear fluids proceeds primarily by passive diffusion but if fluid flow is present, volume flow can occur (Salt and Plontke, 2018). Distribution also includes flow of substances from fluid spaces to extracellular spaces of cochlear tissue compartments, especially in areas where cell layers are not complete or where cells do not possess tight junctions (Salt and Plontke, 2018). Distribution includes all forms of drug movement within the inner ear

(Salt and Plontke, 2018). Distribution may be enhanced by the use of magnetic nanoparticles to cross the RWM and enter the inner ear fluids and tissues. The use of an external magnet can control the delivery of drug packaged in magnetic nanoparticles. After the magnet is taken away, the drug containing nanoparticles can then diffuse through perilymph. Fluorescent magnetic nanoparticles have been shown to traverse the RWM and gain access to the perilymph (Li et al., 2017).

Metabolism is the chemical alteration of drugs administered into the ear. It is also known as biotransformation (Salt and Plontke, 2018). Once a drug enters the inner ear, it can be broken down into substances that are more bioactive or that are inactivated. The intra-tympanic administration of liposomal hyaluronic acid led to the transformation of dexamethasone phosphate, a prodrug, into the active form, dexamethasone (El Kechai et al., 2016). Thus the metabolite may have a greater affinity for its receptors in the inner ear. Changes in physical characteristics of a drug resulting from metabolism can alter its ability to traverse cell membranes and layers in the inner ear. These changes can alter the rate of elimination (Salt and Plontke, 2018).

Elimination includes the processes by which the drug or its metabolites are transferred from the inner ear into other body fluids such as blood or cerebrospinal fluid or transport from the inner ear to the middle ear cavity. From the middle ear cavity a drug administered intra-tympanically can exit be eliminated via the Eustachian tube into the pharynx (Salt and Plontke, 2018). A novel approach to elimination of substances transported into the cochlea is to administer magnetic nanoparticles, then remove them using an external magnet. This has been demonstrated using fluorescently tagged magnetic nanoparticles *in vivo* (Li et al., 2018). Middle ear kinetics of drugs administered intra-tympanically as solutions show rapid decline in concentration within the middle ear cavity, e.g., dexamethasone phosphate, which fell to 10% of the applied concentration at 93 min after injection into the middle ear (Salt and Plontke, 2018). This process could be delayed by the use of slow-release vehicles. The delayed elimination (Hellberg et al., 2013) and prolonged retention of cisplatin for months to years in the cochlea creates challenges for intratympanic protection strategies (Breglio et al., 2017).

Cisplatin Ototoxicity

Cisplatin is frequently used to treat a variety of malignant solid tumors. These include ovarian and testicular cancer, head and neck carcinomas, cervical, bladder, and lung cancer. Although cisplatin is a quite effective antineoplastic drug, dose limiting side effects often occur. Such unintended toxicities include: ototoxicity, neurotoxicity, nephrotoxicity, and bone marrow toxicity. Investigation of potential protective agents to ameliorate cisplatin ototoxicity have not yet yielded an effective drug that has been approved by the United States Food and Drug Administration (FDA). Of great concern is the potential interference of cisplatin efficacy when systemic otoprotective drugs are administered. These otoprotective drugs could neutralize or diminish the anti-tumor effects of cisplatin and may also produce additional side effects, including communication, learning, cognition, and quality of life (Brooks and Knight, 2018). Therefore, numerous preclinical studies have investigated potential protective agents against cisplatin ototoxicity using local therapy, such as intra-tympanic injection. Cisplatin-induced hearing loss is bilateral and permanent. The hearing loss occurs mostly in the high frequencies. It can drastically compromise the quality of life for cancer survivors. Therefore the use of intra-tympanic therapy is attractive since the concentration of putative protective agents will be greater in the basal turn of the cochlea where high frequency hearing is transduced.

Mechanisms Underlying Cisplatin Ototoxicity

Cisplatin ototoxicity and the underlying mechanisms are still being investigated. Several mechanisms have been proposed. These include oxidative stress caused by the production of reactive oxygen species (Kros and Steyger), which can be mediated by activation of a cochlear specific isoform of the enzyme NADPH oxidase (NOX3), and by up regulation of transient receptor potential vanilloid 1 (TRPV1) channels (Mukherjea et al., 2008, 2011; Sheth et al., 2017). Cisplatin mediated damage to mitochondria resulting in cleavage of caspases leading to apoptosis of critical structures in the cochlea (outer hair cells, cells of the stria vascularis and spiral ligament, and spiral ganglion cells); DNA damage with activation of p53 leading to activation of activation of signal transducer and activator of transcription 1 (STAT1) (Zhang et al., 2003; Kaur et al., 2011; Benkafadar et al., 2017; Bhatta et al., 2019), resulting in inflammation and apoptosis (Sheth et al., 2017). Recent reviews of the proposed mechanisms of cisplatin ototoxicity have been published (Karasawa and Steyger, 2015, Sheth et al., 2017, Kros and Steyger, 2018).

Intra-Tympanic Treatments for Cisplatin Ototoxicity

A wide variety of putative protective agents have been reported to ameliorate cisplatin ototoxicity when administered by intra-tympanic injection. A short list of some successful otoprotective agents administered intra-tympanically prior to cisplatin treatment *in vivo* have been categorized as inhibitors, biologicals, siRNA, and dexamethasone and have been listed below:

- Kenpaullone is an inhibitor of multiple kinases, including cyclin-dependent kinase 2 (CDK2). Significant otoprotection was demonstrated in both mice and rats. Mice receiving intra-tympanic kenpaullone demonstrated significant reductions of ABR threshold elevation, at frequencies of 16 and 32 kHz. Morphology of OHCs in the 32 kHz region showed significant protection in kenpaullone treated mice. Even more robust findings were demonstrated in rats. Intra-tympanic kenpaullone provided complete protection against cisplatin ototoxicity in the rat. These findings support the hypothesis that CDK2 inhibition by kenpaullone ameliorates cisplatin ototoxicity by inhibiting mitochondrial ROS production and also preventing cochlear cell death mediated by caspase-3/7 (Teitz et al., 2018).

- Copper sulfate, a copper transporter-1 inhibitor, when administered intra-tympanically 30 min prior to intraperitoneal cisplatin in mice showed significant protection against threshold shifts in ABR using click stimuli and pure tones at 8, 16, and 32 kHz. However, concerns were expressed about the toxicity of copper sulfate. This led to the suggestion that other less toxic inhibitors of CTR1 should be developed and tested (More et al., 2010).
- Thiosulfate, an antioxidant was administered as thiosulphate-hyaluronan gel into the tympanic cavity of guinea pigs 3 h prior to intravenous cisplatin injection. This resulted in high concentrations of thiosulfate in the perilymph of scala tympani and it protected against cochlear hair cell loss from cisplatin. Levels of thiosulfate in blood were kept low, avoiding potential chelation of cisplatin in the blood that could interfere with the anti-tumor efficacy of cisplatin (Berglin et al., 2011).
- KR-22332 (3-amino-3-(4-fluoro-phenyl)-1H-quinoline-2, 4-dione) is a novel compound that suppresses ROS. Intra-tympanic administration of KR-22332 in rats protected against cisplatin induced ABR threshold shift to click stimuli. This compound inhibited cisplatin-induced up regulation of NOX3 in the cochlea and reduced the activation of p53, MAP kinases, caspase 3 and tumor necrosis factor-α (TNF-alpha), and TUNEL expression in rat cochlea. KR-22332 may ameliorate cisplatin ototoxicity by reducing the generation of ROS and by preventing mitochondrial dysfunction (Shin et al., 2013).
- Antioxidant vitamins such as vitamin E and vitamin C have been tested for protection against cisplatin ototoxicity. Trolox, a water-soluble form of alpha-tocopherol is an antioxidant. It was applied locally on the round window of guinea pigs treated with cisplatin. Trolox administered in combination with cisplatin prevented ABR threshold elevations and protected against the loss of hair cells (Teranishi and Nakashima, 2003). Another study in rats looked at the effect of intra-tympanic application of vitamin E solution followed by cisplatin administration 30 min later. Significant protection against cisplatin induced ABR threshold shifts was seen in rats (Paksoy et al., 2011). Another strategy employed the intra-tympanic administration of vitamin E polymeric nanoparticles in rats treated with cisplatin. Rats pretreated with vitamin E nanoparticles had significant protection against cisplatin-induced ABR threshold shifts at 12, 20, and 32 (Martin-Saldana et al., 2017). Vitamin C administered by intra-tympanic injection protected against cisplatin-induced decrease in DPOAE amplitudes in rats treated with cisplatin (Celebi et al., 2013).
- Melatonin is a hormone secreted by the pineal gland that has antioxidant properties. It has both indirect antioxidant and direct free radical scavenger activity. Rats treated with intra-tympanic melatonin showed improved ABR thresholds for clicks, 4, 6, and 8 kHz and threshold shifts for DPOAE. Staining for TNF-alpha was diminished in melatonin treated rats receiving cisplatin (Demir et al., 2015).
- Capsaicin is a spicy capsaicinoid, a natural product produced by hot chili peppers, Capsicum fruits. This alkaloid has been used for its analgesic and anti-inflammatory actions (Lavorgna et al., 2019), Capsaicin activates TRPV1 pain receptors, and can produce rapid desensitization of TRPV1. The intra-tympanic administration of capsaicin in rats 24 h prior to cisplatin reduced ABR threshold shifts. Capsaicin appears to prevent cisplatin ototoxicity by increasing the expression of cannabinoid 2 receptors (CB2R) in the cochlea leading to increased activation of pro-survival transcription factor signal transducer and activator of transcription (STAT3) (Bhatta et al., 2019).
- JWH-015 (2-methyl-1-propyl-1H-indol-3-yl)-1-naphthalenylmethanone) is a cannabinoid receptor 2 (CB2) agonist. Pretreatment with intra-tympanic JWH-015, 30 min prior to cisplatin reduced ABR threshold shifts at 8, 16, and 32 kHz and also protected against the loss of OHCs in rats. In addition, this CB2R agonist prevented cisplatin-induced loss of ribbon synapses on inner hair cells (IHCs) and prevented loss of Na^+/K^+-ATPase immunoreactivity in the stria vascularis (Ghosh et al., 2018).
- Pifithrin-alpha is an inhibitor of p53. Pifithrin-alpha was applied on the RWM of the chinchilla prior to the local application of cisplatin. The cochleae that were pretreated with pifithrin were significantly protected from cisplatin-induced increase in ABR threshold shifts at 1,2,4,8, and 16 kHz (Parhizkar and Rybak, 2003).
- R-PIA (R-phenylisopropyladenosine) is an adenosine A1 receptor agonist. Intra-tympanic administration of R-PIA in rats prior to cisplatin reduced cisplatin-induced ABR threshold elevation and OHCs were preserved. This protection was associated with reduced NOX3 expression, STAT1 activation, TNF-α levels, and apoptosis in the cochlea (Kaur et al., 2016).
- D-methionine and L-methionine are amino acids with antioxidant properties and both of these compounds have been shown to protect against cisplatin ototoxicity in preclinical studies. D-methionine applied to the RWM provided complete protection against cisplatin applied to the round window in chinchillas. ABR thresholds and OHCs were completely preserved in animals pretreated with D-methionine (Korver et al., 2002). In a study using guinea pigs, osmotic pumps were implanted to provide continuous administration of D-methionine, sodium thiosulfate, fibroblast growth factor-2, or brain-derived neurotrophic factor in animals treated with cisplatin. Guinea pigs receiving D-methionine demonstrated better OAEs on the 3th and 5th day of a 5 day regimen of cisplatin administration. On 5th and 6th day of the treatment, D-methionine failed to provide protection. It appears that the additional dosing of cisplatin overpowered the effectiveness of D-methionine

on those later 2 days. The other agents provided no significant protection (Wimmer et al., 2004). The efficacy of L-methionine against cisplatin ototoxicity was investigated in rats. Local application of L-methionine prior to cisplatin provided complete protection against cisplatin-induced ABR threshold shifts and preserved the integrity of OHCs against damage by cisplatin (Li et al., 2001).

- L-N-acetylcysteine (L NAC) is a sulfhydryl compound that can neutralize cisplatin and function as an antioxidant. A 2% solution of L-NAC was administered by intra-tympanic injection in guinea pigs treated with cisplatin. Pretreatment with L-NAC preserved DPOAEs that were otherwise severely affected by cisplatin. This same study successfully utilized lactated Ringer's solution by intra-tympanic injection prior to cisplatin administration. The latter solution was also effective in preserving DPOAEs in cisplatin treated guinea pigs (Choe et al., 2004). A later study showed that intra-tympanic administration of L-NAC was harmful and exacerbated cisplatin ototoxicity in the guinea pig. However, this latter study utilized extremely high concentrations of L-NAC (20%) and this proved to be toxic. Animals receiving this high dose of L-NAC showed severe disruption of OHC stereocilia (Nader et al., 2010). It appears that a more dilute solution of L-NAC is a better preparation to use for intra-tympanic injection to ameliorate cisplatin ototoxicity.
- TNF-alpha antagonist, etanercept, when administered intra-tympanically in rats protected against OHC damage and cisplatin-induced hearing loss. ABR threshold shifts were significantly reduced in rats treated with etanercept 30 min prior to cisplatin. Scanning electron microscopy of etanercept pre-treated animals showed significant protection against cisplatin induced OHC damage (Kaur et al., 2011).
- RNA silencing has been successfully employed using intra-tympanic delivery for protection against cisplatin ototoxicity. In a rat model of cisplatin ototoxicity, it was shown than intra-tympanic administration of siRNA to knock down TRPV1 protected against cisplatin-induced hearing loss and damage to outer hair cells in the cochlea (Mukherjea et al., 2008). It was hypothesized that protection was afforded by reducing down-stream targets, such as the cochlear specific NADPH oxidase -3 (NOX3) enzyme, and STAT-1. Indeed, the intra-tympanic injection of siRNA directed against NOX3 (Mukherjea et al., 2011) or STAT-1 siRNA (Kaur et al., 2011) were each protective against cisplatin induced hearing loss and outer hair cell damage. NOX3 activation results in reactive oxygen species upregulation and STAT-1 can promote inflammation and apoptosis in the cochlea as a result of cisplatin's ototoxic effect. Such deleterious effects can be prevented by the use of these siRNAs.
- Dexamethasone is a glucocorticoid that appears to offer protection against cisplatin ototoxicity by several mechanisms. These include the down-regulation of pro-inflammatory genes that regulate the expression of cytokines; the inhibition of apoptosis; the up-regulation of antioxidant enzymes that could antagonize the effects of ROS (Hazlitt et al., 2018).
  - Successful attenuation of cisplatin ototoxicity has been reported in various animal models treated with intra-tympanic dexamethasone. The animals tested include: mouse (Hill et al., 2008), aged mouse (Parham, 2011), rat (Paksoy et al., 2011), and guinea pig (Shafik et al., 2013). Intratympanic dexamethasone delivered 1 day before cisplatin treatment did not protect against cisplatin ototoxicity. However, intra-tympanic dexamethasone administered 1 h before cisplatin provided significant preservation of cochlear structure and function (Shafik et al., 2013). The efficacy of intra-tympanic dexamethasone solution in protecting against cisplatin ototoxicity in various experimental animal models has been rather inconsistent. Results appear to depend on the dose of both dexamethasone and cisplatin and the species of experimental animals (Hazlitt et al., 2018). Therefore, other formulations have been explored for providing sustained release of steroid or increase in penetration into the cochlea, such as the incorporation of dexamethasone into nanoparticles.
  - Dexamethasone OTO-104 contains micronized dexamethasone in a poloxamer based hydrogel. This formulation was found to be much more effective than dexamethasone solution alone (Fernandez et al., 2016). A single intra-tympanic injection of 6% OTO-104, provided nearly total protection against cisplatin ototoxicity in guinea pigs receiving acute injection of cisplatin. On the other hand intra-tympanic dexamethasone solution offered no protection. OTO-104 was also very effective in prevention of hearing loss associated with chronic administration of cisplatin (Fernandez et al., 2016).
  - Dexamethasone has also been delivered intra-tympanically as nanoparticles. Dexamethasone-PEG-PLA nanoparticles provided significant otoprotection against cisplatin induced ABR threshold shifts at 4 and 8 kHz but not at 16 or 24 kHz in guinea pigs (Sun et al., 2015). Dexamethasone polymeric nanoparticles also protected against cisplatin ototoxicity in rats (Martin-Saldana et al., 2017). Dexamethasone treatment by bullostomy (intra-tympanic administration) successfully reduced hearing loss in all frequencies (from 8 to 32 kHz) tested by auditory steady-state responses (ASSR) (Martin-Saldana et al., 2017).
  - Dexamethasone-A666 nanoparticles administered intra-tympanically protected guinea pigs against cisplatin-induced cochlear outer hair cell damage and hearing loss (Wang et al., 2018). This latter study used A666-peptides that were shown to bind to prestin in outer hair cells. This formulation effectively delivered dexamethasone into outer hair cells and was significantly more effective than intra-tympanic injection of free dexamethasone or dexamethasone

incorporated into nanoparticles without A666 (Wang et al., 2018).

- Prednisolone was found to reduce cisplatin induced ABR threshold elevations in mice. Intra-tympanic magnetically delivered prednisolone-loaded nanoparticles resulted in significantly lower elevations of ABR threshold, particularly at the higher frequencies (16 and 32 kHz) compared with intra-tympanic methylprednisolone solution or empty magnetic nanoparticles (Ramaswamy et al., 2017).

We have summarized the studies reporting intra-tympanic drug delivery that protect against cisplatin ototoxicity in **Table 1**.

Noise Induced Hearing Loss and Underlying Mechanisms

Noise induced hearing loss (NIHL) is a global burden with an estimated 16% of the adult population being affected, with significant regional variations (Nelson et al., 2005; Oishi and Schacht, 2011; Basner et al., 2014; Masterson et al., 2018). NIHL is not only characterized by increased thresholds in hearing, speech processing and tinnitus but also associated with sleep disorders, cardiovascular diseases and cognitive decline (Gates et al., 2000; Ohlemiller, 2008; Kumar et al., 2012; Bressler et al., 2017; Cunningham and Tucci, 2017; Le Prell and Clavier, 2017; Munzel et al., 2018).

The sensitivity to noise varies with the intensity and duration of exposure and the mammalian species tested. Auditory threshold shifts after noise exposure can cause either a temporary threshold shift (TTS) or shifts that do not revert back to baseline are known as permanent threshold shifts (PTS) (Kujawa and Liberman, 2009). Permanent hearing loss or PTS occurs when the noise exposure exceeds the capacity of the cochlea to recover. Permanent damage can be inflicted upon various cochlear tissues, including hair cells, spiral ganglion neurons and the lateral wall (stria vascularis and spiral ligament). Intense noise can cause mechanical damage that can result in the mixing of endolymph and perilymph causing high levels of potassium to kill hair cells (Kurabi et al., 2017). NIHL could be caused by a number of molecular events in the cochlea. Acoustic trauma can lead to the production of reactive oxygen species (Kros and Steyger) in the cochlea. ROS can remain in the cochlea for up to 10 days after noise exposure (Yamane et al., 1995). ROS may be generated by enzymes activated by noise exposure, including NADPH oxidases. ROS can oxidize lipids to form vasoactive lipid peroxidation molecules like isoprostanes (Ohinata et al., 2000). These toxic products may reduce cochlear blood flow. ROS can also lead to the formation of inflammatory cytokines that can cause cochlear damage. These include interleukin-6 and tumor necrosis factor-alpha (Kurabi et al., 2017). Reactive nitrogen species (RNS) are also formed in the cochlea of animals subjected to high levels of noise. These products include nitro tyrosine and peroxynitrite (Ohinata et al., 2000). The latter toxic free radical is formed by the reaction of nitric oxide (NO) with superoxide. Toxic noise exposure can produce accumulation of calcium in the inner ear tissues. Excess calcium may cause ROS release from mitochondria and can upregulate mitogen activated kinase (MAPK) including c-Jun-N-terminal kinase (JNK) and other cellular stress molecules. These downstream molecules can lead to OHC apoptosis or necrosis (Kurabi et al., 2017).

Intra-Tympanic Treatments Against Noise Trauma

Protective agents have been reported to ameliorate NIHL when administered by intra-tympanic injection. The following is a short list of some successful otoprotective agents administered intra-tympanically *in vivo*. Interestingly, some of these inhibitors were also protective against cisplatin induced hearing loss. Most otoprotective agents used are either inhibitors of cellular pathways, antioxidants, anti-inflammatory compounds, siRNA trophic factors or dexamethasone and have been listed below:

- A cell-permeable inhibitor of JNK mediated apoptosis, AM-111, was administered on the RWM (in a hyaluronic acid gel formulation or osmotic mini-pump) 1 or 4 h after impulse noise exposure in chinchillas. Three weeks after traumatic noise exposure the PTS were significantly less in animals receiving AM-111 even when it was administered 4 h after noise exposure (Coleman et al., 2007). D-JNKI-1 was found to block the mitogen-activated protein kinase/JNK-mediated activation of a mitochondrial death pathway. D-JNKi-1 administered intra-tympanically to guinea pigs exposed to acoustic trauma also provided excellent protection. The majority of hair cells were preserved in the area of maximum noise damage and resulted in almost no permanent hearing loss. Treatment was effective even when administered up to 12 h after noise exposure. These findings strongly suggest that the mitogen-activated protein kinase/JNK signaling pathway plays a critical role in producing hair cell death from acoustic trauma (Wang et al., 2007).
  - A novel and intriguing refinement of the intra-tympanic delivery of D-JNKi-1 to the cochlea of mice was recently reported. Mice underwent intra-tympanic application of a chitosan glycerophosphate (CGP)-hydrogel system containing targeted and untargeted D-JNKi-1 containing multifunctional nanoparticles (MFNPs) or empty MFNPs. Targeting was directed to the protein prestin in OHCs. Two days after round window application of the hydrogel the mice were exposed to acoustic trauma. ABR threshold shifts at 14 days after noise exposure were significantly lower for 4 and 8 kHz stimuli in mice treated with targeted MFNPs containing D-JNKi-1 compared to untargeted D-JNKi-l MFNPs but protection was similar at 16, 24 and 32 kHz. At these frequencies, both targeted and untargeted D-JNKi-l-MFNPs provided partial protection that did not significantly differ from each other (Kayyali et al., 2018).

TABLE 1 | This table summarizes pertinent studies demonstrating amelioration of cisplatin-induced ototoxicity using intra-tympanic therapy.

Drug	Animalmodel	Mechanism	References
Kenpaullone	Mouse, Rat	Cyclin-dependent kinase-2 inhibitor	Teitz et al., 2018
Etanercept	Rat	TNF-alpha inhibitor	Kaur et al., 2011
Copper sulfate	Mouse	CTR1 inhibitor	More et al., 2010
Thiosulfate-hyaluronan gel	Guinea pig	Platinum chelator	Berglin et al., 2011
KR 22332 (3-amino-3-(4-fluoro-phenyl)-1H-quinoline-2,4-dione)	Rat	Suppresses ROS	Shin et al., 2013
Trolox	Guinea pig	Antioxidant	Teranishi and Nakashima, 2003
Vitamin E	Rat	Antioxidant	Paksoy et al., 2011
Vitamin E polymeric nanoparticles	Rat		Martin-Saldana et al., 2017
Vitamin C	Rat	Antioxidant	Celebi et al., 2013
Melatonin	Rat	Antioxidant	Demir et al., 2015
Capsaicin	Rat	CB2R upregulation increase STAT3/STAT1	Bhatta et al., 2019
Dexamethasone	Rat	Anti-inflammatory	Paksoy et al., 2011; Özel et al., 2016
	Mouse		Hill et al., 2008
	Aged mouse		Parham, 2011
	Guinea pig		Murphy and Daniel, 2011; Shafik et al., 2013
Dexamethasone-PEG-PLA nanoparticles	Guinea pig		Sun et al., 2015
Dexamethasone polymeric nanoparticles	Rat		Martin-Saldana et al., 2017
Dexamethasone-A666 nanoparticles	Guinea pig		Wang et al., 2018
Dexamethasone OTO-104	Guinea pig	Antioxidant	Fernandez et al., 2016
Prednisolone magnetic nanoparticles	Mouse	Anti-inflammatory	Ramaswamy et al., 2017
JWH-015	Rat	CB2R upregulation	Ghosh et al., 2018
Pifithrin-alpha	Chinchilla	p53 inhibitor	Parhizkar and Rybak, 2003
R-PIA	Rat	Adenosine A1R	Kaur et al., 2016
D-methionine	Chinchilla	Antioxidant	Korver et al., 2002
	Guinea pig		Wimmer et al., 2004
L-methionine	Rat	Antioxidant	Li et al., 2001
L-N-acetylcysteine	Guinea pig	Antioxidant	Choe et al., 2004
Lactated Ringer's	Guinea pig	–	Choe et al., 2004
TRPV1 siRNA	Rat	Decrease ROS	Mukherjea et al., 2008
NOX3 siRNA	Rat	Decrease ROS	Mukherjea et al., 2011
STAT1 siRNA	Rat	Anti-inflammatory	Kaur et al., 2011

- Rosmarinic acid is a polyphenol that is found in aqueous extracts of spearmint. It has demonstrated antioxidant, anti-inflammatory and neuroprotective properties (Falcone et al., 2019). Rats were exposed to acoustic trauma and underwent ABR measurements before and up to 30 days afterward. One group was treated with systemic rosmarinic acid and a second treatment group was administered intra-tympanic rosmarinic acid. Significant protection against ABR threshold shifts was seen in both treatment groups compared with controls. Less OHC loss and decreased evidence of superoxide production and lipid peroxidation was ascertained using dihydroethidium and 8-isoprostane immunostaining, respectively. These findings strongly suggest that adminstration of rosmarinic acid by both routes of administration protected the hearing and preserved the cochlea of rats exposed to noise trauma (Fetoni et al., 2018).
- Peroxisome proliferator-activated receptors (PPARs) function as lipid sensors and help to regulate redox balance by inhibiting ROS and upregulating antioxidant genes. Pioglitazone is a PPAR-gamma agonist that has been shown to reduce inflammation in patients with type two diabetes and coronary artery disease. This drug seemed to have favorable properties to test as a protective agent against noise trauma. Rats were administered pioglitazone in a temperature sensitive gel intra-tympanically 1 h after acoustic trauma. Pioglitazone significantly protected against threshold shifts in the ABR and significantly reduced the loss of OHCs. These findings were associated with a reduction in superoxide anion expression and lipid peroxidation (8-isoprostane). Anti-inflammatory effects of pioglitazone were demonstrated by its blockade of noise induced upregulation of pNFkB and interleukin 1b (IL-1b). Thus, pioglitazone protection against traumatic noise injury to the cochlea by both anti-oxidant and anti-inflammatory effects (Paciello et al., 2018).
- Caroverine is an antagonist of two glutamate receptors, N-methyl-D-aspartate (NMDA) and alpha-amino-3-hydroxy-5-methyl-4-isoxazolepropionic acid (AMPA). Caroverine was applied onto the RWM with gelfoam in

guinea pigs, followed by noise exposure. ABR threshold shifts were significantly lower in caroverine treated animals (Chen et al., 2004).

- Edaravone is a free radical scavenger and antioxidant. Edaravone solid lipid nanoparticles, were delivered to guinea pigs by intra-tympanic injection. Noise exposure resulted in ABR threshold shifts and induced ROS formation. Edaravone reduced the ABR threshold shift and ROS production in noise-exposed animals compared with controls. Edaravone solid lipid nanoparticles show protective effects against noise-induced hearing loss. However, guinea pigs treated with edaravone had no significant protection of OHCs. More experiments will be needed to see if edaravone could be useful in protecting cochlear tissues from noise injury (Gao et al., 2015).
- Kenpaullone is an inhibitor of CDK2. When kenpaullone was injected intra-tympanically in mice had significantly better ABR thresholds and wave 1 amplitudes than controls. In animals treated with this agent, the presynaptic ribbon density at D14 after the acoustic damage was diminished. These data support the hypothesis that kenpaullone protects against noise-induced hearing loss in mice. It is interesting to note that kenpaullone also protected against cisplatin (see above) (Teitz et al., 2018).
- RNA silencing: Noise exposed mice suffered permanent ABR threshold shifts, loss of OHCs and cochlear synapses. G9a (KMT1C, EHMT2) is an important histone lysine methyltransferase encoded by the human *EHMT2* gene and responsible for histone H3 lysine 9 dimethylation (H3K9me2). The intra-tympanic administration of siRNA against G9a to silence the *EHMT2* gene 72 h prior to noise exposure significantly reduced ABR threshold shifts and resulted in greater survival of OHCs compared to treatment with the control siRNA. These data suggest that pretreatment with siG9a partially ameliorates noise-induced permanent hearing loss via the inhibition of G9a (Xiong et al., 2019).

  - Noise exposure activates two key enzymes in the cochlea of mice: phosphorylated AMP-activated protein kinase-alpha-1 (AMPK-alpha-1) and its upstream kinase, liver kinase B1 (LKB1) in the cochlea. Pretreatment with intra-tympanic siRNA against AMPK-alpha-1 prior to noise exposure inhibited the expression of this enzyme and significantly reduced ABR threshold shifts and loss of OHCs and loss of synaptic ribbons at IHCs. Furthermore, inhibition of LKB1 by intra-tympanic siRNA reduced the noise-induced increase in phosphorylation of AMPK-alpha-1 in OHCs, reduced the loss of IHC synaptic ribbons and OHCs, and protected against ABR threshold shifts. These findings provide interesting new approach to prevent noise-induced hearing loss and cochlear synaptopathy (Hill et al., 2016).

- Neurotrophins have been used successfully for preservation of IHC pre and post-synaptic ribbon synapses: Guinea pigs were exposed for 2 h to 4 to 8 kHz noise at 95 dB. Auditory brainstem responses to pure-tone pips were acquired preoperatively, and at 1 and 2 weeks' post exposure. Immediately after noise exposure neurotrophins (brain-derived neurotrophic factor and neurotrophin-3) were applied to the RWM. ABR amplitude growth recovered in the ears of neurotrophin-treated guinea pigs using 16 kHz tones. Significantly more presynaptic ribbons, post-synaptic glutamate receptors, and co-localized ribbon synapse were seen after neurotrophin treatment. These findings supported the hypothesis that the local application of neurotrophins to the round window immediately after noise exposure will prevent noise-induced "hidden hearing loss" (Sly et al., 2016).

  - Even more exciting is the report that synapses may regenerate with intra-tympanic treatment with NT-3 after noise exposure. Mice exposed to noise ("neuropathic noise") that resulted in loss of up to 50% of synapses in the base of the cochlea within 24 h were treated with intra-tympanic neurotrophic-3 (NT-3 in a poloxamer gel) 24 h after noise exposure. Interestingly, this treatment was associated with regeneration of both pre- and post-synaptic elements at the junction of the IHC and cochlear nerve. Not only did the mice show structural recovery of these synapses, but they also demonstrated functional recovery by restoration of ABR wave 1 suprathreshold amplitudes. These findings have significant potential for healing "hidden hearing loss" in humans (Suzuki et al., 2016).

- Dexamethasone is the most frequently tested glucocorticosteroid by intra-tympanic injection to protect against noise-induced hearing loss. Rats were exposed to noise at 110 dB for 25 min and DPOAE measurements were performed before and after noise exposure. DPOAE measurements were performed before and 7 and 10 days after noise trauma. Rats treated with intra-tympanic dexamethasone had significantly better hearing than controls (Gumrukcu et al., 2018). Guinea pigs receiving intra-tympanic dexamethasone demonstrated significantly smaller ABR threshold shifts and decreased OHC loss compared with controls. They also had significant reduction in malondialdehyde concentration in the cochlea. This suggests that dexamethasone provided antioxidant effects in the treated ears (Chi et al., 2011). Another study showed short-term protection against hearing loss in guinea pigs with intra-tympanic dexamethasone. Animals received dexamethasone by intra-tympanic injection 2 h prior to white noise exposure. ABR thresholds were better and hair cell loss was reduced by this treatment. However, the major flaw of this study is that ABR thresholds and cochlear histology were performed only 2 h after noise exposure (Heinrich et al., 2016). Another study using guinea pigs tested the efficacy of dexamethasone administered intra-tympanically 2 h prior to white noise exposure. One group received dexamethasone solution and

TABLE 2 | This table summarizes pertinent studies of amelioration of noise-induced hearing loss using intra-tympanic therapy.

Drug	Animal model	Mechanism	References
AM-111 (D-JNKi-1)	Chinchilla	Anti-apoptotic	Coleman et al., 2007
d-JNKI-1	Guinea pig	Anti-apoptotic	Wang et al., 2007
D-JNKi-1 multifunctional	Mouse	Anti-apoptotic	Kayyali et al., 2018
Methylprednisolone	Guinea pig, Rat	Anti-inflammatory	Zhou et al., 2009; Ozdogan et al., 2012
Dexamethasone	Guinea pig	Anti-inflammatory	Chi et al., 2011; Heinrich et al., 2016
	Mouse		Han et al., 2015
	Rat		Gumrukcu et al., 2018
Dexamethasone (OTO-104)	Guinea pig		Harrop-Jones et al., 2016
Dexamethasone ultrasonic microbubbles	Guinea pig		Shih et al., 2018
Caroverine	Guinea pig	Glutamate antagonism	Chen et al., 2004
Kenpaullone	Mouse	Cyclin-dependent kinase-2 inhibitor	Teitz et al., 2018
Edavarone solid lipid nanoparticles	guinea pig	Antioxidant	Gao et al., 2015
BDNF + NT3	Guinea pig	Synapse regeneration	Sly et al., 2016
NT3	Mouse	Synapse regeneration	Suzuki et al., 2016
Pioglitazone	Rat	Anti-inflammatory, Antioxidant	Paciello et al., 2018
Rosmarinic acid	Rat	Antioxidant	Fetoni et al., 2018
AMPK-alpha1 siRNA	Mouse	*AMPK-alpha 1*	Hill et al., 2016
LKB1 siRNA	Mouse	*LKB1*	Hill et al., 2016
G9a siRNA	Mouse	*EHMT2*	Xiong et al., 2019

a second group was provided dexamethasone microbubbles with ultrasound irradiation. Compared with controls, dexamethasone in both groups provided protection against hair cell loss and auditory threshold shifts. However, significantly greater protection was afforded to the guinea pigs pretreated with ultrasound delivered microbubbles (Shih et al., 2018).

- Interesting findings were reported in a study of noise exposed mice. Animals were exposed to 110 db white noise for 60 min in a single exposure. One group received intraperitoneal dexamethasone injection (IP) daily for five consecutive days, while another cohort was given intra-tympanic injection of dexamethasone on days one and four after noise exposure. Mice in both treatment groups showed improved ABR thresholds but no apparent improvement in DPOAEs. Interestingly, better preservation of organ of Corti ultrastructure was observed in mice receiving IP drug than in those who were administered dexamethasone by intra-tympanic injection. On the other hand, efferent synapses were damaged in control (noise only), and in both groups treated with dexamethasone. However, there was better preservation of synapses of efferent terminals on OHCs in the group treated with intra-tympanic steroids (Han et al., 2015).
- In efforts to provide sustained release of dexamethasone for prolonged otoprotection against noise the efficacy of OTO-104 was investigated both prior to and following acute acoustic trauma. OTO-104 is a poloxamer-based hydrogel containing micronized dexamethasone. Guinea pigs received a single intra-tympanic injection of OTO-104 and were assessed in a model of acute acoustic trauma. Doses of at least 2.0% OTO-104 offered significant protection against hearing loss induced by noise exposure when administered 1 day prior to trauma and up to 3 days afterward. Otoprotection remained effective even with higher degrees of trauma. In contrast, the administration of a dexamethasone sodium phosphate solution did not protect against noise-induced hearing loss. Activation of the classical nuclear glucocorticoid and mineralocorticoid receptor pathways was required for otoprotection by OTO-104. The sustained release features of OTO-104 provided greater protection than the solution (Harrop-Jones et al., 2016).
- Methylprednisolone was administered intra-tympanically to guinea pigs exposed to impulse noise. Animals receiving this treatment had significantly better ABR thresholds at 4 weeks compared with those treated with saline. Significantly better preservation of hair cells was observed in the cochleae of guinea pigs receiving intra-tympanic methylprednisolone compared to those treated with saline (Zhou et al., 2009). Intra-tympanic methylprednisolone injection in rats administered following acoustic trauma was shown to reduce OHC loss. Although DPOAE measurement within the first week demonstrated significantly better amplitudes in the treated rats compared to controls at 2 weeks, there was no significant difference in DPOAE amplitudes between the treated and control group (Ozdogan et al., 2012).

We have summarized the studies reporting intra-tympanic drug delivery that protect against NIHL in **Table 2**.

CONCLUSION

Studies described in the above review highlight some exciting new research on local drug delivery using intra-tympanic administration of substances to ameliorate ototoxicity of cisplatin and noise-induced hearing loss. These are two very important causes of permanent sensorineural hearing loss for which there are currently no approved treatments on the market. The reports that are discussed include the proposed mechanisms for protection against these two major causes of hearing loss in humans.

The advantages of local delivery include targeted effects on the inner ear while minimizing systemic toxicity or interference with cisplatin antitumor efficacy and the ability to deliver sufficient amount of protective agent within the inner ear while by-passing the blood-labyrinth barrier (BLB), a major obstacle to effective protection delivered by systemic administration. The use of intra-tympanic injection in humans is minimally invasive and can generally be performed in the office under local anesthesia. The exploration of methods to extend the duration of release of protective agents and the investigation of round window permeation enhancers can provide higher concentrations of protectant molecules in the cochlea following intra-tympanic administration. The use of nanoparticles incorporating protective agents to target prestin in outer hair cells is very innovative and exciting. Although the regeneration of hair cells in the cochlea of humans has not been demonstrated, the regeneration of synapses on IHCs in animals after noise-induced synaptopathy using locally applied neurotrophins appears feasible. Future research is likely to reveal new mechanisms and exciting and novel treatments for sensorineural hearing loss.

AUTHOR CONTRIBUTIONS

LR conceived the study. LR and AD wrote the manuscript. DM and VR critiqued and revised the manuscript.

REFERENCES

Basner, M., Babisch, W., Davis, A., Brink, M., Clark, C., Janssen, S., et al. (2014). Auditory and non-auditory effects of noise on health. *Lancet* 383, 1325–1332. doi: 10.1016/s0140-6736(13)61613-x

Benkafadar, N., Menardo, J., Bourien, J., Nouvian, R., François, F., Decaudin, D., et al. (2017). Reversible p53 inhibition prevents cisplatin ototoxicity without blocking chemotherapeutic efficacy. *EMBO Mol. Med.* 9, 7–26. doi: 10.15252/emmm.201606230

Berglin, C. E., Pierre, P. V., Bramer, T., Edsman, K., Ehrsson, H., Eksborg, S., et al. (2011). Prevention of cisplatin-induced hearing loss by administration of a thiosulfate-containing gel to the middle ear in a guinea pig model. *Cancer Chemother. Pharmacol.* 68, 1547–1556. doi: 10.1007/s00280-011-1656-2

Bhatta, P., Dhukhwa, A., Sheehan, K., Al Aameri, R. F. H., Borse, V., Ghosh, S., et al. (2019). Capsaicin protects against cisplatin ototoxicity by changing the STAT3/STAT1 ratio and activating cannabinoid (CB2) receptors in the cochlea. *Sci. Rep.* 9:4131. doi: 10.1038/s41598-019-40425-9

Breglio, A. M., Rusheen, A. E., Shide, E. D., Fernandez, K. A., Spielbauer, K. K., McLachlin, K. M., et al. (2017). Cisplatin is retained in the cochlea indefinitely following chemotherapy. *Nat. Commun.* 8:1654. doi: 10.1038/s41467-017-01837-1

Bressler, S., Goldberg, H., and Shinn-Cunningham, B. (2017). Sensory coding and cognitive processing of sound in Veterans with blast exposure. *Hear. Res.* 349, 98–110. doi: 10.1016/j.heares.2016.10.018

Brooks, B., and Knight, K. (2018). Ototoxicity monitoring in children treated with platinum chemotherapy. *Int. J. Audiol.* 57, S34–S40. doi: 10.1080/14992027.2017.1355570

Celebi, S., Gurdal, M. M., Ozkul, M. H., Yasar, H., and Balikci, H. H. (2013). The effect of intratympanic vitamin C administration on cisplatin-induced ototoxicity. *Eur. Arch. Otorhinolaryngol.* 270, 1293–1297. doi: 10.1007/s00405-012-2140-2

Chen, Z., Ulfendahl, M., Ruan, R., Tan, L., and Duan, M. (2004). Protection of auditory function against noise trauma with local caroverine administration in guinea pigs. *Hear. Res.* 197, 131–136. doi: 10.1016/j.heares.2004.03.021

Chi, F. L., Yang, M. Q., Zhou, Y. D., and Wang, B. (2011). Therapeutic efficacy of topical application of dexamethasone to the round window niche after acoustic trauma caused by intensive impulse noise in guinea pigs. *J. Laryngol. Otol.* 125, 673–685. doi: 10.1017/S0022215111000028

Choe, W. T., Chinosornvatana, N., and Chang, K. W. (2004). Prevention of cisplatin ototoxicity using transtympanic N-acetylcysteine and lactate. *Otol. Neurotol.* 25, 910–915. doi: 10.1097/00129492-200411000-00009

Coleman, J. K., Littlesunday, C., Jackson, R., and Meyer, T. (2007). AM-111 protects against permanent hearing loss from impulse noise trauma. *Hear. Res.* 226, 70–78. doi: 10.1016/j.heares.2006.05.006

Creber, N. J., Eastwood, H. T., Hampson, A. J., Tan, J., and O'Leary, S. J. (2019). Adjuvant agents enhance round window membrane permeability to dexamethasone and modulate basal to apical cochlear gradients. *Eur. J. Pharm. Sci.* 126, 69–81. doi: 10.1016/j.ejps.2018.08.013

Cunningham, L. L., and Tucci, D. L. (2017). Hearing Loss in Adults. *N. Engl. J. Med.* 377, 2465–2473.

Demir, M. G., Altintoprak, N., Aydin, S., Kosemihal, E., and Basak, K. (2015). Effect of transtympanic injection of melatonin on cisplatin-induced ototoxicity. *J. Int. Adv. Otol.* 11, 202–206. doi: 10.5152/iao.2015.1094

Ding, S., Xie, S., Chen, W., Wen, L., Wang, J., Yang, F., et al. (2019). Is oval window transport a royal gate for nanoparticle delivery to vestibule in the inner ear? *Eur. J. Pharm. Sci.* 126, 11–22. doi: 10.1016/j.ejps.2018.02.031

Dormer, N. H., Nelson-Brantley, J., Staecker, H., and Berkland, C. J. (2019). Evaluation of a transtympanic delivery system in Mus musculus for extended release steroids. *Eur. J. Pharm. Sci.* 126, 3–10. doi: 10.1016/j.ejps.2018.01.020

El Kechai, N., Mamelle, E., Nguyen, Y., Huang, N., Nicolas, V., Chaminade, P., et al. (2016). Hyaluronic acid liposomal gel sustains delivery of a corticoid to the inner ear. *J. Control Release* 226, 248–257. doi: 10.1016/j.jconrel.2016.02.013

Falcone, P. H., Nieman, K. M., Tribby, A. C., Vogel, R. M., Joy, J. M., Moon, J. R., et al. (2019). The attention-enhancing effects of spearmint extract supplementation in healthy men and women: a randomized, double-blind, placebo-controlled, parallel trial. *Nutr. Res.* 64, 24–38. doi: 10.1016/j.nutres.2018.11.012

Fernandez, R., Harrop-Jones, A., Wang, X., Dellamary, L., LeBel, C., and Piu, F. (2016). The sustained-exposure dexamethasone formulation OTO-104 offers effective protection against cisplatin-induced hearing loss. *Audiol. Neurootol.* 21, 22–29. doi: 10.1159/000441833

Fetoni, A. R., Eramo, S. L. M., Di Pino, A., Rolesi, R., Paciello, F., Grassi, C., et al. (2018). The antioxidant effect of rosmarinic acid by different delivery routes in the animal model of noise-induced hearing loss. *Otol. Neurotol.* 39, 378–386. doi: 10.1097/MAO.0000000000001700

Franz, P., Aharinejad, S., Bock, P., and Firbas, W. (1993). The cochlear glomeruli in the modiolus of the guinea pig. *Eur. Arch. Otorhinolaryngol.* 250, 44–50.

Gao, G., Liu, Y., Zhou, C. H., Jiang, P., and Sun, J. J. (2015). Solid lipid nanoparticles loaded with edaravone for inner ear protection after noise exposure. *Chin. Med. J.* 128, 203–209. doi: 10.4103/0366-6999.149202

Gates, G. A., Schmid, P., Kujawa, S. G., Nam, B., and D'Agostino, R. (2000). Longitudinal threshold changes in older men with audiometric notches. *Hear. Res.* 141, 220–228. doi: 10.1016/s0378-5955(99)00223-3

Ghosh, S., Sheth, S., Sheehan, K., Mukherjea, D., Dhukhwa, A., Borse, V., et al. (2018). The Endocannabinoid/Cannabinoid Receptor 2 System Protects Against Cisplatin-Induced Hearing Loss. *Front. Cell. Neurosci.* 12:271. doi: 10.3389/fncel.2018.00271

Goycoolea, M. V. (1992). The round window membrane under normal and pathological conditions. *Acta Otolaryngol. Suppl.* 493, 43–55.

Goycoolea, M. V., and Lundman, L. (1997). Round window membrane. Structure function and permeability: a review. *Microsc. Res. Tech.* 36, 201–211.

Goycoolea, M. V., Muchow, D., and Schachern, P. (1988). Experimental studies on round window structure: function and permeability. *Laryngoscope* 98(6 Pt 2 Suppl. 44), 1–20. doi: 10.1288/00005537-198806001-00002

Gumrukcu, S. S., Topaloglu, I., Salturk, Z., Tutar, B., Atar, Y., Berkiten, G., et al. (2018). Effects of intratympanic dexamethasone on noise-induced hearing loss: an experimental study. *Am. J. Otolaryngol.* 39, 71–73. doi: 10.1016/j.amjoto.2017.10.011

Han, M. A., Back, S. A., Kim, H. L., Park, S. Y., Yeo, S. W., and Park, S. N. (2015). Therapeutic effect of dexamethasone for noise-induced hearing loss: systemic versus intratympanic injection in mice. *Otol. Neurotol.* 36, 755–762. doi: 10.1097/MAO.0000000000000759

Harrop-Jones, A., Wang, X., Fernandez, R., Dellamary, L., Ryan, A. F., LeBel, C., et al. (2016). The sustained-exposure dexamethasone formulation OTO-104 offers effective protection against noise-induced hearing loss. *Audiol. Neurootol.* 21, 12–21. doi: 10.1159/000441814

Hazlitt, R. A., Min, J., and Zuo, J. (2018). Progress in the Development of Preventative Drugs for Cisplatin-Induced Hearing Loss. *J. Med. Chem.* 61, 5512–5524. doi: 10.1021/acs.jmedchem.7b01653

Heinrich, U. R., Strieth, S., Schmidtmann, I., Stauber, R., and Helling, K. (2016). Dexamethasone prevents hearing loss by restoring glucocorticoid receptor expression in the guinea pig cochlea. *Laryngoscope* 126, E29–E34. doi: 10.1002/lary.25345

Hellberg, V., Wallin, I., Ehrsson, H., and Laurell, G. (2013). Cochlear pharmacokinetics of cisplatin: an in vivo study in the guinea pig. *Laryngoscope* 123, 3172–3177. doi: 10.1002/lary.24235

Hill, G. W., Morest, D. K., and Parham, K. (2008). Cisplatin-induced ototoxicity: effect of intratympanic dexamethasone injections. *Otol. Neurotol.* 29, 1005–1011. doi: 10.1097/MAO.0b013e31818599d5

Hill, K., Yuan, H., Wang, X., and Sha, S. H. (2016). Noise-induced loss of hair cells and cochlear synaptopathy are mediated by the activation of AMPK. *J. Neurosci.* 36, 7497–7510. doi: 10.1523/JNEUROSCI.0782-16.2016

Juhn, S. K., Meyerhoff, W. L., and Paparella, M. M. (1981). Clinical application of middle ear effusion analyses. *Laryngoscope* 91, 1012–1015.

Karasawa, T., and Steyger, P. S. (2015). An integrated view of cisplatin-induced nephrotoxicity and ototoxicity. *Toxicol. Lett.* 237, 219–227. doi: 10.1016/j.toxlet.2015.06.012

Kaur, T., Borse, V., Sheth, S., Sheehan, K., Ghosh, S., Tupal, S., et al. (2016). Adenosine A1 receptor protects against cisplatin ototoxicity by suppressing the NOX3/STAT1 inflammatory pathway in the cochlea. *J. Neurosci.* 36, 3962–3977. doi: 10.1523/JNEUROSCI.3111-15.2016

Kaur, T., Mukherjea, D., Sheehan, K., Jajoo, S., Rybak, L. P., and Ramkumar, V. (2011). Short interfering RNA against STAT1 attenuates cisplatin-induced ototoxicity in the rat by suppressing inflammation. *Cell Death Dis.* 2:e180. doi: 10.1038/cddis.2011.63

Kayyali, M. N., Wooltorton, J. R. A., Ramsey, A. J., Lin, M., Chao, T. N., Tsourkas, A., et al. (2018). A novel nanoparticle delivery system for targeted therapy of noise-induced hearing loss. *J. Control Release* 279, 243–250. doi: 10.1016/j.jconrel.2018.04.028

King, E. B., Salt, A. N., Eastwood, H. T., and O'Leary, S. J. (2011). Direct entry of gadolinium into the vestibule following intratympanic applications in Guinea pigs and the influence of cochlear implantation. *J. Assoc. Res. Otolaryngol.* 12, 741–751. doi: 10.1007/s10162-011-0280-5

Korver, K. D., Rybak, L. P., Whitworth, C., and Campbell, K. M. (2002). Round window application of D-methionine provides complete cisplatin otoprotection. *Otolaryngol. Head Neck Surg.* 126, 683–689. doi: 10.1067/mhn.2002.125299

Kros, C. J., and Steyger, P. S. (2018). Aminoglycoside- and cisplatin-induced ototoxicity: mechanisms and otoprotective strategies*. *Cold Spring Harb. Perspect. Med.* a033548. doi: 10.1101/cshperspect.a033548

Kujawa, S. G., and Liberman, M. C. (2009). Adding insult to injury: cochlear nerve degeneration after temporary noise-induced hearing loss. *J. Neurosci.* 29, 14077–14085. doi: 10.1523/jneurosci.2845-09.2009

Kumar, U. A., Ameenudin, S., and Sangamanatha, A. V. (2012). Temporal and speech processing skills in normal hearing individuals exposed to occupational noise. *Noise Health* 14, 100–105. doi: 10.4103/1463-1741.97252

Kurabi, A., Keithley, E. M., Housley, G. D., Ryan, A. F., and Wong, A. C. (2017). Cellular mechanisms of noise-induced hearing loss. *Hear. Res.* 349, 129–137. doi: 10.1016/j.heares.2016.11.013

Lavorgna, M., Orlo, E., Nugnes, R., Piscitelli, C., Russo, C., and Isidori, M. (2019). Capsaicin in hot chili peppers: in vitro evaluation of its antiradical, antiproliferative and apoptotic activities. *Plant Foods Hum. Nutr.* 74, 164–170. doi: 10.1007/s11130-019-00722-0

Le Prell, C. G., and Clavier, O. H. (2017). Effects of noise on speech recognition: challenges for communication by service members. *Hear. Res.* 349, 76–89. doi: 10.1016/j.heares.2016.10.004

Li, G., Frenz, D. A., Brahmblatt, S., Feghali, J. G., Ruben, R. J., Berggren, D., et al. (2001). Round window membrane delivery of L-methionine provides protection from cisplatin ototoxicity without compromising chemotherapeutic efficacy. *Neurotoxicology* 22, 163–176. doi: 10.1016/s0161-813x(00)00010-3

Li, L., Chao, T., Brant, J., O'Malley, B. Jr., Tsourkas, A., and Li, D. (2017). Advances in nano-based inner ear delivery systems for the treatment of sensorineural hearing loss. *Adv. Drug Deliv. Rev.* 108, 2–12. doi: 10.1016/j.addr.2016.01.004

Li, W., Hartsock, J. J., Dai, C., and Salt, A. N. (2018). Permeation enhancers for intratympanically-applied drugs studied using fluorescent dexamethasone as a marker. *Otol. Neurotol.* 39, 639–647. doi: 10.1097/MAO.0000000000001786

Martin-Saldana, S., Palao-Suay, R., Aguilar, M. R., Ramirez-Camacho, R., and San Roman, J. (2017). Polymeric nanoparticles loaded with dexamethasone or alpha-tocopheryl succinate to prevent cisplatin-induced ototoxicity. *Acta Biomater.* 53, 199–210. doi: 10.1016/j.actbio.2017.02.019

Masterson, E. A., Themann, C. L., and Calvert, G. M. (2018). prevalence of hearing loss among noise-exposed workers within the health care and social assistance sector, 2003 to 2012. *J. Occup. Environ. Med.* 60, 350–356. doi: 10.1097/JOM.0000000000001214

More, S. S., Akil, O., Ianculescu, A. G., Geier, E. G., Lustig, L. R., and Giacomini, K. M. (2010). Role of the copper transporter, CTR1, in platinum-induced ototoxicity. *J. Neurosci.*30, 9500–9509. doi: 10.1523/JNEUROSCI.1544-10.2010

Mukherjea, D., Jajoo, S., Sheehan, K., Kaur, T., Sheth, S., Bunch, J., et al. (2011). NOX3 NADPH oxidase couples transient receptor potential vanilloid 1 to signal transducer and activator of transcription 1-mediated inflammation and hearing loss. *Antioxid. Redox Signal.* 14, 999–1010. doi: 10.1089/ars.2010.3497

Mukherjea, D., Jajoo, S., Whitworth, C., Bunch, J. R., Turner, J. G., Rybak, L. P., et al. (2008). Short interfering RNA against transient receptor potential vanilloid 1 attenuates cisplatin-induced hearing loss in the rat. *J. Neurosci.* 28, 13056–13065. doi: 10.1523/JNEUROSCI.1307-08.2008

Munzel, T., Sorensen, M., Schmidt, F., Schmidt, E., Steven, S., Kroller-Schon, S., et al. (2018). The adverse effects of environmental noise exposure on oxidative stress and cardiovascular risk. *Antioxid. Redox. Signal.* 28, 873–908. doi: 10.1089/ars.2017.7118

Murphy, D., and Daniel, S. J. (2011). Intratympanic dexamethasone to prevent cisplatin ototoxicity: a guinea pig model. *Otolaryngol Head Neck Surg.* 145, 452–457. doi: 10.1177/0194599811406673

Nader, M. E., Theoret, Y., and Saliba, I. (2010). The role of intratympanic lactate injection in the prevention of cisplatin-induced ototoxicity. *Laryngoscope* 120, 1208–1213. doi: 10.1002/lary.20892

Nelson, D. I., Nelson, R. Y., Concha-Barrientos, M., and Fingerhut, M. (2005). The global burden of occupational noise-induced hearing loss. *Am. J. Ind. Med.* 48, 446–458. doi: 10.1002/ajim.20223

Nyberg, S., Abbott, N. J., Shi, X., Steyger, P. S., and Dabdoub, A. (2019). Delivery of therapeutics to the inner ear: the challenge of the blood-labyrinth barrier. *Sci. Transl. Med.* 11:eaao0935. doi: 10.1126/scitranslmed.aao0935

Ohinata, Y., Miller, J. M., Altschuler, R. A., and Schacht, J. (2000). Intense noise induces formation of vasoactive lipid peroxidation products in the cochlea. *Brain Res.* 878, 163–173. doi: 10.1016/s0006-8993(00)02733-5

Ohlemiller, K. K. (2008). Recent findings and emerging questions in cochlear noise injury. *Hear. Res.* 245, 5–17. doi: 10.1016/j.heares.2008.08.007

Oishi, N., and Schacht, J. (2011). Emerging treatments for noise-induced hearing loss. *Expert Opin. Emerg. Drugs* 16, 235–245. doi: 10.1517/14728214.2011.552427

Ozdogan, F., Ensari, S., Cakir, O., Ozcan, K. M., Koseoglu, S., Ozdas, T., et al. (2012). Investigation of the cochlear effects of intratympanic steroids administered following acoustic trauma. *Laryngoscope* 122, 877–882. doi: 10.1002/lary.23185

Özel, H. E., Özdoğan, F., Gürgen, S. G., Esen, E., Genç S., and Selçuk, A. (2016). Comparison of the protective effects of intratympanic dexamethasone and methylprednisolone against cisplatin-induced ototoxicity. *J. Laryngol. Otol.* 130, 225–234. doi: 10.1017/S0022215115003473

Paciello, F., Fetoni, A. R., Rolesi, R., Wright, M. B., Grassi, C., Troiani, D., et al. (2018). pioglitazone represents an effective therapeutic target in preventing oxidative/inflammatory cochlear damage induced by noise exposure. *Front. Pharmacol.* 9:1103. doi: 10.3389/fphar.2018.01103

Paksoy, M., Ayduran, E., Sanli, A., Eken, M., Aydin, S., and Oktay, Z. A. (2011). The protective effects of intratympanic dexamethasone and vitamin E on cisplatin-induced ototoxicity are demonstrated in rats. *Med. Oncol.* 28, 615–621. doi: 10.1007/s12032-010-9477-4

Parham, K. (2011). Can intratympanic dexamethasone protect against cisplatin ototoxicity in mice with age-related hearing loss? *Otolaryngol. Head Neck Surg.* 145, 635–640. doi: 10.1177/0194599811409304

Parhizkar, N., and Rybak, L. (2003). "Round Window Application of the P53 Inhibitor Pifithrin-Alpha provides complete protection against Cisplatin Ototoxicity," in *Proceedings of the 26th Annual Midwinter Research Meeting of The Association for Research in Otolaryngology*, Florida, FL.

Piu, F., Wang, X., Fernandez, R., Dellamary, L., Harrop, A., Ye, Q., et al. (2011). OTO-104: a sustained-release dexamethasone hydrogel for the treatment of otic disorders. *Otol. Neurotol.* 32, 171–179. doi: 10.1097/MAO.0b013e3182009d29

Qi, W., Ding, D., Zhu, H., Lu, D., Wang, Y., Ding, J., et al. (2014). Efficient siRNA transfection to the inner ear through the intact round window by a novel proteidic delivery technology in the chinchilla. *Gene. Ther.* 21, 10–18. doi: 10.1038/gt.2013.49

Ramaswamy, B., Roy, S., Apolo, A. B., Shapiro, B., and Depireux, D. A. (2017). Magnetic nanoparticle mediated steroid delivery mitigates cisplatin induced hearing loss. *Front. Cell. Neurosci.* 11:268. doi: 10.3389/fncel.2017.00268

Salt, A. N., and Hirose, K. (2018). Communication pathways to and from the inner ear and their contributions to drug delivery. *Hear. Res.* 362, 25–37. doi: 10.1016/j.heares.2017.12.010

Salt, A. N., and Plontke, S. K. (2009). Principles of local drug delivery to the inner ear. *Audiol. Neurootol.* 14, 350–360. doi: 10.1159/000241892

Salt, A. N., and Plontke, S. K. (2018). Pharmacokinetic principles in the inner ear: influence of drug properties on intratympanic applications. *Hear. Res.* 368, 28–40. doi: 10.1016/j.heares.2018.03.002

Shafik, A. G., Elkabarity, R. H., Thabet, M. T., Soliman, N. B., and Kalleny, N. K. (2013). Effect of intratympanic dexamethasone administration on cisplatin-induced ototoxicity in adult guinea pigs. *Auris Nasus Larynx* 40, 51–60. doi: 10.1016/j.anl.2012.05.010

Sheehan, K., Sheth, S., Mukherjea, D., Rybak, L. P., and Ramkumar, V. (2018). Trans-tympanic drug delivery for the treatment of ototoxicity*. *J. Vis. Exp.* 56564. doi: 10.3791/56564

Sheth, S., Mukherjea, D., Rybak, L. P., and Ramkumar, V. (2017). Mechanisms of cisplatin-induced ototoxicity and otoprotection. *Front. Cell. Neurosci.* 11:338. doi: 10.3389/fncel.2017.00338

Shi, X. (2016). Pathophysiology of the cochlear intrastrial fluid-blood barrier (review). *Hear. Res.* 338, 52–63. doi: 10.1016/j.heares.2016.01.010

Shih, C. P., Chen, H. C., Lin, Y. C., Chen, H. K., Wang, H., Kuo, C. Y., et al. (2018). Middle-ear dexamethasone delivery via ultrasound microbubbles attenuates noise-induced hearing loss. *Laryngoscope* doi: 10.1002/lary.27713 [Epub ahead of print].

Shin, Y. S., Song, S. J., Kang, S. U., Hwang, H. S., Choi, J. W., Lee, B. H., et al. (2013). A novel synthetic compound, 3-amino-3-(4-fluoro-phenyl)-1H-quinoline-2,4-dione, inhibits cisplatin-induced hearing loss by the suppression of reactive oxygen species: in vitro and in vivo study. *Neuroscience* 232, 1–12. doi: 10.1016/j.neuroscience.2012.12.008

Sly, D. J., Campbell, L., Uschakov, A., Saief, S. T., Lam, M., and O'Leary, S. J. (2016). Applying neurotrophins to the round window rescues auditory function and reduces inner hair cell synaptopathy after noise-induced hearing loss. *Otol. Neurotol.* 37, 1223–1230. doi: 10.1097/MAO.0000000000001191

Sun, C., Wang, X., Zheng, Z., Chen, D., Wang, X., Shi, F., et al. (2015). A single dose of dexamethasone encapsulated in polyethylene glycol-coated polylactic acid nanoparticles attenuates cisplatin-induced hearing loss following round window membrane administration. *Int. J. Nanomed.* 10, 3567–3579. doi: 10.2147/IJN.S77912

Suzuki, J., Corfas, G., and Liberman, M. C. (2016). Round-window delivery of neurotrophin 3 regenerates cochlear synapses after acoustic overexposure. *Sci. Rep.* 6:24907. doi: 10.1038/srep24907

Tanaka, K., and Motomura, S. (1981). Permeability of the labyrinthine windows in guinea pigs. *Arch. Otorhinolaryngol.* 233, 67–73.

Teitz, T., Fang, J., Goktug, A. N., Bonga, J. D., Diao, S., Hazlitt, R. A., et al. (2018). CDK2 inhibitors as candidate therapeutics for cisplatin- and noise-induced hearing loss. *J. Exp. Med.* 215, 1187–1203. doi: 10.1084/jem.20172246

Teranishi, M. A., and Nakashima, T. (2003). Effects of trolox, locally applied on round windows, on cisplatin-induced ototoxicity in guinea pigs. *Int. J. Pediatr. Otorhinolaryngol.* 67, 133–139. doi: 10.1016/s0165-5876(02)00353-1

Wang, J., Ruel, J., Ladrech, S., Bonny, C., van de Water, T. R., and Puel, J. L. (2007). Inhibition of the c-Jun N-terminal kinase-mediated mitochondrial cell death pathway restores auditory function in sound-exposed animals. *Mol. Pharmacol.* 71, 654–666. doi: 10.1124/mol.106.028936

Wang, X., Chen, Y., Tao, Y., Gao, Y., Yu, D., and Wu, H. (2018). A666-conjugated nanoparticles target prestin of outer hair cells preventing cisplatin-induced hearing loss. *Int. J. Nanomed.* 13, 7517–7531. doi: 10.2147/IJN.S170130

Wimmer, C., Mees, K., Stumpf, P., Welsch, U., Reichel, O., and Suckfull, M. (2004). Round window application of D-methionine, sodium thiosulfate, brain-derived neurotrophic factor, and fibroblast growth factor-2 in cisplatin-induced ototoxicity. *Otol. Neurotol.* 25, 33–40. doi: 10.1097/00129492-200401000-00007

Xiong, H., Long, H., Pan, S., Lai, R., Wang, X., Zhu, Y., et al. (2019). Inhibition of histone methyltransferase g9a attenuates noise-induced cochlear synaptopathy and hearing loss. *J. Assoc. Res. Otolaryngol.* 20, 217–232. doi: 10.1007/s10162-019-00714-6

Yamane, H., Nakai, Y., Takayama, M., Iguchi, H., Nakagawa, T., and Kojima, A. (1995). Appearance of free radicals in the guinea pig inner ear after noise-induced acoustic trauma. *Eur. Arch. Otorhinolaryngol.* 252, 504–508. doi: 10.1007/bf02114761

Zhang, L., Xu, Y., Cao, W., Xie, S., Wen, L., and Chen, G. (2018). Understanding the translocation mechanism of PLGA nanoparticles across round window membrane into the inner ear: a guideline for inner ear drug delivery based on nanomedicine. *Int. J. Nanomed.* 13, 479–492. doi: 10.2147/IJN.S154968

Zhang, M., Liu, W., Ding, D., and Salvi, R. (2003). Pifithrin-alpha suppresses p53 and protects cochlear and vestibular hair cells from cisplatin-induced apoptosis. *Neuroscience* 120, 191–205. doi: 10.1016/s0306-4522(03)00286-0

Zhou, Y., Zheng, H., Shen, X., Zhang, Q., and Yang, M. (2009). Intratympanic administration of methylprednisolone reduces impact of experimental intensive impulse noise trauma on hearing. *Acta Otolaryngol.* 129, 602–607. doi: 10.1080/00016480802342424

Zou, J., Pyykko, I., and Hyttinen, J. (2016). Inner ear barriers to nanomedicine-augmented drug delivery and imaging. *J. Otol.* 11, 165–177. doi: 10.1016/j.joto.2016.11.002

16

Inner Ear Therapeutics: An Overview of Middle Ear Delivery

*Jaimin Patel[1], Mikhaylo Szczupak[1], Suhrud Rajguru[1,2], Carey Balaban[3] and Michael E. Hoffer[1,4]**

[1] Department of Otolaryngology, University of Miami Miller School of Medicine, Miami, FL, United States, [2] Department of Biomedical Engineering, University of Miami, Coral Gables, FL, United States, [3] Department of Otolaryngology and Biomedical Engineering, University of Pittsburgh, Pittsburgh, PA, United States, [4] Department of Neurological Surgery, University of Miami Miller School of Medicine, Miami, FL, United States

***Correspondence:**
Michael E. Hoffer
michael.hoffer@miami.edu

There are a variety of methods to access the inner ear and many of these methods depend on utilizing the middle ear as a portal. In this approach the middle ear can be used as a passive receptacle, as part of an active drug delivery system, or simply as the most convenient way to access the inner ear directly in human subjects. The purpose of this volume is to examine some of the more cutting-edge approaches to treating the middle ear. Before considering these therapies, this manuscript provides an overview of some therapies that have been delivered through the middle ear both in the past and at the current time. This manuscript also serves as a review of many of the methods for accessing the inner ear that directly utilize or pass though the middle ear. This manuscript provides the reader a basis for understanding middle ear delivery, the basis of delivery of medicines via cochlear implants, and examines the novel approach of using hypothermia as a method of altering the responses of the inner ear to damage.

Keywords: transtympanic, intratympanic, middle ear, cochlea, labyrinthine

INTRODUCTION/OVERVIEW

Accessing the inner ear can be challenging due to its location and because direct access to the cochlea can result in hearing loss and/or balance disorders. As such, investigators and clinicians have attempted to access the inner ear via the middle ear since it is easier to reach both though the tympanic membrane (in the clinic) or through the middle ear itself (via a surgical approach). Using the middle ear as a route to the inner ear, however, still allows for a plethora of approaches to the inner ear itself. In this chapter we highlight some of the most important approaches the middle ear affords you when accessing the inner ear.

Initially we examine a technique that places an active substance in the middle ear to produce the desired effect in the inner ear. This is by far the most common type of approach to the inner ear and can be accomplished by flooding the middle ear with medication by simply injecting the fluid into the middle ear through the tympanic membrane in clinic. The nomenclature for this approach can be confusing since it appears as transtympanic, intratympanic, middle ear delivery, and a variety of other jargon. For the purposes of this overview chapter we will use the terminology "transtympanic" to refer to the procedure where a needle is passed through the tympanic membrane and allowed to fill the middle ear with medication. This approach can be used to treat a variety of disorders with different medications (only a few are highlighted in this overview chapter). A number of additional tweaks to this technique have been employed to obtain greater distribution of medication to the inner ear. These include delivery devices (some of which have appeared and been abandoned over time and others of which are just emerging onto the market), integrating the substance of interest into a biodegradable compound that is injected or surgically placed into the middle ear to slowly release doses over time. With some variation, all of these achieve the same goal of getting the active ingredient in contact with the inner ear. All of these approaches, again, can be used for an array of disorders and with an assortment of compounds. Finally, pharmaceuticals are not the only modality that can impact the inner ear. Our lab is examining how to utilize the middle ear to deliver therapeutic hypothermia to the inner ear as a countermeasure against inner ear trauma from a variety of sources. This chapter provides an overview of therapies that utilize the middle ear as a highway to the inner ear, which are the fundamental pathways for understanding how to best treat inner ear disorders.

TRANSTYMPANIC DRUG THERAPY

The anatomical configuration of the ear can be separated into three components: external, middle and inner ear. Pathologies arising in the inner ear are difficult to treat due to anatomical and systemic barriers. Anatomically, the inner ear is housed in the petrous bone, one of the densest bones of the human body, with limited access through the orifice of the external auditory canal. Systemically, the blood-labyrinthine barrier limits the delivery of medicine to the inner ear, similar to that of the blood brain barrier (Glueckert et al., 2018).

Transtympanic injection was first described in 1879 by Liel as a method for treating Eustachian Tube Dysfunction (Liel, 1879). The technique has been used for a variety of conditions over last 150 years and continues to be one of the most accessible routes for delivering local therapeutics to the inner ear (Mader et al., 2018). To better understand the mechanism of how this occurs, we have to address factors in both the middle and the inner ear. The middle ear is composed of the tympanic cavity with the ossicles as well as the Eustachian tube that drains into the nasopharynx. For the purpose of inner ear medication delivery, the critical portions of the middle ear are the oval window and the round window. When therapeutics are injected through the tympanic membrane (or through a hole in the tympanic membrane) the middle ear serves as the reservoir for the drug. The inner ear houses the organ of hearing, the cochlea, and the organs of balance, the vestibule and the semicircular canals (El Kechai et al., 2015). The cochlea is intricately connected to the middle ear via the two natural fenestrations of the perilympathic space: the oval window and the round window. These openings act in concert to allow fluid in the inner ear to propagate and allow audition to occur. These two windows and their associated membranes are gateways to make drug therapy into the inner ear possible (Glueckert et al., 2018) and allow the medications to reach both the hearing and balance organs of the inner ear.

ROUND WINDOW MEMBRANE PERMEABILITY

The round window membrane (RWM) in humans consists of three layers: (1) an outer epithelial layer facing the middle ear continuous with the promontory; (2) a middle connective tissue layer; (3) an inner cellular layer that interfaces with the scala tympani (ST). Despite the three layers, studies have shown that the round window behaves as if it is semi-permeable. The epithelium of the outer layer has characteristic microvilli which are indicative of absorptive capabilities of the RWM. In addition, the inner layer lacks continuity in the basement membrane with loose junctions suggesting open passages for substances to transverse the tertiary layer into the ST. In addition, the inner layer has shown to contain pinocytotic vesicles with amorphous substances, possibly perilymph, suggesting an active role in the transfer of substances between the RWM and the ST (Goycoolea and Lundman, 1997). Moreover, detailed anatomic observations of the RWM indicates that the epithelia of the outer and inner layer are metabolically active. They both contain secretory granules, endoplasmic reticulum, and golgi within in the cells supporting a bifunctional purpose of absorption and/or secretion (Richardson et al., 1971; Miriszlai et al., 1978; Salt et al., 2012). Therefore, the RWM is an ideal gateway to deliver drugs into the inner ear.

The factors that influence the permeability of the RWM include the molecule's size, liposolubility, electrical charge and the thickness of the membrane, to list a few. Therefore, substances that are smaller in molecular size, higher in liposolubility and positive in electrical charge will more easily diffuse into the ST via the RWM (Swan et al., 2008). Of note, transport of negatively charged nanoparticles has been reported (Youm et al., 2016). Additionally, the RWM has shown to be highly sensitive to manipulation in an effort to increase the diffusion rate of substances. Mikulec et al. (2008) demonstrated that the RWM permeability can be increased through introducing dry suctioning near the membrane along with preservatives such as benzyl alcohols and increasing osmolality of the substance. Other experiments altering the permeability of the RWM included use of local anesthetics, endotoxins, exotoxins, and histamine (Salt and Plontke, 2009). These external forces do not cause permanent damage to the RWM, but all impact the outer layer, likely making it the key layer in facilitating substances through the RWM (Goycoolea, 2001). The exact mechanism of how transmembrane transport continues to be incompletely understood. Our limited knowledge suggests that passive diffusion, facilitated diffusion through carriers, active transport, and phagocytosis may all play a role in the transmigration of substances across the RWM. This suggests that the mode of transport may be specific to the properties of each respective molecule (Salt and Plontke, 2009). It is important to remember that access to the round window can be affected by many factors that include adhesions, mucoperiosteal folds, and bone dust. Moreover the RWM itself can be thickened (Crane et al., 2005). All of these factors affect the ability of medicinews to reach the inner ear.

OVAL WINDOW

As the oval window is covered by the stapes footplate, less investigation has been done on the oval window as a route of delivering drugs. Studies have shown that the oval window may play a role in facilitating inner ear diffusion of medication, however, quantification of the entry remains problematic since the bony footplate can impedes pure oval window delivery mechanisms (Mikulec et al., 2009; Salt et al., 2012; King et al., 2013).

DRUG DISTRIBUTION IN THE INNER EAR

Following entry into the ST, the next challenge is to ensure distribution of the drug within the inner ear. This geometrically intricate structure has large fluid filled extracellular spaces, termed scalae, containing the inner ear fluid, perilymph. Perilymph is ionically similar to that of fluids in other extracellular spaces. The two large spaces containing perilymph include scala tympani (ST) and scala vestibuli (SV). The two scalae run parallel to one another in the spiral fashion of the cochlea, interconnected at the helicotrema, the cochlear apex. Between the two large scalae lies the scala media (SM), which contains the cellular machinery for audition. The scala media houses the endolymph, a unique fluid, high in potassium. Endolymph provides the ideal environment to transduce mechanical motion into electrical potential by the hair cells and their supporting structures (Swan et al., 2008).

The process of drug distribution has been subdivided into "radial" (with transport through the modiolus, the central core of the cochlea), and "longitudinal" (as if the cochlear spiral is unwound and fluid is flowing in a linear fashion between the parallel scalae and connected at the helicotrema) (Ohyama et al., 1988). One example of radial distribution was shown in 1991 by Salt et al. (1991) in which substances were found in the highest concentration at the basal turn and at the vestibular system after transmigrating the RWM. The mechanism behind this was believed to be that substances traveled between the extracellular spaces via the spiral ligament in the modiolus. With respect to longitudinal distribution, a number of factors come into play before a substance can theoretically achieve uniform distribution. In contrast to other extracellular fluids, the perilymph does not flow or is not actively stirred (Ohyama et al., 1988; Salt and Plontke, 2005). As a result, the drug distribution is slow and dependent on passive diffusion. The rate at which a molecule will passively diffuse in perilymph is dependent upon the diffusion coefficient, as the perilymph is in essence stagnant. A number of physical properties determine the diffusion coefficient of a molecule. Studies have shown that molecular weight is the most important factor (Salt, 2005). Another crucial aspect to drug distribution is clearance of the drug, which is the removal of a substance from the extracellular space into the capillary beds or the modiolus, metabolized in the perilymph or bound with tissue. Therefore, the relationship between a drug's diffusion capacity and clearance rate is key to determining its distributive quality. Consequently, to design an evenly distributed drug, the ideal configuration is a small molecule that is cleared slowly (Salt and Ma, 2001). A number of different medications and modalities have been engineered to ensure adequate delivery of medication to the inner ear.

TRANSTYMPANIC TREATMENT MODALITIES

Transtympanic injections are the simplest approach to delivering medicine to the inner ear, however, not the most efficient. This method has a number of variables unaccounted for, such as the clearances of the solution by the Eustachian tube, prolonged direct contact with the RWM, and effective transport through the RWM. Different drug delivery modalities and devices have been developed to overcome these challenges. The two well studied devices include the Silverstein Microwick® and the Microcather (μ*Cat*®). The Silverstein Microwick® is an absorbable polyvinyl acetate wick that is inserted through a myringotomy and placed overlying the round window. The myringotomy is kept open with a ventilation tube allowing the patient to instill the drug solution through the external auditory canal themselves. The solution is absorbed by the wick, reducing Eustachian tube clearance, and ensures direct contact with the RWM for effective passive diffusion (Silverstein et al., 2004). The Microcather (μ*Cat*®) is designed with an external and internal compartment. The external end contains biluminal ports, one for infusion and the other for withdrawal of fluid, while the internal end has a inflatable bulbous tip. This device is inserted after a tympanomeatal flap has been raised, where the bulbous tip is place within the round window niche and the biluminal end exits out of the external auditory canal. This end is connected to various pumping systems for drug infusions such as micropumps and osmotic pumps (Swan et al., 2008). This system provided more control of the amount of medicine instilled into the area of the round window but was associated with a risk of hearing loss in some centers (Thomsen et al., 2000) Osmotic pumps have been used to test a number of therapies for many inner ear disease in animal models and has been reviewed by Pararas et al. (2012).

The previous two devices do require exposing the middle ear for treatment making them more invasive. So forth, research in developing different injectable solutions was done to overcome the barriers of the middle ear. One such solution is hydrogels. Hydrogels are solutions with high viscosity and unique properties that allow environmental triggers to release drugs into the surrounding area (Mader et al., 2018). The viscous nature of the solution helps reduce Eustachian tube clearance, consequently increasing the residence time in the middle ear. This in turn supports increased RMW exposure time. For example, Poloxamer 407 is a hydrogel that is temperature sensitive. At room temperature it is an injectable liquid, but once it resides at body temperature within the middle ear, it gelifies allowing adequate drug exposure time (Wang et al., 2009). These drug-hydrogel solutions have been used both clinically and in animal studies (El Kechai et al., 2015). Recently, one has completed two Phase 3 clinical trials. The company Otonomy has created OTIVIDEX, a sustained-exposure formulation of transtympanic injectable dexamethasone for the treatment of Meniere's disease. This drug-hydrogel has shown to have significant benefits in patients with Meniere's disease (Mader et al., 2018).

Nanoparticular injection systems have also garnered attention recently for otologic purposes. These nanocarriers are of interest due to their ability to permeate the RWM and deliver their payload to targeted tissues. Some well-studied nanocarriers include liposomes, superparamagnetic iron oxide nanoparticles (SPIONs), and PLGA nanoparticles to name a few (Ge et al., 2007; Pritz et al., 2013; Bozzuto and Molinari, 2015). Liposomes are small phospholipid bilayer structures with an aqueous core. Due to their bilayer property, a liposome can encapsulate both hydrophobic and hydrophilic substances. This helps facilitate transport of substances through the RWM efficiently, while being able carry either type of substance. In addition, they allow surface modification with PEG, antibodies, peptides, carbohydrates, chitosan, hyaluronic acid and folic acid (Bozzuto and Molinari, 2015). Poly (lactic-co-glycolic acid) (PLGA) nanoparticles are biodegradable polymers versatile and safe enough for parenteral administration (Kumari et al., 2010). Different PLGA polymers have different properties allowing them to encapsulate hydrophobic and hydrophilic molecules while allowing surface modification with PEGylation, antibody ligands and chitosan adsorption (Grottkau et al., 2013). PLGA nanoparticle's adaptability and diversity in modification makes them an interesting drug delivery system for inner ear disease. SPIONs are Fe_3O_4 particles that are magnetized by an external magnetic field to control the migration of particles through the RWM. These particles do not encapsulate molecules; therefore, they contain a polymeric layer where PLGA nanoparticles are bound carrying the drug payload (Ge et al., 2007). This is a novel delivery mechanism where we can magnetically control the delivery of medication into the inner ear. Through continued research, a number of different nanoparticles, hydrogels, and substances are being engineered to ensure adequate and targeted therapy to the inner ear with the safe, non-invasive approach of transtympanic injections.

TRANSTYMPANIC USE OF MEDICATION

A variety of drugs have been used to tackle some of the common diseases that affect the inner ear. Some examples include corticosteroids, aminoglycoside antibiotics, antioxidants, anesthetics, and neurotrophins. Even vectors for gene therapy have been introduced through transtympanic injections (Kanzaki, 2018). The most common transtympanic drugs includes corticosteroids and aminoglycosides as they treat a number of common diseases, such as sudden sensorineural hearing loss (SSNHL), tinnitus, and Meniere's disease. Therefore, these two classes of medications will be discussed in detail.

As a medication class, steroids are known for their immunosuppressive qualities and in this case, electrolyte altering properties as well (Fukushima et al., 2002). The exact mechanism of action is still elusive but a number of known properties of this class of agent likely play a role in the ear as well and these include the following: 1) suppression of irritability or hypersensitivity of the sensory cells in the inner ear; 2) reduction of immune-mediated inflammation/autoimmune dysfunction; and/or 3) direct effect on the inner ear neuroepithelium (Yilmaz et al., 2005). SSNHL is debilitating to patients and steroids are the first line of treatment. Despite a paucity of high level evidence supporting the use of steroids for SSNHL, oral steroids are the standard of care for this disorder. A number of studies have suggested that oral steroids are equally as effective as transtympanic steroids, however, there are side effects associated with long term use of oral steroids (Hong et al., 2009; Dispenza et al., 2011; Rauch et al., 2011; Filipo et al., 2013). Additionally, transtympanic delivery can achieve a 100-fold higher concentration of steroids in the perilymph versus systemic delivery without the severe side effects (Bird et al., 2007). Clinical trials combining systemic and transtympanic versus transtympanic alone has shown to have no significant difference (Tsounis et al., 2018). So forth, there continues to be variations in an exact protocol on how to treat SSNHL. There are discrepancies on the frequency of injections, treatment length, and the ideal steroid of choice. Ultimately, the clinician's judgment about the choice of therapy should be patient centered, airing on the side of risk profile and cost efficiency (Stachler et al., 2012; Bear and Mikulec, 2014).

In recent years there have been five prospective, randomized, controlled trials with blinding, investigating the use of transtympanic steroids for the treatment of tinnitus. For the three studies comparing transtympanic steroid infusion to saline, there was not a statistically significant difference between the two groups with both producing a placebo-like improvement (Araujo et al., 2005; Topak et al., 2009; Choi et al., 2013). Another study that compared transtympanic dexamethasone or prednisolone to oral carbamazepine, showed no difference in tinnitus control rates among the groups (She et al., 2009). The remaining study, which only included patients that developed symptoms of tinnitus within the previous 3 months, was the only one to demonstrate a statistically significant difference between the two groups that received transtympanic steroids compared to the group that did not (25.8% and 25.0% vs. 9.8%, $p < 0.05$) (Shim et al., 2011). These works are not without limitations such as the low concentrations of dexamethasone employed (Araujo et al., 2005; Choi et al., 2013) as well as the small sample sizes (Chandrasekhar, 2014). The latter is inherent to studies of this design as it is difficult to conduct randomized, controlled trials with the number of patients Sakata et al. (1996) did near the end of the 20th century.

Meniere's disease (MD) causes devastating vertigo attacks with roaring tinnitus and aural fullness. As the disease progresses hearing loss is also inevitable (Syed et al., 2015). An algorithm on treatment of MD has evolved over time (Nevoux et al., 2018). Up to eighty percent of patients are either cured or in remission especially from vertigo from first line therapy, which includes lifestyle change, low salt diet, and diuretics (Claes and Van de Heyning, 2000). The remaining patients are treated conservatively with transtympanic steroids. Improvement in MD with steroids has been hypothesized to occur if hydrops is due to inflammation or autoimmune factors (Foster, 2015). Transtympanic steroids have been shown to improve both frequency and severity of vertigo spells compared to placebo at 24 months after treatment (Nevoux et al., 2018). Patel et al. (2016) reports two injections of methylprednisolone given 2 weeks apart is effective as gentamicin for the treatment of refractory MD, without the ototoxicity (Patel et al., 2016). Following the treatment protocol, refractory MD is treated with local destructive medical treatment with transtympanic gentamicin (TTG). However, gentamicin is not without risk. TTG is recommended if hearing function is already impaired as it is severely ototoxic. Based on a meta-analysis by Syed et al. (2015), a "titration" protocol of TTG (40 mg/ml) until disappearance of vertigo has been described (Syed et al., 2015). This protocol is in an effort to preserve hearing through directed therapy over exposing the patient to systemic gentamicin.

INTRACOCHLEAR TREATMENT

The next step in inner ear therapy is direct delivery to the root of the problem. Intracochlear administration is delivering the drug directly to the cochlea thus avoiding the middle ear barriers, such as the RWM and the Eustachian tube. While this modality involves direct inner ear administration the middle ear is usually the route to access the inner ear. The general modalities of introducing intracochlear medications includes direct injection, osmotic pumps, a constant infusion system, cochlear implant coating, and microfluidic reciprocating reservoir (El Kechai et al., 2015). As of this date, not all of these have been translated into human use.

Clinically, intracochlear injections are only possible using a surgical approach. Access is established through a cochleostomy either through the RWM or through the basal turn of the cochlea where a needle is inserted, and the drug is delivered. This method's inherent problem is the possibility of a leak at the injection site. Experiments have been done to control the fluid efflux with internal and external sealing procedures which show promising results (Plontke et al., 2016). An osmotic pump utilizes the osmotic gradient between the cannister containing the drug and the perilymph to drive the drug through the cannula and into the cochlea at a rate determined by the device. A number of drugs and gene vectors have been delivered through this mechanism in animal models (Borenstein, 2011).

The constant infusion system employs two points of entry, one in the cochlea and one in the posterior semicircular canal. The cochleostomy is at the basal turn and has an infusion pump through a cannula which supplies the drug at a predetermined rate. The inherent problem of a leak is threat with this technique. The canalostomy, near the SV, provides a fluid outlet to reduce concentration gradient within the perilymph enhancing, drug diffusion to the apex (Borkholder et al., 2010). An additional hinderance to this delivery method is the low rate of clearance of cochlear fluid, hence a limited volume of drug can be introduced through the pump in a given time span. To address this limitation, the reciprocating microfluidic reservoir was developed to provide a net zero volume delivery system that infused and withdrew a constant volume of drug in a cyclical fashion. Strategically, the infusion portion of the cycle lasts a few seconds and a total drug concentration in 1 μL is delivered. This fluid mixture is cycled through the cochlea through a withdraw port and into the device to be cycled through the infusion port in a cyclical fashion. This ensures adequate mixture and delivery by controlling the variables of flow and clearance rate of the cochlear fluid (Tandon et al., 2016).

The most logical method of intracochlear drug administration is through a cochlear implant. Patients that can qualify for this invasive procedure have profound hearing loss making it an ideal situation to implant a device directly into the inner ear. This device is placed surgically through a cochleostomy or through the RWM. This convenient situation allows the opportunity to deliver drugs to patients for a number of different applications. Some possible pathways include coating the device in biodegradable eluting polymers or integrating an active infusion pump within the device (Borenstein, 2011). One current effort to utilize this opportunity is to reduce the histological trauma of inserting the implant (Eshraghi et al., 2005). Different experiments have been conducted to reduce the inflammation and fibrosis of tissue, most applying the coating capabilities of the device with biodegradable polymers. El Kechai et al. (2015) has reviewed these thoroughly. With regards to an active pump integration, cochlear implant catheters have been combined with intracochlear implants in animal models, up to 15 mm of insertion, to test delivering a single bolus of iodine concurrently with the insertion of the device (Ibrahim et al., 2011). This method shows promise with delivery of iodine without leak or radiologic damage to the inner ear. However, further work needs to be done to determine the efficacy between different drugs and the quantity of the bolus injectable without damaging the delicate structures of the inner ear.

RECENT ADVANCES

Recent advances in novel inner ear therapeutics include different drug modalities, the robust application of genetic manipulation through viral vectors, and even hypothermic inner ear treatments. One particular study shows the inhibition of cochlear N-methyl-D-aspartate (NMDA) receptors with AM-101, a small novel antagonist, to treat tinnitus triggered by glutamate excitotoxicity. Clinical trials with this inhibitor showed that 3 transtympanic injections over 3 consecutive days of 0.81 mg/ml of AM-101 demonstrated a significant and dose dependent improvement in tinnitus (Staecker et al., 2015). N-Acetylcysteine (NAC), a low molecular weight agent with significant otoprotective qualities has also been tested clinically. Transtympanic injections have been studied with this agent to combat the ototoxic side effects of cisplatin, a well-known phenomenon from this chemotherapeutic agent. A 10% NAC solution was injected transtympanically prior to the infusion of cisplatin versus the control and the pure tone audiometry was measured. The study concluded that control patients had a significant reduction at 8000 HZ showing that NAC may play a role in otoprotection against ototoxic elements (Riga et al., 2013). With regards to autoimmune inner ear disease, a clinical trial with transtympanic TNF-alpha inhibitor (infliximab) was shown to improve hearing and reduce disease relapse (Van Wijk et al., 2006). As the next frontier of medicine is genetic manipulation, the inner ear is an ideal location to utilize this technology. Kanzaki (2018) has thoroughly reviewed the literature with regards to the application of viral vectors targeting the inner ear. Predominantly this technology is still in its early phase with animal models. However, as further studies are conducted, the ideal vision is to allow Otolaryngologists the ability to deliver targeted therapy to different types of inner ear cells based on the pathological presentation of the patient. Furthermore, as previously mentioned in the intracochlear treatment section, cochlear implant insertion can cause significant damage to the inner ear, particularly loss of residual hearing. Tamames et al. (2016) has created an animal model to test a custom probe that is infused with cooled fluorocarbon adjacent to the middle turn of the cochlea prior to implant insertion, as a means to protect the inner ear. Their work has demonstrated that rats with normothermic cochlea had significant loss of residual hearing compared to the hypothermic group due to implant trauma. Histologic studies confirmed the findings with significant loss of outer hair cells in the normothermic group. They showed this method to be feasible in human temporal bones with the cochlea cooling down 4 to 6 °C with their custom designed probe. This novel method to combat implant insertion trauma is promising to further our efforts of inner ear therapeutics.

CONCLUSION

Inner ear therapeutics are undergoing tremendous progress with a wide range of drug selection and different delivery methods. The anatomical intricacies of the ear employ a difficult challenge to drug delivery, however, through the advancements of knowledge and technology we have been able to locally deliver medication to the inner ear. Transtympanic injections are relatively simple procedures performed routinely by Otolaryngologists. This simple procedure has a complex physiological mechanism that is not yet fully understood. However, through further experimentation and novel pharmaceutical design the goal of treating inner ear disease is possible. As our understanding of the oval window, RWM, inner ear pharmacokinetics, drug distribution and mechanisms continue to grow, so will our applicability to better patient outcomes. With more invasive procedures such as intracochlear therapies, the development of miniaturized devices as a means to deploy therapies and even cooling the cochlea are promising ventures. With the future of medicine being targeted therapies, genetics may be the next avenue in clinical trials for inner ear disease. However, with our current understanding, further research is necessary to address the pharmaceutical and physiological challenges to safely and efficaciously treat all inner ear diseases.

AUTHOR CONTRIBUTIONS

JP prepared the manuscript. MS collected the data and prepared the manuscript. SR collected the data and edited the manuscript. CB edited the manuscript. MH prepared the manuscript and edited the manuscript.

REFERENCES

Araujo, M. F., Oliveira, C. A., and Bahmad, F. M. Jr. (2005). Intratympanic dexamethasone injections as a treatment for severe, disabling tinnitus: does it work? *Arch. Otolaryngol. Head Neck Surg.* 131, 113–117.

Bear, Z. W., and Mikulec, A. A. (2014). Intratympanic steroid therapy for treatment of idiopathic sudden sensorineural hearing loss. *Mol. Med.* 111, 352–356.

Bird, P. A., Begg, E. J., Zhang, M., Keast, A. T., Murray, D. P., and Balkany, T. J. (2007). Intratympanic versus intravenous delivery of methylprednisolone to cochlear perilymph. *Otol. Neurotol.* 28, 1124–1130. doi: 10.1097/mao.0b013e31815aee21

Borenstein, J. T. (2011). Intracochlear drug delivery systems. *Expert. Opin. Drug Deliv.* 8, 1161–1174. doi: 10.1517/17425247.2011.588207

Borkholder, D. A., Zhu, X., Hyatt, B. T., Archilla, A. S., Livingston, W. J. III, and Frisina, R. D. (2010). Murine intracochlear drug delivery: reducing concentration gradients within the cochlea. *Hear. Res.* 268, 2–11. doi: 10.1016/j.heares.2010.04.014

Bozzuto, G., and Molinari, A. (2015). Liposomes as nanomedical devices. *Int. J. Nanomed.* 10, 975–999. doi: 10.2147/IJN.S68861

Chandrasekhar, S. S. (2014). In reference to intratympanic dexamethasone injection for refractory tinnitus: prospective placebo-controlled study. *Laryngoscope* 124:E255.

Choi, S. J., Lee, J. B., Lim, H. J., In, S. M., Kim, J. Y., Bae, K. H., et al. (2013). Intratympanic dexamethasone injection for refractory tinnitus: prospective placebo-controlled study. *Laryngoscope* 123, 2817–2822. doi: 10.1002/lary.24126

Claes, J., and Van de Heyning, P. H. (2000). A review of medical treatment for Meniere's disease. *Acta Otolaryngol. Suppl.* 544, 34–39.

Crane, B. T., Minor, L. B., Della Santina, C. C., and Carey, J. P. (2005). Middle ear exploration in patients with Ménière's disease who have failed outpatient intratympanic gentamicin therapy.Otol Neurotol 2009; 30: 619-24; Penha, R and Escada,P. Round-window anatomical considerations in intratympanic drug therapy for inner-ear diseases. *Int. Tinnitus J.* 11, 31–33.

Dispenza, F., Amodio, E., De Stefano, A., Gallina, S., Marchese, D., Mathur, N., et al. (2011). Treatment of sudden sensorineural hearing loss with transtympanic injection of steroids as single therapy: a randomized clinical study. *Eur. Arch. Otorhinolaryngol.* 268, 1273–1278. doi: 10.1007/s00405-011-1523-0

El Kechai, N., Agnely, F., Mamelle, E., Nguyen, Y., Ferrary, E., and Bochot, A. (2015). Recent advances in local drug delivery to the inner ear. *Int. J. Pharm.* 494, 83–101. doi: 10.1016/j.ijpharm.2015.08.015

Eshraghi, A. A., Polak, M., He, J., Telischi, F. F., Balkany, T. J., and Van De Water, T. R. (2005). Pattern of hearing loss in a rat model of cochlear implantation trauma. *Otol. Neurotol.* 26, 442–447; discussion 447.

Filipo, R., Attanasio, G., Russo, F. Y., Viccaro, M., Mancini, P., and Covelli, E. (2013). Intratympanic steroid therapy in moderate sudden hearing loss: a randomized, triple-blind, placebo-controlled trial. *Laryngoscope* 123, 774–778. doi: 10.1002/lary.23678

Foster, C. A. (2015). Optimal management of Meniere's disease. *Ther. Clin. Risk Manag.* 11, 301–307. doi: 10.2147/TCRM.S59023

Fukushima, M., Kitahara, T., Uno, Y., Fuse, Y., Doi, K., and Kubo, T. (2002). Effects of intratympanic injection of steroids on changes in rat inner ear aquaporin expression. *Acta Otolaryngol.* 122, 600–606. doi: 10.1080/000164802320396268

Ge, X., Jackson, R. L., Liu, J., Harper, E. A., Hoffer, M. E., Wassel, R. A., et al. (2007). Distribution of PLGA nanoparticles in chinchilla cochleae. *Otolaryngol. Head Neck Surg.* 137, 619–623. doi: 10.1016/j.otohns.2007.04.013

Glueckert, R., Johnson Chacko, L., Rask-Andersen, H., Liu, W., Handschuh, S., and Schrott-Fischer, A. (2018). Anatomical basis of drug delivery to the inner ear. *Hear. Res.* 368, 10–27. doi: 10.1016/j.heares.2018.06.017

Goycoolea, M. V. (2001). Clinical aspects of round window membrane permeability under normal and pathological conditions. *Acta Otolaryngol.* 121, 437–447. doi: 10.1080/000164801300366552

Goycoolea, M. V., and Lundman, L. (1997). Round window membrane. structure function and permeability: a review. *Microsc. Res. Tech.* 36, 201–211. doi: 10.1002/(sici)1097-0029(19970201)36:3<201::aid-jemt8>3.0.co;2-r

Grottkau, B. E., Cai, X., Wang, J., Yang, X., and Lin, Y. (2013). Polymeric nanoparticles for a drug delivery system. *Curr. Drug Metab.* 14, 840–846. doi: 10.2174/138920021131400105

Hong, S. M., Park, C. H., and Lee, J. H. (2009). Hearing outcomes of daily intratympanic dexamethasone alone as a primary treatment modality for ISSHL. *Otolaryngol. Head Neck Surg.* 141, 579–583. doi: 10.1016/j.otohns.2009.08.009

Ibrahim, H. N., Bossard, D., Jolly, C., and Truy, E. (2011). Radiologic study of a disposable drug delivery intracochlear catheter. *Otol. Neurotol.* 32, 217–222. doi: 10.1097/MAO.0b013e3182040c47

Kanzaki, S. (2018). Gene delivery into the inner ear and its clinical implications for hearing and balance. *Molecules* 23:E2507. doi: 10.3390/molecules23102507

King, E. B., Salt, A. N., Kel, G. E., Eastwood, H. T., and O'Leary, S. J. (2013). Gentamicin administration on the stapes footplate causes greater hearing loss and vestibulotoxicity than round window administration in guinea pigs. *Hear. Res.* 304, 159–166. doi: 10.1016/j.heares.2013.07.013

Kumari, A., Yadav, S. K., and Yadav, S. C. (2010). Biodegradable polymeric nanoparticles based drug delivery systems. *Colloids Surf. B Biointerf.* 75, 1–18. doi: 10.1016/j.colsurfb.2009.09.001

Liel, W. (1879). On intratympanic injections in catarrhal affections of the middle ear. *Br. Med. J.* 2:364. doi: 10.1136/bmj.2.975.364

Mader, K., Lehner, E., Liebau, A., and Plontke, S. K. (2018). Controlled drug release to the inner ear: concepts, materials, mechanisms, and performance. *Hear. Res.* 368, 49–66. doi: 10.1016/j.heares.2018.03.006

Mikulec, A. A., Hartsock, J. J., and Salt, A. N. (2008). Permeability of the round window membrane is influenced by the composition of applied drug solutions and by common surgical procedures. *Otol. Neurotol.* 29, 1020–1026. doi: 10.1097/MAO.0b013e31818658ea

Mikulec, A. A., Plontke, S. K., Hartsock, J. J., and Salt, A. N. (2009). Entry of substances into perilymph through the bone of the otic capsule after intratympanic applications in guinea pigs: implications for local drug delivery in humans. *Otol. Neurotol.* 30, 131–138. doi: 10.1097/mao.0b013e318191bff8

Miriszlai, E., Benedeczky, I., Csapo, S., and Bodanszky, H. (1978). The ultrastructure of the round window membrane of the cat. *ORL J. Otorhinolaryngol. Relat. Spec.* 40, 111–119. doi: 10.1159/000275393

Nevoux, J., Barbara, M., Dornhoffer, J., Gibson, W., Kitahara, T., and Darrouzet, V. (2018). International consensus (ICON) on treatment of Meniere's disease. *Eur. Ann. Otorhinolaryngol. Head Neck Dis.* 135, S29–S32. doi: 10.1016/j.anorl.2017.12.006

Ohyama, K., Salt, A. N., and Thalmann, R. (1988). Volume flow rate of perilymph in the guinea-pig cochlea. *Hear. Res.* 35, 119–129. doi: 10.1016/0378-5955(88)90111-6

Pararas, E. E., Borkholder, D. A., and Borenstein, J. T. (2012). Microsystems technologies for drug delivery to the inner ear. *Adv. Drug Deliv. Rev.* 64, 1650–1660. doi: 10.1016/j.addr.2012.02.004

Patel, M., Agarwal, K., Arshad, Q., Hariri, M., Rea, P., Seemungal, B. M., et al. (2016). Intratympanic methylprednisolone versus gentamicin in patients with unilateral Meniere's disease: a randomised, double-blind, comparative effectiveness trial. *Lancet* 388, 2753–2762. doi: 10.1016/S0140-6736(16)31461-1

Plontke, S. K., Hartsock, J. J., Gill, R. M., and Salt, A. N. (2016). Intracochlear drug injections through the round window membrane: measures to improve drug retention. *Audiol. Neurootol.* 21, 72–79. doi: 10.1159/000442514

Pritz, C. O., Dudas, J., Rask-Andersen, H., Schrott-Fischer, A., and Glueckert, R. (2013). Nanomedicine strategies for drug delivery to the ear. *Nanomedicine* 8, 1155–1172. doi: 10.2217/nnm.13.104

Rauch, S. D., Halpin, C. F., Antonelli, P. J., Babu, S., Carey, J. P., Gantz, B. J., et al. (2011). Oral vs intratympanic corticosteroid therapy for idiopathic sudden sensorineural hearing loss: a randomized trial. *JAMA* 305, 2071–2079. doi: 10.1001/jama.2011.679

Richardson, T. L., Ishiyama, E., and Keels, E. W. (1971). Submicroscopic studies of the round window membrane. *Acta Otolaryngol.* 71, 9–21. doi: 10.3109/00016487109125327

Riga, M. G., Chelis, L., Kakolyris, S., Papadopoulos, S., Stathakidou, S., Chamalidou, E., et al. (2013). Transtympanic injections of N-acetylcysteine for the prevention of cisplatin induced ototoxicity: a feasible method with promising efficacy. *Am. J. Clin. Oncol.* 36, 1–6. doi: 10.1097/COC.0b013e31822e006d

Sakata, E., Itoh, A., and Itoh, Y. (1996). Treatment of cochlear-tinnitus with dexamethasone infusion into the tympanic cavity. *Int. Tinnitus J.* 2, 129–135.

Salt, A. N. (2005). Pharmacokinetics of drug entry into cochlear fluids. *Volta. Rev.* 105, 277–298.

Salt, A. N., King, E. B., Hartsock, J. J., Gill, R. M., and O'Leary, S. J. (2012). Marker entry into vestibular perilymph via the stapes following applications to the round window niche of guinea pigs. *Hear. Res.* 283, 14–23. doi: 10.1016/j.heares.2011.11.012

Salt, A. N., and Ma, Y. (2001). Quantification of solute entry into cochlear perilymph through the round window membrane. *Hear. Res.* 154, 88–97. doi: 10.1016/s0378-5955(01)00223-4

Salt, A. N., Ohyama, K., and Thalmann, R. (1991). Radial communication between the perilymphatic scalae of the cochlea. II: estimation by bolus injection of tracer into the sealed cochlea. *Hear. Res.* 56, 37–43. doi: 10.1016/0378-5955(91)90151-x

Salt, A. N., and Plontke, S. K. (2005). Local inner-ear drug delivery and pharmacokinetics. *Drug Discov. Today* 10, 1299–1306. doi: 10.1016/s1359-6446(05)03574-9

Salt, A. N., and Plontke, S. K. (2009). Principles of local drug delivery to the inner ear. *Audiol. Neurootol.* 14, 350–360. doi: 10.1159/000241892

She, W., Dai, Y., Du, X., Chen, F., Ding, X., and Cui, X. (2009). Treatment of subjective tinnitus: a comparative clinical study of intratympanic steroid injection vs. *oral carbamazepine. Med. Sci. Monit.* 15, I35–I39.

Shim, H. J., Song, S. J., Choi, A. Y., Hyung Lee, R., and Yoon, S. W. (2011). Comparison of various treatment modalities for acute tinnitus. *Laryngoscope* 121, 2619–2625. doi: 10.1002/lary.22350

Silverstein, H., Thompson, J., Rosenberg, S. I., Brown, N., and Light, J. (2004). Silverstein microWick. *Otolaryngol. Clin. North Am.* 37, 1019–1034. doi: 10.1016/j.otc.2004.04.002

Stachler, R. J., Chandrasekhar, S. S., Archer, S. M., Rosenfeld, R. M., Schwartz, S. R., Barrs, D. M., et al. (2012). Clinical practice guideline: sudden hearing loss. *Otolaryngol.Head Neck Surg.* 146, S1–S35.

Staecker, H., Maxwell, K. S., Morris, J. R., van de Heyning, P., Morawski, K., Reintjes, F., et al. (2015). Selecting appropriate dose regimens for AM-101 in the intratympanic treatment of acute inner ear tinnitus. *Audiol. Neurootol.* 20, 172–182. doi: 10.1159/000369608

Swan, E. E., Mescher, M. J., Sewell, W. F., Tao, S. L., and Borenstein, J. T. (2008). Inner ear drug delivery for auditory applications. *Adv. Drug Deliv. Rev* 60, 1583–1599. doi: 10.1016/j.addr.2008.08.001

Syed, M. I., Ilan, O., Nassar, J., and Rutka, J. A. (2015). Intratympanic therapy in Meniere's syndrome or disease: up to date evidence for clinical practice. *Clin. Otolaryngol.* 40, 682–690. doi: 10.1111/coa.12449

Tamames, I., King, C., Bas, E., Dietrich, W. D., Telischi, F., and Rajguru, S. M. (2016). A cool approach to reducing electrode-induced trauma: localized therapeutic hypothermia conserves residual hearing in cochlear implantation. *Hear. Res.* 339, 32–39. doi: 10.1016/j.heares.2016.05.015

Tandon, V., Kang, W. S., Robbins, T. A., Spencer, A. J., Kim, E. S., McKenna, M. J., et al. (2016). Microfabricated reciprocating micropump for intracochlear drug delivery with integrated drug/fluid storage and electronically controlled dosing. *Lab. Chip* 16, 829–846. doi: 10.1039/c5lc01396h

Thomsen, J., Charabi, S., and Tos, M. (2000). Preliminary results of a new delivery system for gentamicin to the inner ear in patients with Meniere's disease. *Eur. Arch. Otorhinolaryngol.* 257, 362–365. doi: 10.1007/s004059900219

Topak, M., Sahin-Yilmaz, A., Ozdoganoglu, T., Yilmaz, H. B., Ozbay, M., and Kulekci, M. (2009). Intratympanic methylprednisolone injections for subjective tinnitus. *J. Laryngol. Otol.* 123, 1221–1225. doi: 10.1017/S0022215109990685

Tsounis, M., Psillas, G., Tsalighopoulos, M., Vital, V., Maroudias, N., and Markou, K. (2018). Systemic, intratympanic and combined administration of steroids for sudden hearing loss. a prospective randomized multicenter trial. *Eur. Arch. Otorhinolaryngol.* 275, 103–110. doi: 10.1007/s00405-017-4803-5

Van Wijk, F., Staecker, H., Keithley, E., and Lefebvre, P. P. (2006). Local perfusion of the tumor necrosis factor alpha blocker infliximab to the inner ear improves autoimmune neurosensory hearing loss. *Audiol. Neurootol.* 11, 357–365. doi: 10.1159/000095897

Wang, X., Dellamary, L., Fernandez, R., Harrop, A., Keithley, E. M., Harris, J. P., et al. (2009). Dose-dependent sustained release of dexamethasone in inner ear cochlear fluids using a novel local delivery approach. *Audiol. Neurootol.* 14, 393–401. doi: 10.1159/000241896

Yilmaz, I., Yilmazer, C., Erkan, A. N., Aslan, S. G., and Ozluoglu, L. N. (2005). Intratympanic dexamethasone injection effects on transient-evoked otoacoustic emission. *Am. J. Otolaryngol.* 26, 113–117. doi: 10.1016/j.amjoto.2004.11.001

Youm, I., Musazzi, U. M., Gratton, M. A., Murowchick, J. B., and Youan, B. C. (2016). Label-free ferrocene-loaded nanocarrier engineering for in vivo cochlear drug delivery and imaging. *J. Pharm. Sci.* 105, 3162–3171. doi: 10.1016/j.xphs.2016.04.012

17

Local Delivery of Therapeutics to the Inner Ear: The State of the Science

Caroline R. Anderson[1,2†], Carol Xie[1,2†], Matthew P. Su[1,2], Maria Garcia[1,2], Helen Blackshaw[1,2] and Anne G. M. Schilder[1,2*]*

[1] *evidENT, Ear Institute, University College London, London, United Kingdom,*

[2] *NIHR University College London Hospitals Biomedical Research Centre, London, United Kingdom*

***Correspondence:**
Caroline R. Anderson
caroline.anderson@ucl.ac.uk
Anne G. M. Schilder
a.schilder@ucl.ac.uk*

† Joint first authors

Background: Advances in the understanding of the genetic and molecular etiologies of inner ear disorders have enabled the identification of therapeutic targets and innovative delivery approaches to the inner ear. As this field grows, the need for knowledge about effective delivery of therapeutics to the inner ear has become a priority. This review maps all clinical and pre-clinical research published in English in the field to date, to guide both researchers and clinicians about local drug delivery methods in the context of novel therapeutics.

Methods: A systematic search was conducted using customized strategies in Cochrane, pubmed and EMBASE databases from inception to 30/09/2018. Two researchers undertook study selection and data extraction independently.

Results: Our search returned 12,200 articles, of which 837 articles met the inclusion criteria. 679 were original research and 158 were reviews. There has been a steady increase in the numbers of publications related to inner ear therapeutics delivery over the last three decades, with a sharp rise over the last 2 years. The intra-tympanic route accounts for over 70% of published articles. Less than one third of published research directly assesses delivery efficacy, with most papers using clinical efficacy as a surrogate marker.

Conclusion: Research into local therapeutic delivery to the inner ear has undergone a recent surge, improving our understanding of how novel therapeutics can be delivered. Direct assessment of delivery efficacy is challenging, especially in humans, and progress in this area is key to understanding how to make decisions about delivery of novel hearing therapeutics.

Keywords: drug delivery, inner ear, novel therapeutics, systematic review, intratympanic, intracochlear

INTRODUCTION

Rationale

Recent advances in the understanding of the varied genetic and molecular etiologies of inner ear dysfunction have enabled the identification of multiple potential therapeutic targets (Müller and Barr-Gillespie, 2015; Mittal et al., 2017). This has accelerated the development of a range of novel therapeutics, from small molecule drugs to gene and cell therapies, several of which are starting to enter the clinical trial domain (Schilder et al., 2018)[1],[2]. Whilst significant progress has been achieved with regards to therapeutic identification and development, the most effective mechanisms of therapeutic delivery to the inner ear have yet to be determined. The importance of delivery cannot be understated; the success of any novel therapeutic depends on selection of the most suitable method for the pharmacokinetic profile of the individual agent, and the balance of risks associated with delivery against the potential benefit of the treatment (Salt and Plontke, 2009; Plontke and Salt, 2018).

The inner ear poses a unique pharmacokinetic and pharmacodynamic challenge due to its anatomical location, epithelial barriers and the relatively unstirred nature of the perilymph (Salt, 2002). Local delivery is an attractive option as it overcomes concerns regarding toxicity or side effects associated with systemic administration (Plontke et al., 2014; Salt and Plontke, 2018), allowing higher concentrations to reach the inner ear (Liu et al., 2018). It can be broadly divided into intra-tympanic or intra-cochlear routes, each with many options for delivery method and therapeutic formulation (Liu et al., 2018; Peppi et al., 2018; Salt and Plontke, 2018). Middle ear approaches, such as transtympanic injection, rely on simple diffusion through the epithelial barriers of the round and/or oval window (Salt and Plontke, 2018). This can lead to the formation of concentration gradients, with variable concentrations reaching more apical regions of cochlea, and potentially insufficient levels of the therapeutic reaching the basal regions (Salt et al., 2007; Liu et al., 2014; Li et al., 2018; Salt and Plontke, 2018). Delivery using sustained release formulations, magnetically targeted delivery, and nanoparticles (Pyykkö and Jing Zou, 2013; Shapiro et al., 2014; Pyykkö et al., 2016) aims to overcome these problems, but they remain a significant concern. Intra-cochlear therapeutic delivery offers the best control of delivery at the cost of the highest risk to hearing, although the problem of base-apex gradient formation remains (Hahn et al., 2012; Salt et al., 2017). Cochlear implant (CI) associated delivery presents a unique opportunity to develop this route for a subset of patients (Hochmair et al., 2006; Budenz et al., 2012; Roemer et al., 2016; Plontke et al., 2017).

At present there is a limited understanding of how delivery method, therapeutic agent and formulation, and disease process interact. This makes choosing a delivery method for a given therapeutic a major challenge faced by all involved in the development, production and administration of novel therapeutics, including discovery scientists, clinicians, industry, regulators, and patients. There is little to guide these stakeholders as to the best delivery method for a given therapeutic in a given patient group. A systematic review of the available literature is therefore necessary in order to collate and make accessible the currently available information.

Aims

The aims of this paper are to map all research undertaken so far in the field of local delivery of therapeutics to the inner ear, and to signpost to information to support decisions about delivery methods in the context of novel therapeutics.

Objectives

- To identify all relevant literature on local delivery of therapeutics to the inner ear.
- To understand the ways in which delivery methods are tested, and delivery efficacy assessed.
- To understand how the field of local therapeutic delivery to the inner ear has evolved, by exploring trends in publication type, experimental design, therapeutic classes and delivery methods.
- To identify which local delivery routes and methods have been tested in the pre-clinical and clinical research settings.
- To create searchable tables of the current literature on local delivery of therapeutics to the inner ear to signpost interested parties to the work that is most relevant to them.

METHODS

Study Design

A systematic review of the published scientific literature.

Systematic Review Protocol

The review protocol was registered with PROSPERO and is available from http://www.crd.york.ac.uk/PROSPERO/display_record.php?ID=CRD42018105903.

Search Strategy

The search strategy was designed using key words for inner ear therapeutic delivery and customized for each database (available in **Supplementary Material Section 1**) with assistance provided by the University College London Ear Institute & Action on Hearing Loss Libraries. No restriction was placed on study design. The search was restricted to English language articles.

TABLE 1 | Inclusion and exclusion criteria.

Inclusion criteria	Exclusion criteria
Any study design	Studies reporting only intra-uterine delivery to otocyst
Local delivery of therapeutic to inner ear target	Studies reporting only *in vitro* work
Intact inner ear architecture and anatomy	Studies reporting only explant culture delivery
	Mechanical models
	Computer generated data
	Letters to the editor/Editorials/Expert opinion without references
	Articles not in English

[1] *Safety, Tolerability and Efficacy for CGF166 in Patients With Unilateral or Bilateral Severe-to-profound Hearing Loss—Full Text View—ClinicalTrials.gov.* Available online at: https://clinicaltrials.gov/ct2/show/NCT02132130 (accessed July 20, 2018).

[2] *ISRCTN-ISRCTN59733689: A First-in-Human Study of the Safety and Efficacy of a New Drug, a Gamma Secretase Inhibitor, to Treat People With Sensorineural Hearing Loss.* Available online at: http://www.isrctn.com/ISRCTN59733689 (accessed December 23, 2018).

TABLE 2 | Categorization of extracted data in local therapeutic delivery to the inner ear.

Study design

Study type	Experimental model/review type	Assessment of delivery method	Disease model
Original research	Human, *in vivo*	Direct assessment via pharmaco-kinetics	Meniere's Disease
			Sudden sensorineural hearing loss
			Ototoxicity
		Indirect assessment via functional effects	CI-outcome improvement
	Human temporal bone		Autoimmune inner ear disease
			Genetic hearing loss
	Animal, *in vivo*		Tinnitus
		Assessing feasibility	Other
			Multiple
			None
Review	Meta-analysis		
	Systematic review		
	Narrative review		

Delivery

Route	Approach	Delivery method
Intra-tympanic	Non-surgical	Transtympanic injection
		Tympanostomy tube
	Surgical	Bullostomy (animals)
		Micropump or catheter
		Endoscope-assisted
		Stapes surgery*
Intra-cochlear/labyrinthine	Round or oval window	Injection
		Stapes surgery
		Micropump or catheter
		Cochlear implant
	Cochleostomy	Injection
		Micropump or catheter
		Cochlear implant
	Canalostomy	Injection
	Endolymphatic sac	
Other		Iontophoresis
		Post-auricular injection

Therapeutic category and formulation

Formulation	Agent delivered
Solutions and suspensions	Clinically used small molecules
Sustained release	Experimental small molecules
	Biopharmaceuticals
Nano-scale	
Viral vectors	Other
	Multiple
	None

**Stapedectomy, followed by placing therapy on oval window.*

Data Sources, Studies Sections, and Data Extraction

Pubmed, Embase and the Cochrane library were searched from inception to May 30th, 2017. The search was updated on September 30th 2018 and the results combined with the initial search.

Study Selection

Titles and abstracts were screened for inclusion independently by two review authors, with discrepancies resolved by full text review and discussion within the study team.

All studies and reviews of local delivery of therapeutics to the inner ear in human or animal models, where the architectural structure of the inner ear was maintained, were included. Studies that included only systemic therapeutic administration, data on *in vitro* experiments, animal explants, mechanical models and models utilizing computer-generated data were excluded. Inclusion and exclusion criteria are summarized in **Table 1**.

Data Extraction

Two authors carried out full text review and data extraction independently, with discrepancies resolved by discussion within the study team. During full text review, papers were identified as original research or review articles. Data extracted from review articles was limited to the type of review; narrative, systematic, or systematic with meta-analysis. Data extracted from original research articles was year of publication, experimental model (animal or human, living or temporal bone), method of assessment of efficacy of delivery, delivery method(s), therapeutic agent, therapeutic formulation, and underlying disorder targeted or treated.

Data Categorization

Extracted data was grouped as shown in **Table 2**.

Categorization of the method of assessment of delivery efficacy was designed to aid understanding of how research is designed. Studies directly investigating the efficacy of delivery (e.g., by concentration in perilymph, or presence or absence of a delivered substance in the target tissue) were classified as "direct assessment of delivery efficacy via pharmacokinetics." Studies investigating the functional, toxic or clinical effects of a therapeutic agent delivered to the inner ear were classified as "indirect assessment of delivery efficacy via functional effects" (as an indirect marker of delivery method efficacy). Studies

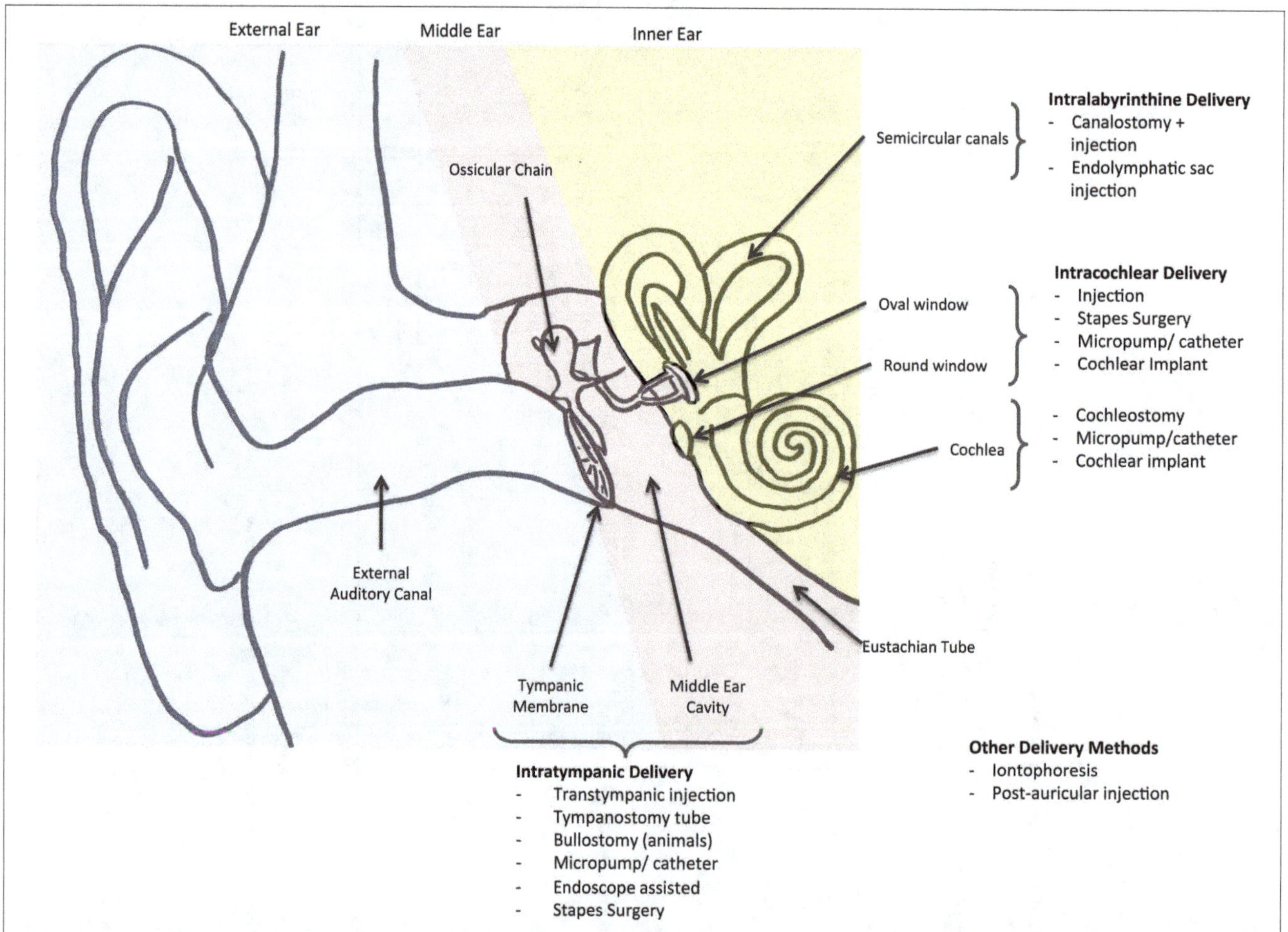

FIGURE 1 | Schematic figure summarizing the structure of the inner ear and delivery routes.

focusing on the practicalities and/or adverse effects of a proposed delivery method or therapeutic formulation, without measuring the efficacy of delivery, were classified as "assessing feasibility."

Delivery methods were categorized by route, approach, and method, as shown in **Table 2,** and in schematic form in **Figure 1**.

Formulation was defined as the combination of therapeutic and any other substance that affects the pharmacokinetic profile of that therapeutic (Kulkarni and Shaw, 2016). They were categorized as solutions and suspensions, sustained release formulations, nano-scale formulations and viral vectors (Fukui and Raphael, 2013; Kulkarni and Shaw, 2016; Pyykkö et al., 2016; Kim, 2017; Liu et al., 2018). These categories are defined with examples in **Table 3**. Therapeutics were categorized as clinically used small molecules, experimental small molecules, biopharmaceuticals, other, multiple, and none, as defined in **Table 4** (Nakagawa and Ito, 2005; Budenz et al., 2012; Fukui and Raphael, 2013; Liu, 2014)[3].

This categorization was designed to allow combinations of delivery methods, therapeutic agents and formulations to be considered together. For example, a study evaluating transtympanic injection of a liquid form drug and a study evaluating transtympanic injection of a gel containing nanoparticles containing the same drug would both be classed broadly as intra-tympanic injections, but would be differentiated in the formulation category to allow for the fact that this may alter delivery efficacy.

Data Analysis

Data was managed in Microsoft Excel and analyzed in R. The annual number of publications in the field was counted as a whole and for each subcategory. Total numbers of publications across each subcategory were counted and displayed as both a total number and a list of references for those publications.

RESULTS

Search Results

Combining the searches from May 30th, 2017 and September 30th 2018 yielded a total of 12,201 records. Removing duplicates left 6,468 unique entries. Title and abstract screening excluded 5,600 articles, with a further 31 excluded during full text screening, leaving a total of 837 papers included in this review (**Figure 2**).

Numbers of Publications

Of the 837 papers, 679 were original research papers and 158 were reviews. Review papers were primarily narrative reviews (131/158, 82.9%). Systematic reviews accounted for 18 papers, and meta-analysis for 9 papers (**Table 5**). Of the original research papers, 315 (46.4%) studied humans and 364 (53.6%) studied animals.

Eight studies (1.2%) directly assessed delivery efficacy via pharmacokinetics to the live human inner ear, with a further three directly assessing delivery efficacy in human temporal bones. Animal experimental models were used in 177 (26.0%) papers to directly assess delivery efficacy via pharmacokinetics. The majority of papers used functional effects as an indirect marker of delivery efficacy; 296 (43.6%) studies in humans and 158 (23.2%) in animals. Feasibility of delivery methods, without assessment of delivery efficacy, was assessed in 8 (1.2%) human studies and 29 (4.3%) animal studies.

TABLE 3 | Categorization of formulations used in therapeutic delivery to the inner ear with definitions and examples.

Formulation category	Definition	Examples
Solutions and suspensions	Soluble therapeutic agent dissolved in solvent or a less soluble agent suspended as particles in the solvent (Kulkarni and Shaw, 2016)	Dexamethasone suspension in 0.9% saline; dexamethasone-phosphate solution in saline
Sustained release formulations	Combination of therapeutic with any substance designed to prolong the exposure of the therapeutic agent to the inner ear (Liu et al., 2013)	Hydrogels, polymers, poloxamers, gelfoam microwick®
Nano-scale formulations	Particles 1–100 nm in size in at least one dimension (Pyykkö et al., 2016). Includes nano-scale formulations placed in a sustained release formulation	Nanoparticles, magnetic nanoparticles, liposomes, polymersomes
Viral vectors	Viruses used to deliver normal genes into cells, in place of missing or faulty genes (Fukui and Raphael, 2013)	Adeno-associated virus (AAV), adenovirus

The most common disease studied was Meniere's disease (or endolymphatic hydrops) with 164 (24.2%) original research papers looking at local therapeutic delivery in this context. Next was idiopathic sudden sensorineural hearing loss (ISSNHL) in 98 (14.4%) studies, followed by ototoxicity with 87 (12.8%) studies.

Four hundred and eighty two (70.9%) original studies investigated intra-tympanic delivery methods, 175 (25.7%) intra-cochlear delivery methods, 19 (2.8%) a combination of the two, and 3 (0.4%) other delivery methods.

Solution and suspension formulations were used in 472 (69.5%) papers, sustained release formulations for 99 (14.6%), nanoscale in 41 (6.0%), and viral vectors in 50 (7.4%). Seventeen papers studied other or multiple formulations.

Clinically used small molecules were studied in 340 (50.1%) publications, experimental small molecules in 106 (15.6%), and biopharmaceuticals in 143 (21.1%). Fifty papers studied combinations or empty formulations.

Trends in Publications

The annual number of publications in the field of local therapeutic delivery to the inner ear has increased steadily over the last three decades, with a sharp increase over the last 5 years (**Figure 3A**). Of the 679 original research articles 226 have been published in the last 5 years. Remarkably, there have been 56 reviews published in the last 5 years.

[3]*Documentation and Sources-DrugBank*. Available online at: https://www.drugbank.ca/documentation#drug-cards (accessed January 26, 2019).

TABLE 4 | Categorization of therapeutics locally delivered to the inner ear with definitions.

Therapeutic category	Subcategory	Class	Definition
Clinically used small molecules		Corticosteroids Aminoglycosides	Low molecular weight drugs (900 daltons), produced by chemical synthesis and delivered to the inner ear in clinical practice[3]
Experimental small molecules	Therapeutic agents	Local anesthetics Bisphosphonates Antioxidants Antivirals Apoptosis inhibitors NMDA receptor antagonists	Low molecular weight drugs (900 daltons), produced by chemical synthesis and ***not*** delivered to the inner ear in clinical practice[3]
	Toxic agents		Low molecular weight drugs (900 daltons), produced by chemical synthesis[3]. Designed to impair inner ear function thus allowing assessment of delivery
	Contrast media, dyes and fluorescently tagged molecules		Low molecular weight drugs (900 daltons), produced by chemical synthesis[3]. Used for assessment of delivery rather than for therapeutic benefit
Biopharmaceuticals	Protein based therapies	Neurotrophins	Proteins with a biological origin that induce the survival, development and function of neurons[3]
		Monoclonal antibodies	Laboratory produced antibodies, with a biological origin, designed to recognize and bind specific receptors (Liu, 2014)
	Gene correction therapies		Therapies with a biological origin that deliver normal genes into cells, in place of missing or faulty genes (Fukui and Raphael, 2013)
	Cell therapies		Cell transplantation to the inner ear for either regeneration or drug delivery (Nakagawa and Ito, 2005)
Other			
Multiple			Studies using combinations of above classes
None			Empty vehicle delivery, or feasibility studies

Trends in experimental design are seen in **Figure 3B.** There has been a sharp increase in the number of animal studies published, while human studies have increased more gradually. The early human work indirectly assessing delivery via functional effects relates almost exclusively to transtympanic injections of corticosteroids and aminoglycosides. Direct assessment of delivery methods via pharmacokinetics accounts for around half of animal studies year on year.

Trends in delivery routes are seen in **Figure 3C.** Transtympanic delivery methods outnumber intracochlear methods year on year.

The trend in category of therapeutic administered is shown in **Figure 3D**. Clinically used small molecules (corticosteroids and aminoglycosides) account for the majority of publications each year, the majority of which are case series. The number of papers delivering experimental small molecules and biopharmaceuticals has increased steadily, reflecting development in the field.

Delivery Methods

The delivery methods used in original research papers identified by this study are seen in **Table 6,** with numbers of publications organized by therapeutic formulation and experimental model. An identical table is found in **Supplementary Material** giving the reference numbers of papers referred to within each cell of the table (**Supplementary Table 1**).

Reference Tables

Cross-referenced tables have been formed to allow identification of papers looking at any combination of delivery method, therapeutic class/formulation, and disease model. Reviews are tabulated separately. All are available in **Supplementary Material.**

DISCUSSION

Summary of Main Findings

In this review we provide a comprehensive overview of all research activity in the field of local therapeutic delivery to the inner ear, and show how this activity has increased over the last two decades. Though our categorization systems, we reveal how delivery methods are developed and assessed, and our cross referenced tables highlight the complexity in the way that delivery methods combine with formulations and therapeutic agents.

Categorization of the studies by method of assessment of delivery has exposed for the first time a relative lack of research into direct delivery efficacy, especially in humans, with most studies looking at clinical efficacy. Direct assessment of delivery efficacy is critical to understanding how to deliver therapeutics. Without this understanding, it becomes impossible to tell if an absence of a clinical effect is due to therapeutic failure or delivery failure, which has significant implications for both pre-clinical

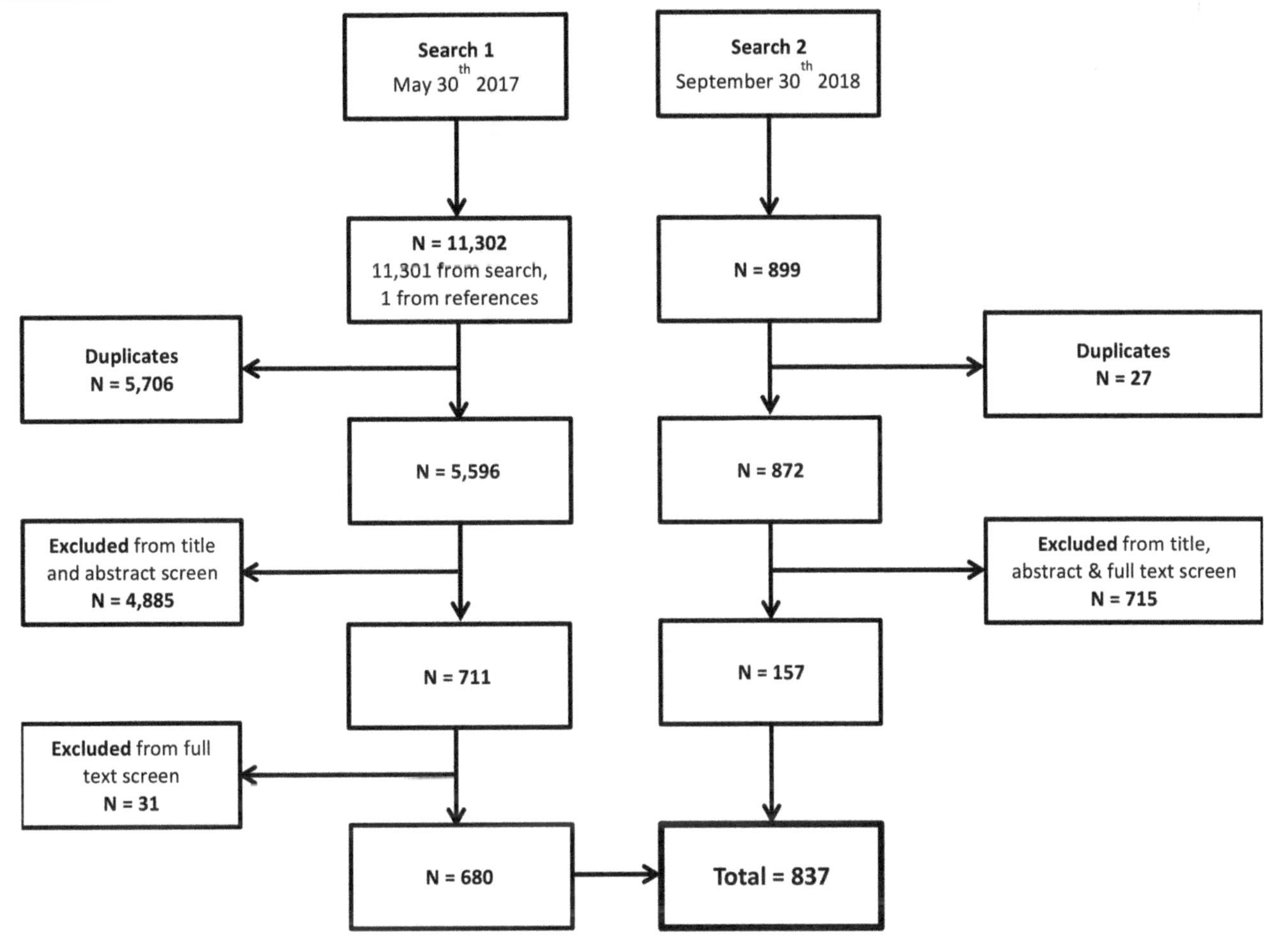

FIGURE 2 | Flow diagram of search results.

TABLE 5 | Study design and assessment of delivery method.

Study type	Assessment of delivery method	Human	Animal	Both	Total
Original research	Direct assessment	11	177	0	188
	Indirect assessment	296	158	0	454
	Feasibility	8	29	0	37
	Total	315	364	0	679
Meta-analysis		9	0	0	9
Systematic review		18	0	0	18
Narrative review		35	29	68	132

work and trials of novel therapeutics. Given the difficulties in assessing delivery directly in humans (found in this review to be limited to imaging of compounds with a contrast effect, or tissue/perilymph sampling alongside operative management of a pathological ear), more work is needed into understanding how the animal work in this area translates to humans. Computer modeling has potential to assist with this but at present is limited to interpretation of experimental data (Salt, 2002).

Original research outputs have increased steeply over the last decade, reflecting increased interest and funding into hearing. Animal models have been used in over half of the original research studies included in this systematic review, with a growing trend. This reflects the increasing number of novel therapeutics in pre-clinical development, and to some extent, the challenges of locally delivering therapeutics in humans. Whilst animal models play a vital role in the development of delivery

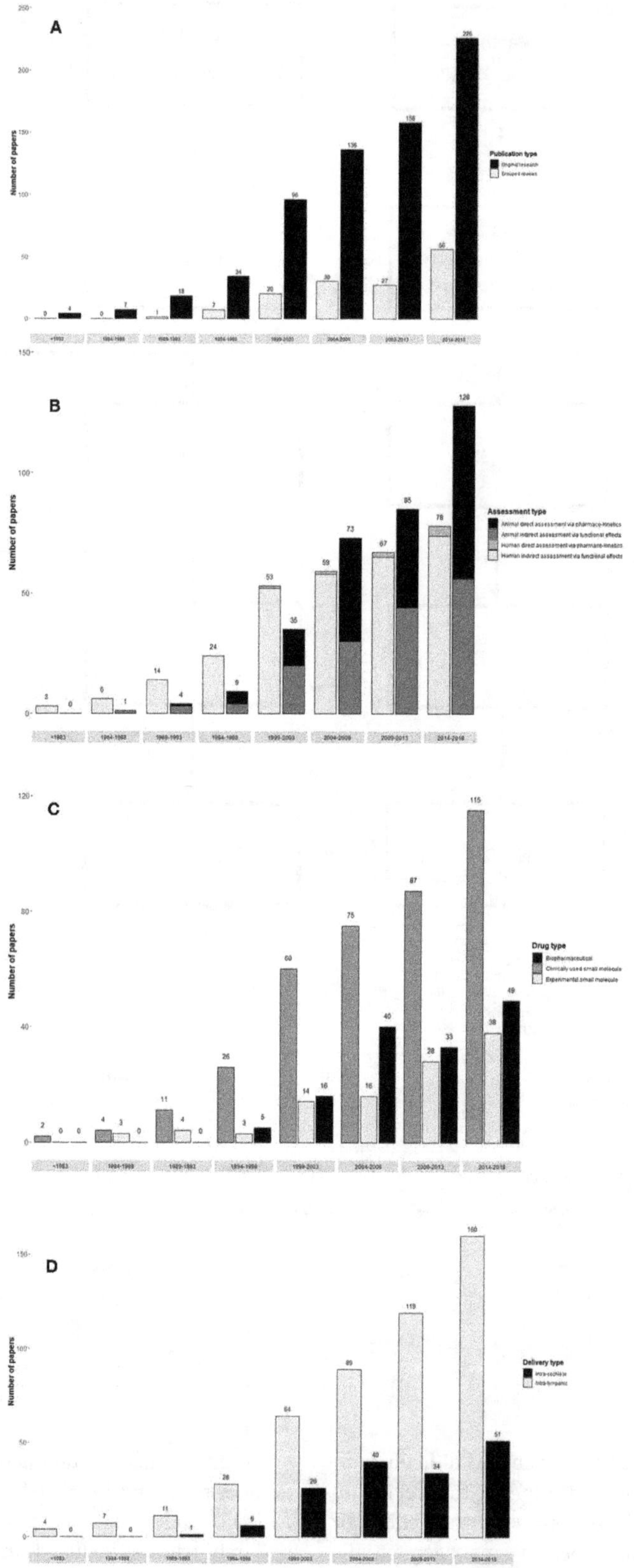

FIGURE 3 | Trends in publication of studies on local delivery to the inner ear. **(A)** Publications per 5 years by study type (original research or review). **(B)** Original research publications of per 5 years by method of assessment of delivery efficacy (direct assessment via pharmacokinetics or indirect assessment via functional

(Continued)

FIGURE 3 | effects, excluding feasibility studies where delivery efficacy is not assessed). **(C)** Original research publications per 5 years by intratympanic and intracochlea delivery routes in both humans and animals (excluding "other" delivery routes). **(D)** Original research publications per 5 years by therapeutic class (clinically used small molecule, experimental small molecule, or biopharmaceutical) in both humans and animals. [n.b. **(A–D)** runs from top to bottom of figure panel].

TABLE 6 | Total numbers of original studies for each delivery method arranged by formulation, in humans (living and temporal bone models), and animals.

Delivery			Formulation									Total
Route	**Approach**	**Delivery method**	**Solution**		**Sustained release**		**Nano-scale**		**Viral vector**		**Other/multiple**	
			Human	**Animal**	**Human**	**Animal**	**Human**	**Animal**	**Human**	**Animal**		
Intra-tympanic	Non-surgical	Transtympanic Injection	203	63	7	14	–	10	–	–	2	299
		Tympanostomy Tube	6	–	11	–	–	–	–	–	–	17
	Surgical	Bullostomy (animal only)	–	1	–	2	–	2	–	–	–	5
		Micropump or catheter	27	7	–	–	–	2	–	–	2	38
		Endoscope-assisted	–	–	–	–	–	–	–	–	–	0
		Stapes surgery	–	1	–	2	–	–	–	–	–	3
	Other		2	15	10	30	1	16	–	–	4	78
	Multiple		27	4	4	1	–	1	–	–	5	42
Intra-cochlear/labyrinthine	Round or oval window	Injection	1	17	–	1	–	1	–	26	–	46
		Stapes surgery	–	–	–	–	–	–	–	–	–	0
		Micropump or catheter	–	32	–	–	–	–	–	–	–	32
		Cochlear implant	–	2	–	7	–	–	–	–	–	9
	Cochleostomy	Injection	–	20	–	3	–	2	–	15	–	40
		Micropump or catheter	–	14	–	1	–	1	–	1	–	17
		Cochlear implant	–	–	–	1	–	–	–	–	–	1
	Canalostomy	Injection	5	4	–	–	–	–	–	8	–	17
	Endolymphatic sac	Injection	–	–	–	–	–	–	–	–	–	0
	Other		–	–	–	1	–	–	–	–	–	1
	Multiple		4	8	–	–	–	–	–	–	–	12
Other		Iontophoresis	1	1	–	–	–	–	–	–	–	2
		Post-auricular injection	1	–	–	–	–	–	–	–	–	1
Combination				6	–	4	–	5	–	–	4	19

This table is mirrored by ***Supplementary Table 1****, in which cells contain reference numbers of each study in place of total numbers.*

methods, and the testing of novel inner ear therapeutics (Frisina et al., 2018), their applicability to humans is unclear (Denayer et al., 2014; Le Prell et al., 2016; Frisina et al., 2018). There remain significant challenges in translating from animals to humans due to differences in anatomy (thinner bone overlying cochlea; Mikulec et al., 2009), size (smaller cochlea allows greater diffusion; Salt, 2008), and disease models (ISSNHL difficult to replicate).

There is a significant body of literature on aminoglycosides and steroids as intra-tympanic treatments for Meniere's disease and ISSNHL, respectively. Whilst this is expected for treatments in clinical use, the large number of papers that continue to be published investigating the efficacy of these drugs suggests that either published information is not of high enough quality to draw conclusions, or is not being disseminated widely enough. In either case, it emphasizes the need for appropriately powered studies with accessible results as novel therapeutics move to trials and beyond.

This review has gone beyond previous systematic reviews in the field, which have focused on assessing the efficacy of single delivery techniques and therapeutic agents in humans. Here we have mapped the large number of delivery methods available, which have been tested with a range of therapeutic agents and formulations, in order to signpost readers from different backgrounds to the information most relevant to them. Intra-tympanic delivery routes dominate the field. This in large part reflects clinical acceptance of intra-tympanic injections resulting from the work described above. Furthermore, small molecules account for the majority of therapeutics delivered locally to the inner ear (447/680, 65.7%), and these agents are mostly suitable for intra-tympanic administration. Intra-cochlear delivery, whilst currently almost essential for cell and gene based therapeutic modalities, carries much higher risks, and has only recently started to be tested in humans (Nakagawa and Ito, 2005)[1]. The observed imbalance in research across these delivery routes therefore indicates how the field has developed, and is developing, rather than representing a gap in research into intra-cochlear delivery methods.

Limitations

Some limitations of this study merit discussion. Firstly, we did not set out to extract data on the methodological quality, or to extract and meta-analyze results of individual publications. We did not therefore aim to make recommendations on which delivery method should be used for a given experimental model, therapeutic, or disease, although we do enable studies containing this information to be identified.

Secondly, we did not include gray literature in this paper. In a fast moving field, this inevitably means we have not captured ongoing, or very recently completed studies.

Finally, the extraction of data about delivery method and formulation is highly complex, with multiple sub-categories required (e.g., intra-tympanic injection, through tympanostomy tube, of hydrogel) to ensure the exact nature of a delivery method was captured. This opens the possibility of misclassification, which we mitigated by ensuring two authors extracted all data independently, and that any discrepancies or difficult classifications were discussed within the review team.

CONCLUSIONS

Research into local therapeutic delivery to the inner ear has undergone a recent surge, improving our understanding of how novel therapeutics can be delivered. The way in which a therapeutic should be delivered, however, remains somewhat elusive, limited by the difficulty in directly researching the efficacy of delivery to the human inner ear.

The majority of research so far focuses on clinical efficacy of administered therapies. Our knowledge about the efficacy of delivery methods in humans remains limited, and this has the potential to limit how we assess the effectiveness of novel therapeutics.

As the field of inner ear therapeutics develops, it is crucial that research into delivery methods considers both the relationships between therapeutic agent, formulation, delivery method and disease, and the translational challenges that exist when moving from animal to human work. Collaboration between lab scientists, computer scientists, clinicians, industry, and patients will be key to overcoming these challenges, and tailoring delivery methods to novel therapeutics to maximize the chances of success in clinical trials.

AUTHOR CONTRIBUTIONS

CA, CX, HB, and AS designed the study. CX ran the systematic searches. CA, CX, MS, MG, and HB determined study inclusion/exclusion and extracted data. CA, CX, and MS performed data analysis. CA, CX, MS, MG, HB, and AS wrote the manuscript.

REFERENCES

Budenz, C. L., Pfingst, B. E., and Raphael, Y. (2012). The use of neurotrophin therapy in the inner ear to augment cochlear implantation outcomes. *Anat. Rec.* 295, 1896–1908. doi: 10.1002/ar.22586

Denayer, T., Stöhr, T., and Van Roy, M. (2014). Animal models in translational medicine: validation and prediction. *New Horiz. Transl. Med.* 2, 5–11. doi: 10.1016/j.nhtm.2014.08.001

Frisina, R. D., Budzevich, M., Zhu, X., Martinez, G. V., Walton, J. P., and Borkholder, D. A. (2018). Animal model studies yield translational solutions for cochlear drug delivery. *Hear. Res.* 368, 67–74. doi: 10.1016/j.heares.2018.05.002

Fukui, H., and Raphael, Y. (2013). Gene therapy for the inner ear. *Hear. Res.* 297, 99–105. doi: 10.1016/j.heares.2012.11.017

Hahn, H., Salt, A. N., Biegner, T., Kammerer, B., Delabar, U., Hartsock, J. J., et al. (2012). Dexamethasone levels and base-to-apex concentration gradients in the scala tympani perilymph after intracochlear delivery in the guinea pig. *Otol. Neurotol.* 33, 660–665. doi: 10.1097/MAO.0b013e318254501b

Hochmair, I., Nopp, P., Jolly, C., Schmidt, M., Schößer, H., Garnham, C., et al. (2006). MED-EL cochlear implants: state of the art and a glimpse into the future. *Trends Amplif.* 10, 201–219. doi: 10.1177/1084713806296720

Kim, D.-K. (2017). Nanomedicine for inner ear diseases: a review of recent *in vivo* studies. *Biomed. Res. Int.* 2017:3098230. doi: 10.1155/2017/3098230

Kulkarni, V. S., and Shaw, C. (2016). "Chapter 1-Introduction," in *Essential Chemistry for Formulators of Semisolid and Liquid Dosages*, eds V. S. Kulkarni and C. Shaw (Boston, MA: Academic Press), 1–4. Available online at: http://www.sciencedirect.com/science/article/pii/B9780128010242000017 (accessed January 22, 2019).

Le Prell, C. G., Fulbright, A., Spankovich, C., Griffiths, S. K., Lobarinas, E., Campbell, K. C., et al. (2016). Dietary supplement comprised of β-carotene, vitamin C, vitamin E, and magnesium: failure to prevent music-induced temporary threshold shift. *Audiol. Neurotol. Extra* 6, 20–39. doi: 10.1159/000446600

Li, W., Hartsock, J. J., Dai, C., and Salt, A. N. (2018). Permeation enhancers for intratympanically-applied drugs studied using fluorescent dexamethasone as a marker. *Otol. Neurotol.* 39, 639–647. doi: 10.1097/MAO.0000000000001786

Liu, H., Feng, L., Tolia, G., Liddell, M. R., Hao, J., and Li, S. K. (2014). Evaluation of intratympanic formulations for inner ear delivery: methodology and sustained release formulation testing. *Drug Dev. Ind. Pharm.* 40, 896–903. doi: 10.3109/03639045.2013.789054

Liu, H., Hao, J., and Li, K. S. (2013). Current strategies for drug delivery to the inner ear. *Acta Pharm. Sinica B* 3, 86–96. doi: 10.1016/j.apsb.2013.02.003

Liu, J. K. H. (2014). The history of monoclonal antibody development – Progress, remaining challenges and future innovations. *Ann. Med. Surg.* 3, 113–116. doi: 10.1016/j.amsu.2014.09.001

Liu, X., Li, M., Smyth, H., and Zhang, F. (2018). Otic drug delivery systems: formulation principles and recent developments. *Drug Dev. Ind. Pharm.* 44, 1395–1408. doi: 10.1080/03639045.2018.1464022

Mikulec, A. A., Plontke, S. K., Hartsock, J. J., and Salt, A. N. (2009). Entry of substances into perilymph through the bone of the otic capsule after intratympanic applications in guinea pigs: implications for local drug delivery in humans. *Otol. Neurotol.* 30, 131–138. doi: 10.1097/MAO.0b013e318191bff8

Mittal, R., Nguyen, D., Patel, A. P., Debs, L. H., Mittal, J., Yan, D., et al. (2017). Recent advancements in the regeneration of auditory hair cells and hearing restoration. *Front. Mol. Neurosci.* 10:236. doi: 10.3389/fnmol.2017.00236

Müller, U., and Barr Gillespie, P. G. (2015). New treatment options for hearing loss. *Nat. Rev. Drug Discov.* 14, 346–365. doi: 10.1038/nrd4533

Nakagawa, T., and Ito, J. (2005). Cell therapy for inner ear diseases. *Curr. Pharm. Des.* 11, 1203–1207. doi: 10.2174/1381612053507530

Peppi, M., Marie, A., Belline, C., and Borenstein, J. T. (2018). Intracochlear drug delivery systems: a novel approach whose time has come. *Expert Opin. Drug Deliv.* 15, 319–324. doi: 10.1080/17425247.2018.1444026

Plontke, S. K., Glien, A., Rahne, T., Mäder, K., and Salt, A. N. (2014). Controlled release dexamethasone implants in the round window niche for salvage treatment of idiopathic sudden sensorineural hearing loss. *Otol. Neurotol.* 35, 1168–1171. doi: 10.1097/MAO.0000000000000434

Plontke, S. K., Götze, G., Rahne, T., and Liebau, A. (2017). Intracochlear drug delivery in combination with cochlear implants. *HNO* 65(suppl. 1), 19–28. doi: 10.1007/s00106-016-0285-9

Plontke, S. K., and Salt, A. N. (2018). Local drug delivery to the inner ear: principles, practice, and future challenges. *Hear. Res.* 368, 1–2. doi: 10.1016/j.heares.2018.06.018

Pyykkö, I., and Jing Zou, Y. Z. (2013). Nanoparticle based inner ear therapy. *World J. Otorhinolaryngol.* 3, 114–133. doi: 10.5319/wjo.v3.i4.114

Pyykkö, I., Zou, J., Schrott-Fischer, A., Glueckert, R., and Kinnunen, P. (2016). "An overview of nanoparticle based delivery for treatment of inner ear disorders," in *Auditory and Vestibular Research: Methods and Protocols (Methods in Molecular Biology)*, ed B. Sokolowski (New York, NY: Springer New York), 363–415.

Roemer, A., Köhl, U., Majdani, O., Klöß, S., Falk, C., Haumann, S., et al. (2016). Biohybrid cochlear implants in human neurosensory restoration. *Stem Cell Res. Ther.* 7:148. doi: 10.1186/s13287-016-0408-y

Salt, A., Hartsock, J., Gill, R., Smyth, D., Kirk, J., and Verhoeven, K. (2017). Perilymph pharmacokinetics of marker applied through a cochlear implant in guinea pigs. *PLoS ONE* 12:e0183374. doi: 10.1371/journal.pone.0183374

Salt, A. N. (2002). "Simulation of methods for drug delivery to the cochlear fluids," in *Advances in Oto-Rhino-Laryngology*, eds D. Felix and E. Oestreicher (Basel: KARGER), 140–148. Available online at: https://www.karger.com/Article/FullText/59251 (accessed July 20, 2018).

Salt, A. N. (2008). Dexamethasone concentration gradients along scala tympani after application to the round window membrane. *Otol. Neurotol.* 29, 401–406. doi: 10.1097/MAO.0b013e318161aaae

Salt, A. N., and Plontke, S. K. (2009). Principles of local drug delivery to the inner ear. *Audiol. Neurootol.* 14, 350–360. doi: 10.1159/000241892

Salt, A. N., and Plontke, S. K. (2018). Pharmacokinetic principles in the inner ear: influence of drug properties on intratympanic applications. *Hear. Res.* 368, 28–40. doi: 10.1016/j.heares.2018.03.002

Salt, A. N., Sirjani, D. B., Hartsock, J. J., Gill, R. M., and Plontke, S. K. (2007). Marker retention in the cochlea following injections through the round window membrane. *Hear. Res.* 232:78–86. doi: 10.1016/j.heares.2007.06.010

Schilder, A. G. M., Blackshaw, H., Lenarz, T., Warnecke, A., Lustig, L. R., and Staecker, H. (2018). Biological therapies of the inner ear: what otologists need to consider. *Otol. Neurotol.* 39, 135–137. doi: 10.1097/MAO.0000000000001689

Shapiro, B., Kulkarni, S., Nacev, A., Sarwar, A., Preciado, D., and Depireux, D. A. (2014). Shaping magnetic fields to direct therapy to ears and eyes. *Annu. Rev. Biomed. Eng.* 16, 455–481. doi: 10.1146/annurev-bioeng-071813-105206

18

Stem Cell Based Drug Delivery for Protection of Auditory Neurons in a Guinea Pig Model of Cochlear Implantation

Verena Scheper[1,2,3], Andrea Hoffmann[3,4], Michael M. Gepp[5,6], André Schulz[5], Anika Hamm[3,4], Christoph Pannier[1], Peter Hubka[3,7], Thomas Lenarz[1,2,3] and Jana Schwieger[1,3]*

[1] Department of Otolaryngology, Hannover Medical School, Hanover, Germany, [2] Cluster of Excellence 'Hearing4all', German Research Foundation, Bonn, Germany, [3] Lower Saxony Centre for Biomedical Engineering, Implant Research and Development (NIFE), Hanover, Germany, [4] Department of Orthopaedic Surgery, Hannover Medical School, Hanover, Germany, [5] Fraunhofer Institute for Biomedical Engineering IBMT, Sulzbach, Germany, [6] Fraunhofer Project Center for Stem Cell Process Engineering, Würzburg, Germany, [7] Department of Experimental Otology, Hannover Medical School, Hanover, Germany

Correspondence:
Verena Scheper
scheper.verena@mh-hannover.de

Background: The success of a cochlear implant (CI), which is the standard therapy for patients suffering from severe to profound sensorineural hearing loss, depends on the number and excitability of spiral ganglion neurons (SGNs). Brain-derived neurotrophic factor (BDNF) has a protective effect on SGNs but should be applied chronically to guarantee their lifelong survival. Long-term administration of BDNF could be achieved using genetically modified mesenchymal stem cells (MSCs), but these cells should be protected – by ultra-high viscous (UHV-) alginate ('alginate-MSCs') – from the recipient immune system and from uncontrolled migration.

Methods: Brain-derived neurotrophic factor-producing MSCs were encapsulated in UHV-alginate. Four experimental groups were investigated using guinea pigs as an animal model. Three of them were systemically deafened and (unilaterally) received one of the following: (I) a CI; (II) an alginate-MSC-coated CI; (III) an injection of alginate-embedded MSCs into the scala tympani followed by CI insertion and alginate polymerization. Group IV was normal hearing, with CI insertion in both ears and a unilateral injection of alginate-MSCs. Using acoustically evoked auditory brainstem response measurements, hearing thresholds were determined before implantation and before sacrificing the animals. Electrode impedance was measured weekly. Four weeks after implantation, the animals were sacrificed and the SGN density and degree of fibrosis were evaluated.

Results: The MSCs survived being implanted for 4 weeks *in vivo*. Neither the alginate-MSC injection nor the coating affected electrode impedance or fibrosis. CI insertion with and without previous alginate injection in normal-hearing animals resulted in increased hearing thresholds within the high-frequency range. Low-frequency hearing loss was additionally observed in the alginate-injected and implanted cochleae, but not in those treated only with a CI. In deafened animals, the alginate-MSC coating of the CI significantly prevented SGN from degeneration, but the injection of alginate-MSCs did not.

Conclusion: Brain-derived neurotrophic factor-producing MSCs encapsulated in UHV-alginate prevent SGNs from degeneration in the form of coating on the CI surface, but not in the form of an injection. No increase in fibrosis or impedance was detected. Further research and development aimed at verifying long-term mechanical and biological properties of coated electrodes *in vitro* and *in vivo*, in combination with chronic electrical stimulation, is needed before the current concept can be tested in clinical trials.

Keywords: spiral ganglion neuron, functionalized cochlear implant, biological functionalization, hydrogel, encapsulation, coating, injection, genetically modified cells

INTRODUCTION

The cochlear implant (CI) is the standard treatment for unilateral and bilateral severe to profound sensorineural hearing loss, both in adults and children. More than 350,000 deaf individuals have already received cochlear implantations worldwide (NIDCD, 2017). In this device, acoustic signals are detected by a microphone, converted into electrical signals and transmitted transcutaneously to an implanted receiver. The signal is decoded and delivered via an electrode array implanted into the scala tympani of the cochlea to the auditory nerve. The entire frequency range of the acoustic signal is split into different frequency bands and allocated to the different contacts, mimicking the physiological tonotopic organization of the cochlea (Lenarz and Scheper, 2015).

The loss of hair cells associated with deafness is followed by retraction of the peripheral nerve fibers in both the animal model (Zilberstein et al., 2012) and in humans (Liu et al., 2015; Whitlon, 2017), and then by degeneration of spiral ganglion neuron (SGN) cell bodies (Liu et al., 2015). This secondary degeneration is highly dependent on the cause of hearing loss and the cochlear structures affected. However, the number of SGNs is crucial for the success of cochlear implantation (Seyyedi et al., 2014). Thus, the prevention of progressive SGN degeneration is a major goal of CI research. The electrical stimulation of SGNs by the CI may (*per se*) reduce the degeneration of SGNs via depolarization-induced neurotrophic signaling pathways (Hansen et al., 2001; Scheper et al., 2009; Leake et al., 2013). The extent to which electrical stimulation alone is able to protect SGNs from degeneration *in vivo* (Li et al., 1999; Agterberg et al., 2010) is unknown, as is the dependence of the protective mechanism of electrical stimulation on various factors such as the onset and duration or stimulation parameters used (Araki et al., 1998; Leake et al., 1999).

In addition to electrical stimulation via the CI, neuroprotective effects on SGNs have also been demonstrated for the application of exogenous neurotrophic factors both *in vitro* (Hegarty et al., 1997) and *in vivo* (Scheper et al., 2009; Leake et al., 2011). The neuroprotective effect of neurotrophic factors persists a few weeks after cessation of neurotrophic treatment (Maruyama et al., 2008; Agterberg et al., 2009). However, neurotrophic therapies may require ongoing administration if a lifelong survival effect is to be achieved in human patients (Gillespie et al., 2003; Gillespie and Shepherd, 2005). Various systems delivering neurotrophins and other drugs locally to the inner ear are under investigation (El Kechai et al., 2015; Nguyen et al., 2017; Mäder et al., 2018; Hao and Li, 2019). For human use, however, most approaches – if intended for continuous application – are not practicable due to the fact that the application has to be repeated [single injection via needle or catheter-based (Prenzler et al., 2018)], or the device or matrix has to be refilled periodically [osmotic pumps (Brown et al., 1993), or intratympanic hydrogels applied to the round window (Wang et al., 2011)].

Cell-based drug delivery is an alternative approach to chronically treating inner ear neurons. Inoculation of the inner ear with appropriate viral vectors, in order to transduce cochlea cells to over-express a desired neurotrophic factor (Geschwind et al., 1996; Kanzaki et al., 2002), allows long-term stable application without a permanent opening of the cochlea. However, there are several safety concerns (David and Doherty, 2017), such as control of neurotrophic factor dosage, choice of transfection site/volume and, where appropriate, options for preventing expression of factors after transduction (Sacheli et al., 2013).

Another approach to supplying inner ear neurons with cell-based neurotrophic factor is the implantation of autologous, allogenic, or xenogenic cells. Implanted cells can either be genetically engineered to overexpress a desired protein or (*per se*) to produce factors at a neuroprotective concentration. Fibroblasts induced to produce brain-derived neurotrophic factor (BDNF), a neurotrophin, have been shown to protect SGNs from degeneration in guinea pigs (Warnecke et al., 2012; Gillespie et al., 2015). However, implanted cells need to be entrapped into a matrix to avoid uncontrolled migration and to shield them from the host's immune system (Warnecke et al., 2012). Gillespie et al. (2015) solved this problem by encapsulating fibroblasts into a non-biodegradable, biocompatible alginate matrix (Immupel^{TM}, Living Cell Technologies Limited). The same hydrogel was used to encapsulate Schwann cells genetically modified to overexpress the neurotrophins BDNF or neurotrophin 3 (NT-3). These entrapped cells supported SGN survival in an *in vitro* model of deafness (Pettingill et al., 2008) and, in the case of the BDNF-producing Schwann cells, protected SGNs in a guinea pig model (Pettingill et al., 2011).

Choroid plexus cells that natively produce neuroprotective factors to protect inner ear neurons were implanted in deafened cats using unspecified alginate capsules (Skinner et al., 2009; Wise et al., 2011). The encapsulated choroid plexus cells were harvested from pigs and produced a cocktail of various neurotrophic factors including GDNF, BDNF, and VEGF (Skinner et al., 2009). These cells did not protect neurons from degeneration in the animal model used. Combined with electrical stimulation by the CI, however, capsule implantation resulted in improved neuronal survival (Wise et al., 2011). In general, microspheres have the disadvantage that they cannot be easily explanted and replaced, which – considering the timescale of lifelong implantation – is likely to be necessary in human CI users. This constraint can be overcome with cells encapsulated in explantable matrixes such as hollow-fiber membrane capsules equipped with a tether for removal. While these devices have already been successfully used in deafened guinea pigs for SGN protection (Fransson et al., 2018), they induced an increase in foreign-body reaction in deafened cats (Konerding et al., 2017). An alternative approach to the implanting of cells for chronic drug delivery to the inner ear neurons involves adhesion of the cells onto the CI surface. Using ultra-high viscous alginate (UHV-alginate) made of the brown algal species *Lessonia nigrescens* and *Lessonia trabeculata*, it has been shown that coating the CI with this alginate is possible (Schwieger et al., 2018). It has also been demonstrated that BDNF-overexpressing murine fibroblasts survive in the UHV-alginate and release BDNF at a concentration that is neuroprotective *in vitro* (Hütten et al., 2013). Since gaining approval for use in humans of murine fibroblasts as xenogeneic cells may be difficult, a human cell source may prove more beneficial. Human mesenchymal stem cells (MSCs) are a promising alternative for lifelong factor delivery. Genetically modified MSCs overexpressing BDNF are shown to produce BDNF at a neuroprotective concentration *in vitro* (Schwieger et al., 2018). When these cells, too, are encapsulated in UHV-alginate, they rescue SGNs from degeneration *in vitro*. Here we investigate the potential neuroprotective effect of MSCs incorporated into a UHV-alginate matrix in deafened guinea pigs. CI electrodes are coated with the cell-UHV-alginate hydrogel layers and implanted into the scala tympani. Additionally, the UHV-alginate-MSC matrix was injected into the scala tympani and gelled instead of being used to coat the CI. Injection into the inner ear was an approach used not only in deafened animals, but also in hearing animals, to investigate the effect of injection on hearing ability.

MATERIALS AND METHODS

Animals and Experimental Conditions

Adult male t Dunkin-Hartley guinea pigs (N = 43, weight 300–500 g, Charles River Laboratories, Sulzfeld, Germany) were kept in a temperature- and humidity-controlled room, exposed to a 24-h light-dark cycle (14 h/10 h) with free access to food and water.

All animals were normal hearing, this having been proven by initial measurement of the acoustically evoked auditory brainstem response (AABR, see below). The guinea pigs were randomly divided into five experimental groups. Twenty-six animals were systemically deafened (see below). Deafening was verified after 1 week by AABR measurements, and these animals were randomly assigned to one of three experimental groups unilaterally implanted with the following: a cochlear implant (CI) (N = 8; one ear deaf: deaf; one ear deaf and CI inserted: deaf-CI), a CI with alginate-mesenchymal stem cell (MSC) coating (N = 10; one ear deaf: not analyzed; one ear deaf with alginate-MSC-coated CI: deaf-alginate-C) or an alginate-MSC injection into the scala tympani followed by the CI insertion (N = 8; one ear deaf: not analyzed; one ear deaf with alginate injection: *deaf-alginate-I*). The 17 remaining, non-deafened, normal-hearing animals were either directly sacrificed after verification of normal hearing (*NH;* N = 9) or received a bilateral CI implantation with an additional unilateral alginate-MSC injection (N = 8; one ear normal hearing with CI: *NH-CI*; one ear normal hearing with CI and MSC-UHV-alginate injection: *NH-alginate-I*). **Figure 1** illustrates the experimental conditions (A) and the time line (B).

The purpose of the various experimental conditions is to provide information on:

(1) Spiral ganglion neuron (SGN) density in normal-hearing ears: NH.
(2) Influence of CI insertion on SGN density and hearing status in normal-hearing ears: *NH-CI.*
(3) SGN density after deafening: *deaf.*
(4) Effect of CI insertion on SGN density in deafened animals: *deaf-CI.*
(5) Neuroprotective potential of CI coated with UHV-alginate containing brain-derived neurotrophic factor- (BDNF-)overexpressing MSCs: *deaf-alginate-C* versus *deaf-CI.*
(6) Neuroprotective potential of UHV-alginate containing BDNF-overexpressing MSCs injected into the inner ear with subsequent CI insertion: *deaf-alginate-I* versus *deaf-CI.*
(7) Influence on hearing threshold of UHV-alginate injection with subsequent CI insertion: *NH-alginate-I.*
(8) Assessment of which application method (coating versus injection) is more favorable: *deaf-alginate-C* versus *deaf-alginate-I.*

Deafening, AABR measurement, inner ear surgery and perfusion were performed under general anesthesia with medetomidine hydrochloride (0.2 mg/kg, intramuscular; CP-Pharma Handelsgesellschaft, Burgdorf, Germany), midazolam (1 mg/kg, intramuscular; Ratiopharm, Ulm, Germany) and fentanyl (0.025 mg/kg, intramuscular; Janssen-Cilag, Neuss, Germany). Animals were placed on a heating pad to maintain the body temperature at 37–38°C. They subcutaneously received 0.05 mg/kg atropine (B. Braun, Melsungen, Germany) to reduce bronchial secretion and salivation, 0.2 mg meloxicam/kg

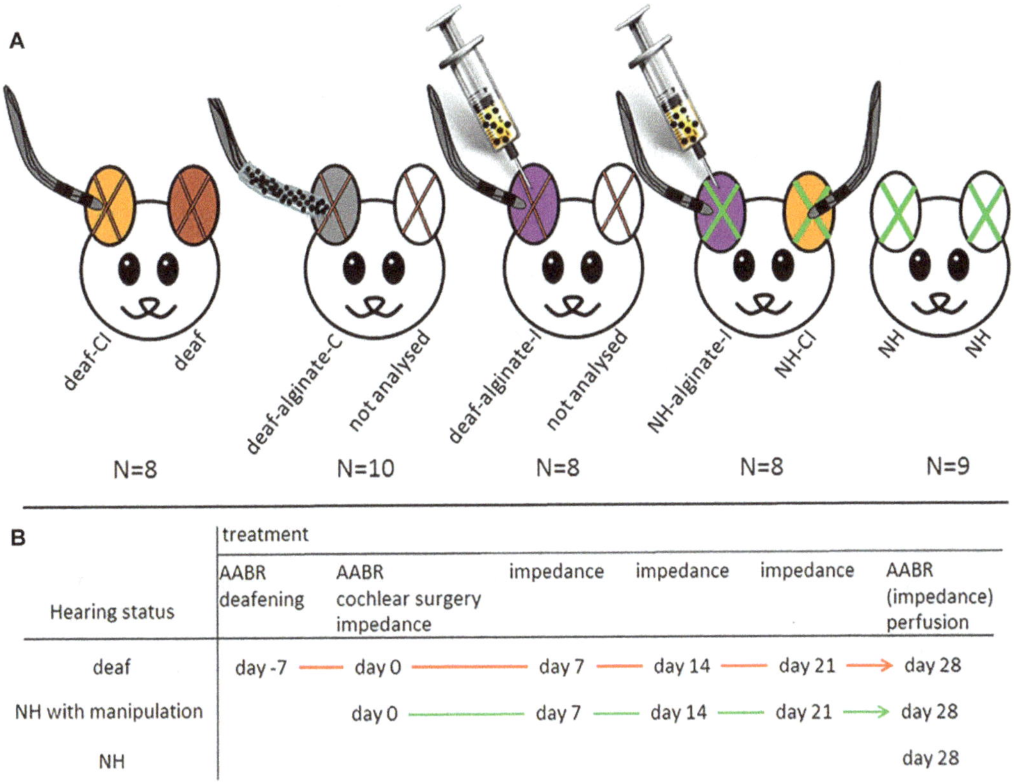

FIGURE 1 | (A) Illustration of experimental groups: red X: deafened ears; green X: normal-hearing ears; color code for ears: orange: deafened (red X) or normal-hearing (green X) ears with cochlear implant: *deaf-CI and NH-CI*; red: deafened ear without further treatment, included in group *deaf*; gray: deaf and implantation of CI with UHV-alginate-MSC coating: *deaf-alginate-C*; white with red x: contralateral ears of those treated with factor-releasing cells. Since it cannot be ruled out that the factor has an effect on contralateral neurons, theses ears were not included in the analysis. Violet: animals first received an alginate-MSC injection using a microcatheter system (provided by MED-EL Corp.) inserted 3 mm deep into the scala tympani. After injection the catheter was removed, a normal CI was inserted and the polymerization solution for alginate crosslinking was applied for 30 min at the round window niche. Violet with red X: *deaf-alginate-I*; violet with green X: normal hearing with CI and UHV-alginate-MSC injection: *NH-alginate-I*, while with green X: normal hearing; *NH*. **(B)** illustrates the time line of the experiments for each treatment condition.

(Boehringer Ingelheim, Ingelheim am Rhein, Germany) for analgesia, and 2 × 4 ml Ringer's solution including 5% glucose (both from B. Braun) per 300 g body weight, 10 mg enrofloxacin/kg (Bayer Vital, Leverkusen, Germany) for prophylactic antibiotic therapy. Areas to be incised were locally infiltrated with prilocaine (Xylonest 1%, AstraZeneca).

The anesthesia was antagonized by injecting atipamezole (1 mg/kg; Zoetis, Parsippany, United States), flumazenil (0.1 mg/kg; Hexal, Holzkirchen, Germany) and naloxone (0.03 mg/kg, Ratiopharm).

AABR Measurement

Acoustic stimulation and recording of the auditory brainstem response (AABR) signals were performed using an Audiology Lab system (Otoconsult, Frankfurt a. M., Germany) in a soundproof booth. To detect general auditory system thresholds, acoustic clicks (duration: 50 μs) were used. For detection of frequency-specific acoustic thresholds, tone bursts (duration: 6 ms with 2 ms rising/falling ramps) at frequencies of 1, 2, 4, 8, 16, and 32 kHz with 1 octave step were used. The acoustic stimuli were presented by a calibrated loudspeaker (DT48, BeyerDynamic, Heilbronn, Germany) via a plastic cone placed in the outer ear canal.

The AABR signals were recorded using subcutaneous electrodes. The signals were amplified, band-pass filtered and recorded at a sampling rate of 100 kHz. The signals were analyzed using custom-made software in MATLAB (Mathworks, Natick, MA, United States). The signals were averaged and smoothed using the Savitzky–Golay FIR filter (frame length: 1 ms; polynomial order: 5). The hearing thresholds were determined by visual inspection of AABR signals. The lowest stimulus intensity at which AABR signals could be detected was taken to be a hearing threshold for the relevant stimulus configuration.

Only animals with initial normal hearing (thresholds of <40 dB SPL) were included into the study.

Additional AABR measurements were performed in all animals 1 week after the deafening procedure on experimental day 0 to verify deafness, and in all animals on experimental day 28. In normal-hearing animals, frequency-specific stimulation was performed on day 0 and day 28 (following click measurement) to identify the frequency-specific impact of cochlear manipulation.

The threshold shift was calculated as the difference between the initial hearing threshold and the hearing threshold after deafening or after cochlear implantation in the normal-hearing animals. Where the AABR threshold could not be identified up to the maximum click level [0 dB att. (=120 dB SPL)], the threshold shift was defined as the difference between the AABR threshold at initial measurement and the maximum click level.

Deafening

Directly after verification of normal hearing by AABR measurement, 26 animals were systemically deafened by subcutaneous injection of kanamycin (400 mg/kg; Kanamycin Sulfate, BioChemica, AppliChem GmbH, Darmstadt, Germany) and subsequent infusion of furosemide (100 mg/kg; Diuren, WDT, Garbsen, Germany) into the external jugular vein (Meyer et al., 2012), which has been shown to eliminate the majority of both inner and outer hair cells (Versnel et al., 2007). The success of the procedure was determined after 1 week by click-evoked AABR measurement. A click AABR threshold shift of 50 dB after the ototoxic treatment was set as the limit for indication of a successful deafening (Meyer et al., 2012). A click AABR threshold shift of 50 dB after the ototoxic treatment was set as the limit for indication of successful deafening (Meyer et al., 2012).

Preparation of Genetically Modified MSCs

The expression of human BDNF (entire coding sequence including signal peptide: Warnecke et al., 2012) was under the control of a spleen focus-forming virus (SFFV) promoter in a lentiviral vector that also mediated red fluorescence using the marker protein tdTomato (red). Subsequently, after lentivirus production, hMSCs from one selected donor were seeded at 3,000 cells/cm^2, passage 4 or 5, and were infected with the BDNF-lentivirus including 8 μg/ml polybrene. In order to subsequently downgrade the cells to S1 level, the cells were cultured and expanded for 11 days before being harvested with trypsin/EDTA solution. The medium used for expansion of MSCs ('MSC medium') was Dulbecco's Modified Eagle's Medium (1 g/l glucose, Biochrom, FG0415) supplemented with 10% (v/v) fetal calf serum (FCS, not heat-inactivated, Thermo Fisher Scientific, Schwerte, Germany, 'HyClone', SV30160.03), 25 mM HEPES (Biochrom, Berlin, Germany), 1% (100 U/ml/100 μg/ml) penicillin/streptomycin (Biochrom, Berlin, Germany) and 2 ng/ml human recombinant FGF 2 (from *Escherichia coli*, PeproTech, Hamburg, Germany).

Preparation of UHV-Alginate-MSC Injections and CI Coating

For injection into the inner ear, 1 ml UHV-alginate solution (0.65% (w/v%) in isotonic 0.9% sodium chloride solution (B. Braun), provided by Fraunhofer IBMT, Sulzbach, Germany, now commercially available from Alginatec GmbH, Riedenheim, Germany) was mixed with 250,000 BDNF-producing MSCs. The alginate-MSC solution was freshly prepared during surgery; immediately following its preparation, it was injected into the scala tympani using a catheter system provided by MED-EL, Innsbruck, Austria. Two catheter types were used, one with a yellow conus and an outer diameter of 0.38 mm, and one with a transparent conus and an outer diameter of 0.64 mm. The thinner catheter had a more flexible consistency and was more difficult to insert, but was still the first choice as its insertion is hypothetically less traumatizing than that of the transparent catheter system.

The cochlear implants were kindly provided by MED-EL Corp., Innsbruck, Austria. They consisted of a connector, a reference and an active electrode. The active electrode array had two electrode contacts and a marker point to guide insertion at a depth of 3 mm from the tip (**Figure 2**). The electrode arrays were precoated with poly-L-Lysine (pLL, Sigma-Aldrich, Taufkirchen, Germany), after which they were dipped into 300 μl alginate-MSC solution containing about 500,000 MSCs before subsequently being transferred into a 20 mM $BaCl_2$ solution (with 115 mM NaCl and 5 mM L-histidine) to achieve crosslinking of the UHV-alginate-MSC layer, and finally washed with saline solution (0.9% w/v, B. Braun, Melsungen, Germany). In total, four alginate-MSC layers were applied, followed by three outer layers with cell-free alginate to protect the MSCs from the host immune system and to avoid migration of cells (**Figure 3**).

Cochlear Surgery

Cochlear implantation was performed in all experimental groups except the NH group. Either a CI (coated or uncoated) was immediately inserted, or one was inserted following insertion of a catheter for purposes of alginate-MSC injection.

The middle ear cavity was opened using a postauricular approach, the cochlea visualized and the round window membrane incised. The CI electrode array was inserted into the scala tympani until the marker point reached the round window niche. Where alginate-MSC was injected (groups: *deaf-alginate-I* and *NH-alginate-I*), a catheter was inserted 3 mm into the scala tympani and the alginate-MSC matrix was injected until the surgeon observed flushing of the medium (pink color) that exited the cochlear while the bony cochlea capsule was being rinsed. The catheter was withdrawn while injection continued, and subsequently the CI was inserted. After CI insertion, the round window niche was filled with TABOTAMP® (Ethicon SARL, Neuchatel, Switzerland) and about two drops of $BaCl_2$ were placed on the material using a syringe to induce gelation of the cell-containing UHV-alginate. After 30 min, the TABOTAMP®/$BaCl_2$ layer was removed. The CI was secured in place and the bulla fenestration site closed using Tetric EvoFlow® (ivoclar vivadent, Schaan, Liechtenstein) in all implantation groups. The reference electrode was placed extratympanically on the bony wall of the bulla and the wound was sutured in two layers.

Impedance Measurement

Electrode impedances were measured in all implanted animals using a standard MED-EL PULSARci100 stimulator with a HD-CIS 750 pps coding strategy to generate biphasic monopolar pulse

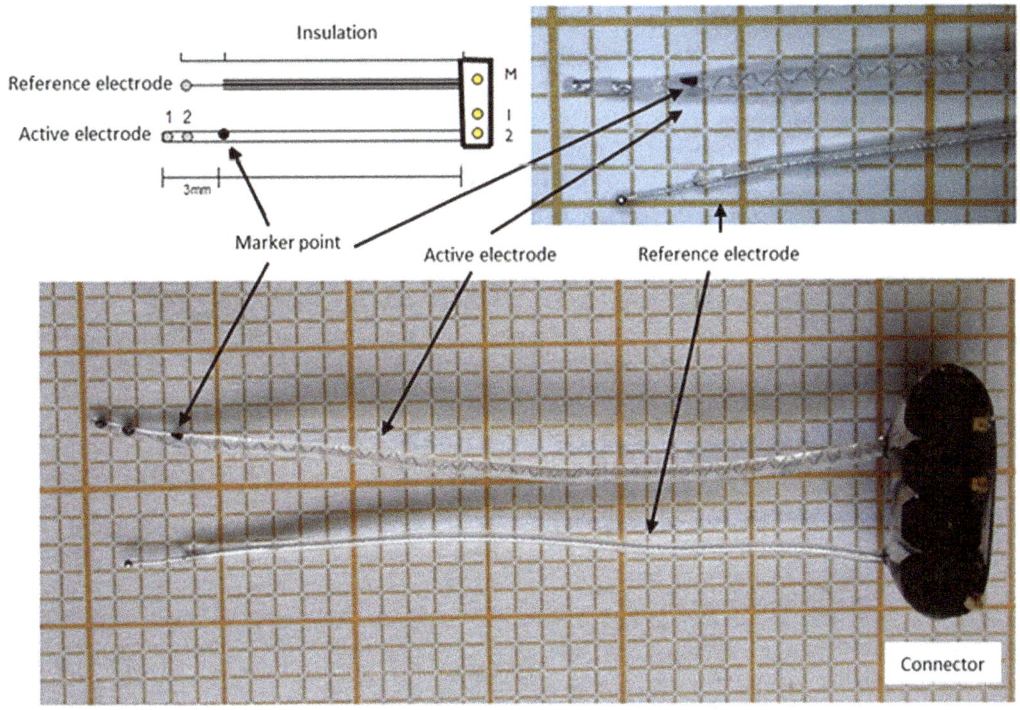

FIGURE 2 | Cochlear implant electrode. The electrodes consisted of a connector, a reference electrode and an active electrode with two contacts and a marker point to determine the insertion depth.

trains with a charge of 16 nC, as previously described (Wilk et al., 2016). Starting with the first (apical) contact, impedance was measured three times, followed by three subsequent impedance measurements at the second contact (basal). For data analysis purposes, the mean of the three measurements was taken for each contact (Wilk et al., 2016). *In vivo* measurement of electrode impedance was performed directly after CI insertion and 7, 14, 21, and 28 days postsurgically.

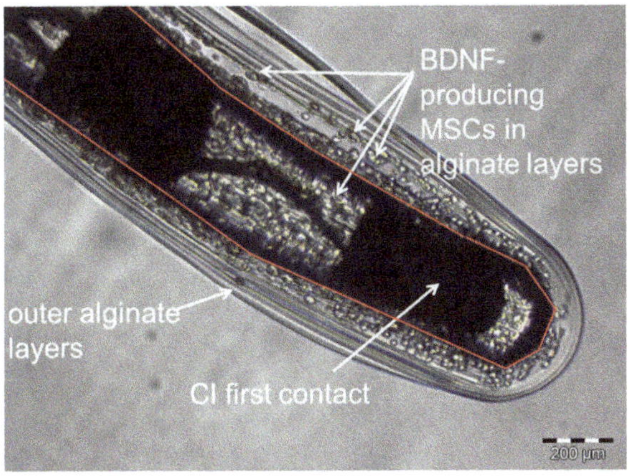

FIGURE 3 | Representative image of a UHV-alginate-MSC-coated cochlear implant. The photograph is taken from the tip of the array. The red layer depicts the boundary between CI surface and alginate coating. The first electrode contact is marked. BDNF-producing MSCs are visible all around the electrode array. The electrode was coated by dip-coating with four inner layers of alginate containing MSCs and three outer layers of cell-free alginate.

In addition to *in vivo* measurements, the impedance of $n = 3$ electrode arrays was measured *ex vivo* to investigate whether the coating has an impact on electrode impedance. The first measurement without alginate coating was performed directly prior to coating with pLL in phosphate-buffered saline (PBS), because pLL is diluted 1:10 in PBS. The second impedance measurement (without coating) was performed in the MSC medium, and the final measurement (following coating with alginate-MSCs) was carried out in the MSC medium.

Preparation of Specimen for Histological Analysis

After the final AABR and impedance measurement, the animals received a second injection of the initial anesthesia and were euthanized by transcardial perfusion. Temporal bones were removed (Hütten et al., 2014) and the implant was secured in place at the round window niche using Tetric EvoFlow® (ivoclar vivadent). The duration of fixation was prolonged overnight followed by decalcification for about 3 weeks in 10% ethylenediamine tetraacetic acid-disodium salt (EDTA, Sigma-Aldrich Chemie GmbH, Steinheim, Germany). After

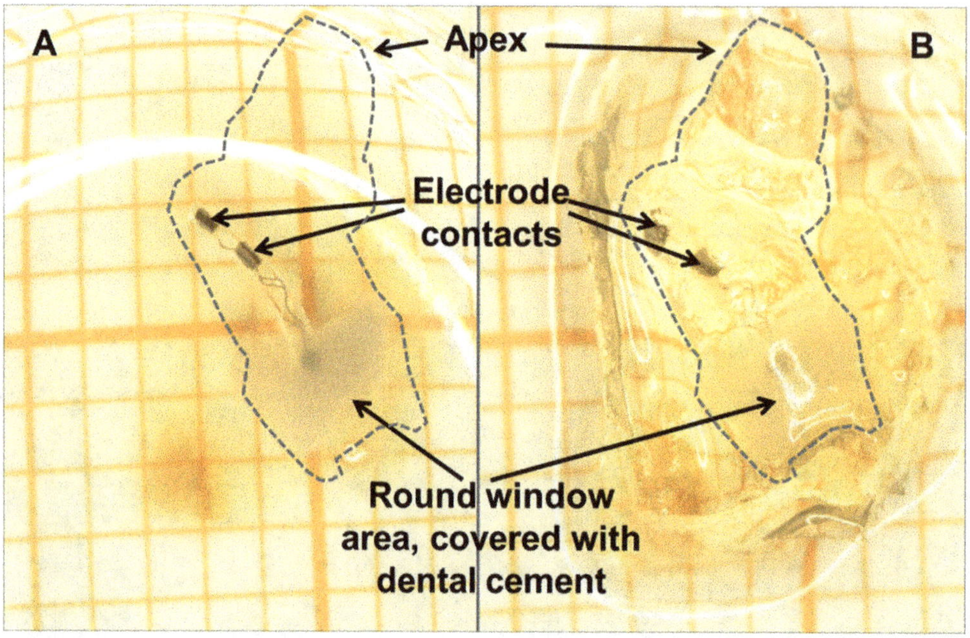

FIGURE 4 | The same cleared cochlea (dashed line) with CI *in situ* in methyl salicylate, benzyl benzoate (MSBB) **(A)** and without MSBB **(B)**, illustrating the total transparency of decalcified cochleae positioned in MSBB **(A)** suitable for confocal laser scanning microscopy of SGNs. The electrode is secured in place at the round window niche with dental cement.

dehydration with ethanol, the cochleae were cleared in Spalteholz solution [methyl salicylate, benzyl benzoate (MSBB); **Figure 4**], placed in self-made glass chambers (Wrzeszcz et al., 2013) and microscopically analyzed.

SGN Density

Using a Leica TSC SP8 confocal laser scanning microscope and the tissue's PFA-induced autofluorescence, images were generated at a speed of 400 Hz and 2048 pixels × 2048 pixels with a fivefold object lens or 1024 pixels × 1024 pixels with a 10-fold object lens. Following the previously published protocol, the cochlea was scanned and the images were exported and further processed using ImageJ software (Wrzeszcz et al., 2013). The area of Rosenthal's canal was traced and the SGNs were automatically counted in the traced area using the Image-based Tool for Counting Nuclei (ITCN) plug-in (Center for Bio-Image Informatics[1]). SGN count was performed on five subsequent images of cochlear cross-sections. The number of SGNs divided by the measured cross-sectional area of Rosenthal's canal gives the SGN density (cells/10,000 μm^2). The mean SGN density of the total cochlear length, including all cross-sections of Rosenthal's canal, was analyzed. The mean SGN density of the (lower and upper) basal turn was also analyzed, but separately.

Fibrosis

Fibrosis was visually evaluated for one representative image per area to be analyzed. Since no fibrosis was detectable apically from the electrode tip, two areas of the scala tympani were analyzed where the electrode was located. One was the basal part of the cochlea including the area near the round window, and the other was the area of the scala tympani where the electrode tip was located. A subjective evaluation was performed using a ranking system. Scores for subjective ranking were assigned as follows: score 0: no connective tissue; score 1: thin film of fibrosis directly on the electrode surface; score 2: thin fibrous cloudy structures around the electrode; score 3: more prominent cloudy structures around the electrode; score 4: almost the entire investigated area of the scala tympani is filled with fibrous tissue.

Alginate and Cell Analysis

In one middle ear of the deaf-alginate-MSC injected group, crosslinked alginate was found in the middle ear cavity on experimental day 28 when the specimen preparation was performed. This alginate was transferred into the cell medium and microscopically (CKX53 + Camera XM10, Olympus) analyzed for detection of fluorescent marker protein producing MSCs. Cells with fluorophore expression were deemed to be surviving cells.

Statistical Analysis

The data were statistically analyzed using the GraphPad Prism® 5 program.

The relevant data sets (AABR threshold and threshold shift, SGN density, impedances and connective tissue score) were tested for normal distribution of the values, the D'Agostino and Pearson omnibus normality test being used for this purpose. Click-evoked AABR threshold and threshold shift, electrode impedances and SGN densities exhibited normal distribution.

[1] https://imagej.nih.gov/ij/plugins/itcn.html

To compare click-evoked AABR threshold shifts between groups and impedances between groups, an unpaired *t*-test was performed. For the purpose of analyzing frequency-specific AABR thresholds on day 0 and day 28, as well as impedance over time, paired *t*-tests were performed.

Spiral ganglion neurons density was then analyzed by applying Bartlett's Test for Equality of Variances to the sample sets. With a *p*-value of 0.9833, the variances of the SGN densities of all groups were homogeneous. An ANOVA was performed and subsequently the Bonferroni multiple comparison test was used to analyze the variance of independent samples.

The scores yielded by the connective tissue analysis were not distributed normally. The Kruskal–Wallis test was performed to compare these scores between groups, and the Wilcoxon matched-pairs test was used to compare basal and apical fibrosis within one experimental group.

The significance levels determined were defined as follows:

- $p > 0.05$ = not significantly different (ns).
- $p < 0.05$ = significantly different (*).
- $p < 0.01$ = highly significantly different (**).
- $p < 0.001$ = most significantly different (***).

In the following sections, the data are represented as mean ± standard error of mean (SEM) for each experimental group.

RESULTS

AABR

A reference AABR using click stimuli was performed in all animals prior to their inclusion into the study to confirm that physiological hearing function was present. All animals' hearing threshold (based on click-evoked potentials) was 80 dB att. (=40 dB SPL) or lower, and therefore all animals showed normal hearing as defined by previous studies.

An additional AABR measurement was performed on experimental day 0 in animals 1 week after treatment with kanamycine and furosemide, the aim being to verify the success of the deafening method. All animals receiving ototoxic drugs were deaf and therefore underwent cochlear implantation.

To investigate whether alginate injection may have an impact on residual hearing in implanted subjects, click- and frequency-specific hearing thresholds were analyzed for normal-hearing animals unilaterally provided with a cochlear implant (*NH-CI*), and contralaterally injected with alginate-embedded mesenchymal stem cells (MSCs) followed by CI insertion (*NH-alginate-I*).

Using click-evoked AABR, a mean threshold shift (difference between day 0 threshold before surgery and day 28 threshold before perfusion) of 23.75 ± 19.78 dB SPL was detected in *NH-CI* ears. The same animals received a contralateral injection of UHV-alginate-MSCs; a CI was subsequently inserted and the UHV-alginate was crosslinked for 30 min using $BaCl_2$. These ears had a threshold shift of 35.00 ± 21.21 dB SPL (*NH-alginate-I*). No statistically significant differences in mean hearing loss between both experimental groups were observed (**Figure 5**).

Analysis of frequency-specific thresholds revealed a significant increase in high-frequency thresholds (8, 16, and 32 kHz) in both experimental conditions, namely both CI insertion and alginate injection followed by cochlear implantation (**Figure 6**). At 32 kHz, the mean threshold shift after 28 days of implantation was 44 ± 17 dB (NH-CI) and 48 ± 13 dB (NH-alginate-I).

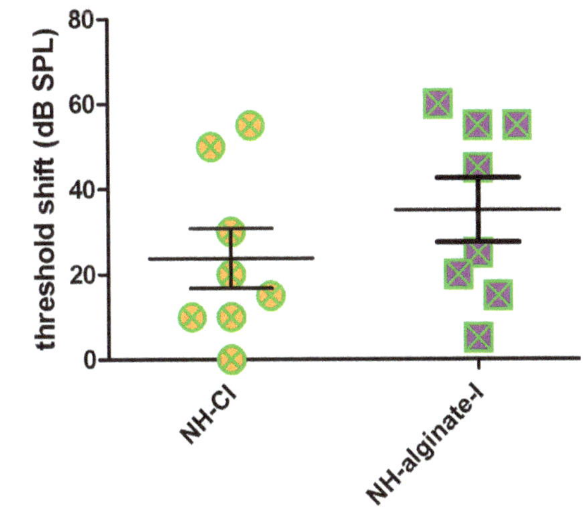

FIGURE 5 | The mean hearing threshold shift (click-evoked) of normal-hearing ears implanted with an uncoated cochlear implant (NH-CI) or of normal-hearing ears receiving an alginate-MSC injection followed by insertion of an uncoated cochlear implant (NH-alginate-I) did not differ 28 days after implantation. Each data point represents the threshold shift of click-evoked AABR in one ear.

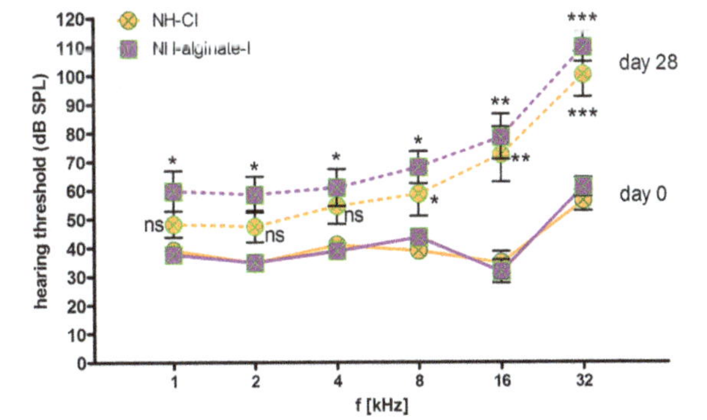

FIGURE 6 | Frequency-specific hearing thresholds in normal-hearing ears. The data shown are means ± SEM of data for all ears ($n = 8$) within the various experimental groups. Continuous lines: day 0 thresholds before implantation. Dashed lines: Thresholds 28 days after implantation. Orange: Normal hearing with CI (NH-CI); purple: Normal hearing with alginate-MSC injection and subsequent CI insertion (NH-alginate-I). Significant differences between initial hearing thresholds and the thresholds determined after 28 days of implantation are depicted above (NH-alginate-I) or below (NH-CI) the experimental condition in question. In both experimental groups, the hearing threshold at the higher frequencies (8, 16, and 32 kHz) increased significantly after implantation. At 4–1 kHz, cochlear implantation did not affect the threshold significantly, but alginate injection with subsequent CI insertion resulted in a significantly increased threshold at all frequencies. ns = not significat; *$p < 0.05$; **$p < 0.01$; ***$p < 0.001$.

With increasing distance from the round window, the threshold shift decreased in both conditions, from 37 ± 26 dB (NH-CI) and 47 ± 25 dB (NH-alginate-I) at 16 kHz to 20 ± 23 dB (NH-CI) and 24 ± 21 dB (NH-alginate-I) at 8 kHz, and 13 ± 19 dB (NH-CI) and 22 ± 22 dB (NH-alginate-I) at 4 kHz; in NH-CI treated ears, no significant difference in hearing thresholds (compared with the initial condition) was observed. At the lowest frequencies (i.e., 1 and 2 kHz), the hearing threshold on day 0 and day 28 in UHV-alginate-injected and cochlear-implanted ears (NH-alginate-I) - but not in only cochlear-implanted ears (NH-CI) - differed significantly (NH-CI mean threshold at 1 kHz: d0 39 dB and d28 48 dB; at 2 kHz: d0 35 dB and d28 47 dB; NH-alginate-I mean threshold at 1 kHz: d0 38 dB and d28 60 dB; at 2 kHz: d0 35 dB and d28 58 dB).

SGN Survival

In normal-hearing guinea pigs (NH, n = 9 animals, n = 18 ears), a mean neuronal density of 23.31 ± 0.34 spiral ganglion neurons (SGN)/10,000 μm^2 was detected. Implantation of a CI or injection of UHV-alginate-MSCs followed by CI insertion in normal-hearing/non-deafened animals did not affect the SGN density compared with NH when the total cochlea is analyzed (NH-CI: 22.67 ± 0.48 SGN/10,000 μm^2, n = 8; NH-alginate-I: 22.87 ± 0.65 SGN/10,000 μm^2; n = 8; **Figure 7A**) or when the lower and upper basal region of the cochlea is investigated (**Figure 7B**) (ANOVA, total cochlea: $p = 0.57$; basal: $p = 0.64$).

The analysis of variance of the mean SGN densities in deafened ears showed highly significant differences both for the total cochlear ($p = 0.0005$) and for the basal region ($p < 0.0001$) when compared with NH. Applying the Bonferroni multiple comparison test, the mean SGN densities of the deafened groups were tested for difference. The deafening procedure resulted in a significantly reduced mean SGN density of 10.91 ± 0.52 SGN/10,000 μm^2 over the entire length of the cochlea (**Figure 8A**). With 13.84 ± 0.56 surviving SGN/10,000 μm^2, CI insertion evidently did not change neuronal survival compared with the non-implanted deafened ears, if measurements over the entire length of the cochlea are included. Four weeks after implantation of alginate-MSC-coated CIs into deafened ears, the SGNs were significantly protected compared with deafened controls (deaf-alginate-C: 16.30 ± 0.64 SGN/10,000 μm^2 vs. deaf: 10.91 ± 0.52 SGN/10,000 μm^2, $p < 0.05$). The injection of MSC-containing alginate (deaf-alginate-I: 11.61 ± 1.54 SGN/10,000 μm^2) did not affect SGN survival compared with the deafened, or deafened and CI-implanted, ears, but resulted in significantly lower SGN survival than where ears were implanted with an alginate-MSC-coated CI.

Focusing on the basal cochlear region (lower basal and upper basal cross-section of Rosenthal's canal) where injection and implantation takes place, even more prominent differences are evident between the treatment strategies (**Figure 8B**). Cochlear implantation (*per se*) resulted in better SGN preservation than no intervention at all (deaf-CI: 14.10 ± 0.60 SGN/10,000 μm^2 vs. 10.46 ± 0.50 SGN/10,000 μm^2, $p < 0.01$). Protection of SGNs from degeneration by coating the CI with MSC-containing alginate resulted, in the basal cochlear region, in a SGN density of 16.36 ± 0.048 SGN/10,000 μm^2, and was significantly improved compared with all other conditions ($p < 0.001$). No difference was observed between cochlear-implanted ears and those receiving an alginate injection before cochlear implantation (deaf-CI: 14.10 ± 0.60 SGN/10,000 μm^2 vs. deaf-alginate-I: 11.64 ± 0.98 SGN/10,000 μm^2; ns).

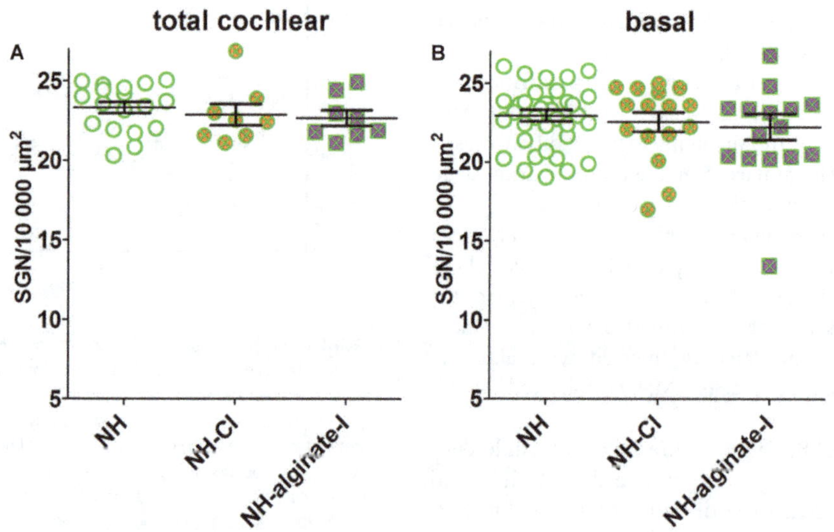

FIGURE 7 | Mean spiral ganglion neuron density in normal-hearing ears without further intervention (NH; n = 9 animals, i.e., n = 18 ears), with cochlear implantation (NH-CI; n = 8 ears) and with injection of alginate-MSCs followed by CI insertion (NH-alginate-I; n = 8 ears) did not differ over the entire length of the cochlea **(A)** and for the basal region (lower and upper basal turn) **(B)**. Each data point in **(A)** represents the mean SGN density of one animal over the full length of the cochlea. Each data point in B represents the mean SGN density of the lower basal or upper basal cochlear turn of one experimental animal. ns = not significat; **$p < 0.01$; ***$p < 0.001$.

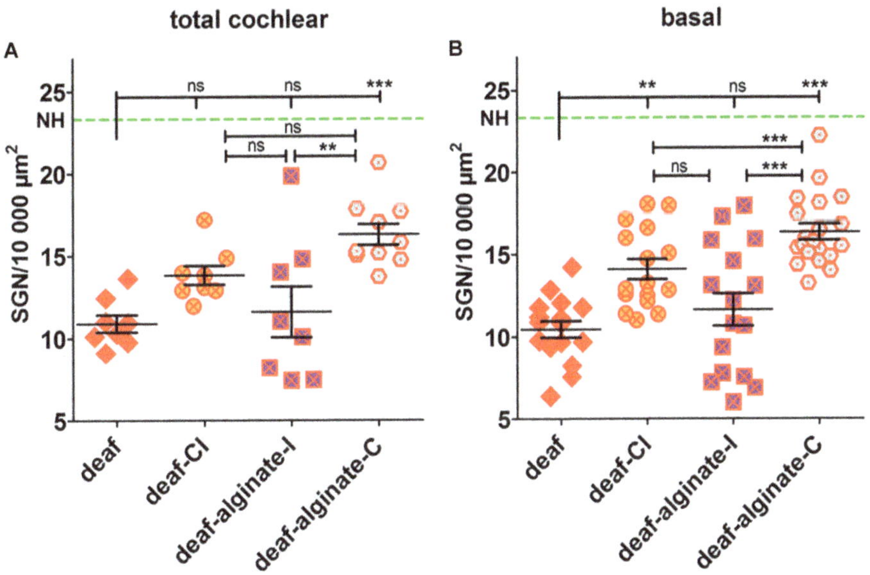

FIGURE 8 | The SGN density (number of surviving SGNs in 10,000 μm^2) was influenced by the different interventions tested when data were collected for the total length of the cochlea **(A)** and, even more markedly, when the basal cochlear region was analyzed separately **(B)**. The deafening procedure resulted in a significantly reduced SGN density compared with the normal-hearing control (NH, green dashed line). Cochlear implantation preserved SGNs from degeneration in the basal region. Coating the CI with alginate-MSCs (deaf-alginate-C) significantly preserved the SGNs from degeneration in deafened animals; the injection (deaf-alginate-I), however, did not. Each data point in **(A)** represents the mean SGN density of one animal over the full length of the cochlea. Each data point in **(B)** is the mean SGN density of the lower basal or upper basal cochlear turn of one experimental animal. ns = not significat; $^{**}p < 0.01$; $^{***}p < 0.001$.

Impedance

To investigate whether coating with alginate-MSCs had an impact on electrode impedance, coated electrodes had to be measured in the MSC medium to avoid damage to these cells and alginate destruction. Comparative measurements were made of the electrode impedance of arrays placed in the MSC medium and those placed in PBS: for both electrode contacts, impedance was found to be lower in PBS than in the MSC medium (**Figure 9A**; those data are not included in **Figure 9B**). Electrode impedances of contacts in the MSC medium were not affected by alginate-MSC coating as compared with impedance of the same contact before coating (**Figure 9B**; mean of contact 1 and 2 for uncoated in PBS: 2.38 ± 0.19 kΩ versus alginate-MSCs coated in medium: 2.77 ± 0.11 kΩ). In contrast to impedances measured *ex vivo* in the MSC medium, impedances measured *in vivo* directly after surgery were significantly increased (4.36 ± 0.20 kΩ, $p < 0.001$).

Change over time in impedance *in vivo* did not differ between experimental groups. This is mainly due to the high variability in each group (**Supplementary Figure S1**).

Comparison of final electrode impedances on experimental day 28 revealed a statistically not significant tendency toward increased impedance at contact 2 (basal) in comparison with contact 1 (tip) in all groups. No differences in electrode impedance between groups were found (**Figure 10**).

Fibrosis

Fibrosis around the electrode array was visible in all cochleae analyzed. No fibrosis was detectable apically from the electrode tip. None of the ears showed an absence of fibrosis (score 0), and none was affected by massive fibrosis with a score of 4. **Figure 11** includes representative images for scores 1, 2, and 3. No difference between alginate-injected cochleae or cochleae with insertion of alginate-coated CI or uncoated CI was observed (**Figure 11**).

Alginate and Cell Analysis

The explanted alginate from one animal after 28 days of injection included living MSCs (**Figure 12**).

DISCUSSION

To determine the neuroprotective effect of brain-derived neurotrophic factor endogenously overexpressed from infected mesenchymal stem cells (MSCs), two different application methods were evaluated in systemically deafened guinea pigs. The BDNF-overexpressing MSCs were encapsulated in a UHV-alginate matrix and were either injected into the scala tympani or used to coat the cochlear implant array.

Neuroprotection

Cochlear implantation resulted in significantly increased spiral ganglion neuron survival in the basal region compared with deafened ears that were not further treated (**Figure 8**). A greater decrease in SGN density was to be expected due to the fact that the cochlear-implanted ears were locally manipulated, in contrast to the deafened ears which were not opened at all. It is possible, however, that merely the activation of the electrode for the purpose of the weekly impedance measurement itself resulted

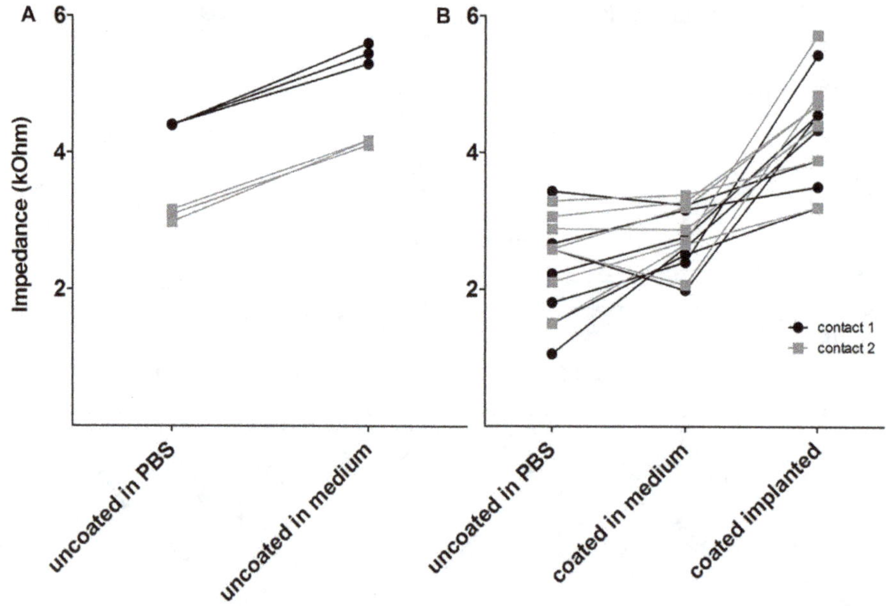

FIGURE 9 | Electrode impedance on electrode contact 1 (apical) and 2 (basal) in PBS and MSC medium before coating **(A)** and after coating **(B)** in medium and *in vivo* (coated implanted). Electrode impedance of uncoated contacts was increased in MSC medium compared with PBS **(A)**. The coating did not affect impedance but after implantation, all impedances were increased **(B)**.

in a neuroprotective effect. It is known that electrical stimulation may have a protective effect on auditory neurons (Scheper et al., 2009; Leake et al., 2013; Shepherd et al., 2018). The electric fields increase gene expression for, and synthesis of, growth factors (Aaron et al., 2004), which may lead to neuroprotection through autocrine and paracrine neurotrophic signaling (Hansen et al., 2001). To date, exact parameters for electrical stimulation of the SGNs that result in reliable neuroprotection have not been defined. There are indications that even only short-term electrical stimulation may lead to increased SGN survival. This application of 'short-term' stimulation was for 2.3 h during weekly electrical ABR measurements in guinea pigs (Mitchell et al., 1997), and for 8–88 h over a period of 8.5–9.6 months in cats (Konerding et al., 2017). It may be that, by contrast, neuronal protection in the present study was initiated by electrical stimulation during impedance measurement, which is very brief and involves only a matter of seconds. This is a very interesting finding which should be investigated further in future projects.

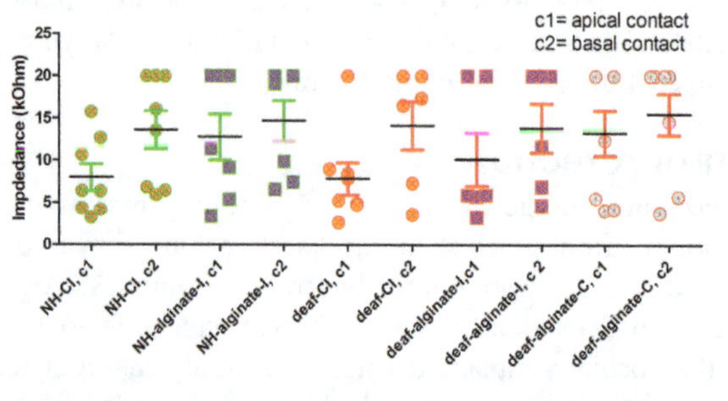

FIGURE 10 | Electrode impedance on experimental day 28 did not differ between experimental groups.

Coating the CI with alginate containing MSCs that continuously secrete BDNF additionally increased SGN survival in deafened animals compared to cochlear implantation without alginate-MSC functionalization (**Figure 8**). This effect is significant for the basal region ($p < 0.001$). Compared with deafened-only ears, this effect is evident in terms of the mean SGN density of the entire cochlea, and also if the focus is on the basal region only. This coating would therefore seem to be a feasible method of applying BDNF-overexpressing MSCs into the inner ear for chronic growth factor therapy. It is known from previous *in vitro* experiments that 50 ng/ml exogenous, recombinant human BDNF is optimal in order to preserve murine SGNs from degeneration, and that lower concentrations result in lower numbers of surviving neurons (Wefstaedt et al., 2005). To date, *in vivo* BDNF delivery has involved an osmotic pump or carrier matrices that deliver it into the inner ear or onto the round window. Ramekers et al. (2015) used pumps with a flow rate of 0.25 μl/h filled with 100 μg/ml BDNF, resulting in a calculated total quantity of BDNF infused into guinea pig cochleae after 28 days of about 17 μg. The same concentration of BDNF, i.e., 100 μg/ml, delivered into the inner ear using a pump was examined as to its biological effect by Miller (in combination with FGF) and by Miller et al. (2007) and Agterberg et al. (2009). Other studies have used much lower concentrations in guinea pigs [50 ng/ml pump-based delivery (Miller et al., 1997), or gelfoam cubes (1 $mm^{3)}$ infiltrated with 6 μg BDNF/ml saline placed on the round window (Havenith et al., 2010)] or rat [5.4 μg/ml pump-based delivery (McGuinness and Shepherd, 2005)] which also effectively preserved SGNs from degeneration.

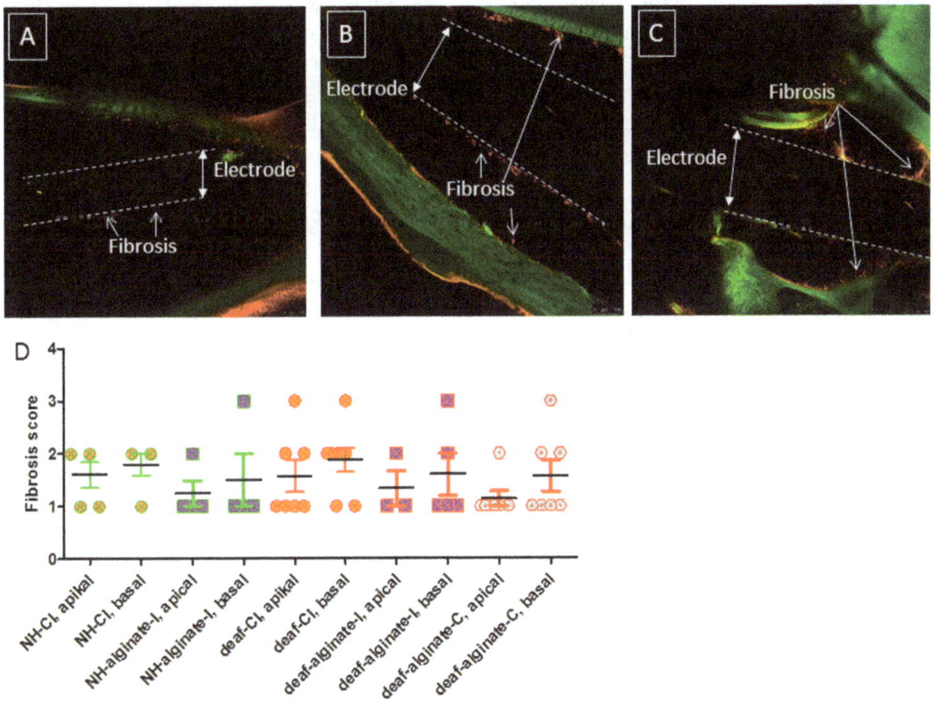

FIGURE 11 | Fibrosis score of implanted ears for all experimental groups. Representative images of scores 1 **(A)**, 2 **(B)**, and 3 **(C)** are given. No images of score 0 and score 4 are shown, since all cochleae were affected to some extent by fibrosis and none of them was densely packed with fibrotic tissue. The extent of fibrosis did not differ between groups **(D)**.

We know that the BDNF produced by the encapsulated hMSCs and released from the UHV-alginate was in the pg/ml-range and protected SGNs from degeneration *in vitro* (Schwieger et al., 2018). Although we did not measure the amount of BDNF released from the alginate coating *in vivo*, we speculate that the BDNF concentration in the inner ear was also in the pg/ml-range. If this is indeed the case, then our study reports a neuroprotective effect using a very low dose of BDNF compared with experiments described in the literature. It must be noted, however, that all these previous studies reported the BDNF concentration in the primed pumps or matrixes but did not measure the final concentration in the perilymph. There are initial reports on the pharmacokinetics of glucocorticoids (Salt and Plontke, 2018), but relevant studies regarding growth factor uptake, distribution and stability in the inner ear are still pending. It remains virtually impossible to state which BDNF concentration is required *in vivo* to achieve significant protection of SGN, since relevant pharmacokinetic studies are lacking. It should also be mentioned that there are indications that endogenous growth factors, as used in the present study, may be more potent for neuronal protection than exogenous factors, due to increased bioactivity of the endogenously produced growth factor. For erythropoietin (EPO), a profound structural difference between human endogenous and various pharmaceutical preparations of human recombinant erythropoietins have been shown (Reichel, 2011), which may lead to different biological activity. This effect may also apply for endogenous and recombinant BDNF. Before translating any approach for growth factor delivery into clinical practice, well-planned and well-performed studies on their pharmacokinetics are a prerequisite.

In contrast to coating the CI with alginate-MSCs, injection of the alginate-MSC matrix with subsequent CI insertion did not affect SGN density compared to deafened-only ears (**Figure 8**).

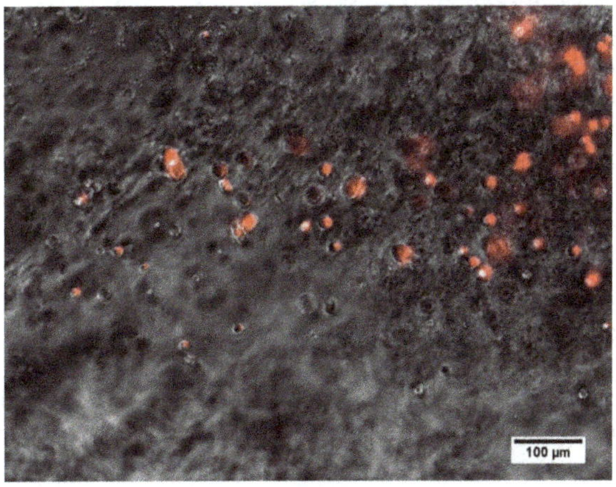

FIGURE 12 | Alginate including spherical MSCs explanted from the middle ear 28 days after injection and crosslinking in an animal. Several MSCs still produce the red fluorescence marker protein tdTomato, which is associated with the genetic modification for BDNF-overexpression and is an indicator for living cells.

Since increased SGN survival was observed in the basal region of ears implanted with a CI, it would appear that alginate injection diminishes the effect of cochlear implantation. The reduced SGN survival observed in the injected alginate-MSC cohort (compared to the cohort with alginate-MSC coating on the electrode array) is caused by the injection technique. Although histological analysis did not include seeking for trauma of the inner ear structures, we know from the electrophysiological data that there is a functional impact on the inner ear that is mediated by injection of alginate-MSCs. Since we did not observe a difference in fibrous tissue growth between the groups, we speculate that the reason for the absence of a neuroprotective effect is not increased tissue trauma but physical impact on the delicate inner ear structures.

Residual Hearing

To investigate whether the hearing threshold may be influenced by alginate-MSC injection, we provided one experimental group with unilateral CI and alginate-MSC injection combined with subsequent CI insertion in the contralateral ear. Cochlear implantation resulted in a shift of 23 ± 20 dB SPL in click-evoked AABR threshold levels. In comparison to CI insertion with previous alginate injection, where the threshold increased by 35 ± 21 dB, no significant differences were detectable (**Figure 5**). However, the recording of click stimuli gives the lowest threshold detectable over the entire frequency range of the cochlea. To investigate whether there are differences between the high- (CI and alginate injection) and the low-frequency regions of the ear (no manipulation, region of physiologically functioning cochlear in patients with residual hearing), frequency-specific thresholds were measured. In both implantation modes – with and without additional alginate injection – high-frequency (32, 16, and 8 kHz) hearing ability was significantly reduced compared with the initial thresholds measured before cochlear manipulation. At 4–1 kHz, cochlear implantation did not modify the threshold significantly, but alginate injection with subsequent CI insertion resulted – across all frequencies – in a significantly increased threshold (**Figure 6**). Hearing preservation after cochlear implantation is affected by factors including insertion depth, length and mechanical characteristics of the electrode in use, surgical technique used (Lenarz and Scheper, 2015), insertion angle (Helbig et al., 2018) as well as insertion trauma, foreign-body reaction, electrode-neuron interfacing, and long-term stability of electrode position and function (Lenarz and Scheper, 2015). The high-frequency threshold increase observed in this study may be due to the presence of the CI inside the scala tympani, the insertion angle or depth, as well as to fibrous tissue growth around the electrode. It can, however, be stated that this high-frequency hearing loss is not clinically relevant, since the most important prerequisite for cochlear implantation is high-frequency hearing loss. Furthermore, we observed a significant low frequency threshold shift in all animals receiving an alginate injection. This loss of hearing in a cochlear region where no manipulation was performed may be due to the filling of the scala tympani with viscous alginate. This may lead to interference with the pressure wave in the perilymph or with basilar membrane movement, which may in turn lead to decreased activation of the high-frequency areas of the inner ear.

We did not investigate a potential effect of alginate-MSC-coated CIs on the hearing threshold. It cannot be ruled out that such coating affects the hearing ability by inducing additional swelling, for example in general, alginate hydrogels are osmotically active and swell in, for example, low-pH environments or in hypotonic solutions (Bajpai and Sharma, 2004). The alginate hydrogel used in this study was produced using isoosmolaric reagents (storage solution and cross-linked solution). In a previous study, Ehrhart et al. (2013) demonstrated the stable volume (low swelling behavior) of such UHV-alginate hydrogels in isoosmolaric media over time. However, for reasons of patient safety, the swelling behavior in perilymph has to be investigated in detail in future studies.

Alginate and Cell Analysis *in situ*

The injection of alginate-MSCs was visually monitored and discontinued as soon as the surgeon observed the phenol-red-colored alginate (due to the matrix formed with the MSC medium) exiting the cochlea. There was, however, one individual in which UHV-alginate was found in the middle ear cavity. By means of microscopic analysis, it was proven that the MSCs survived (as indicated by red fluorescence) in alginate for 28 days *in vivo* (**Figure 12**).

No information about the alginate-MSCs located in the scala tympani is generated by the present study, due to the fact that dehydration is a prerequisite for preparation of specimens for histological analysis of SGNs. This is not only the case for the method used in this study, but also for established procedures such as paraffin or plastic embedding (Scheper et al., 2017). Dehydration erases the alginate, so that the MSCs no longer remain *in situ* and cannot be visualized in the scala tympani. If electrodes had been explanted to evaluate the coating, it would not have been possible to compare fibrosis between CI-explanted ears and other ears where the electrode remained *in situ*; this is because it cannot be ruled out that, together with the electrode, fibrous tissue is additionally translocated or even extracted from the scala. Potential future studies could involve implanting additional animals, focusing only on investigation of alginate coating stability. Alternatively, the electrode array could be left *in situ*, and parts of the bony cochlear wall removed in order to investigate the electrode and its coating *in situ*, with subsequent dehydration for histological processing.

Fibrosis

The amount of fibrosis around the implanted arrays did not differ between the experimental groups, suggesting that the alginate – whether in the form of coating or an injection – does not increase the activation of the host immune system. It has previously been shown that the UHV-alginate is biocompatible (Schneider et al., 2005; Zimmermann et al., 2007), and here we show for the first time that this is also the case for application in the inner ear.

Electrode Impedance – Effect of Coating

Electrode impedance of uncoated contacts was increased in the MSC medium compared with PBS. These measurements were started in PBS, with three consecutive measurements performed;

only afterwards were impedance levels measured in the MSC medium, again three times. Electrode impedance decreases after activation in an animal model (Wilk et al., 2016) and in humans (Hu et al., 2017). Therefore, the impedances were expected to be lower in the MSC medium than in PBS. Since the medium is protein-rich, these proteins may have attached to the contact surface and increased impedance levels. Since the coated electrodes in the MSC medium had the same impedance levels as uncoated electrodes in PBS, it can be speculated that, with this coating, protein attachment was prevented, so that it positively influenced electrode impedance. After implantation, all impedance levels of the coated electrodes were significantly higher; this finding was expected, since it is well known that electrode impedance rises after implantation (Paasche et al., 2006) compared with impedance measured *ex vivo*.

Electrode Impedance – Effect of Experimental Condition Over Time

Electrode impedance levels were measured weekly in all implanted ears over the experimental period of 28 days (**Supplementary Figure S1**). Changes in impedance over time did not differ between groups, suggesting that where the coating or scala tympani fills with the alginate-MSC matrix, this may not have a negative effect on electrode impedance.

CONCLUSION

Coating of the electrode array with BDNF-producing mesenchymal stem cells embedded in UHV-alginate has the effect of protecting spiral ganglion neurons from degeneration in systemically deafened animals. Such coating is superior to alginate-MSC injection, which did not affect the SGNs and which resulted in increased hearing loss compared with cochlear implantation alone in normal-hearing animals.

Further research and development are needed before this concept can be tested in clinical trials. Additional studies are needed into how long MSCs survive *in vivo* in the alginate coating, and into whether the neuroprotective effect can be sustained for longer periods. Additionally, chronic electrical stimulation should simultaneously be applied: to mimic the situation in CI patients, and to investigate the influence of electrical stimulation on MSCs, coating stability and the combined effect of electrical stimulation and MSC-produced BDNF on SGNs.

ETHICS STATEMENT

All animal procedures were performed in accordance with the European Council directive (2010/63/EU). The protocol was approved by the Local Institutional Animal Care and Research Advisory Committee (IACUC) and permitted by the local authority [Lower Saxony State Office for Consumer Protection, Food Safety, and Animal Welfare Service (LAVES); approval number 17/2396].

AUTHOR CONTRIBUTIONS

VS, TL, and AHo conceived and designed the experiments. MG and AS produced the UHV-alginate used in the study. AHo and AHa isolation, expansion, transduction, and characterization of MSCs. VS, JS, and PH performed *in vivo* experiments. VS, JS, and CP participated in the processing of the cochleae for histology. CP blinded to the different groups and performed the CLSM and analyzed these data. PH designed and implemented software for AABR analysis. VS and PH analyzed the AABR data. JS impedance data. VS and JS wrote the first version of the manuscript. All authors participated in the reviewing and rewriting of the manuscript. All authors read and approved the final manuscript.

ACKNOWLEDGMENTS

The authors would like to thank Roland Hessler at MED-EL, Innsbruck, Austria, for providing the electrode arrays.

REFERENCES

Aaron, R. K., Boyan, B. D., Ciombor, D. M., Schwartz, Z., and Simon, B. J. (2004). Stimulation of growth factor synthesis by electric and electromagnetic fields. *Clin. Orthop. Relat Res.* 419, 30–37. doi: 10.1097/00003086-200402000-00006

Agterberg, M. J., Versnel, H., de Groot, J. C., van den Broek, M., and Klis, S. F. (2010). Chronic electrical stimulation does not prevent spiral ganglion cell degeneration in deafened guinea pigs. *Hear. Res.* 269, 169–179. doi: 10.1016/j.heares.2010.06.015

Agterberg, M. J., Versnel, H., van Dijk, L. M., de Groot, J. C., and Klis, S. F. (2009). Enhanced survival of spiral ganglion cells after cessation of treatment with brain-derived neurotrophic factor in deafened guinea pigs. *J. Assoc. Res. Otolaryngol.* 10, 355–367. doi: 10.1007/s10162-009-0170-2

Araki, S., Kawano, A., Seldon, L., Shepherd, R. K., Funasaka, S., and Clark, G. M. (1998). Effects of chronic electrical stimulation on spiral ganglion neuron survival and size in deafened kittens. *Laryngoscope* 108, 687–695. doi: 10.1097/00005537-199805000-00012

Bajpai, S. K., and Sharma, S. (2004). Investigation of swelling/degradation behaviour of alginate beads crosslinked with Ca2+ and Ba2+ ions. *React. Funct. Polym.* 59, 129–140. doi: 10.1016/j.reactfunctpolym.2004.01.002

Brown, J. N., Miller, J. M., Altschuler, R. A., and Nuttall, A. L. (1993). Osmotic pump implant for chronic infusion of drugs into the inner ear. *Hear. Res.* 70, 167–172. doi: 10.1016/0378-5955(93)90155-t

David, R. M., and Doherty, A. T. (2017). Viral vectors: the road to reducing genotoxicity. *Toxicol. Sci.* 155, 315–325. doi: 10.1093/toxsci/kfw220

Ehrhart, F., Mettler, E., Bose, T., Weber, M. M., Vasquez, J. A., and Zimmermann, H. (2013). Biocompatible coating of encapsulated cells using ionotropic gelation. *PLoS One* 8:e73498. doi: 10.1371/journal.pone.0073498

El Kechai, N., Agnely, F., Mamelle, E., Nguyen, Y., Ferrary, E., and Bochot, A. (2015). Recent advances in local drug delivery to the inner ear. *Int. J. Pharm.* 494, 83–101. doi: 10.1016/j.ijpharm.2015.08.015

Fransson, A., Tornoe, J., Wahlberg, L. U., and Ulfendahl, M. (2018). The feasibility of an encapsulated cell approach in an animal deafness model. *J. Control. Release* 270, 275–281. doi: 10.1016/j.jconrel.2017.12.014

Geschwind, M. D., Hartnick, C. J., Liu, W., Amat, J., Van De Water, T. R., and Federoff, H. J. (1996). Defective HSV-1 vector expressing BDNF in auditory ganglia elicits neurite outgrowth: model for treatment of neuron loss following cochlear degeneration. *Hum. Gene Ther.* 7, 173–182. doi: 10.1089/hum.1996.7.2-173

Gillespie, L. N., Clark, G. M., Bartlett, P. F., and Marzella, P. L. (2003). BDNF-induced survival of auditory neurons in vivo: cessation of treatment leads to accelerated loss of survival effects. *J. Neurosci. Res.* 71, 785–790. doi: 10.1002/jnr.10542

Gillespie, L. N., and Shepherd, R. K. (2005). Clinical application of neurotrophic factors: the potential for primary auditory neuron protection. *Eur. J. Neurosci.* 22, 2123–2133. doi: 10.1111/j.1460-9568.2005.04430.x

Gillespie, L. N., Zanin, M. P., and Shepherd, R. K. (2015). Cell-based neurotrophin treatment supports long-term auditory neuron survival in the deaf guinea pig. *J. Control. Release* 198, 26–34. doi: 10.1016/j.jconrel.2014.11.026

Hansen, M. R., Zha, X. M., Bok, J., and Green, S. H. (2001). Multiple distinct signal pathways, including an autocrine neurotrophic mechanism, contribute to the survival-promoting effect of depolarization on spiral ganglion neurons in vitro. *J. Neurosci.* 21, 2256–2267. doi: 10.1523/jneurosci.21-07-02256.2001

Hao, J., and Li, S. K. (2019). Inner ear drug delivery: recent advances, challenges, and perspective. *Eur. J. Pharm. Sci.* 126, 82–92. doi: 10.1016/j.ejps.2018.05.020

Havenith, S., Versnel, H., Agterberg, M. J., de Groot, J. C., Sedee, R. J., Grolman, W., et al. (2010). Spiral ganglion cell survival after round window membrane application of brain-derived neurotrophic factor using gelfoam as carrier. *Hear. Res.* 272, 168–177. doi: 10.1016/j.heares.2010.10.003

Hegarty, J. L., Kay, A. R., and Green, S. H. (1997). Trophic support of cultured spiral ganglion neurons by depolarization exceeds and is additive with that by neurotrophins or cAMP and requires elevation of [Ca2+]i within a set range. *J. Neurosci.* 17, 1959–1970. doi: 10.1523/jneurosci.17-06-01959.1997

Helbig, S., Adel, Y., Leinung, M., Stover, T., Baumann, U., and Weissgerber, T. (2018). Hearing preservation outcomes after cochlear implantation depending on the angle of insertion: indication for electric or electric-acoustic stimulation. *Otol. Neurotol.* 39, 834–841. doi: 10.1097/MAO.0000000000001862

Hu, H.-C., Chen, J. K.-C., Tsai, C.-M., Chen, H.-Y., Tung, T.-H., and Li, L. P. (2017). Evolution of impedance field telemetry after one day of activation in cochlear implant recipients. *PLoS One* 12:e0173367. doi: 10.1371/journal.pone.0173367

Hütten, M., Dhanasingh, A., Hessler, R., Stöver, T., Esser, K. H., Möller, M., et al. (2014). In vitro and in vivo evaluation of a hydrogel reservoir as a continuous drug delivery system for inner ear treatment. *PLoS One* 9:e104564. doi: 10.1371/journal.pone.0104564

Hütten, M., Ehrhart, F., Zimmermann, H., Reich, U., Esser, K. H., Lenarz, T., et al. (2013). UHV-alginate as matrix for neurotrophic factor producing cells - a novel biomaterial for cochlear implant optimization to preserve inner ear neurons from degeneration. *Otol. Neurotol.* 34, 1127–1133. doi: 10.1097/MAO.0b013e3182804949

Kanzaki, S., Stover, T., Kawamoto, K., Prieskorn, D. M., Altschuler, R. A., Miller, J. M., et al. (2002). Glial cell line-derived neurotrophic factor and chronic electrical stimulation prevent VIII cranial nerve degeneration following denervation. *J. Comp. Neurol.* 454, 350–360. doi: 10.1002/cne.10480

Konerding, W. S., Janssen, H., Hubka, P., Tornoe, J., Mistrik, P., Wahlberg, L., et al. (2017). Encapsulated cell device approach for combined electrical stimulation and neurotrophic treatment of the deaf cochlea. *Hear. Res.* 350, 110–121. doi: 10.1016/j.heares.2017.04.013

Leake, P. A., Hradek, G. T., Hetherington, A. M., and Stakhovskaya, O. (2011). Brain-derived neurotrophic factor promotes cochlear spiral ganglion cell survival and function in deafened, developing cats. *J. Comp. Neurol.* 519, 1526–1545. doi: 10.1002/cne.22582

Leake, P. A., Hradek, G. T., and Snyder, R. L. (1999). Chronic electrical stimulation by a cochlear implant promotes survival of spiral ganglion neurons after neonatal deafness. *J. Comp. Neurol.* 412, 543–562. doi: 10.1002/(SICI)1096-9861(19991004)412:4<543::AID-CNE1>3.0.CO;2-3

Leake, P. A., Stakhovskaya, O., Hetherington, A., Rebscher, S. J., and Bonham, B. (2013). Effects of brain-derived neurotrophic factor (BDNF) and electrical stimulation on survival and function of cochlear spiral ganglion neurons in deafened, developing cats. *J. Assoc. Res. Otolaryngol.* 14, 187–211. doi: 10.1007/s10162-013-0372-5

Lenarz, T., and Scheper, V. (2015). "Preserving residual hearing in cochlear implant patients," in *Free Radicals in ENT Pathology*, eds J. Miller, C. G. Le Prell, and L. Rybak (New York, NY: Humana Press), 423–443.

Li, L., Parkins, C. W., and Webster, D. B. (1999). Does electrical stimulation of deaf cochleae prevent spiral ganglion degeneration? *Hear. Res.* 133, 27–39. doi: 10.1016/s0378-5955(99)00043-x

Liu, W., Edin, F., Atturo, F., Rieger, G., Lowenheim, H., Senn, P., et al. (2015). The pre- and post-somatic segments of the human type I spiral ganglion neurons - structural and functional considerations related to cochlear implantation. *Neuroscience* 284, 470–482. doi: 10.1016/j.neuroscience.2014.09.059

Mäder, K., Lehner, E., Liebau, A., and Plontke, S. K. (2018). Controlled drug release to the inner ear: concepts, materials, mechanisms, and performance. *Hear. Res.* 368, 49–66. doi: 10.1016/j.heares.2018.03.006

Maruyama, J., Miller, J. M., and Ulfendahl, M. (2008). Glial cell line-derived neurotrophic factor and antioxidants preserve the electrical responsiveness of the spiral ganglion neurons after experimentally induced deafness. *Neurobiol. Dis.* 29, 14–21. doi: 10.1016/j.nbd.2007.07.026

McGuinness, S. L., and Shepherd, R. K. (2005). Exogenous BDNF rescues rat spiral ganglion neurons in vivo. *Otol. Neurotol.* 26, 1064–1072. doi: 10.1097/01.mao.0000185063.20081.50

Meyer, H., Stover, T., Fouchet, F., Bastiat, G., Saulnier, P., Baumer, W., et al. (2012). Lipidic nanocapsule drug delivery: neuronal protection for cochlear implant optimization. *Int. J. Nanomed.* 7, 2449–2464. doi: 10.2147/IJN.S29712

Miller, J. M., Chi, D. H., O'Keeffe, L. J., Kruszka, P., Raphael, Y., and Altschuler, R. A. (1997). Neurotrophins can enhance spiral ganglion cell survival after inner hair cell loss. *Int. J. Dev. Neurosci.* 15, 631–643. doi: 10.1016/s0736-5748(96)00117-7

Miller, J. M., Le Prell, C. G., Prieskorn, D. M., Wys, N. L., and Altschuler, R. A. (2007). Delayed neurotrophin treatment following deafness rescues spiral ganglion cells from death and promotes regrowth of auditory nerve peripheral processes: effects of brain-derived neurotrophic factor and fibroblast growth factor. *J. Neurosci. Res.* 85, 1959–1969. doi: 10.1002/jnr.21320

Mitchell, A., Miller, J. M., Finger, P. A., Heller, J. W., Raphael, Y., and Altschuler, R. A. (1997). Effects of chronic high-rate electrical stimulation on the cochlea and eighth nerve in the deafened guinea pig. *Hear. Res.* 105, 30–43. doi: 10.1016/s0378-5955(96)00202-x

Nguyen, K., Kempfle, J. S., Jung, D. H., and McKenna, C. E. (2017). Recent advances in therapeutics and drug delivery for the treatment of inner ear diseases: a patent review (2011-2015). *Expert. Opin. Ther. Patents* 27, 191–202. doi: 10.1080/13543776.2017.1252751

NIDCD (2017). *Cochlear Implants, Vol. Publication No. 00-4798.* Bethesda, MD: National Institute of Health/National Institute on Deafness and Other Communication Disorders.

Paasche, G., Bockel, F., Tasche, C., Lesinski-Schiedat, A., and Lenarz, T. (2006). Changes of postoperative impedances in cochlear implant patients: the short-term effects of modified electrode surfaces and intracochlear corticosteroids. *Otol. Neurotol.* 27, 639–647. doi: 10.1097/01.mao.0000227662.88840.61

Pettingill, L. N., Minter, R. L., and Shepherd, R. K. (2008). Schwann cells genetically modified to express neurotrophins promote spiral ganglion neuron survival in vitro. *Neuroscience* 152, 821–828. doi: 10.1016/j.neuroscience.2007.11.057

Pettingill, L. N., Wise, A. K., Geaney, M. S., and Shepherd, R. K. (2011). Enhanced auditory neuron survival following cell-based BDNF treatment in the deaf guinea pig. *PLoS One* 6:e18733. doi: 10.1371/journal.pone.0018733

Prenzler, N. K., Salcher, R., Timm, M., Gaertner, L., Lenarz, T., and Warnecke, A. (2018). Intracochlear administration of steroids with a catheter during human cochlear implantation: a safety and feasibility study. *Drug Deliv. Transl. Res.* 8, 1191–1199. doi: 10.1007/s13346-018-0539-z

Ramekers, D., Versnel, H., Strahl, S. B., Klis, S. F. L., and Grolman, W. (2015). Temporary neurotrophin treatment prevents deafness-induced auditory nerve degeneration and preserves function. *J. Neurosci.* 35, 12331–12345. doi: 10.1523/JNEUROSCI.0096-15.2015

Reichel, C. (2011). The overlooked difference between human endogenous and recombinant erythropoietins and its implication for sports drug testing and pharmaceutical drug design. *Drug Test. Anal.* 3, 883–891. doi: 10.1002/dta.388

Sacheli, R., Delacroix, L., Vandenackerveken, P., Nguyen, L., and Malgrange, B. (2013). Gene transfer in inner ear cells: a challenging race. *Gene Ther.* 20, 237–247. doi: 10.1038/gt.2012.51

Salt, A. N., and Plontke, S. K. (2018). Pharmacokinetic principles in the inner ear: influence of drug properties on intratympanic applications. *Hear. Res.* 368, 28–40. doi: 10.1016/j.heares.2018.03.002

Scheper, V., Hessler, R., Hütten, M., Wilk, M., Jolly, C., Lenarz, T., et al. (2017). Local inner ear application of dexamethasone in cochlear implant models is safe for auditory neurons and increases the neuroprotective effect of chronic electrical stimulation. *PLoS One* 12:e0183820. doi: 10.1371/journal.pone.0183820

Scheper, V., Paasche, G., Miller, J. M., Warnecke, A., Berkingali, N., Lenarz, T., et al. (2009). Effects of delayed treatment with combined GDNF and continuous electrical stimulation on spiral ganglion cell survival in deafened guinea pigs. *J. Neurosci. Res.* 87, 1389–1399. doi: 10.1002/jnr.21964

Schneider, S., Feilen, P. J., Brunnenmeier, F., Minnemann, T., Zimmermann, H., Zimmermann, U., et al. (2005). Long-term graft function of adult rat and human islets encapsulated in novel alginate-based microcapsules after transplantation in immunocompetent diabetic mice. *Diabetes Metab. Res. Rev* 54, 687–693. doi: 10.2337/diabetes.54.3.687

Schwieger, J., Hügl, S., Hamm, A., Lenarz, T., Hoffmann, A., Rau, T., et al. (2018). *BDNF-Producing Human Mesenchymal Stem Cells in An Alginate-Matrix: Neuroprotection and Cochlear Implant Coating Stability in Vitro*. Poster presented at the Laryngo-Rhino-Otologie Vol. 97. Thieme, Lübeck, 382.

Seyyedi, M., Viana, L. M., and Nadol, J. B. (2014). Within-subject comparison of word recognition and spiral ganglion cell count in bilateral cochlear implant recipients. *Otol. Neurotol.* 35, 1446–1450. doi: 10.1097/MAO.0000000000000443

Shepherd, R. K., Carter, P. M., Enke, Y. L., Wise, A. K., and Fallon, J. B. (2018). Chronic intracochlear electrical stimulation at high charge densities results in platinum dissolution but not neural loss or functional changes in vivo. *J. Neural Eng.* 16:026009. doi: 10.1088/1741-2552/aaf66b

Skinner, S. J., Geaney, M. S., Lin, H., Muzina, M., Anal, A. K., Elliott, R. B., et al. (2009). Encapsulated living choroid plexus cells: potential long-term treatments for central nervous system disease and trauma. *J. Neural Eng.* 6:065001. doi: 10.1088/1741-2560/6/6/065001

Versnel, H., Agterberg, M. J., de Groot, J. C., Smoorenburg, G. F., and Klis, S. F. (2007). Time course of cochlear electrophysiology and morphology after combined administration of kanamycin and furosemide. *Hear. Res.* 231, 1–12. doi: 10.1016/j.heares.2007.03.003

Wang, X., Dellamary, L., Fernandez, R., Ye, Q., LeBel, C., and Piu, F. (2011). Principles of inner ear sustained release following intratympanic administration. *Laryngoscope* 121, 385–391. doi: 10.1002/lary.21370

Warnecke, A., Sasse, S., Wenzel, G. I., Hoffmann, A., Gross, G., Paasche, G., et al. (2012). Stable release of BDNF from the fibroblast cell line NIH3T3 grown on silicone elastomers enhances survival of spiral ganglion cells in vitro and in vivo. *Hear. Res.* 289, 86–97. doi: 10.1016/j.heares.2012.04.007

Wefstaedt, P., Scheper, V., Lenarz, T., and Stover, T. (2005). Brain-derived neurotrophic factor/glial cell line-derived neurotrophic factor survival effects on auditory neurons are not limited by dexamethasone. *Neuroreport* 16, 2011–2014. doi: 10.1097/00001756-200512190-00008

Whitlon, D. S. (2017). Drug discovery for hearing loss: phenotypic screening of chemical compounds on primary cultures of the spiral ganglion. *Hear. Res.* 349, 177–181. doi: 10.1016/j.heares.2016.07.019

Wilk, M., Hessler, R., Mugridge, K., Jolly, C., Fehr, M., Lenarz, T., et al. (2016). Impedance changes and fibrous tissue growth after cochlear implantation are correlated and can be reduced using a dexamethasone eluting electrode. *PLoS One* 11:e0147552. doi: 10.1371/journal.pone.0147552

Wise, A. K., Fallon, J. B., Neil, A. J., Pettingill, L. N., Geaney, M. S., Skinner, S. J., et al. (2011). Combining cell-based therapies and neural prostheses to promote neural survival. *Neurotherapeutics* 8, 774–787. doi: 10.1007/s13311-011-0070-0

Wrzeszcz, A., Reuter, G., Nolte, I., Lenarz, T., and Scheper, V. (2013). Spiral ganglion neuron quantification in the guinea pig cochlea using confocal laser scanning microscopy compared to embedding methods. *Hear. Res.* 306, 145–155. doi: 10.1016/j.heares.2013.08.002

Zilberstein, Y., Liberman, M. C., and Corfas, G. (2012). Inner hair cells are not required for survival of spiral ganglion neurons in the adult cochlea. *J. Neurosci.* 32, 405–410. doi: 10.1523/JNEUROSCI.4678-11.2012

Zimmermann, H., Shirley, S. G., and Zimmermann, U. (2007). Alginate-based encapsulation of cells: past, present, and future. *Curr. Diab. Rep.* 7, 314–320. doi: 10.1007/s11892-007-0051-1

19

Comparison of the Pharmacokinetic Properties of Triamcinolone and Dexamethasone for Local Therapy of the Inner Ear

Alec Nicholas Salt[1], Jared James Hartsock[1], Jennifer Hou[2] and Fabrice Piu[2]*

[1] *Department of Otolaryngology, Washington University School of Medicine, St. Louis, MO, United States,*

[2] *Otonomy Inc., San Diego, CA, United States*

***Correspondence:**
Alec Nicholas Salt
alecsalt@wustl.edu*

Some forms of triamcinolone may provide alternate options for local therapy of the inner ear in addition to the steroids currently in use. We compared the perilymph pharmacokinetics of triamcinolone-acetonide, triamcinolone, and dexamethasone, each delivered as crystalline suspensions to guinea pigs. Triamcinolone-acetonide is a widely used form of the drug with molecular properties that allow it to readily permeate biological barriers. When applied intratympanically triamcinolone-acetonide entered perilymph rapidly but was also found to be eliminated rapidly from perilymph. The rapid rate of elimination severely limits the apical distribution of the drug when applied locally, making it unsuitable for use in the ear. In contrast, triamcinolone, rather than triamcinolone-acetonide, is a more polar form of the molecule, with higher aqueous solubility but calculated to pass less-readily through biological boundaries. Perilymph concentrations generated with intratympanic applications of triamcinolone were comparable to those with triamcinolone-acetonide but elimination measurements showed that triamcinolone was retained in perilymph longer than triamcinolone-acetonide or dexamethasone. The slower elimination is projected to result in improved distribution of triamcinolone toward the cochlear apex, potentially allowing higher drug levels to reach the speech frequency regions of the human ear. These measurements show that triamcinolone could constitute an attractive additional treatment option for local therapy of auditory disorders.

Keywords: intratympanic therapy, Meniere's disease, idiopathic sudden sensorineural hearing loss, dexamethasone, triamcinolone, triamcinolone acetonide

INTRODUCTION

Treatment of the inner ear with a locally applied steroid has become a widely accepted therapy for Meniere's disease, idiopathic sudden sensorineural hearing loss and immune-related hearing loss. The choice of which steroid and what concentration to use has largely been established empirically based except for a limited few pioneering studies where drug kinetics (dexamethasone and methylprednisolone) were compared in animals (Parnes et al., 1999) and in humans (Bird et al., 2007, 2011). Currently, steroids that have been used for local inner ear therapy

Abbreviations: LSCC, lateral semi-circular canal; RW, round window; ST, scala tympani; SV, scala vestibuli.

include dexamethasone-phosphate (Liebau et al., 2017); dexamethasone (Lambert et al., 2016); methylprednisolone-succinate (Rauch et al., 2011; Liebau et al., 2017); and triamcinolone-acetonide (Jumaily et al., 2017; Dahm et al., 2019).

We recently reported that dexamethasone-phosphate, the most common form of dexamethasone used for local treatment of the ear, has properties that make it quite unsuitable for local therapy of the ear (Salt et al., 2018). The polar phosphate group that makes the drug more soluble also makes this form of the drug substantially less permeable though the RW membrane than native dexamethasone, limiting the amount entering. Within the ear it is then metabolized to the active form, dexamethasone, which is highly permeable through the blood-labyrinth barrier and is rapidly lost from perilymph. The high rate of dexamethasone elimination limits how far the drug spreads apically along the ear (Plontke et al., 2008; Salt et al., 2018). As a result, concentrations reaching the speech frequency regions of the human are calculated to be low (Liebau et al., 2017). Large gradients along the ear will persist even when higher doses of dexamethasone-phosphate are given (Alexander et al., 2015).

A second problem exists when the steroid is applied to the middle ear as a solution. For dexamethasone-phosphate, loss from the middle ear occurs rapidly. Measurement of the solution remaining in the RW niche of guinea pigs demonstrated a decline in concentration with a half-time of approximately 28 min (Salt et al., 2018). This rate occurred in anesthetized recumbent animals which did not lose volume through the Eustachian tube. The rate of loss is likely to be even higher in the conscious animal in normal posture in which fluid in the middle ear is cleared by the ciliated ventral epithelium to the Eustachian tube (Thompson and Tucker, 2013). The residence time of drug in the middle ear has a major influence on the perilymph concentration of drug achieved (Salt and Plontke, 2005). A longer drug residence time in the middle ear can be achieved by delivering the drug as a suspension. Measurable perilymph concentrations of dexamethasone were achieved for over 3 months after intratympanic application of dexamethasone suspension (Wang et al., 2009; Piu et al., 2011). Both triamcinolone-acetonide and triamcinolone exhibit low aqueous solubility making them suitable for delivery to the middle ear as a suspension. We therefore evaluated the pharmacokinetics of different formulations these two compounds in perilymph and compared them with comparable measurements with dexamethasone which were previously reported (Salt et al., 2012, 2018).

The ability of molecules to pass through biological barriers such as the blood-brain barrier and the gut has been shown to depend on their lipid solubility and polar properties (Egan et al., 2000; Daina and Zoete, 2016). A plot of lipid solubility (WLOGP) against the polar surface area (TPSA) shows that molecules with properties within a specific range can pass certain biological boundaries, as shown in **Figure 1**. The gut is permeable to molecules within a specific range (gray ellipse) while the blood-brain barrier is more restrictive, only permeable to molecules within a more limited range (yellow ellipse) (Daina and Zoete, 2016). The degree to which inner ear barriers, specifically those between the middle ear and perilymph and between perilymph and blood, compare to these better-studied boundaries remains to be determined. Nevertheless, molecules with properties located toward the lower right side of the plot (large, hydrophilic, and polar) are expected to pass through membranous biological boundaries less easily than molecules located toward upper left side of the plot (small, lipophilic, and non-polar). The plot shows the molecular properties calculated by SwissADME[1] (Daina et al., 2017) for triamcinolone-acetonide and triamcinolone, compared to those of dexamethasone-phosphate and dexamethasone. Triamcinolone-acetonide is more lipophilic than dexamethasone while triamcinolone is more polar and less lipophilic.

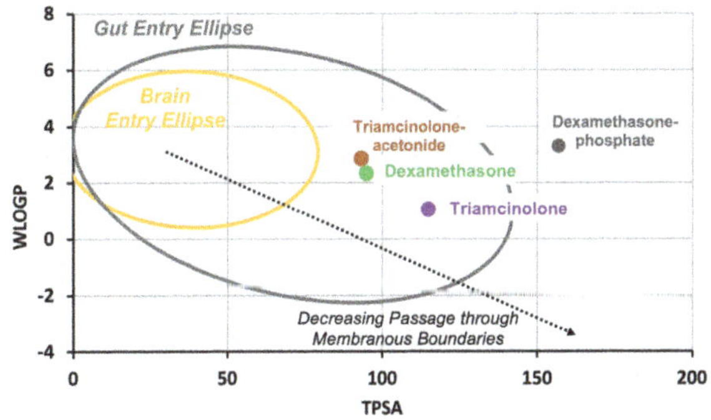

FIGURE 1 | Molecular properties compared for common forms of dexamethasone and triamcinolone. WLOGP is a calculated index of lipid solubility for the drug and TPSA represents the surface area of the molecule occupied by polar groups. Large, polar, hydrophilic molecules (lower right of plot) typically have high aqueous solubility but do not readily pass through membranous biological boundaries. In contrast, small, non-polar lipophilic molecules (upper left of plot) pass more readily through biological boundaries but have lower aqueous solubility. The yellow ellipse indicates the range of properties for molecules that pass through the blood brain barrier and the gray ellipse indicates the range of properties for molecules that pass into the body through the gut (Daina and Zoete, 2016). Dexamethasone-phosphate is larger and more polar than dexamethasone, giving it higher aqueous solubility but limiting passage through biological boundaries. Triamcinolone-acetonide is calculated to pass boundaries more readily than dexamethasone while triamcinolone is calculated to pass less readily.

MATERIALS AND METHODS

Animals

The study used 32 pigmented, NIH-strain guinea pigs weighing 400–600 g. Experiments were performed under protocol 20160053, approved by the Institutional Animal Care and Use Committee of Washington University. Animal use followed policies in accordance with the United States Department of Agriculture and National Institutes of Health guidelines for the handling and use of laboratory animals.

In non-recovery perilymph sampling experiments, animals were first anesthetized with 100 mg/kg sodium thiobutabarbital (Inactin, Sigma, St. Louis, MO, United States). A tracheal cannula was inserted and the animal was maintained on 0.8 to 1.2% isoflurane in oxygen using a mechanical ventilator. End-tidal CO_2 level was maintained close to 5% by adjustment

[1] http://www.swissadme.ch

of the tidal volume of the ventilator. Heart rate and oxygen saturation were monitored throughout the experiment. Core body temperature was maintained at 38°C with a thermistor-controlled heating blanket.

The ear was exposed by opening the lateral portion of the auditory bulla. This gave access to the LSCC and to the RW niche. Drug solutions were either applied to the RW niche or injected into perilymph of the lateral SCC. In all experiments, perilymph was sampled from the lateral SCC. In some experiments as detailed below, triamcinolone-acetonide or triamcinolone suspension was applied intratympanically as a recovery procedure, followed by perilymph sampling 1 or 3 days afterward.

Drug Delivery: Application to the Round Window Niche

In non-recovery experiments, the lateral bulla was opened and suspensions of triamcinolone-acetonide or triamcinolone were applied to the RW niche with a hand-held micropipetter. A 20 μL volume was applied, sufficient to fill the entire niche and stapes area of the guinea pig, with excess overflowing toward the anterior bulla.

Drug formulations were:

(1) Triamcinolone-acetonide 40 mg/mL injectable crystalline suspension (Kenalog-40: Bristol-Myers Squibb, Princeton, NJ, United States). Kenalog-40 also contains 0.99% benzyl alcohol as a preservative (in higher concentrations shown to increase permeability of the RW membrane and stapes; Li et al., 2018) and 0.04% polysorbate-80 (Tween-80), an emulsifier. This formulation was applied to two animals. The aqueous solubility of triamcinolone-acetonide is reported to be 42 μg/mL (Drugbank)[2]. We measured aqueous solubility by taking a 1:1 dilution of the supernatant over the suspension after it had settled for at least 24 h. The concentration in the supernatant, corrected for dilution, was 26.5 μg/mL; *SD* 1.7; $n = 4$.

(2) Triamcinolone-acetonide (Spectrum Chemicals, New Brunswick, NJ, United States) 60 mg/mL crystalline suspension in PBS with 17% Poloxamer 407 (Spectrum Chemicals). This formulation was applied to five animals.

(3) Triamcinolone (Sigma, St. Louis, MO, United States) 40 mg/mL suspension in PBS with 17% Poloxamer 407. This formulation was applied to 12 animals. Aqueous solubility of triamcinolone is reported to be 80 μg/mL (PubChem)[3]. The concentration of the supernatant over the suspension was measured to be 81.05 μg/mL; *SD* 29.4; $n = 4$).

Drug Delivery: Intratympanic Injection

The procedure for intratympanic injection of drug suspension in poloxamer gel is described elsewhere in detail (Salt et al., 2011). The guinea pig was anesthetized with isoflurane (0.8–1.2% in oxygen) and buprenorphine (0.05 mg/kg) given for analgesia. The head of the animal was positioned against a foam pad on a head-holder with its nose vertically upward, held in position by a Velcro strap. A speculum was placed in the right ear, allowing the tympanic membrane to be visualized. A hypodermic needle held in a manipulator was used to make two perforations in the tympanic membrane, one anterior to the umbo as a vent and a second posterior to the umbo for injection. Drug injection through the latter perforation was performed from a blunt-tipped 26G needle, bent 90 degrees and attached to a syringe mounted on a syringe pump (Ultrapump; World Precision Instruments, Sarasota, FL).

Perilymph was sampled from the LSCC either 1 or 3 days after the application of the drug formulation. Triamcinolone-acetonide suspension was applied in three animals followed by perilymph sampling 1 day later. Triamcinolone suspension was applied in 6 animals followed by perlilymph sampling 1 day ($n = 4$) or 3 days ($n = 2$) later.

Drug Delivery: Injection Into the Lateral Semi-Circular Canal

The rates of elimination of triamcinolone or triamcinolone-acetonide from perilymph were measured by first loading the perilymph with drug solution as detailed in Salt et al. (2012). At varying times after application (zero, 1 or 2 h) perilymph was sampled from the LSCC for analysis to establish how much drug remained in perilymph. The injected solution consisted of the supernatant over the suspension as described above, diluted 1:1 in a bicarbonate-buffered artificial perilymph. Triamcinolone-acetonide solution was applied in four animals and triamcinolone solution was applied in 12 animals.

Sequential Sampling From the Lateral Semi-Circular Canal

Sequential sampling of perilymph makes it possible to quantify drug concentration gradients along the perilymphatic spaces (Mynatt et al., 2006; Salt et al., 2012). The LSCC was prepared for perilymph sampling by first removing the mucosa and cleaning the bone and with saline and cotton swabs. The bone overlying the canal was thinned with a dental burr and a thin layer of cyanoacrylate glue (Permabond 101; Permabond, Pottstown, PA, United States) was applied. A covering of two-part silicone adhesive (Kwik-Cast, World Precision Instruments, Sarasota, FL, United States), was applied to this surface, built up at the edges to form a hydrophobic cup. This allowed perilymph to be collected free of contamination of drug solution in the rest of the bulla.

Sampling commenced by making a 30–40 μm fenestration in the silicone-coated canal wall with a 30° House stapes pick (N1705 80, Bausch and Lomb Inc.). The perilymph emerging from the perforation accumulated on the hydrophobic surface of the silicone where it was collected in hand-held, blunt tipped capillary tubes (VWR 53432-706), marked to a nominal volume of 1 μL. Twenty individual samples were collected from each animal, each taking 1–2 min. The exact volume of each sample was determined by measuring the sample length under a calibrated dissecting microscope. The 20 samples were paired consecutively and each pair added to 50 μL of 1:1 methanol:water diluent, resulting in 10 diluted samples, each containing 2 μL perilymph and 50 μL diluent. Samples were stored frozen at −80°C until analysis.

[2]https://www.drugbank.ca/

[3]http://pubchem.ncbi.nlm.nih.gov

Analysis of Samples

Samples were analyzed using high-pressure liquid chromatography combined with mass spectrometry detection (Wang et al., 2011). HPLC operators were blinded to the experimental conditions and to the origin of the samples. The LLOQ for triamcinolone was 0.2–1 ng/mL and the LLOQ for triamcinolone-acetonide was 0.28 ng/mL. In experiments where triamcinolone was applied to the ear only triamcinolone was measured. In experiments where triamcinolone acetonide was applied, both triamcinolone-acetonide and triamcinolone were measured.

Quantitative Simulation of Sequential Sample Data

A computer program simulating the inner ear fluids (which can be downloaded from)[4] can be set to replicate all aspects of the experiments performed in this study in great detail. For intratympanic applications, calculations include known entry sites from the middle ear into perilymph of the guinea pig, including the RW, stapes and through the thin bone at the apex. Drug distribution through the fluid and tissue spaces of the entire inner ear is calculated based on defined diffusion coefficients and elimination rates. Simulation of drug injections into the lateral SCC and the sequential sampling procedure takes into account the induced volume flows. In the perilymph sampling procedure, the specific volumes and collection times for each of the samples are replicated. Rates of elimination were adjusted to best fit the calculated sample concentrations from the model to the measured sample data, allowing the kinetic properties of the drugs to be compared quantitatively.

RESULTS

Triamcinolone-Acetonide Kinetics

Triamcinolone-acetonide suspension was applied to the RW niche for 60 min before perilymph was sampled. **Figure 2** shows the perilymph levels measured when the triamcinolone-acetonide suspension was applied as a liquid (green) or gel (blue) formulation. Perilymph concentrations were found to be lower than found in previous studies with a dexamethasone suspension (red dashed line; from Salt et al., 2018). It is important to note that these are results using dexamethasone suspension, which differ considerably from the commonly used solution of dexamethasone-phosphate. The average across all 40 samples for triamcinolone-acetonide was 0.71 ug/mL compared to 2.16 ug/mL for dexamethasone. Although perilymph triamcinolone-acetonide concentrations were lower than those for dexamethasone by a factor of 3.1×, this is largely explained by differences in the middle ear concentration of the two drugs. Triamcinolone-acetonide has 3.6× lower aqueous solubility (26.5 ug/mL) compared to dexamethasone (94.2 ug/mL), so there will be a lower concentration driving entry into perilymph. Although both triamcinolone and triamcinolone-acetonide were measured in the samples, the vast majority of the drug was present in perilymph as triamcinolone-acetonide. In 37 of the 40 samples triamcinolone concentration was unmeasurable, but in three of the samples a low concentration of triamcinolone was present, averaging just 1.4% of the total drug concentration.

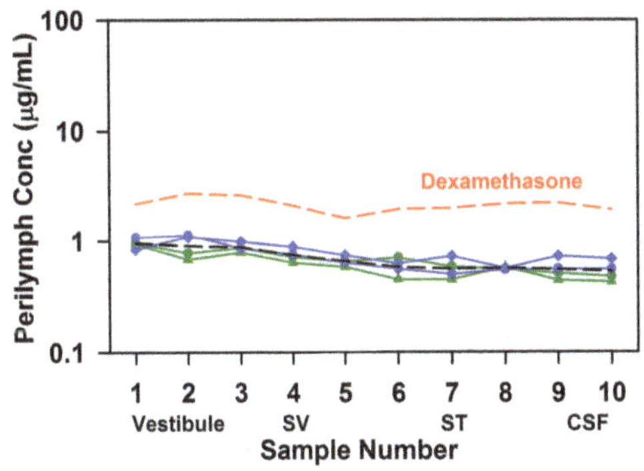

FIGURE 2 | Perilymph triamcinolone-acetonide concentrations achieved 1 h after application of triamcinolone-acetonide suspension to the RW niche of guinea pigs. Perilymph was collected as 10 × 2 uL sequential samples from the LSCC, each of which was analyzed independently. Early samples originate from the vestibule, followed by SV and ST in sequence. In two experiments the drug suspension was applied as a liquid (green curves) and in two experiments in poloxamer gel (blue curves), with similar results. The group mean (four experiments) is shown as a black dotted line. For comparison the group mean results of similar experiments applying dexamethasone suspension (Salt et al., 2018) are shown as the red dotted line.

In separate experiments the rate of triamcinolone-acetonide elimination from perilymph was quantified by loading perilymph by injection from a pipette sealed into the lateral SCC. **Figure 3A** shows the measured perilymph concentrations from four experiments, two sampled immediately after loading and two measured at 2 h after loading. Concentrations shown are the sum of triamcinolone-acetonide and triamcinolone in each sample. These studies show that triamcinolone-acetonide elimination occurred extremely rapidly, falling to 5–10% of the applied concentration within 2 h. The declining curve for perilymph seen with zero delay time was also consistent with rapid elimination. It shows the injection rate was insufficient to load the ear uniformly with drug, due to the high ongoing elimination rate during injection. Simulations fitted to the perilymph measurements provide the most quantitative way to compare kinetics across drugs. Elimination rates that best-fitted the measured data (dotted lines) were half times of 34 min in SV and 12 min in ST. These are the most rapid rates of drug elimination from perilymph we have ever measured. **Figure 3B** (solid lines) shows the calculated perilymph distribution of triamcinolone-acetonide at the three sampling times. Also shown on the plot for comparison (dotted lines) is the calculated distribution for dexamethasone at the same times, using a ST elimination half-time of 46 min and a SV elimination half-time of 91 min (Salt et al., 2018). Elimination of triamcinolone-acetonide occurs far faster than that of dexamethasone. The metabolism of triamcinolone-acetonide to triamcinolone was also apparent in the data from canal injection experiments,

[4]http://oto.wustl.edu/saltlab

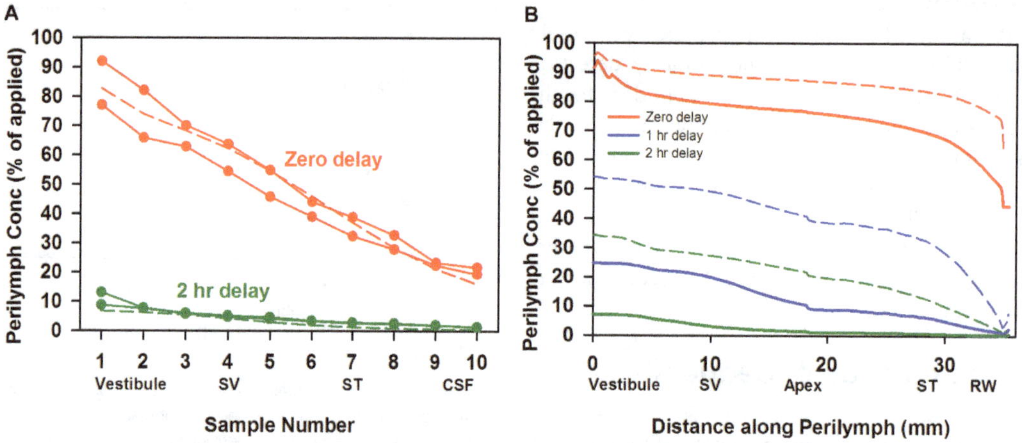

FIGURE 3 | (A) Elimination measurement of triamcinolone-acetonide. Solid lines with symbols are individual experiments in which triamcinolone-acetonide concentrations of perilymph samples obtained by sequential sampling were measured either immediately (zero delay; red curves, $n = 2$) or 2 h (green curves, $n = 2$) after perilymph loading. Dotted lines show calculated sample concentrations derived by simulation with elimination half time 12 min for ST and 34 min for SV, parameters which best fit the data set. **(B)** Solid lines show the calculated distribution of triamcinolone-acetonide along the perilymphatic space at zero (red), 1 h (blue), and 2 h (green) delay after loading calculated using the same kinetic parameters. For comparison curves based on a best fit to dexamethasone sampling data are shown dotted (ST elimination: 46 min; SV elimination 91 min; Salt et al., 2018). Triamcinolone-acetonide is lost more rapidly from perilymph than dexamethasone, faster than any other substance measured to date.

with triamcinolone making up 10.5% of the total in zero delay experiments and 63.3% of the total after 2 h. The accumulation of triamcinolone proportion with time provided the first indication that triamcinolone was better retained in perilymph than triamcinolone-acetonide.

Triamcinolone Kinetics

A suspension of triamcinolone was applied to the RW niche either in acute experiments with sampling 1 or 3 h after application to the RW niche, or as recovery experiments with sampling 1 or 3 days after intratympanic injection. The measured perilymph concentrations are summarized in **Figure 4**. A relatively uniform perilymph concentration over the time period was observed. Even after 3 days, triamcinolone crystals were visible in the RW niche and the perilymph concentration was maintained. The average concentrations for each of the groups (averaging all samples) were 1.52 µg/mL ($n = 3$; 1 h); 0.71 µg/mL ($n = 3$; 3 h); 0.72 ($n = 4$; 1 day); and 1.07 ($n = 2$, 3 days). Significance testing with two way ANOVA indicated that perilymph levels at 1 h were significantly higher than at 3 h and 1 day (Bonferroni, $P < 0.001$). It is also notable that the perilymph concentrations of triamcinolone were quite similar to those observed above with triamcinolone-acetonide, and even more so when normalized for middle ear concentration differences for the two forms of triamcinolone.

The rate of elimination of triamcinolone from perilymph was measured by loading perilymph by injection from a pipette sealed into the LSCC. The results of six experiments in which perilymph was sampled after zero delay ($n = 1$), 1 hr delay ($n = 3$); or 2 h delay ($n = 2$) are summarized in **Figure 5**. The data show that triamcinolone is retained well in perilymph, with initial vestibular samples at 70% of the applied drug concentration after 2 h. Dotted lines show the best fit of the kinetic model to the data set, with elimination half times of 278 min in SV and 700 min in ST. In **Figure 5B** the calculated distribution of triamcinolone along the perilymphatic spaces for the three time periods (solid lines) is compared with the distribution of dexamethasone (dotted lines). It is apparent that triamcinolone is retained in perilymph much better than triamcinolone-acetonide and dexamethasone, consistent with the more polar properties of this form of the molecule.

Based on the kinetic parameters for entry into perilymph from the middle ear and elimination from perilymph to the vasculature derived in this study, we are able to project how the two forms of triamcinolone might compare with the distribution of dexamethasone in the human cochlea. In each case, the drug can be applied as a suspension so the concentration in the middle ear is assumed constant over the 24 h period calculated, with the dissolved (free) concentration based on the aqueous solubility of the compound. The calculated perilymph concentrations as a function of distance along the cochlea and of time are shown in **Figure 6**.

As triamcinolone-acetonide is lost very rapidly from perilymph it will not spread far apically before being lost. Dexamethasone distributes further along the cochlea but does not reach apical regions in appreciable concentration. In contrast triamcinolone is calculated to distribute throughout the length of the human cochlea as a result of the lower rate of elimination from perilymph.

DISCUSSION

The elimination of locally applied drugs from perilymph has a major influence on effective local drug therapy of the inner ear. If elimination occurs more rapidly than the drug diffuses

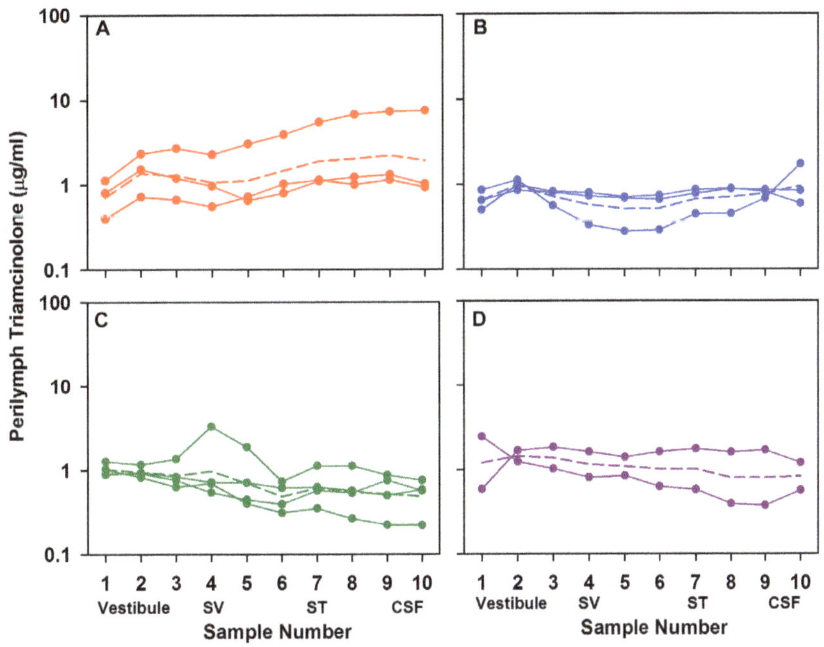

FIGURE 4 | Perilymph triamcinolone concentrations measured 1 h **(A)**, 3 h **(B)**, 1 day **(C)**, and 3 days **(D)** after application of triamcinolone suspension to the RW niche of guinea pigs. Perilymph was collected as 10×2 μL sequential samples each of which was analyzed independently. Each curve shows the measured data from a single animal. Animal numbers in each group were 3, 3, 4, and 2, respectively. For each group the mean is shown as a dotted line.

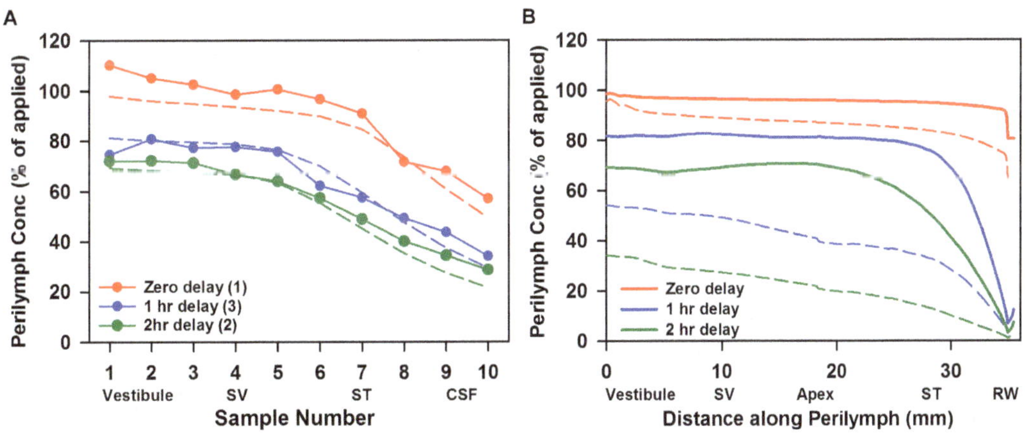

FIGURE 5 | (A) Elimination measurement of triamcinolone. Solid lines with symbols are the group means of the number of experiments indicated in which triamcinolone concentrations of perilymph samples obtained by sequential sampling were measured either immediately (zero delay; red curve, $n = 1$), 1 h (blue curve, $n = 3$), or 2 h (green curve, $n = 2$) after perilymph loading. Dotted lines show calculated sample concentrations derived by simulation with elimination half time 700 min for ST and 278 min for SV; parameters which best fit this data set. **(B)** Solid lines show the distribution of triamcinolone along the perilymphatic space at zero, 1 and 2 h delay after loading calculated using the same parameters. For comparison, curves calculated based on a best fit to dexamethasone sampling data are shown dotted (ST elimination: 46 min; SV elimination 91 min; Salt et al., 2018).

along the scala, this may limit the distribution of the drug along the cochlea. The influence of elimination also depends on the cochlear dimensions of the species under study. For a given drug, concentration gradients along the ear as a result of elimination will be substantially smaller in short cochleas, such as those of mice, and greater in longer cochleas, such as those of humans.

Measurement of elimination from perilymph was performed here by loading the fluid and tissue spaces of the inner ear with drug and then following the subsequent decline of drug with time by taking fluid samples at varying delay times after loading. This method overcomes difficulties with other application methods where drug gradients in the ear may exist. If drug gradients exist, decline of drug concentration due to distribution into regions of lower concentration cannot be differentiated from the decline due to elimination. Triamcinolone-acetonide was shown to be rapidly eliminated from perilymph while triamcinolone

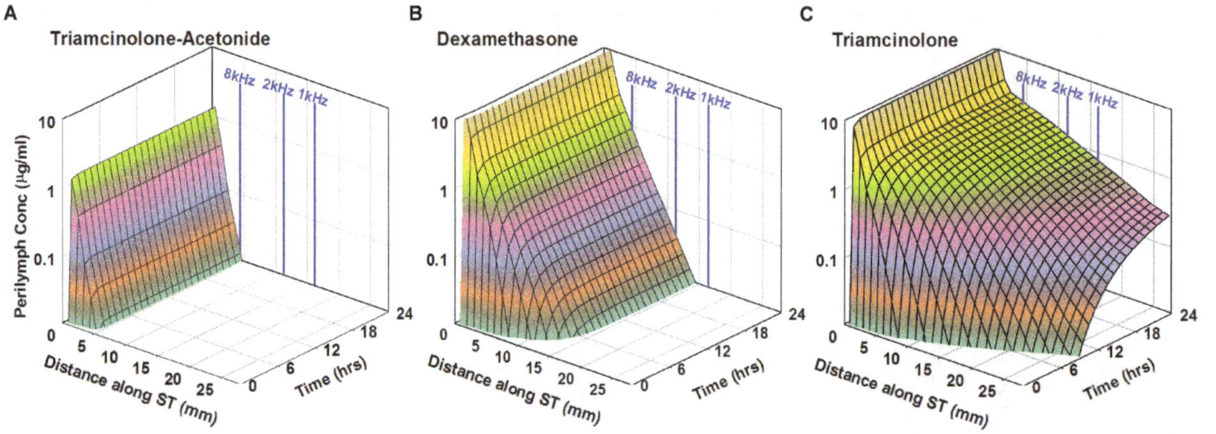

FIGURE 6 | Simulation of intratympanic applications of triamcinolone-acetonide suspension **(A)**, dexamethasone suspension **(B)**, and triamcinolone suspension **(C)** to the human ear. Entry and elimination kinetics are based on perilymph measurements in guinea pigs. ST elimination half-times were 12, 44, and 700 min for triamcinolone-acetonide, dexamethasone, and triamcinolone, respectively. Triamcinolone-acetonide and dexamethasone only distribute apically to a limited degree before reaching a steady state, unlike triamcinolone which reaches the cochlear apex.

had completely different characteristics and was retained well. Elimination of dexamethasone occurred at an intermediate rate. The measured elimination characteristics are consistent with the polar properties of the three molecules influencing passage across biological lipid membrane boundaries. In the case of elimination measurements, the molecular properties likely influence their ability to pass through cell membranes of the capillary endothelial cells (Salt and Hirose, 2018).

An interesting observation from this study is that while elimination differed markedly between triamcinolone-acetonide (fast) and triamcinolone (slow), the perilymph levels measured with RW niche applications were similar for both drugs. Simulations (not shown) indicate that perilymph concentration of drug depends on the rate of entry from the middle ear, balanced against the losses from perilymph due to elimination to blood and from interactions with cerebrospinal fluid. A similar perilymph level can result from fast entry with fast elimination (as in the case of triamcinolone-acetonide) or from slower entry with a slower rate of elimination (as in the case of triamcinolone). This raises an intriguing idea as it suggests that measured perilymph concentrations resulting from intratympanic applications cannot be easily interpreted in terms of the underlying perilymph pharmacokinetics. The similar perilymph levels observed here with triamcinolone and triamcinolone-acetonide gave no indication that the underlying kinetics in perilymph were completely different. In order to understand the perilymph kinetics additional measurements, such as measurement of elimination as performed here is required.

Our pharmacokinetic measurements suggest that triamcinolone should be considered as a potential therapy for auditory disorders where steroid therapy is indicated. Specifically, triamcinolone has pharmacokinetic properties that are predicted to allow it to reach apical cochlear regions of the human ear in higher concentration, potentially allowing all frequency regions to be treated. The choice of steroid for use in the clinic is, however, complex and based on many factors other than pharmacokinetic studies in animals. For instance, relative potencies at the target receptors are critical. Triamcinolone has been reported to have 660× lower potency than dexamethasone, while triamcinolone-acetonide may have 2–6× higher potency than dexamethasone at the glucocorticoid receptor (Mayer et al., 1974; Pratt et al., 1975; Yeakley et al., 1980; Grossmann et al., 2004; Nehmé et al., 2009). Potency estimates vary with many factors, however, including species, tissue and application duration (Giannopoulos and Keichline, 1981; Nehmé et al., 2009). Relative steroid potency remains unmeasured for tissues of the human inner ear. The relative affinity of mineralocorticoid receptors to the different steroids is also unknown. Another major factor concerns the difference between the concentrations of steroid in the tissues compared to those in perilymph and the factors contributing to tissue absorption. Although dexamethasone time courses have been compared in tissues and plasma with systemic dosing (Cherlet et al., 2005; Li et al., 2017) and in vitreous humor and retina tissues for the eye with local delivery (Chang-Lin et al., 2011), neither of these systems exhibit concentration gradients comparable to those seen in the ear. The cochlear tissue concentrations of steroid resulting from different perilymph distributions therefore remain unknown. It is possible that for some therapies of the ear, such as the treatment of Meniere's disease, the spatial distribution of drug may not be a limiting factor and treatment of vestibular and basal cochlear tissue may be sufficient. In animals, triamcinolone-acetonide therapy.

So in some cases, there may be limited benefit to a more apical distribution of drug along the cochlea. It therefore becomes important to evaluate how patients with auditory disorders respond to triamcinolone therapy. Unfortunately, human pilot studies with triamcinolone have been hampered by the lack of an available formulation approved for intravenous use, as exists for triamcinolone-acetonide. As triamcinolone-acetonide has higher potency for systemic delivery it has replaced the use of triamcinolone, so comparable formulations of triamcinolone are no longer available. Nevertheless, for the treatment of auditory disorders, a drug which can provide apical regions with substantially higher concentration would seem desirable and potentially allow all frequency regions of the human ear to be treated.

The three drugs compared here were all delivered to the middle ear as crystalline suspensions, which dissolve slowly over a period of weeks. Unlike solutions, where drug is lost rapidly from the middle ear, suspensions provide a depot effect, increasing the duration of the drug time course in perilymph. Such a "depot," influence has previously been reported for both triamcinolone-acetonide (Ye et al., 2007; Honeder et al., 2014) and for dexamethasone (Wang et al., 2009, 2011).

Our studies show that the requirements for an effective steroid for inner ear therapy are very different from those for intravenous or oral therapies. With local therapy the ease of passage through membranous boundaries, such as the RW membrane and blood-perilymph barrier, influence the spatial distribution of drug. The physical properties of the molecule that determine membrane permeability (such as lipophilicity and polarity) therefore play an important role in the cochlear distribution of drug. With systemic delivery, the molecular form is of lesser importance if the drug is metabolized to an active form in organs such as the liver. We have previously shown that the molecular properties of dexamethasone-phosphate make it quite unsuitable for local therapy of the ear (Salt et al., 2018). The present study shows that triamcinolone-acetonide, a more potent form of triamcinolone in widespread clinical use, also does not have appropriate kinetic properties for local treatment of the ear. In contrast, the more polar triamcinolone appears better suited. We conclude that the properties that make a drug suitable for local use in the ear are completely different from those that make the drug suitable for intravenous or oral use.

A key factor to improve drug distribution along the length of the ear is to reduce the rate of elimination. The triamcinolone molecule is almost identical to dexamethasone, differing by one non-polar CH_3 group in dexamethasone which is replaced by a polar OH group in triamcinolone. As can be seen in our measurements, this modest increase in polar properties markedly increases retention in perilymph, thus predicting the drug to be distributed more evenly along the ear. One possible confounding factor could have been that the reduced passage through membranous boundaries would limit entry from the middle ear. The perilymphatic measurements with local applications showed that any reduction in entry from the middle ear is largely offset by reduced rate of elimination, so that the measured perilymph concentration of triamcinolone was similar to that of triamcinolone-acetonide (**Figures 2, 4**).

CONCLUSION

In conclusion, the studies described herein suggest that administration to the middle ear of a triamcinolone suspension yields an attractive pharmacokinetic profile in the perilymph. These measurements show that triamcinolone could provide an additional treatment option for local therapy of auditory disorders.

ETHICS STATEMENT

Experiments were performed under protocol 20160053, approved by the Institutional Animal Care and Use Committee of Washington University. Animal use followed policies in accordance with the United States Department of Agriculture and National Institutes of Health guidelines for the handling and use of laboratory animals.

AUTHOR CONTRIBUTIONS

AS and FP conceived and designed the study. JJH and JH collected, organized, and analyzed the data. AS wrote the first draft of the manuscript. All authors contributed to manuscript revision, read, and approved the submitted version.

ACKNOWLEDGMENTS

The content is solely the responsibility of the authors and does not necessarily represent the official views of the National Institutes of Health.

REFERENCES

Alexander, T. H., Harris, J. P., Nguyen, Q. T., and Vorasubin, N. (2015). Dose effect of intratympanic dexamethasone for idiopathic sudden sensorineural hearing Loss: 24 mg/mL Is Superior to 10 mg/mL. *Otol. Neurotol.* 36, 1321–1327. doi: 10.1097/MAO.0000000000000834

Bird, P. A., Begg, E. J., Zhang, M., Keast, A. T., Murray, D. P., and Balkany, T. J. (2007). Intratympanic versus intravenous delivery of methylprednisolone to cochlear perilymph. *Otol. Neurotol.* 28, 1124–1130. doi: 10.1097/mao.0b013e31815aee21

Bird, P. A., Murray, D. P., Zhang, M., and Begg, E. J. (2011). Intratympanic versus intravenous delivery of dexamethasone and dexamethasone sodium phosphate to cochlear perilymph. *Otol. Neurotol.* 32, 933–936. doi: 10.1097/MAO.0b013e3182255933

Chang-Lin, J. E., Attar, M., Acheampong, A. A., Robinson, M. R., Whitcup, S. M., Kuppermann, B. D., et al. (2011). Pharmacokinetics and pharmacodynamics of a sustained-release dexamethasone intravitreal implant. *Invest Ophthalmol. Vis. Sci.* 52, 80–86. doi: 10.1167/iovs.10-5285

Cherlet, M., De Baere, S., Croubels, S., and De Backer, P. (2005). Quantitative determination of dexamethasone in bovine plasma and tissues by liquid chromatography–atmospheric pressure chemical ionization–tandem mass spectrometry. *Analytica Chimica Acta* 529, 361–369. doi: 10.1016/j.aca.2004.07.014

Dahm, V., Nieratschker, M., Riss, D., Kaider, A., Auinger, A., and Honeder, C. (2019). Intratympanic triamcinolone acetonide as treatment option for idiopathic sudden sensorineural hearing loss. *Otol. Neurotol.* 40, 720–727. doi: 10.1097/MAO.0000000000002283

Daina, A., Michielin, O., and Zoete, V. (2017). SwissADME: a free web tool to evaluate pharmacokinetics, drug-likeness and medicinal chemistry friendliness of small molecules. *Sci. Rep.* 7:42717. doi: 10.1038/srep42717

Daina, A., and Zoete, V. (2016). A BOILED-Egg To predict gastrointestinal absorption and brain penetration of small molecules. *ChemMedChem* 11, 1117–1121. doi: 10.1002/cmdc.201600182

Egan, W. J., Merz, K. M. Jr., and Baldwin, J. J. (2000). Prediction of drug absorption using multivariate statistics. *J. Med. Chem.* 43, 3867–3877. doi: 10.1021/jm000292e

Giannopoulos, G., and Keichline, D. (1981). Species-related differences in steroid-binding specificity of glucocorticoid receptors in lung. *Endocrinology.* 108, 1414–1419. doi: 10.1210/endo-108-4-1414

Grossmann, C., Scholz, T., Rochel, M., Bumke-Vogt, C., Oelkers, W., Pfeiffer, A. F., et al. (2004). Transactivation via the human glucocorticoid and mineralocorticoid receptor by therapeutically used steroids in CV-1 cells: a comparison of their glucocorticoid and mineralocorticoid properties. *Eur. J. Endocrinol.* 151, 397–406. doi: 10.1530/eje.0.1510397

Honeder, C., Engleder, E., Schöpper, H., Gabor, F., Reznicek, G., Wagenblast, J., et al. (2014). Sustained release of triamcinolone acetonide from an intratympanically applied hydrogel designed for the delivery of high glucocorticoid doses. *Audiol. Neurootol.* 19, 193–202. doi: 10.1159/000358165

Jumaily, M., Faraji, F., and Mikulec, A. A. (2017). Intratympanic triamcinolone and dexamethasone in the treatment of ménière's syndrome. *Otol. Neurotol. Mar.* 38, 386–391. doi: 10.1097/mao.0000000000001311

Lambert, P. R., Carey, J., Mikulec, A. A., and LeBel, C. (2016). Otonomy ménière's study group. intratympanic sustained-exposure dexamethasone thermosensitive gel for symptoms of ménière's disease: randomized phase 2b safety and efficacy trial. *Otol. Neurotol.* 37, 1669–1676. doi: 10.1097/mao.0000000000001227

Li, W., Hartsock, J. J., Dai, C., and Salt, A. N. (2018). Permeation enhancers for intratympanically-applied drugs studied using fluorescent dexamethasone as a marker. *Otol. Neurotol.* 39, 639–647. doi: 10.1097/MAO.0000000000001786

Li, X., DuBois, D. C., Song, D., Almon, R. R., Jusko, W. J., and Chen, X. (2017). Modeling combined immunosuppressive and anti-inflammatory effects of dexamethasone and naproxen in rats predicts the steroid-sparing potential of naproxen. *Drug Metab Dispos.* 45, 834–845. doi: 10.1124/dmd.117.075614

Liebau, A., Pogorzelski, O., Salt, A. N., and Plontke, S. K. (2017). Hearing changes after intratympanically applied steroids for primary therapy of sudden hearing loss: a meta-analysis using mathematical simulations of drug delivery protocols. *Otol. Neurotol.* 38, 19–30. doi: 10.1097/mao.0000000000001254

Mayer, M., Kaiser, N., Milholland, R. J., and Rosen, F. (1974). The binding of dexamethasone and triamcinolone acetonide to glucocorticoid receptors in rat skeletal muscle. *J. Biol. Chem.* 249, 5236–5240.

Mynatt, R., Hale, S. A., Gill, R. M., Plontke, S. K. R., and Salt, A. N. (2006). Demonstration of a longitudinal concentration gradient along scala tympani by sequential sampling of perilymph from the cochlear apex. *J. Assoc. Res. Otolaryngol.* 7, 182–193. doi: 10.1016/j.jneumeth.2005.10.008

Nehmé, A., Lobenhofer, E. K., Stamer, W. D., and Edelman, J. L. (2009). Glucocorticoids with different chemical structures but similar glucocorticoid receptor potency regulate subsets of common and unique genes in human trabecular meshwork cells. *BMC Med. Genomics* 2:58. doi: 10.1186/1755-8794-2-58

Parnes, L. S., Sun, A. H., and Freeman, D. J. (1999). Corticosteroid pharmacokinetics in the inner ear fluids: an animal study followed by clinical application. *Laryngoscope.* 109, 1–17. doi: 10.1097/00005537-199907001-00001

Piu, F., Wang, X., Fernandez, R., Dellamary, L., Harrop, A., Ye, Q., et al. (2011). OTO-104: a sustained-release dexamethasone hydrogel for the treatment of otic disorders. *Otol. Neurotol.* 32, 171–179. doi: 10.1097/MAO.0b013e3182009d29

Plontke, S. K., Biegner, T., Kammerer, B., Delabar, U., and Salt, A. N. (2008). Dexamethasone concentration gradients along scala tympani after application to the round window membrane. *Otol. Neurotol.* 29, 401–406. doi: 10.1097/mao.0b013e318161aaae

Pratt, W. B., Kaine, J. L., and Pratt, D. V. (1975). The kinetics of glucocorticoid binding to the soluble specific binding protein of mouse fibroblasts. *J. Biol. Chem.* 250, 4584–4591.

Rauch, S. D., Halpin, C. F., Antonelli, P. J., Babu, S., Carey, J. P., Gantz, B. J., et al. (2011). Oral vs intratympanic corticosteroid therapy for idiopathic sudden sensorineural hearing loss: a randomized trial. *JAMA* 305, 2071–2079. doi: 10.1001/jama.2011.679

Salt, A. N., Hartsock, J. J., Gill, R. M., Piu, F., and Plontke, S. K. (2012). Perilymph pharmacokinetics of markers and dexamethasone applied and sampled at the lateral semi-circular canal. *J. Assoc. Res. Otolaryngol.* 13, 771–783. doi: 10.1007/s10162-012-0347-y

Salt, A. N., Hartsock, J. J., Piu, F., and Hou, J. (2018). Dexamethasone and dexamethasone phosphate entry into perilymph compared for middle ear applications in guinea Pigs. *Audiol. Neurootol.* 23, 245–257. doi: 10.1159/000493846

Salt, A. N., Hartsock, J. J., Plontke, S. K., LeBel, C., and Piu, F. (2011). Distribution of dexamethasone and preservation of inner ear function following intratympanic delivery of a gel-based formulation. *Audiol. Neurotol.* 16, 323–335. doi: 10.1159/000322504

Salt, A. N., and Hirose, K. (2018). Communication pathways to and from the inner ear and their contributions to drug delivery. *Hear Res.* 362, 25–37. doi: 10.1016/j.heares.2017.12.010

Salt, A. N., and Plontke, S. K. (2005). Local inner-ear drug delivery and pharmacokinetics. *Drug Discov. Today.* 10, 1299–1306. doi: 10.1016/s1359-6446(05)03574-9

Thompson, H., and Tucker, A. S. (2013). Dual origin of the epithelium of the mammalian middle ear. *Science.* 22, 1453–1456. doi: 10.1126/science.1232862

Wang, X., Dellamary, L., Fernandez, R., Harrop, A., Keithley, E. M., Harris, J. P., et al. (2009). Dose-dependent sustained release of dexamethasone in inner ear cochlear fluids using a novel local delivery approach. *Audiol. Neurootol.* 14, 393–401. doi: 10.1159/000241896

Wang, X., Dellamary, L., Fernandez, R., Ye, Q., LeBel, C., and Piu, F. (2011). Principles of inner ear sustained release following intratympanic administration. *Laryngoscope.* 121, 385–391. doi: 10.1002/lary.21370

Ye, Q., Tillein, J., Hartmann, R., Gstoettner, W., and Kiefer, J. (2007). Application of a corticosteroid (*Triamcinolon*) protects inner ear function after surgical intervention. *Ear. Hear.* 28, 361–369. doi: 10.1097/01.aud.0000261655.30652.62

Yeakley, J. M., Balasubramanian, K., and Harrison, R. W. (1980). Comparison of glucocorticoid-receptor binding kinetics with predictions from a biomolecular model. *J. Biol. Chem.* 255, 4182–4188.

Permissions

All chapters in this book were first published by Frontiers; hereby published with permission under the Creative Commons Attribution License or equivalent. Every chapter published in this book has been scrutinized by our experts. Their significance has been extensively debated. The topics covered herein carry significant findings which will fuel the growth of the discipline. They may even be implemented as practical applications or may be referred to as a beginning point for another development.

The contributors of this book come from diverse backgrounds, making this book a truly international effort. This book will bring forth new frontiers with its revolutionizing research information and detailed analysis of the nascent developments around the world.

We would like to thank all the contributing authors for lending their expertise to make the book truly unique. They have played a crucial role in the development of this book. Without their invaluable contributions this book wouldn't have been possible. They have made vital efforts to compile up to date information on the varied aspects of this subject to make this book a valuable addition to the collection of many professionals and students.

This book was conceptualized with the vision of imparting up-to-date information and advanced data in this field. To ensure the same, a matchless editorial board was set up. Every individual on the board went through rigorous rounds of assessment to prove their worth. After which they invested a large part of their time researching and compiling the most relevant data for our readers.

The editorial board has been involved in producing this book since its inception. They have spent rigorous hours researching and exploring the diverse topics which have resulted in the successful publishing of this book. They have passed on their knowledge of decades through this book. To expedite this challenging task, the publisher supported the team at every step. A small team of assistant editors was also appointed to further simplify the editing procedure and attain best results for the readers.

Apart from the editorial board, the designing team has also invested a significant amount of their time in understanding the subject and creating the most relevant covers. They scrutinized every image to scout for the most suitable representation of the subject and create an appropriate cover for the book.

The publishing team has been an ardent support to the editorial, designing and production team. Their endless efforts to recruit the best for this project, has resulted in the accomplishment of this book. They are a veteran in the field of academics and their pool of knowledge is as vast as their experience in printing. Their expertise and guidance has proved useful at every step. Their uncompromising quality standards have made this book an exceptional effort. Their encouragement from time to time has been an inspiration for everyone.

The publisher and the editorial board hope that this book will prove to be a valuable piece of knowledge for researchers, students, practitioners and scholars across the globe.

List of Contributors

Pernilla Videhult Pierre
Division of Audiology, Department of Clinical Science, Intervention and Technology, Karolinska Institutet, Stockholm, Sweden

Anette Fransson, Marta Alina Kisiel and Göran Laurell
Department of Surgical Sciences, Uppsala University, Uppsala, Sweden

Peter Damberg and Sahar Nikkhou Aski
Karolinska Experimental Research and Imaging Center, Karolinska University Hospital, Stockholm, Sweden

Mats Andersson and Lotta Hällgren
Division of Bioscience and Materials, RISE Research Institutes of Sweden, Södertälje, Sweden

Debashree Mukherjea
Department of Otolaryngology, School of Medicine, Southern Illinois University, Springfield, IL, United States

Leonard P. Rybak
Department of Otolaryngology, School of Medicine, Southern Illinois University, Springfield, IL, United States
Department of Pharmacology, School of Medicine, Southern Illinois University, Springfield, IL, United States

Asmita Dhukhwa and Vickram Ramkumar
Department of Pharmacology, School of Medicine, Southern Illinois University, Springfield, IL, United States

Eric C. Bielefeld
Department of Speech and Hearing Science, The Ohio State University, Columbus, OH, United States

Megan J. Kobel
Department of Speech and Hearing Science, The Ohio State University, Columbus, OH, United States
Department of Otolaryngology-Head & Neck Surgery, The Ohio State University Wexner Medical Center, Columbus, OH, United States

Gail Ishiyama
Department of Neurology, David Geffen School of Medicine at UCLA, Los Angeles, CA, United States

Ivan A. Lopez, Dora Acuna and Akira Ishiyama
Department of Head and Neck Surgery, David Geffen School of Medicine at UCLA, Los Angeles, CA, United States

Puspanjali Bhatta
Department of Pharmacology, Southern Illinois University School of Medicine, Springfield, IL, United States

Sandeep Sheth
Department of Pharmaceutical Sciences, College of Pharmacy, Larkin University, Miami, FL, United States

Krishi Korrapati, Coral Tieu and Debashree Mukherjea
Department of Otolaryngology, Southern Illinois University School of Medicine, Springfield, IL, United States

Chaitanya Mamillapalli
Department of Internal Medicine, Southern Illinois University School of Medicine, Springfield, IL, United States

Caroline R. Anderson, Carol Xie, Matthew P. Su, Maria Garcia, Helen Blackshaw and Anne G. M. Schilder
evidENT, Ear Institute, University College London, London, United Kingdom
NIHR University College London Hospitals Biomedical Research Centre, London, United Kingdom

Gilda M. Kalinec and Federico Kalinec
Department of Head and Neck Surgery, David Geffen School of Medicine, University of California, Los Angeles, Los Angeles, CA, United States

Lucy Gao, Whitaker Cohn, Julian P. Whitelegge and Kym F. Faull
Pasarow Mass Spectrometry Laboratory, Department of Psychiatry and Biobehavioral Sciences, Jane and Terry Semel Institute for Neuroscience and Human Behavior, David Geffen School of Medicine, University of California, Los Angeles, Los Angeles, CA, United States

Sara Talaei, Michael E. Schnee and Ksenia A. Aaron
Department of Otolaryngology-Head and Neck Surgery, Stanford University School of Medicine, Stanford, CA, United States

Anthony J. Ricci
Department of Otolaryngology-Head and Neck Surgery, Stanford University School of Medicine, Stanford, CA, United States
Department of Molecular and Cellular Physiology, Stanford University School of Medicine, Stanford, CA, United States

Amit Wolfovitz, Rasim Yilmazer, Ayca Baskadem Yilmazer, Esperanza Bas, Peter Ashman, Jonathan Roell, Rahul Mittal and Jeenu Mittal
Department of Otolaryngology, University of Miami Hearing Research Laboratory, Miller School of Medicine, Miami, FL, United States

Adrien A. Eshraghi
Department of Otolaryngology, University of Miami Hearing Research Laboratory, Miller School of Medicine, Miami, FL, United States
Department of Neurological Surgery, Miller School of Medicine, Miami, FL, United States
Department of Biomedical Engineering, University of Miami, Miami, Coral Gables, FL, United States

Jorge Bohorquez
Department of Biomedical Engineering, University of Miami, Miami, Coral Gables, FL, United States

Carolyn Garnham, Roland Hessler and Daniel Sieber
MED-EL Hearing Implants, Innsbruck, Austria

Christoph Pannier
Department of Otolaryngology, Hannover Medical School, Hanover, Germany

Verena Scheper and Thomas Lenarz
Department of Otolaryngology, Hannover Medical School, Hanover, Germany
Cluster of Excellence 'Hearing4all', German Research Foundation, Bonn, Germany
Lower Saxony Centre for Biomedical Engineering, Implant Research and Development (NIFE), Hanover, Germany

Andrea Hoffmann and Anika Hamm
Lower Saxony Centre for Biomedical Engineering, Implant Research and Development (NIFE), Hanover, Germany
Department of Orthopaedic Surgery, Hannover Medical School, Hanover, Germany

Jana Schwieger
Department of Otolaryngology, Hannover Medical School, Hanover, Germany
Lower Saxony Centre for Biomedical Engineering, Implant Research and Development (NIFE), Hanover, Germany

André Schulz
Fraunhofer Institute for Biomedical Engineering IBMT, Sulzbach, Germany

Michael M. Gepp
Fraunhofer Institute for Biomedical Engineering IBMT, Sulzbach, Germany
Fraunhofer Project Center for Stem Cell Process Engineering, Würzburg, Germany

Peter Hubka
Lower Saxony Centre for Biomedical Engineering, Implant Research and Development (NIFE), Hanover, Germany
Department of Experimental Otology, Hannover Medical School, Hanover, Germany

Ildar I. Sadreev
Department of Medicine, Faculty of Medicine, Imperial College, London, United Kingdom

George W. S. Burwood, Samuel M. Flaherty and Ian J. Russell
Sensory Neuroscience Research Group, School of Pharmacy and Biomolecular Sciences, University of Brighton, Brighton, United Kingdom

Jongrae Kim
School of Mechanical Engineering, Institute of Design, Robotics and Optimisation, Aerospace Systems Engineering, University of Leeds, Leeds, United Kingdom

Timur I. Abdullin
Department of Biochemistry, Biotechnology and Pharmacology, Institute of Fundamental Medicine and Biology, Kazan Federal University, Kazan, Russia

Andrei N. Lukashkin
Sensory Neuroscience Research Group, School of Pharmacy and Biomolecular Sciences, University of Brighton, Brighton, United Kingdom
Centre for Regenerative Medicine and Devices, University of Brighton, Brighton, United Kingdom

Christopher Rathnam and Sy-Tsong Dean Chueng
Department of Chemistry and Chemical Biology, Rutgers, The State University of New Jersey, Piscataway, NJ, United States

Yu-Lan Mary Ying
Department of Otolaryngology Head and Neck Surgery, Rutgers New Jersey Medical School, Newark, NJ, United States

Ki-Bum Lee
Department of Chemistry and Chemical Biology, Rutgers, The State University of New Jersey, Piscataway, NJ, United States
Stem Cell Research Center and Keck Center for Collaborative Neuroscience, Rutgers, The State University of New Jersey, Piscataway, NJ, United States

Kelvin Kwan
Stem Cell Research Center and Keck Center for Collaborative Neuroscience, Rutgers, The State University of New Jersey, Piscataway, NJ, United States
Department of Cell Biology and Neuroscience, Rutgers, The State University of New Jersey, Piscataway, NJ, United States

David N. Furness
School of Life Sciences, Keele University, Keele, United Kingdom

Marie-Josée Duran
Fondation Pour l'Audition, Paris, France

Ralph Holme
Action on Hearing Loss, London, United Kingdom

Jay C. Buckey
Space Medicine Innovations Laboratory, Center for Hyperbaric Medicine, Department of Medicine, Geisel School of Medicine at Dartmouth, Lebanon, NH, United States

Jaimin Patel and Mikhaylo Szczupak
Department of Otolaryngology, University of Miami Miller School of Medicine, Miami, FL, United States

Suhrud Rajguru
Department of Otolaryngology, University of Miami Miller School of Medicine, Miami, FL, United States
Department of Biomedical Engineering, University of Miami, Coral Gables, FL, United States

Carey Balaban
Department of Otolaryngology and Biomedical Engineering, University of Pittsburgh, Pittsburgh, PA, United States

Michael E. Hoffer
Department of Otolaryngology, University of Miami Miller School of Medicine, Miami, FL, United States
Department of Neurological Surgery, University of Miami Miller School of Medicine, Miami, FL, United States

Yin Ren
Department of Otolaryngology, Harvard Medical School, Boston, MA, United States
Eaton Peabody Laboratories, Department of Otolaryngology, Massachusetts Eye and Ear, Boston, MA, United States

Lukas D. Landegger
Department of Otolaryngology, Harvard Medical School, Boston, MA, United States
Eaton Peabody Laboratories, Department of Otolaryngology, Massachusetts Eye and Ear, Boston, MA, United States
Department of Otolaryngology, Vienna General Hospital, Medical University of Vienna, Vienna, Austria

Konstantina M. Stankovic
Department of Otolaryngology, Harvard Medical School, Boston, MA, United States
Eaton Peabody Laboratories, Department of Otolaryngology, Massachusetts Eye and Ear, Boston, MA, United States
Program in Speech and Hearing Bioscience and Technology, Harvard Medical School, Boston, MA, United States
Harvard Program in Therapeutic Science, Harvard University, Boston, MA, United States

Kathie M. Bishop
Otonomy Inc, San Diego, CA, United States

Alec Nicholas Salt and Jared James Hartsock
Department of Otolaryngology, Washington University School of Medicine, St. Louis, MO, United States

Jennifer Hou and Fabrice Piu
Otonomy Inc, San Diego, CA, United States

Index

www.ingramcontent.com/pod-product-compliance
Lightning Source LLC
LaVergne TN
LVHW082220200926
848484LV00008B/2278